THE JUNIOR DOCTOR SURVIVAL GUIDE

Paul Watson MBBS, DipSurgAnat

General Surgery Registrar, Austin Hospital,
Melbourne, VIC, Australia

Joseph M O'Brien MBBS, BMedSc(Hons)

General Medical Registrar, Austin Health,
Melbourne, VIC, Australia

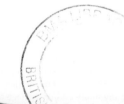

ELSEVIER

ELSEVIER

Elsevier Australia. ACN 001 002 357
(a division of Reed International Books Australia Pty Ltd)
Tower 1, 475 Victoria Avenue, Chatswood, NSW 2067

Notice

Knowledge and best practice in this field are constantly changing. As new research and experience broaden our understanding, changes in research methods, professional practices, or medical treatment may become necessary.

Practitioners and researchers must always rely on their own experience and knowledge in evaluating and using any information, methods, compounds, or experiments described herein. In using such information or methods they should be mindful of their own safety and the safety of others, including parties for whom they have a professional responsibility.

With respect to any drug or pharmaceutical products identified, readers are advised to check the most current information provided (i) on procedures featured or (ii) by the manufacturer of each product to be administered, to verify the recommended dose or formula, the method and duration of administration, and contraindications. It is the responsibility of practitioners, relying on their own experience and knowledge of their patients, to make diagnoses, to determine dosages and the best treatment for each individual patient, and to take all appropriate safety precautions.

To the fullest extent of the law, neither the Publisher nor the authors, contributors, or editors, assume any liability for any injury and/or damage to persons or property as a matter of product liability, negligence or otherwise, or from any use or operation of any methods, products, instructions, or ideas contained in the material herein.

National Library of Australia Cataloging-in-Publication Data

Watson, Paul, author.
    The junior doctor survival guide / Paul Watson; Joseph M. O'Brien.
    9780729542258 (paperback)
    Includes index.
    Physicians–Vocational guidance.
        Clinical medicine–Handbooks, manuals, etc.
        Medicine–Practice.
O'Brien, Joseph M., author.

Senior Content Strategist: Larissa Norrie
Content Development Specialist: Lauren Santos
Senior Project Manager: Anitha Rajarathnam
Edited by Linda Littlemore
Proofread by Melissa Faulkner
Design by Georgette Hall
Index by Innodata Indexing
Typeset by Toppan Best-set Premedia Limited
Printed in China

CONTENTS

PREFACE

We all live in the ocean of medicine. On our best days the water is still and clear. Sometimes the waves build, crashing over us. We need only put up our hands and someone will lift us from the storm. Remember to keep your head above the water and offer a hand to those who are being battered by the waves.

With great pleasure we present the *Junior Doctor Survival Guide*, a companion to the new students, interns and residents beginning their incredible journeys as medical practitioners. We wrote this text from the perspective of giving handover to you, our colleagues, regarding the daily life of the fledgling junior doctor.

There is a strong focus on the practical nature of working within the hospital system, learning the day-to-day job requirements often overlooked by formal medical education. Most interns spend more time worrying about how to order investigations, put on a backslab and properly document patient plans than they do about the minutiae of specialist practice. This is where we come in.

The prevocational years of medicine are greatly influenced by the hand of experience. It takes time to adjust to the inner workings of a hospital and becoming a busy, young professional. This text is the sum of our collective experiences, a series of tips and tricks for surviving that initial foray into the great unknown.

With a large number of concise chapters (and hopefully a bit of levity) we hope this book can provide a framework for you to build your own skills and knowledge with the wisdom to pass what you learn to others.

Paul Watson
Joseph O'Brien
thewelljuniordoctor@gmail.com

CONTRIBUTORS

Kelsey Broom MD, BBiomedSc
Resident Medical Officer, Queensland Health
QLD, Australia

Kerry Jewell MBBS, BMedSc(Hons)
Medical Registrar, Austin Health
Melbourne, VIC, Australia

Todd Galvin Manning MBBS, DipSurgAnat, DipLapSurg
Research Fellow, MS (Urol) Candidate,
Department of Surgery (Urology), University of Melbourne, Austin Health;
Department of Anatomy and Developmental Biology, Monash University;
Young Urology Researchers Organisation (YURO),
Melbourne, VIC, Australia;
British Urology Researchers in Surgical Training (BURST),
United Kingdom

Joseph M O'Brien MBBS, BMedSc(Hons)
General Medical Registrar, Austin Health,
Melbourne, VIC, Australia

Rami Shenouda MBBS, DipSurgAnat
Emergency Registrar, Alfred Health
Melbourne, VIC, Australia

Paul Watson MBBS, DipSurgAnat
General Surgery Registrar, Austin Hospital,
Melbourne, VIC, Australia

Lachlan Wight MBBS, DipSurgAnat
Orthopaedic Registrar, Barwon Health
Geelong, VIC, Australia

REVIEWERS

Anna Bondorovsky MD, BSc (Anatomy & Histology and Physiology)
Hospital Medical Officer, The Royal Women's Hospital
Parkville, VIC

David A Kandiah MBChB(Hons), MClinEd, MPH, MHL, MBA, PhD, MRCP(UK)
FRACP
Clinical Professor, University of Western Australia
Perth, WA

Benjamin Kwan MBBS, BSc(Med), FRACP
Staff Specialist, Sutherland Hospital
Caringbah, NSW

Kate Lord MBBS, BSc(Hons)
Physician Trainee, Austin Health and Northern Health
Melbourne, VIC

Hareeshan Nandakoban MBBS, FRACP
Network Director of Physician Education and Renal Staff Specialist, Liverpool Hospital
Liverpool, NSW

Yogendra Narayan MPH, MHA, Grad Cert PSM, DSM, FRACMA
Specialist Medical Administrator, Medical and Dental Workforce Services, Western Sydney
Local Health District
NSW

Louisa Ng MBChB, MD, FAFRM (RACP)
Rehabilitation Physician, Supervisor of Intern Training and Deputy Director of RMH
Clinical School, Royal Melbourne Hospital
Parkville, VIC

Belinda Weich MBChB, FRCAP
Senior Staff Physician, Mackay Base Hospital
Mackay, QLD

Kristen Pearson MBBS, FRACP
Consultant Geriatrician, Northern Health, VIC

ACKNOWLEDGEMENTS

Thanks to my friends and family who have supported me through this grand adventure. A special mention goes to my co-authors, Joe, Kelsey, Lachlan, Kerry, Rami and Todd. To the powerhouse team at Elsevier, Larissa, Lauren, Neli, Anitha and Linda, I thank you for your enthusiasm and superhuman patience! This is dedicated to all the junior doctors who work tirelessly, compassionately and admirably.

Paul Watson

I dedicate my work on this book to my family and friends, for their kindness and devotion. Together they have tolerated complaining and foot-dragging for nearly three years. Thanks go to the Elsevier team who took a gamble on two cocky interns from the country, to my co-authors who generously donated their time and, lastly, to the caffeine and sugar that enabled me to (almost) meet deadlines.

Joseph M O'Brien

ABBREVIATIONS, ACRONYMS, MNEMONICS

Clinical abbreviations and acronyms

ABBREVIATION/ ACRONYM	EXPANSION	NOTES
−ve	Negative	
/x	Average	
#	Fracture	
Δ	Change	
+ve	Positive	
2°	Secondary to...	
4WF	Four wheel frame	
6MP	6-Mercaptopurine	
A/E	Air entry	
a/w	Associated with	
A&E	Accident and Emergency	
A&O	Alert and oriented	
AAA	Abdominal aortic aneurysm	
AB	Antibody	
ABG	Arterial blood gas	
ABI	Acquired brain injury or ankle-brachial index	
ABP	Ambulatory blood pressure	
ABx	Antibiotics	
ACE-I	Angiotensin-converting enzyme inhibitors	
ACh	Acetylcholine	
AChR	Acetylcholine receptor	
ACL	Anterior cruciate ligament	
ACLS	Advanced cardiac life support	
ACS	Acute coronary syndrome	
ACTH	Adrenocorticotropic hormone	
AD	Alzheimer's disease	
ADF	Augmentin® Duo Forte	Amoxicillin with clavulanic acid, a very common oral antibiotic
ADH	Antidiuretic hormone	

Clinical abbreviations and acronyms—cont'd

ABBREVIATION/ ACRONYM	EXPANSION	NOTES
ADLs	Activities of daily living	I-ADL if independent of ADLs; P-ADLs for personal ADLs; D-ADLs for domestic ADLs
ADT	Androgen deprivation therapy	
AED	Automated external defibrillator or anti-epileptic drug	
AF/A-Fib	Atrial fibrillation	A-Fib is very American
AFB	Acid fast bacilli	
AFP	Alpha-fetoprotein	
AG	Anion gap	
AHI	Apnoea–hypopnoea index	
AIDP	Acute inflammatory demyelinating polyradiculoneuropathy	
AIDS	Acquired immunodeficiency syndrome	
ALOC	Altered level of consciousness	
ALP	Alkaline phosphatase	
ALS	Advanced life support	
ALT	Alanine aminotransferase	
AKA	Above knee amputation	
AKI	Acute kidney injury	
Alb	Albumin	
ALL	Acute lymphoblastic leukaemia	Sometimes denoted as B-ALL or T-ALL depending on the cells involved
ALP	Alkaline phosphatase	
ALT	Anterolateral thigh flap or alanine aminotransferase	
AMA	Antimitochondrial antibodies	
AMAN	Acute motor axonal neuropathy	
AMI	Acute myocardial infarction	
AML	Acute myeloid leukaemia	
AMSAN	Acute sensorimotor axonal neuropathy	
ANA	Antinuclear antibody	

continued

Clinical abbreviations and acronyms—cont'd

ABBREVIATION/ ACRONYM	EXPANSION	NOTES
ANCA	Anti-neutrophil cytoplasmic antibody	
Anti-CCP	Anti-citrullinated protein antibody	
anti-dsDNA	Anti-double-stranded DNA test	
AoCRF	Acute on chronic renal failure	
AP	Anteroposterior	
APC	Argo plasma coagulation	
APO	Acute pulmonary oedema	
APP	As per protocol	
Appt	Appointment	
APR	Acute phase reactants or abdominoperineal resection	Consider context
APTT	Activated partial thromboplastin time	
AR	Aortic regurgitation	
ARB	Angiotensin receptor blocker or alpha-receptor blocker	Consider context
ARDS	Acute respiratory distress syndrome	
ARF	Acute renal failure	Also known as AKI or acute kidney injury
AS	Aortic stenosis	
ASA	Aspirin	From 'acetylsalicylic acid'
ASD	Atrial septal defect	
AST	Aspartate aminotransferase	
aSx	Asymptomatic	
ATN	Acute tubular necrosis	
ATSP	Asked to see patient	
AUC	Area under concentration curve	
AV	Arteriovenous or aortic valve or atrioventricular	Consider the context
AVM	Arteriovenous malformation	
AVN	Avascular necrosis	
AVR	Aortic valve replacement	

Clinical abbreviations and acronyms—cont'd

ABBREVIATION/ ACRONYM	EXPANSION	NOTES
AWS	Alcohol withdrawal scale	
Ax	Assessment	
AXR	Abdominal X-ray	
AZA	Azathioprine	
BAC	Blood alcohol concentration	
BAL	Biphenotypic acute leukaemia or bronchoalveolar lavage	Mixed AML and ALL
BBB	Blood–brain barrier	
BC	Blood culture	
BCC	Basal cell carcinoma	
BCT	Breast conservation therapy	
BD	Twice daily	From the Latin, 'bis die'
beta-HCG	Human chorionic gonadotropin	
BIBA	Brought in by ambulance	
Bilat.	Bilateral	
BiPAP	Bilevel positive airway pressure	
BiV	Biventricular	
BL	Burkitt lymphoma	
BLS	Basic life support	
BMAT	Bone marrow aspirate trephine	Alternatively, BMBx for bone marrow biopsy
BMD	Bone mineral density	
BMI	Body mass index	
BMS	Bare metal stent	
BNO	Bowels not open	
BNP	Brain natriuretic peptide	See 'Investigations'
BO	Bowels open	
BOOP	Bronchiolitis obliterans organising pneumonia	
BP	Blood pressure	
BPD	Borderline personality disorder	
BPH	Benign prostatic hypertrophy or benign prostate hyperplasia	
BPM	Beats (or breaths) per minute	
BPPV	Benign paroxysmal positional vertigo	

continued

Clinical abbreviations and acronyms—cont'd

ABBREVIATION/ ACRONYM	EXPANSION	NOTES
BS	Bowel sounds	
BSA	Body surface area	
BSL/BGL	Blood sugar/glucose level	
Bx	Biopsy	
C-Diff	*Clostridium difficile*	Alternatively, CDT – *Clostridiums difficile* toxin
c/o	Complains of	
Ca	Carcinoma, cancer or calcium	Calcium should be Ca^{2+}
CABG	Coronary artery bypass graft	Pronounced 'CAGs' or 'cabbages'
CAD	Coronary artery disease or carotid artery disease	
CAM	Complementary and alternative medicine	
CAP	Community-acquired pneumonia	
CAS	Carotid artery stenting	
CBC	Complete blood count	Very American
CBD	Common bile duct	
CBF	Cerebral blood flow	
CBWO	Continuous bladder washout	
CCB	Calcium channel blocker	
CCF/CHF	Congestive cardiac failure	H for heart can be substituted for C
CCL	Cardiac catheterisation lab	
CCS-x	Canadian Cardiac Society x	Scored 1–4
CCU	Coronary Care Unit	
CD	Crohn's disease	
CDNH	Chondrodermatitis nodularis helicis	
CDT	Carbohydrate deficient transferrin or *Clostridium difficile* toxin	
CDUS	Carotid duplex ultrasound	
CEA	Carotid endarterectomy or carcinoembryonic antigen	
CF	Cystic fibrosis *or* clear fluids	Consider context

Clinical abbreviations and acronyms—cont'd

ABBREVIATION/ ACRONYM	EXPANSION	NOTES
CHB	Complete heart block	
CIDP	Chronic inflammatory demyelinating polyneuropathy	
CK	Creatine kinase	
CKD	Chronic kidney disease	
CLD	Chronic liver disease	
CLL	Chronic lymphocytic leukaemia	
CLO	Campylobacter-like organism test	
CM	Cardiomyopathy	DCM = dilated
CME	Continuing medical education	
CML	Chronic myeloid leukaemia	
CMML	Chronic myelomonocytic leukaemia	
CMP	Comprehensive metabolic panel; also calcium, magnesium, phosphate	
CMV	Cytomegalovirus	
CN	Cranial nerve	
CNS	Central nervous system	
CO	Carbon monoxide	
CO_2	Carbon dioxide	
COPD/COAD	Chronic obstructive pulmonary disease	A for airways can be substituted for P
CP	Cerebral palsy or chest pain	Consider context
CPAP	Continuous positive airway pressure	
CPB	Cardiopulmonary bypass	
CPP	Cerebral perfusion pressure	
CPR	Cardiopulmonary resuscitation	
Cr	Creatinine	
CR	Controlled release	
CRC	Colorectal cancer	
CrCl	Creatinine clearance	
CRE	Carbapenem-resistant *Enterobacteriaceae*	

continued

Clinical abbreviations and acronyms—cont'd

ABBREVIATION/ ACRONYM	EXPANSION	NOTES
CRF	Chronic renal failure	
CRI	Chronic renal insufficiency	Newer term, replacing CRF
CRP	C-reactive protein	
CRPS	Complex regional pain syndrome	
CRT	Cardiac resynchronisation therapy or chemoradiotherapy	Consider context
CSL	Compound sodium lactate	
CSF	Cerebrospinal fluid	
CT	Computed tomography	No longer CAT as it is no longer 'axial'
CT-C/A/P	CT chest/abdo/pelvis	
CT-KUB	CT Kidneys, ureters, bladder	
CTB	CT brain	
CTPA	Computed tomography pulmonary angiogram	
CTR	Carpal tunnel release	
CTX	Ceftriaxone	
CVA	Cerebrovascular accident	Falling out of favour
CVC	Central venous catheter	Or CVL – central venous line
Cx	Complication or cervix	Consider context
CXR	Chest X-ray	
D/C	Discharge	In both meanings of the word
D/W	Discussion with	
D&C	Dilatation and curettage	
DAI	Diffuse axonal injury	
DALY	Disability-adjusted life year	
DAPT	Dual antiplatelet therapy	
DAT	Direct antibody test	
DBE	Double balloon enteroscopy	
DBP	Diastolic blood pressure	
DCIS	Ductal carcinoma in situ	
DCR	Direct current reversion	
DDx	Differential diagnosis	
DES	Drug-eluting stent	
Dex	Dextrose	

Clinical abbreviations and acronyms—cont'd

ABBREVIATION/ ACRONYM	EXPANSION	NOTES
DEXA	Dual energy X-ray absorptiometry	
DFA	Direct fluorescence antibody	
DHS	Dynamic hip screw	
DI	Diabetes insipidus	
DIC	Disseminated intravascular coagulation	
DIDO	Door-in door-out	
DIEP	Deep inferior epigastric (artery) perforator flap	
DILI	Drug-induced liver injury	
DKA	Diabetic ketoacidosis	
DLB	Dementia with Lewy bodies	
DLBCL	Diffuse large B-cell lymphoma	
DLCO	Diffusing capacity of carbon monoxide	
DM	Diabetes mellitus	Also T1DM or T2DM. ID afterwards refers to insulin dependence
DMARD	Disease-modifying antirheumatic drug	
DNA	Deoxyribonucleic acid	
DNR	Do not resuscitate	More American than Australian
DOS	Diffuse oesophageal spasm	
DPL	Diagnostic peritoneal lavage	Technique not used often in Australia
DRE	Digital rectal examination	
DT	Delirium tremens	
DVT	Deep venous thrombosis	
Dx	Diagnosis	
EBM	Evidence-based medicine	
EBV	Epstein–Barr virus	
ECF	Extracellular fluid	
ECG	Electrocardiogram	Americans use EKG
ECMO	Extracorporeal membrane oxygenation	

continued

Clinical abbreviations and acronyms—cont'd

ABBREVIATION/ ACRONYM	EXPANSION	NOTES
ECOG	Eastern Cooperative Oncology Group	
ECT	Electroconvulsive therapy	
ED	Emergency Department	
EDH	Extradural haemorrhage	
EEG	Electroencephalogram	
EF	Ejection fraction	
eGFR	Estimated glomerular filtration rate	
ELISA	Enzyme-linked immunosorbent assay	
EMD	Electromechanical dissociation	Bad news
EMG	Electromyography	
EMR	Endoscopic mucosal resection	
EN	Enrolled nurse	
ENA	Extractable nuclear antigen antibodies	
ENT	Ear, Nose and Throat (Department)	
EOM	Extraocular muscles	
EP	Electrophysiology	
EPO	Erythropoietin	
EPoA	Enduring power of attorney	Also MPoA (medical), FPoA (financial), and LPoA (lifestyle, or where someone can live)
ER	Oestrogen receptor	
ERCP	Endoscopic retrograde cholangiopancreatography	
ESBL	Extended spectrum beta-lactamase	
ESM	Ejection systolic murmur	
ESR	Erythrocyte sedimentation rate	
ESRF	End-stage renal failure	eGFR <10
ET	Essential thrombocytosis or extraterrestrial	

Clinical abbreviations and acronyms—cont'd

ABBREVIATION/ ACRONYM	EXPANSION	NOTES
EtOH	Alcohol	
ETT	Endotracheal tube	
ETV	Endoscopic third ventriculostomy	
EUA	Examination under anaesthesia	
EUP	Extra-uterine pregnancy	
EUS	Endoscopic ultrasonography	
EVAR	Endovascular aortic repair	
EVD	External ventricular drain	
Ex	Examination	
F/U	Follow up	
FAP	Familial adenomatous polyposis	
FAST	Focused assessment with sonography for trauma	
FB	Foreign body	
FBE	Full blood examination	
FDA	Iron deficiency anaemia	F comes from Fe
Fe	Iron	
FEV	Forced expiration volume	
FF	Free fluids	
FFMN	Fasting from midnight	
FFP	Fresh frozen plasma	
FFR	Fractional flow reserve	Tests pressures across lesions
FHx	Family history	
FI	For investigation	
FiO_2	Fraction of inspired oxygen	
FL	Follicular lymphoma	
FLK	Funny looking kid	Offensive, but you may still see it used
FNA	Fine needle aspirate	
FOBT	Faecal occult blood test	
FOOSH	Fall on outstretched hand	
FRII	Fixed rate insulin infusion	
FSH	Follicle-stimulating hormone	
FTSG	Full thickness skin graft	

continued

Clinical abbreviations and acronyms—cont'd

ABBREVIATION/ ACRONYM	EXPANSION	NOTES
FTT	Failure to thrive	
FUO	Fever unknown origin	
FWB	Full weight bearing	
FWD	Full ward diet	
FWT	Full ward test	
G&H	Group-and-hold	
GA	General anaesthetic	
GABA	Gamma-aminobutyric acid	
GAD	Generalised anxiety disorder	
GB	Gallbladder	
GBM	Glomerular basement membrane	
GBS	Group B Strep or Guillain–Barré syndrome	Consider context
GCA	Giant cell arteritis	
GCS	Glasgow Coma Scale	
GFR	Glomerular filtration rate	
GGT	Gamma-glutamyl transferase	
GH	Growth hormone	
GHB	Gamma-hydroxy butyrate	
GI	Gastrointestinal	
GIT	Gastrointestinal tract	
GN	Glomerulonephritis	
GORD	Gastro-oesophageal reflux disease	GERD in the USA ('esophageal')
GOS	Gastro-oesophageal sphincter	
GP	General practitioner	
Gr$^+$ or Gr$^-$	Gram positive or negative	
GSV	Great saphenous nerve	
GSW	Gunshot wound	
GTN	Glyceryl trinitrate	
GU	Genitourinary or gastric ulcer	Consider context
GVHD	Graft versus host disease	A lowercase 'c' denotes chronic GVHD
Gy	Grays	Measurement of radiation
H&M	Haematemesis and melaena	

Clinical abbreviations and acronyms—cont'd

ABBREVIATION/ ACRONYM	EXPANSION	NOTES
H_1 or H_2	Histamine receptor 1 or 2	
HA	Headache	
HAART	Highly active anti-retroviral therapy	
HAP	Hospital-acquired pneumonia	
HAV	Hepatitis A virus	
Hb	Haemoglobin	
HB	Heart block	For example, 1° HB
HbA_{1c}	Glycated haemoglobin	
HBV	Hepatitis B virus	
HCAP	Healthcare associated pneumonia	
HCC	Hepatocellular carcinoma	
hCG	Human chorionic gonadotropin	
HCO_3^-	Bicarbonate	
HCT	Hydrochlorothiazide or haematocrit	Consider context, often haematocrit is written as Hct
HCV	Hepatitis C virus	
HD	Haemodialysis	
HDL	High density lipoprotein	
HDU	High Dependency Unit	
HDV	Hepatitis D virus	
HE	Hepatic encephalopathy	
HEENT	Head, Eyes, Ears, Nose and Throat (Department)	
HELLP syndrome	Haemolysis/elevated liver enzymes/low platelets	
HEV	Hepatitis E virus	
HFM	Hand, foot and mouth disease	
HFpEF	Heart failure with preserved ejection fraction	
HFrEF	Heart failure with reduced ejection fraction	
HHS	Hyperosmolar hyperglycaemic state	

continued

Clinical abbreviations and acronyms—cont'd

ABBREVIATION/ ACRONYM	EXPANSION	NOTES
HIT	Heparin-induced thrombocytopenia	
HITH	Hospital in the Home	
HITS	Heparin-induced thrombocytopenia syndrome	
HIV	Human immunodeficiency virus	
HL	Hodgkin's lymphoma	
HLA	Human leukocyte antigen	
HOCM	Hypertrophic obstructive cardiomyopathy	Sometimes the O is dropped
HOPC	History of presenting complaint	
HPB	Hepatic-pancreatic-biliary	
HPNCC	Hereditary nonpolyposis colorectal cancer	
HPV	Human papillomavirus	
HR	Heart rate	
HRCT	High resolution computed tomography	
HRT	Hormone replacement therapy	
HS	Heart sounds	
HSP	Henoch–Schönlein purpura	
HSV	Herpes simplex virus	
HTN	Hypertension	Sometimes just HT
HUS	Haemolytic uraemic syndrome	
Hx	History	
HZV	Herpes zoster virus	
I&D	Incision and drainage	
IBD	Inflammatory bowel disease	
IBS	Irritable bowel syndrome	
ICC	Intercostal catheter	
ICD	Implantable cardioverter-defibrillator	
ICF	Intracellular fluid	
ICH	Intracranial haemorrhage	
ICM	Ischaemic cardiomyopathy	

Clinical abbreviations and acronyms—cont'd

ABBREVIATION/ ACRONYM	EXPANSION	NOTES
ICP	Intracranial pressure	
ICS	Intercostal space	
ICU	Intensive Care Unit	
ID	Infectious disease or intellectual disability	Consider context
IDC	Indwelling catheter or infiltrating ductal carcinoma	
IDDM	Insulin dependent diabetes mellitus	Older term
IE	Infective endocarditis	
Ig	Immunoglobulin	
IHC	Immunohistochemistry	
IHD	Ischaemic heart disease	Angina or MIs
ILC	Infiltrating lobular cancer	
ILD	Interstitial lung disease	
IM	Intramuscular or intermedullary nail	
INF	Interferon	
INR	International normalised ratio	
IO	Intraosseous	
IOC	Intraoperative cholangiography	
IPF	Idiopathic pulmonary fibrosis	
IPSS	International prostate symptom score	
IR	immediate release	
ISQ	No change	From Latin, 'in status quo'
IT	Intrathecal	Rarely used
ITP	Idiopathic thrombocytopenia purpura	
IU	International units	
IUCD	Intrauterine contraceptive device	
IV	Intravenous	
IVC	Inferior vena cava	
IVC/IVB	Intravenous cannula/bung	
IVDU	Intravenous drug user	

continued

Clinical abbreviations and acronyms—cont'd

ABBREVIATION/ ACRONYM	EXPANSION	NOTES
IVH	Interventricular haemorrhage	
IVIG	Intravenous immunoglobulin	
IVP	Intravenous pyelogram	
IVT/IVF	Intravenous therapy/fluids	Careful using IVF
Ix	Investigations	
JVP	Jugular venous pressure	
K$^+$	Potassium	KCl is potassium chloride
kg	Kilogram	Measure of mass
kPa	Kilopascal	Measure of pressure
KUB	Kidneys, ureters, bladders	
KVO	Keep vein open	For very slow infusions
L	Litre	
L)	Left	
LA	Lymphadenopathy or left atrium or local anaesthetic	Consider context
LAD	Left anterior descending (artery) or left axis deviation	
LADA	Latent autoimmune diabetes in adults	
LAMA	Long-acting muscarinic agonist	
LBBB	Left bundle branch block	
LBO	Large bowel obstruction	
LCP	Liverpool Care Plan	
LCx	Left circumflex (artery)	
LDH	Lactate dehydrogenase	
LDL	Low density lipoprotein	
LFT	Liver function test	
LHC	Left heart catheterisation	
LIF	Left iliac fossa	
LKM	Liver kidney microsome	
LL	Lower limb	
LLL	Left lower lobe	Denotes auscultation or percussion
LLQ	Left lower quadrant	
LMA	Laryngeal mask airway	

Clinical abbreviations and acronyms—cont'd

ABBREVIATION/ ACRONYM	EXPANSION	NOTES
LMO	Local medical officer	aka GP
LMN	Lower motor neuron	
LMWH	Low-molecular-weight heparin	
LN	Lymph node	
LND	Lymph node dissection	
LOA	Loss of appetite	
LOC	Loss of consciousness	
LOS	Length of stay	
LOW	Loss of weight	
LP	Lumbar puncture	
LRTI	Lower respiratory tract infection	
LUQ	Left upper quadrant	
LUTS	Lower urinary tract symptoms	
LV	Left ventricle	
LVEF	Left ventricular ejection fraction	
LVF	Left ventricular failure	
LVH	Left ventricular hypertrophy	
M&M	Morbidity and mortality	
MAC	*Mycobacterium avium* complex	
MALT	Mucosa-associated lymphoid tissue	
MAOI	Monoamine oxidase inhibitor	
MAP	Mean arterial pressure	
MAPT	Mono-antiplatelet therapy	(i.e. aspirin)
MCA	Middle cerebral artery	
MCH	Mean corpuscular haemoglobin	
M/c/s	Microscopy, culture and sensitivities	
MCL	Mantle cell lymphoma	
MCP	Metacarpophalangeal	
MCPJ	Metacarpalphalangeal joint	
MCS	Microscopy, culture and sensitivity	
MCV	Mean corpuscular volume	
MDD	Major depressive disorder	(i.e. DSM-V name for depression)

continued

Clinical abbreviations and acronyms—cont'd

ABBREVIATION/ ACRONYM	EXPANSION	NOTES
MDI	Metered dose inhaler	
MDM	Multidisciplinary meeting	
MDS	Myelodysplastic syndrome	
MDT	Multidisciplinary team	
MDU	Medical Day Unit	
MELD	Model for end-stage liver disease	
MEN	Multiple endocrine neoplasia	
MET	Medical emergency team	
MFS	Miller Fisher syndrome	
MG	Myasthenia gravis	
Mg^{2+}	Magnesium	$MgSO_4$ is magnesium sulphate
MGUS	Monoclonal gammopathy of unknown significance	
MH	Malignant hyperthermia	
MHx	Medical history	
MI	Myocardial infarction	
MIC	Minimum inhibitory concentration	
MIPPO	Mini-invasive percutaneous plate osteosynthesis	
MM	Multiple myeloma	
mmHg	Millimetres of mercury	Measuring blood pressure
MMSE	Mini Mental State Examination	
MODS	Multi-organ dysfunction syndrome	
MOF	Multi-organ failure	
MR	Mitral regurgitation	
MRA	Magnetic resonance angiography or magnetic resonance arteriography	
MRCP	Magnetic resonance cholangiopancreatography	
MRE	Magnetic resonance enterography	
MRI-B	Magnetic resonance imaging-brain	

Clinical abbreviations and acronyms—cont'd

ABBREVIATION/ ACRONYM	EXPANSION	NOTES
MRSA	Multiple-resistant *Staphylococcus aureus*	
MS	Mitral stenosis or multiple sclerosis	
MSA	Multisystem atrophy	
MSE	Mental state exam	
MSK	Musculoskeletal	
MSM	Men who have sex with men	
MSSA	Methicillin sensitive *Staphylococcus aureus*	
MTP	Metatarsophalangeal	
MTX	Methotrexate	
MuSK	Muscle-specific kinase	
MVA	Motor vehicle accident	
MVP	Mitral valve prolapse	
MVR	Mitral valve replacement	
MWA	Microwave ablation	
Mx	Management	
N&V	Nausea and vomiting	
Na^+	Sodium	NaCl is sodium chloride
NA	Noradrenaline	
NAC	N-Acetylcysteine	
NAD	No abnormality detected	Very common
NAI	Non-accidental injury	
NASH	Non-alcoholic steatohepatitis	
NB	Nota bene	(i.e. take note)
NBM	Nil by mouth	
NCS	Nerve conduction studies	
NEC	Necrotising enterocolitis	
NFR	Not for resuscitation	DNR in the USA – do not resuscitate
NGT	Nasogastric tube	
NHL	Non-Hodgkin's lymphoma	
NIDDM	Non-insulin dependent diabetes mellitus	

continued

Clinical abbreviations and acronyms—cont'd

ABBREVIATION/ ACRONYM	EXPANSION	NOTES
NIHSS	National Institutes of Health Stroke Scale	
NIMC	National inpatient medical chart	
NIV	Non-invasive ventilation	
NKA	No known allergies	
NKDA	No known drug allergies	
NMJ	Neuromuscular junction	
NMS	Neuroleptic malignant syndrome	
NMSC	Non-melanoma skin cancer	
NOAC	Novel oral anticoagulant	
NOF	Neck of femur	
NOK	Next of kin	
NPA	Nasopharyngeal aspirate	(i.e. a nasal swab)
NPH	Normal pressure hydrocephalus	
NQR	Not quite right	
NS	Normal saline	Also N/Saline
NSAID	Non-steroidal anti-inflammatory drug	
NSCLC	Non-small cell lung carcinoma	
NSTEMI	Non-ST elevation myocardial infarction	
NSVT	Non-sustained ventricular tachycardia	
NTD	Neural tube defect	
NVD	Normal vaginal delivery	
NVI	Neurovascular intact	
NWB	Non-weight bearing	
NYHA-x	New York Heart Association x	Scored 1–4
O/E	On examination	
O&G	Obstetrics and Gynaecology	
OA	Osteoarthritis	
OAB	Over active bladder	
OCD	Obsessive compulsive disorder	
OCP	Oral contraceptive pill or ova, cysts and parasites	Consider context

Clinical abbreviations and acronyms—cont'd

ABBREVIATION/ ACRONYM	EXPANSION	NOTES
OD	Overdose	DO NOT use it as 'once daily' on a drug chart!
OGTT	Oral glucose tolerance test	
OHG	Oral hypoglycaemic	
OP	Osteoporosis	
OPC	Outpatient Clinic	
OPD	Outpatient Department	
OPG	Orthopantomogram	Dental X-ray
OR	Operating room	
ORIF	Open reduction internal fixation	
ORS	Oral rehydration solution	
ORT	Oral rehydration therapy	
OSA	Obstructive sleep apnoea	
OT	Occupational therapy	
OTC	Over the counter	Refers to medication
PA	Posteroanterior	
PAA	Popliteal artery aneurysm	
PAC	Premature atrial contraction *or* post acute care or pre-admission clinic	
PAD	Peripheral arterial disease	
PAN	Polyarteritis nodosa	
PAP	Positive airway pressure	
PBC	Primary biliary cirrhosis	
PBS	Pharmaceutical Benefits Scheme	
PCA	Patient-controlled analgesia *or* posterior cerebral artery	
PCI	Percutaneous coronary intervention	Angioplasty
PCKD	Polycystic kidney disease	
PCL	Posterior cruciate ligament	
pCO_2	Partial pressure of carbon dioxide	
PCOS	Polycystic ovarian syndrome	
PCP	*Pneumocystis carinii* pneumonia	Also PJP
PCR	Polymerase chain reaction	

continued

Clinical abbreviations and acronyms—cont'd

ABBREVIATION/ ACRONYM	EXPANSION	NOTES
PCV	Packed cell volume	
PD	Peritoneal dialysis *or* Parkinson's disease	
PE	Pulmonary embolism	
PEA	Pulseless electrical activity	
PEARL	Pupils equal and reactive to light	
PEEP	Positive end expiratory pressure	
PEFR	Peak expiratory flow rate	
PEG	Percutaneous endoscopic gastronomy	
PEP	Post-exposure prophylaxis	
PET	Positron emission tomography	
PFO	Pissed fell over	
PFO	Patent foramen ovale	
PFS	Progression-free survival	
PFTs	Pulmonary function tests	Also known as RFTs – 'respiratory'
PHx	Past history	
PICC	Peripherally-inserted central catheter	
PID	Pelvic inflammatory disease	
PIN	Posterior interosseous nerve	
PJP	*Pneumocystis jiroveci* pneumonia	
PKU	Phenylketonuria	
PLT	Platelet	
PMB	Post-menstrual bleeding	
PML	Progressive multifocal leuconcephalopathy	
PMN	Polymorphonuclear leukocytes	(i.e. neutrophils)
PMR	Polymyalgia rheumatica	
PND	Paroxysmal nocturnal dyspnoea	
PO	Oral	From Latin '*per os*'. Some doctors write oral as 'ō'
pO$_2$	Partial pressure of oxygen	
POA	Power of attorney	

Clinical abbreviations and acronyms—cont'd

ABBREVIATION/ ACRONYM	EXPANSION	NOTES
POP	Plaster of Paris	(i.e. a cast)
PP	Pulse pressure	
PPE	Personal protective equipment	
PPH	Post-partum haemorrhage	
PPI	Proton pump inhibitor or a post-platelet increment	
PPM	Permanent pacemaker	
PRBC	Packed red blood cells	
PR	Per rectum or progesterone receptor	
PRES	Posterior reversible encephalopathy syndrome	
PRN	As required	From Latin, 'pro re nata'
PSA	Prostate-specific antigen	
PSC	Primary sclerosing cholangitis	
PSGN	Post-streptococcal glomerulonephritis	
PSI	pneumonia severity index	
PSP	Progressive supranuclear palsy	
PT	Physiotherapy or prothrombin time	
Pt	Patient	
PTA	Percutaneous transluminal angioplasty	
PTC	Percutaneous hepatic cholangiography	
PTCL	Peripheral T-cell lymphoma	
PTH	Parathyroid hormone	
PTx	Pneumothorax	
PUD	Peptic ulcer disease	
PUO	Pyrexia of unknown origin	
PV	Per vaginam	
PVC	Premature ventricular contraction	
PVD	Peripheral vascular disease	
PVIT	Patient voided in toilet	

continued

Clinical abbreviations and acronyms—cont'd

ABBREVIATION/ ACRONYM	EXPANSION	NOTES
PVR	Post void residual	
PVT	Paroxysmal ventrical tachycardia	
PWB	Partial weight bearing	
PXR	Pelvic X-ray	
py	Pack years	
Q	Perfusion	
QALY	Quality adjusted life year	
QFG	Quantiferon gold	
QID	Four times per day	From Latin, 'quater in die'
QT	Interval measuring the heart's electrical cycle	
R-CHOP	Rituximab, cyclophosphamide, hydroxydaunomycin, oncovin (vincristine), prednisolone	
R)	Right	
R/F	Referral	
R/O	Rule out or removal of	Avoid this if you can
R/V	Review	
RA	Right atrium or rheumatoid arthritis or room air	Consider context
RAAS	Renin–angiotensin–aldosterone system	
RACGP	Royal Australian College of General Practice	
RACP	Royal Australian College of Physicians	
RACS	Royal Australian College of Surgeons	
RAIU	Radioactive iodine uptake	
RAS	Renal artery stenosis	
RBBB	Right bundle branch block	
RBC	Red blood cell	
RCC	Renal cell carcinoma	
RCT	Randomised controlled trial	
RDNS	Royal District Nursing Service	
REM	Rapid eye movement	

Clinical abbreviations and acronyms—cont'd

ABBREVIATION/ ACRONYM	EXPANSION	NOTES
RF	Rheumatoid factor *or* rheumatic fever	
RFFF	Radial forearm free flap	
RFTs	Respiratory function tests	
RHC	Right heart catheterisation	
RIB	Resting in bed	
RLL	Right lower lobe	On auscultation or percussion
RLN	Regional lymph node *or* recurrent laryngeal nerve	
RLQ	Right lower quadrant	
RN	Registered nurse	
RNA	Ribonucleic acid	
RNS	Repetitive nerve stimulation	
ROM	Range of movement	
RoSC	Return of spontaneous circulation	
RPLND	Retroperitoneal lymph node dissection	
RR	Respiratory rate	
RRMS	Relapsing-remitting multiple sclerosis	
RRR	Regular rate and rhythm	
RRT	Renal replacement therapy	
RSI	Rapid sequence induction	
RTA	Renal tubular acidosis	
RTT	Return to theatre	
RUQ	Right upper quadrant	
RV	Right ventricle	
RVF	Right ventricular failure	
RVH	Right ventricular hypertrophy	
Rx	Medication	
RXN	Reaction	
s	Second	
S_1	First heart sound	
S_2	Second heart sound	

continued

Clinical abbreviations and acronyms—cont'd

ABBREVIATION/ ACRONYM	EXPANSION	NOTES
S_3	Third heart sound	
S_4	Fourth heart sound	
SABA	Short acting beta agonist	
SAH	Subarachnoid haemorrhage	
SaO_2	Arterial oxygen saturations	(i.e. 'sats')
SAN	Sinoatrial node	
SARS	Severe acute respiratory syndrome	
S/B	Seen by	(e.g. S/B Gastro consultant)
SBE	Subacute bacterial endocarditis	
SBO	Small bowel obstruction	
SBP	Systolic blood pressure or spontaneous bacterial peritonitis	Consider context
S/C	Subcutaneous	'subcut' is much preferred
SCBU	Special Care Baby Unit	
SCC	Squamous cell carcinoma	
SCLC	Small cell lung carcinoma	
SCM	Sternocleidomastoid	
SDH	Subdural haematoma	
Se	Serum	Common on request slips
SFX	Side effects	
SG	Specific gravity	
SGCT	Seminomatous germ cell tumour	
SHx	Social history	
SIADH	Syndrome of inappropriate antidiuretic hormone secretion	
SIDS	Sudden infant death syndrome	
SIRS	Systemic inflammatory response syndrome	
SIRT	Selective internal radiation therapy	
SJS	Stevens–Johnson syndrome	
SL	Sublingual	
SLE	Systemic lupus erythematosus	
SLN	Sentinel lymph node	
SLR	Straight leg raise	

Clinical abbreviations and acronyms—cont'd

ABBREVIATION/ ACRONYM	EXPANSION	NOTES
SMA	Superior mesenteric artery	
SNAC	Scaphoid non-union advanced collapse	
SNRI	Serotonin and noradrenaline reuptake inhibitor	
SNT	Soft not tender	
SOA	Swelling of ankles	
SOB	Shortness of breath	
SOBOE	Short of breath on exertion	
SOL	Space occupying lesion	
SOOB	Sitting out of bed	
SPC	Suprapubic catheterisation	
SPEP	Serum protein electrophoresis	
SpO_2	Oxygen saturation	
SPS	Single point stick	
SR	Sustained release	Or 'slow' release
SSG	Split skin graft	
SSRI	Serotonin selective reuptake inhibitor	
SSS	Sick sinus syndrome	
STD	Sexually-transmitted disease	Being phased out by STI
STEMI	ST elevation myocardial infarction	
STI	Sexually transmitted infection or soft tissue injury	
Subcut	Subcutaneous	
SV	Stroke volume	
SVT	Supraventricular tachycardia	
SW	Social work	
Sz	Seizure	
T_4	Thyroxine	
T/F	Transfer	
TACE	Transarterial chemoembolisation	
TACO	Transfusion-associated cardiac overload	
TAG	Triacylglycerides	

continued

Clinical abbreviations and acronyms—cont'd

ABBREVIATION/ ACRONYM	EXPANSION	NOTES
TAPP	Transabdominal peritoneal patchplasty	
TAVI	Transcatheter aortic valve replacement	
TB	Tuberculosis	
TBI	Traumatic brain injury	
TBSA	Total body surface area	
TBW	Total body water	
TCA	Tricyclic antidepressant	
TCC	Transitional cell carcinoma	
tCO_2	Plasma total carbon dioxide	
TDS	Three times daily	From Latin, *'ter in die sumendus'*
TEN	Toxic epidermal necrolysis	Sometimes TENS with 'syndrome'
TEPP	Total extraperitoneal patchplasty	
TFCC	Triangular fibrocartilage complex	
TFT	Thyroid function tests	Include T_3 and T_4
TG	Triglycerides	
Tg Ab	Thyroglobulin antibody	
THR	Total hip replacement	
TIA	Transient ischaemic attack	
TIPS	Transjugular intrahepatic portosystemic shunt	
TKR	Total knee replacement	
TM	Timpanic membrane	
TMJ	Temporomandibular joint	
TNF	Tumour necrosis factor	
TOE	Transoesophageal echo	TEE in USA
TOF	Tracheo-oesophageal fistula	
TP	Total protein	
tPA	Tissue plasminogen activator	Sometimes rTPA as it is recombinant
TPN	Total parenteral nutrition	
TPO Ab	Thyroid peroxidase antibody	
TPR	Total peripheral resistance	
TR	Tricuspid regurgitation	

Clinical abbreviations and acronyms—cont'd

ABBREVIATION/ ACRONYM	EXPANSION	NOTES
TRALI	Transfusion-related acute lung injury	
TRUS Bx	Transrectal ultrasound-guided biopsy	
TSH	Thyroid-stimulating hormone	
TSI	Thyroid-stimulating immunoglobulin	
TTE	Transthoracic echo	
TTP	Thrombotic thrombocytopenic purpura	
TUG	Timed 'up and go' test	For assessing strength in the elderly
TURBT	Transurethreal resection of bladder tumour	
TURP	Transurethral resection of prostate	
TV	Transvaginal	
TVT	Tension-free vaginal tape	
Tx	Treatment or therapy	
$T_xN_xM_x$	Tumour–nodes–metastases	
UA	Unstable angina	Also written as USA sometimes
UC	Ulcerative colitis	
UEC	Urea, electrolytes, creatinine	
UFH	Unfractionated heparin	
UGIB	Upper gastrointestinal bleeding	
UL	Upper limb	
ULN	Upper limit of normal	
UMN	Upper motor neuron	
UOP	Urinary output	
Ur	Urea	
URTI	Upper respiratory tract infection	
USA	Unstable angina	
USS	Ultrasound scan	
UTI	Urinary tract infection	
V/Q	Ventilation/perfusion	Refers to a VQ scan
VA	Visual acuity	

continued

Clinical abbreviations and acronyms—cont'd

ABBREVIATION/ ACRONYM	EXPANSION	NOTES
VAP	Ventilator-associated pneumonia	
VATS	Video-assisted thoracic surgery	
VBAC	Vaginal birth after caesarean	
VBG	Venous blood gas	
VC	Vital capacity	
VF	Ventricular fibrillation	
VIP	Vasoactive intestinal peptide	
VL	Viral load	
VLDL	Very low density lipoprotein	
V/Q	Ventilation/perfusion scan	
VRE	Vancomycin resistant Enterococci	
VT	Ventricular tachycardia	
VTE	Venous thromboembolism	
VUR	Vesicoureteral reflux	
vWF	von Willebrand factor	
VZV	Varicella zoster virus	
w/	With	
W/H	Withhold/withheld	
w/o	Without	
WAP	Wandering atrial pacemaker	
WBAT	Weight bear as tolerated	
WBC	White blood cell	
WCC	White cell count	
WLE	Wide local excision	
WNL	Within normal limits	NAD is used preferably
WPW	Wolff–Parkinson–White syndrome	
WR	Ward round	
x/12	Months	
x/24	Hours	Used on IV fluids
x/52	Weeks	
x/60	Minutes	
x/7	Days	
XR	Extended release	If relating to drugs

Clinical abbreviations and acronyms—cont'd

ABBREVIATION/ ACRONYM	EXPANSION	NOTES
XR	X-ray	
XRT	Radiotherapy	
yo	Years old	
YPLL	Years potential life lost	
Zn	Zinc	
Φ	Nil or no	
ψ	Psychiatry	
♂	Male	
♀	Female	

Common and useful medical mnemonics

TOPIC	MNEMONIC	EXPANSION
Causes of pancreatitis	GET SMASHED	Gallstones, ethanol, trauma, steroids, mumps, autoimmune, hypercalcaemia/ hypertriacylglyceridaemia, ERCP, drugs
Cranial nerves	Oh Oh Oh To Touch And Feel Very Good Velvet and Hats	Olfactory, optic, oculomotor, trochlear, trigeminal, abducens, facial, vestibulocochlear, glossopharyngeal, vagus, accessory, hypoglossal
Reversible causes of arrest	6Hs and 5Ts	Hypovolaemia, hypoxia, hypothermia, hyper/hypoglycaemia, hyper/ hypokalaemia and hydrogen ions (acidosis)
		Tension pneumothorax, tamponade, trauma, toxins (drugs and poison), thromboembolic events
Compartment syndrome	6Ps	Pain, paraesthesia, pallor, paralysis, pulselessness, poikilothermia
Management of chest pain	MONASH	Morphine, oxygen, nitrates, aspirin, statin, anti-hypertensives (Note: oxygen is now only used if hypoxemic)
Management of soft tissue injuries	RICE and no HARM	Rest, ice, compression, elevation and no heat, alcohol, running, massage
Emergency principles	DR ABCDE	Danger, response, airway, breathing, circulation, defibrillation, exposure
Responding to shortness of breath	LMNOP	Lasix (frusemide), morphine, nitrates, oxygen, positioning (i.e. sit them up)

SECTION I
GENERAL INFORMATION

CHAPTER 1

WELCOME TO MEDICAL PRACTICE

Joseph M O'Brien and Paul Watson

Starting life as a junior doctor is like moving to a new country. There are strange new customs, an entirely different language (with an acronym for everything!), people of various backgrounds and a whole set of pressures placed upon you that may seem strange and confusing. It takes time to become comfortable working in the surreal environment of a hospital. Where else can you have a conversation about bowel motions and still be considered a normal human being? Progressively, you will learn to navigate your way around the place. Although medical school does its best to teach you the principles of clinical practice, no fresh graduate feels truly prepared.

You will gradually learn to apply the principles you have learned in medical school to the real world. With continued exposure to clinical scenarios, you will build your confidence in each area and – just as you feel truly competent – it will be time for your next rotation! Fortunately, your experiences in past rotations will continue to be of use as you progress through your career.

> Expected errors are made by not knowing,
> Common errors are made by not looking.
> True mistakes are made by not asking.
>
> (An anonymous twist on the classic medical idiom)

The first few rotations will be unfamiliar and scary. Minor clinical decisions seem to be monstrous judgements that could have horrendous consequences – be mindful that your registrars will be watching over your shoulder (even if it doesn't feel like it) and you are never truly unsupported. You should always feel like you are able to approach your senior colleagues for advice – even seasoned consultants need to request help (and some even admit to it!). The dread of asking what you deem a 'silly question' is no match for the regret of having made an avoidable error. Honest and open communication is critical. A wise medical registrar once said, 'Don't lie, don't be lazy, and don't be late and we'll be great friends'.

SECTION I

Starting your career is a genuinely exciting experience and it is best to embrace every opportunity to learn while you have the greatest amount of support. Be enthusiastic, ask questions and get involved. If you don't know how to do something, ask! The best way to compensate for a lack of experience is a genuine abundance of enthusiasm.

Your intern year will not be a breeze. You will be sleep-deprived and hungry approximately 75% of the time. You will lose patients you have grown close to, you will make mistakes, and you may even wonder why you chose this profession at all. Hopefully, the thought of knowing what you are doing is making a difference to patients and their families is reward enough to counter the more difficult times. People may not always remember your name, but they will remember the way you made them feel while you provided their loved one with care long after you've clocked off for the day. We do what we can to work through the rough patches, but know that you are not in it alone – many have trodden the path before you – and there are many resources that support mental health first aid.

This text seeks to offer a guide to the wonderfully diverse and unique world of medicine and surgery. The following chapters will cover a wide range of content, from how to conduct an efficient ward round and carry out emergency assessments to outlining the most salient features of specialist medical and surgical care in both in- and outpatient settings. Written by residents, for residents, *The Junior Doctor Survival Guide* could be thought of as a 'compilation of handover documents', guiding your approach to problems encountered throughout the hospital. When used in combination with current guidelines and the knowledge of your senior clinicians, we hope to have provided a thorough yet focused summary of the required information for getting through your intern year (relatively) intact.

Be punctual, hard-working and honest, but most importantly – be excellent.

CHAPTER 2

THE JUNIOR DOCTOR

Paul Watson

WHAT IS A JUNIOR DOCTOR ANYWAY?

The term 'junior doctor' encompasses interns, residents and registrars, although colloquially it refers to interns and residents. In the Australian hospital system, each health network uses its own terminology in reference to junior doctors, although variations on the term 'medical officer' (e.g. 'house medical officer' [HMO]) are common.

The role of the junior doctor spans three domains:

- the Emergency Department (Chapter 9)
- the inpatient wards (Chapter 21)
- the outpatient clinics (Section V).

At the start of a working year junior doctors are typically allocated four or five rotations to various areas of their health network. Most health networks encompass multiple hospital sites, so it is common to be allocated to an 'external' site for at least one rotation. A hospital 'unit' refers to a department of a hospital. The unit might be split into several 'teams' of medical staff, and each team will have separate inpatient loads and outpatient clinics. Multiple teams within a department are common for General Medicine and General Surgery, whereas specialist units tend to have one team of variable size (e.g. Cardiology or Cardiac Surgery).

The medical staff will typically include those listed in Table 2.1.

UNIT STRUCTURE

The structure of your unit will be covered during orientation or handover. Depending on the workload of the unit, junior doctors will spend the majority of their time on the inpatient ward ensuring daily tasks are completed. Some metropolitan surgical units have upwards of 50 inpatients, ensuring plenty of jobs for the eager junior doctor. Other units (e.g. Rheumatology) may have few inpatients, but a heavy outpatient focus.

The specific role and responsibilities of the junior doctor vary between departments, but the core responsibilities for ward-based jobs remain the same. In the

TABLE 2.1 Medical staff in the hospital setting

Consultants	Supervising clinicians responsible for overseeing management of inpatients, reviewing outpatients and running unit meetings. They ensure the unit operates to hospital and professional standards
Fellows	Qualified specialists who are gaining experience in a sub-specialty area. May have involvement in daily ward activities, research or clinic-based roles
Registrars	Doctors in a specialist training pathway. Responsibilities change depending on area but generally include day-to-day management of inpatients, reviewing outpatients and performing procedures under supervision of consultant staff
Residents and interns	Junior doctors of varying levels of experience, responsible for ensuring daily management plans are implemented. Expected to coordinate discharges with allied health and assist as required with admissions, outpatient clinics and procedures. Interns are those in their first year of clinical practice, and are technically the most junior subtype of resident

Emergency Department (ED) junior doctors take on a more autonomous role with close supervision from consultant staff.

Before commencing a rotation, it is expected that the incoming junior doctor will contact the person whose role they are about to begin to receive a handover. This may be written (often referred to as a rolling handover or 'ROVER') or verbal, preferably in person and on the relevant ward. The handover for inpatient units should cover:

- the practical aspects of the job (e.g. workplace geography [locations of offices, clinics, tea rooms and/or the morning meeting point], pager numbers and the names of other staff members currently on the unit, and don't forget your friendly neighbourhood Allied Health team!)
- the weekly timetable for the department including ward rounds, clinics and unit meetings
- the expected daily jobs for the junior doctors on the ward
- long-term or complex patients
- any regular cover shifts, including the areas to be covered
- common and unique medications and protocols used by the unit (e.g. proton pump inhibitor infusions on Gastroenterology)
- common 'pitfalls' for the rotation (e.g. forgetting to order coagulation studies before surgery)

- useful resources (e.g. specialty guidelines and protocols, books, journal articles or websites)
- any 'quirks' to the job, unit or particular team members (e.g. the consultant who will only read a patient list if it is printed in size 9 Helvetica Neue).

For ED rotations a handover is generally unnecessary, as the department will conduct their own orientation each rotation. Junior doctors in ED are quite well supervised – ED consultants are very good at monitoring their minions (uh, interns).

COMPLETING A ROTATION

The Medical Workforce Unit expect their junior doctors to complete an evaluation form with a senior member of the medical team as a means of assessing their performance. This is a valuable time for you to provide your thoughts regarding your time as part of the team. Feedback is an important aspect of your development as a clinician, and any advice you are given should be taken seriously.

Feedback is a two-way street – senior doctors also periodically require feedback from their junior staff as part of '360° feedback' programs. Although this should be welcomed, on some units there may be resistance as this is a relatively recent concept for older clinicians. If you have a suggestion about how a unit could work better, never be afraid to suggest it – just choose your audience appropriately! You could improve outcomes for future patients and doctors by speaking up.

Internship and residency are early stages in your medical career; therefore, expansive knowledge is not expected. Take the time to ask questions, observe procedures and review patients in ED. Gaining experience is key to furthering your understanding, and an appetite for learning demonstrates your enthusiasm to the team, providing you with further opportunities for teaching. Additionally, if you were provided with a ROVER at the beginning of your rotation it is good form to update it before you rotate onwards.

THE WELL JUNIOR DOCTOR

No junior doctor should have to feel alone. As we begin our transition from medical student to junior doctor we face one of the most significant challenges in our medical careers. I've been there, as have all of your senior colleagues.

It's common to feel overwhelmed during these initial few months as you become accustomed to the daily workings of a hospital. Medicine is a teaching profession, and there are strong cultural and professional traditions of assisting our juniors through their early steps. If you feel stressed, upset or unsure of what needs to be done, speak to your registrar, a person who has a responsibility to support you.

Your fellow junior doctors will have their own unique learning experiences and pressures. Share your stories, debrief with one another, let off some steam. Your internship colleagues may well be around with you for a few years to come, with some familiar faces rotating through different units. Seek advice from these people when you become uncertain, help them when they need a hand and, most importantly, tell them when you're struggling.

The most important person to take care of is yourself. Let someone know that you're having a bad day/week/rotation. When your shift is over, go and be social, make the time to get out of the routine of working, home to sleep and then working again (with occasional eating). If you don't think you can talk to your team or registrar, contact your resident medical officer (RMO) society for support or your director of training.

If you need someone to talk to, email me at thewelljuniordoctor@gmail.com. We'll check every day.

Take care of yourself!

CHAPTER 3

CAREERS

Paul Watson and Joseph M O'Brien

GENERAL CAREER PATHWAYS

All junior doctors in Australia begin their hospital careers as interns. Internship (HMO1) is a general year with compulsory rotations in Medicine, Surgery and Emergency Medicine. During this year your medical registration with the Australian Health Practitioner Regulation Agency (AHPRA) is considered 'provisional', placing restrictions on the scope of your practice. This means that interns may only work in their own hospital network, allowing for structured education, teaching and feedback.

After internship junior doctors are given their general registration, which permits less supervised outside work such as locum positions and private assisting. Some hospital networks in Australia employ junior doctors for their first two postgraduate years.

Training is divided into prevocational and vocational. Prevocational training includes internship and residency positions and exists prior to vocational training, i.e. training years required for specialist qualification. The majority of early prevocational positions are allocated using a centralised computer matching process. Some states, such as New South Wales and Queensland, employ a lottery system to allocate internship. The increasing number of medical student graduates has increased competition for these positions nationwide.

Most positions for junior doctors are titled by the level of experience (in terms of years) and by the 'stream' (e.g. Medical, Surgical or General). For example, a position for a 3rd year postgraduate resident employed within a surgical stream might be 'HMO3 Surgical'. It should be noted that job titles vary greatly between states.

After internship, junior doctors can decide between several options to continue their residency in preparation for specialist or generalist training. There are many different streams for resident positions. Commonly used terms are listed below:

- *Medical*: most Medical (HMO2+) positions are for doctors intending to complete Basic Physician Training (BPT). After gaining a hospital position, residents then contact the Director of Physician Education (DPE) at their hospital network before registering for the training program with the Royal Australian College of Physicians (RACP).

- *Surgical*: Surgical (HMO2+) positions are typically for doctors looking for experience in preparation for applying to the Surgical Education and Training (SET) program. It is becoming common for residents to then take positions as 'unaccredited' surgical registrars before 'accredited' (or, colloquially, 'on-SET') training.

- *General*: these rotations have no specialty focus, instead seeking to give junior doctors a variety of experiences across medicine, surgery and other specialist areas such as obstetrics and psychiatry. These positions are popular with doctors considering GP training.

- *Critical care*: these (HMO2+) positions are suited to doctors interested in anaesthetics, emergency and ICU training. Typically, these years include rotations in ICU, ED or Anaesthetics, and some rotations found in the 'general' stream such as cover/relieving.

This is not an exhaustive list. There are many streams available, including residency streams at dedicated women's health and paediatric hospitals. Health networks offer a variety of senior residency roles for further experience prior to specialist training. Applications for these positions are usually made by direct application to the health network, although some states coordinate the application of junior medical positions through government websites. If you are unsure of the application process for a specific job, contact the Medical Workforce Unit at that particular network.

There are a limited number of vocational training positions offered per year, and selection is usually highly competitive. The relevant boards responsible for training determine how many training positions will be available each year. Surgical departments at hospitals often require more registrars to manage clinical workload and therefore create positions alongside accredited trainees, known as 'unaccredited' (or 'provisional') registrars. These positions do not constitute recognised surgical training to the Royal Australasian College of Surgeons (RACS) but are seen as valuable experience in preparation for future applications to SET. Each training program has different entry requirements, which are subject to change every year. Some training programs now require unaccredited registrar experience prior to applying for SET.

SPECIALIST TRAINING COLLEGES

The following brief descriptions (Table 3.1) outline the 15 medical specialist colleges and their associated specialist qualifications as recognised by the Australian Medical Council (AMC). Specialist training practices are constantly subject to review and major structural changes can be implemented. When researching career pathways you should review the website for the training college on a regular basis for updates.

When considering a specialist pathway there are many additional ways to get information regarding the selection and training process. Consider the following:

TABLE 3.1 Australian Medical Council recognised training colleges

SPECIALTY	SPECIALTY COLLEGE	SPECIALTY AREAS
Physician • **Adult** • **Paediatrics and Child Health**	Royal Australasian College of Physicians (RACP) (https://www.racp.edu.au) Every junior doctor must complete BPT, a 3-year program of mixed residency and registrar responsibilities After the BPT has been completed, further specialist training in medical disciplines can then be undertaken, known as Advanced Training (AT) Junior doctors commence BPT as early as PGY2, with a growing mix of resident and registrar positions over the training period	General Medicine General Paediatrics Cardiology Clinical Genetics Clinical Pharmacology Community Child Health Endocrinology Gastroenterology and Hepatology Geriatric Medicine Haematology Immunology and Allergy Infectious Diseases Intensive Care Medicine Medical Oncology Neonatal/Perinatal Medicine Nephrology Neurology Nuclear Medicine Paediatric Emergency Medicine Palliative Medicine Respiratory and Sleep Medicine Rheumatology RACP also coordinate training for the following recognised specialist fields: Addiction Medicine Public Health Rehabilitation Sexual Health Occupational and Environmental Medicine

continued

TABLE 3.1 Australian Medical Council recognised
training colleges—cont'd

SPECIALTY	SPECIALTY COLLEGE	SPECIALTY AREAS
Surgeon	Royal Australasian College of Surgeons (www.surgeons.org)	Cardiothoracic Surgery General Surgery Neurosurgery Orthopaedic Surgery Otolaryngology – Head and Neck Surgery Paediatric Surgery Plastic and Reconstructive Surgery Urology Vascular Surgery
General Practice	Royal Australian College of General Practice (www.racgp.org.au) Australian College of Rural and Remote Medicine (www.acrrm.org.au)	General Practice Rural and Remote Medicine
Obstetrics and Gynaecology	Royal Australian and New Zealand College of Obstetricians and Gynaecologists (www.ranzcog.edu.au)	Obstetrics and Gynaecology Gynaecological Oncology Maternal–Foetal Medicine Obstetrics and Gynaecological Ultrasound Reproductive Endocrinology and Infertility Urogynaecology
Intensive Care	College of Intensive Care Medicine (www.cicm.org.au)	Intensive Care Medicine
Emergency	Australasian College for Emergency Medicine (https://www.acem.org.au)	Emergency Medicine
Radiology	Royal Australian and New Zealand College of Radiologists (www.ranzcr.edu.au)	Diagnostic Radiology Diagnostic Ultrasound Nuclear Medicine Radiation Oncology

TABLE 3.1 Australian Medical Council recognised training colleges—cont'd

SPECIALTY	SPECIALTY COLLEGE	SPECIALTY AREAS
Pathology	Royal College of Pathologists of Australasia (www.rcpa.edu.au)	General Pathology Anatomical Pathology (including Cytopathology) Chemical Pathology Forensic Pathology Haematology Immunology Microbiology
Ophthalmology	Royal Australian and New Zealand College of Ophthalmologists (https://www.ranzco.edu)	Ophthalmology
Dermatology	Australasian College of Dermatologists (www.dermcoll.edu.au)	Dermatology
Medical Administrators	The Royal Australasian College of Medical Administrators (www.racma.edu.au)	Medical Administration
Psychiatry	Royal Australian and New Zealand College of Psychiatrists (https://www.ranzcp.org) Psychiatry is a minimum of 5 years: 12 months basic adult psychiatry; 24 months elective rotations; and 24 months advanced level electives and subspecialty training	Adult Psychiatry Child and Adolescent Psychiatry Addiction Medicine Consultation–Liaison Psychiatry Forensic Psychiatry Psychiatry of Old Age Psychotherapies
Anaesthetics	Australian and New Zealand College of Anaesthetists (www.anzca.edu.au)	Anaesthesia Pain Medicine
Sports Medicine	Australasian College of Sports Physicians (https://acsp.org.au)	Sports and Exercise Medicine

- Preference a rotation in that specialty, which may include applying for a position in a health network that offers the service.
- Seek out senior clinicians who have recently completed (or are about to complete) the training pathway as mentors. This gives you an opportunity to learn about their workload and lifestyle, network and become involved in research.
  - Once you are more senior yourself, becoming a mentor to those more junior than you can be an enriching experience and a good way to build a referral base for the future.
- Attend conferences as a student or junior doctor to develop an understanding of common research themes. This also gives you insight into sub-specialist practice that you may not have been previously exposed to.
- Skills courses (Chapter 6) offered by colleges will assist in preparing you for practice as a trainee; these courses can usually be completed before training.

Medicine offers a rich variety of career options for the junior doctor, and each rotation has the potential to surprise and inspire. Keep an open mind to new experiences as, even if you don't end up pursuing that particular path, the skills and knowledge further your overall development as a clinician.

CHAPTER 4

PROFESSIONALISM

Paul Watson and Joseph M O'Brien

Medical school curriculums now place huge emphasis on educating students about professionalism. The term 'professionalism' is widely used to describe a variety of expectations regarding the performance of students and doctors in health care settings. The Australian Medical Association (AMA) has outlined a set of principles in their publication of a code of ethics that relate to the conduct of medical professionals. Box 4.1 contains one section of the code, which provides an overview of the concept of workplace professionalism (note that a new code will be released in 2017).

PROFESSIONALISM IN THE WORKPLACE

There are also a number of practical applications of the AMA principles that relate to your daily work as a junior doctor. Your perceived professionalism (and, thereby, reputation) is influenced by a number of factors related to your work performance. Often, medical students and junior doctors feel that professionalism is 'taught to death' and is unnecessarily repeated. However, it is essential to remember that professionalism is not just an attitude, but a competency. Some of the broad areas that apply to junior doctors include:

- Communication
  - Polite, clear and constant communication with your colleagues and patients ensures that everyone is kept aware of issues affecting the team and patient care. Consultants, especially in medical teams where oral presentations of cases are common, will always take note and give feedback on communication skills.
  - Honesty is mandatory in all dealings with colleagues, patients and their families.
  - Communication with the administrative staff of the hospital regarding issues of annual, conference and sick leave also helps plan for staffing of your unit if you're unavailable to work. As in any workplace, the more notice you can give the more chance the unit has to cover your absence.

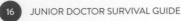

BOX 4.1 AMA Code of Ethics: 2 The doctor and the profession

- Build a professional reputation based on integrity and ability.
- Recognise that your personal conduct may affect your reputation and that of your profession.
- Refrain from making comments which may needlessly damage the reputation of a colleague.
- Report suspected unethical or unprofessional conduct by a colleague to the appropriate peer review body.
- Where a patient alleges unethical or unprofessional conduct by another doctor, respect the patient's right to complain and assist them in resolving the issue.
- Accept responsibility for your psychological and physical wellbeing as it may affect your professional ability.
- Keep yourself up to date on relevant medical knowledge, codes of practice and legal responsibilities.

Adapted from: 'Australian Medical Association, 2006. AMA Code of Ethics. A new code will be released in 2017. <https://ama.com.au/position-statement/ama-code-ethics-2004-editorially-revised-2006>.

- Written communication in the form of documentation is an expectation. This includes ward rounds, phone advice, procedures and discharge summaries.
- Organisation
  - The junior doctor is often tasked with creating patient lists, preparing unit meetings and following up clinical investigations and documentation. Your ability to prioritise tasks, share workload with your colleagues and keep track of daily tasks is essential to the function of your department.
  - An important factor in your ability to be organised relates to how well you prepare at the start of a shift. It seems like commonsense that arriving early, and not late, is key to ensuring a prompt start. If only one person from the team needs to arrive much earlier to prepare a list, a discussion the day before regarding who will take responsibility can help prevent delays. A simple but often overlooked solution.
- Education
  - As soon as you graduate from medical school you're completely responsible for your own education. Teaching is a large part of medical culture; however, medicine is a content heavy profession that is always undergoing revision. Training programs offer curriculums for study but the learning is self-directed.
  - Minor procedures like IV cannulation and suturing are best learned as a student; however, if you're unable to perform these expected minor

skills as a junior doctor, you need to take responsibility to develop and practice.

- Performance
  - As a registered health practitioner your actions are subject to peer scrutiny. Junior doctors are expected to seek feedback on their performance at regular intervals. For interns this is a compulsory aspect of your provisional registration.

The topic of professionalism is vastly more expansive than these four categories. This discussion seeks to demonstrate that your education regarding the standards of professionalism spans your career. As you develop more responsibility as a doctor, the expectations regarding your performance increase. The ability to upgrade your knowledge and skills and their practical implementation have a direct impact on patient care. Failure to develop in line with professional standards throughout your training will potentially lead to a stalled career, and can even result in risk to patient safety. A positive attitude towards your professional development is essential to your growth as a junior doctor. Seek out feedback, as identifying and addressing your shortcomings will increase your confidence in your own performance.

THE JUNIOR DOCTOR AND #SOCIALMEDIA

The ongoing creep of online social media into our lives continues, with the majority of junior doctors having an account with at least one platform (be it Twitter, Facebook, Instagram or 'miscellaneous'). Junior doctors can be tempted to convey their workplace victories, emotions and opinions in the same manner as they do in their personal lives. Unfortunately, this has led to instances where patient confidentiality has been breached, intra-hospital relations have been damaged, and future employment opportunities lost due to unprofessional behaviour in these media. In response, the AMA and many hospitals have developed a social media policy outlining the expectations for junior doctors. A summary of common recommendations includes the following:

- To maintain confidentiality, no patients or situations should be able to be accurately determined by the *sum* of information you post (e.g. don't complain about your 'male ward consultant' in a deidentified manner if there is only one male consultant on that team – you don't have to be the world's greatest detective to decipher that one!).
- Particular caution should be taken in rural areas – obscure connections are more easily made in smaller communities and the ramifications can be greater.
- Anonymity does not make unprofessional behaviour acceptable.
- Don't make defamatory statements. Just don't. If you need to vent, go to a boxing class.

- Avoid forming online relationships (e.g. Facebook friendships) with patients or former patients. Consider creating a professional page, separate to your personal account.

Lastly, remember that potential employers are increasingly screening their candidate's online presence prior to the interview stage. You don't want to miss out on your dream job because the first Google hit on your name is a picture of you up to no good!

CHAPTER 5

COMMUNICATION

Paul Watson

First impressions with colleagues, patients and seniors are largely influenced by your communication skills. The term 'communication skills' refers to more than the classically described verbal and non-verbal communication categories – it encompasses the proficiency and consistency of the junior doctor in conveying information. The effort the junior doctor puts into communication is such a crucial yet underrated factor in the success (or lack thereof) of their interactions with other doctors, students, nurses, allied health staff, patients and visitors.

There are two main domains of communication – verbal and written.

1 Verbal communication includes both face-to-face and over the telephone. The latter has an added layer of complexity, as you are speaking to somebody without the ability to use non-verbal cues to convey information.

2 Written communication is predominantly thorough documentation, and includes:

   o ward notes (Chapter 21)

   o discharge summaries (Chapter 31)

   o operation notes (Chapter 28)

   o discussions held with other units/family members/primary care practices

   o following clinical reviews of patients and clinical procedures.

VERBAL COMMUNICATION

When speaking to someone in person, follow the rules of basic courtesy – be attentive, polite and constructive in your discussions. Arguments with other staff members are seldom helpful and only taint future interactions. You might feel as though you are in the right, but a loud, heated and public exchange does not constitute professional behaviour. If you believe that an important discussion point needs to be raised, allow tempers to cool and return at a later point if the clinical situation allows.

If a situation arises on the ward where you believe that you are unable to have reasonable discussion with other staff members due to (for example) differences of opinion or prior miscommunication, it is best to get your senior involved. This is fairly generic advice but the early involvement of a third party prevents escalation of conflict.

Discussions over the telephone typically take the form of referrals to other medical services. The expectations of the person in this situation are different to a face-to-face discussion. When you call to make a referral it is expected that you are prepared with the relevant, accurate information, present in a logical structure and have easy access to other patient information. The ISBAR system is commonly used in Australian hospitals as a template for presenting complex information (see Chapter 15).

Referrals proceed much more smoothly when the person on the other end of the phone is clear on the clinical status of the patient. The conversation is likely to be more productive if you know the facts of the patient's history and examination and have access to their current medications and results. This organisation gives your colleague the impression that you have given the situation some careful thought, showing respect for their time.

WRITTEN COMMUNICATION

Written communication is the most crucial task of a junior doctor. Your seniors will constantly ask if you have documented key patient events in the notes. It is essential to adopt a practice of documenting every change in your patient's current clinical condition and management plan, as well as discussions with other staff/family. Always begin any note with the date, time and an identification of those present. Your notes need to be legible; the joke of the doctor with the bad handwriting falls flat when the nursing staff must continually call you to interpret your morning notes.

As a future independent clinician, your own notes will provide background to potentially years of complex medical treatment; it is therefore in the patient's best interest that clear, thorough documentation is made that forms an accurate past history. Inpatient documentation is taken seriously: any adverse event at any point of inpatient care will result in careful scrutiny of the documented notes; ensure you document in a professional manner, with relevant clinical information. Slang and uncommon acronyms and abbreviations are best avoided.

There are special forms of documentation that the junior doctor is responsible for (as listed above) that will be covered in later parts of the text, but the principles of written communication remain the same. It is worth noting that, once you have written in a patient's notes, you must always assume that someone has read that entry.

It is unacceptable to alter clinical notes retrospectively without a notation on the time and nature regarding the change to what has been previously documented. This new entry must always be written at the next empty space in the patient's folder, without marking the previous notes. All computer-based patient note systems do not allow alteration to clinical notes for this reason.

Remember that your attitude towards communicating with those around you shapes how your colleagues perceive you as a junior medical professional. A reputation for being argumentative or difficult with unreliable documentation can often outlast changed behaviours.

CHAPTER 6

TEACHING AND EDUCATION

Joseph M O'Brien and Paul Watson

The word 'doctor' originates from the Latin for 'teacher', and the spirit of passing down one's knowledge from one generation of doctors to the next has been an integral part of our profession since before the first 'modern' medical schools were established in Paris in the 1800s.

TEACHING AS A JUNIOR DOCTOR

There are plenty of opportunities for you to share your knowledge with your peers as you progress through medicine. Most universities will have 'vertical education' programs in place, as well as study group mentoring. These range from informal chats over coffee with junior students in your inpatient team (my personal preference) to regularly occurring, university-style tutorials. Teaching junior students on your ward round should not be a long, laborious task – slip knowledge and hints in around what your team is doing. Reviewing a patient with AF? Quiz them quickly about therapeutic anticoagulation! Be friendly and approachable, allocate them roles on your ward round (e.g. getting charts and closing curtains), and make sure they know their professional boundaries when dealing with senior clinicians. Encourage involvement in team activities and remember it is good form for the most senior doctor (which may be you!) to buy the coffee after rounds. Teaching reinforces content you have learned in previous years, improves your communication skills and helps foster professional networks outside your own cohort. Who do you think will be referring patients to you when you are a Ferrari-driving orthopaedic surgeon?

The natural evolution of a senior medical student with a great interest in teaching is to university-employed tutoring. At certain universities this may be possible prior to graduation. Teaching medical students in a professional capacity is a rewarding experience that may lead to a role as a lecturer later in your career. Surgical candidates commonly teach anatomy to medical and other science students at a university level, allowing them to perform dissections and garner further experience while learning to convey the information at an appropriate level, something they are expected to do as part of their oral examinations. Becoming a tenured professor may be your long-term dream, but it requires years of casual and part-time experience before you can work in the world of academia exclusively.

CONTINUING MEDICAL EDUCATION

Your medical education in no way ends once you've walked across that brightly-lit graduation stage – it marks the beginning of the next phase of your life-long learning. A well-known paper stated the 'half-life' of knowledge in medicine is 5 years. This implies that, 5 years after you graduate, *half* of what you learned in medical school will have been superseded. Whether or not this figure is accurate, the fact remains that much will change in medicine over the course of your career. These changes range from minor – for example, new medications are released that are shown clinically to be superior and thus replace our familiar drugs – to large, practice-changing developments in patient management. Who would have imagined 5 years ago that we would be using teleconferencing to thrombolyse stroke patients in rural hospitals?

In Australia we are not only ethically but professionally bound to continue our own education beyond the tertiary level. Continuing medical education (CME) points are awarded for taking part in several activities – publishing research, intern/resident teaching or attending and presenting at conferences. Specialist training programs require registrars to accrue a specified number of CME points over the duration of their program. Hospitals that provide accredited intern positions are required to provide sufficient intern teaching to satisfy your Australian Medical Council training requirements in a year. Experiences vary, but in many hospitals this is protected teaching time where your pager is covered by another doctor. These lectures are usually delivered by consultants in your network and are worth attending when your ward is under control.

Self directed learning is the norm in both university-level and postgraduate studies. Apart from textbooks, many senior students and junior doctors read journals in the fields they are interested in pursuing as specialist exams will have a level of expected knowledge of current literature. Other popular resources include clinical decision support services such as ClinicalKey and websites on the internet, which discuss recent happenings in evidence-based medicine. Investigate the type of examinations you will have to pass in your career and tailor your study methods to match.

There are many courses offered by specialist training bodies to further your skills. For example, the Royal Australasian College of Surgeons offer several programs such as Emergency Management of Severe Trauma (EMST), similar to the international Advanced Trauma Life Support course. These skill courses offer an opportunity to further your education in advanced clinical scenarios. These courses are requirements for all surgical training programs; however, spots are allocated to junior doctors. If you hold a strong interest in surgical training it is worthwhile registering your interest early in your prevocational training as the waiting list for some of these courses can be up to three years.

Lastly, it can be easy to think of ongoing medical education as a purely academic pursuit but do not neglect the procedural aspect of learning. There are many skills to be learned on the wards as a junior doctor from venepuncture to lumbar punctures. It is a good idea (and sometimes enforced by hospitals) to keep a logbook of your clinical skills. Particularly for surgical jobs, these are increasingly requested at interviews and feedback sessions and you do not want to get caught without one!

CHAPTER 7

REPRESENTATION OF JUNIOR DOCTORS

Joseph M O'Brien

There are a number of challenges that face junior doctors as they begin their careers, both individually and as a cohort. Fortunately, this is well-recognised by those who have trodden the path before them and there are a number of groups and important documents in place that advocate for the rights and interests of doctors-in-training. Doctors-in-training (DiT) are junior doctors who have not yet completed their fellowship (e.g. interns, residents and registrars).

THE AUSTRALIAN MEDICAL ASSOCIATION

The Australian Medical Association (AMA) is recognised as the peak membership organisation representing the registered medical practitioners (and medical students) of Australia. Born out of the Australian-based branches of the British Medical Association in 1962, the AMA advocates for the rights of doctors at federal and state levels, protects the independence of doctors, promotes ethical behaviour, informs the government on policy, represents Australia on the World Medical Association Council and supports medical research through their publications, such as the *Medical Journal of Australia*. There are state branches located in each capital city and they operate multiple councils and committees with particular purposes (e.g. the AMA Council of General Practice or the Committee for Healthy Ageing). The AMA has close ties with student groups, such as the Australian Medical Student Association, to advocate for the rights of future doctors.

The AMA also has a number of useful position papers surrounding national health issues such as aged care, mental health and Indigenous health care. Also available are workplace-related papers that guide daily practice such as registration, working conditions and eHealth records. There are even statements on political issues in the media, such as health reform, global warming and doctors' fees.

Of particular interest to junior doctors is the DiT committee. These state-based groups represent doctors-in-training in each Australian state, aiming to improve

CHAPTER 8

FINANCES

Paul Watson

Internship may mark the beginning of full-time employment for the junior doctor. For some, this may involve moving house, possibly out of the family home for the very first time. Junior doctors not only have to contend with increasing responsibility at work, but also over their own financial affairs.

Even as early as medical school you may notice increasing discussion around concepts such as salary packaging, saving receipts for tax deductions and looking into deals offered by various financial and accounting institutions specifically targeted at junior doctors. This chapter seeks to outline some basic concepts of managing money that are common concerns for the junior doctor. The following information is an explanation of how these processes work, not an endorsement of their use. You should seek independent financial advice regarding whether these packages are suitable for you.

SALARY AND PACKAGING OPTIONS

Salary

The gross salary you are paid each pay cycle is calculated according to the number of hours worked at base rate with the addition of overtime, penalty rates and other allowances as per the doctors-in-training agreement for your state. Before this amount is deposited in your account, income tax and, if required, Higher Education Loan Program (HELP) amounts are withheld along with any other agreed deductions resulting in your net pay. The amount of income tax and HELP withheld amounts are based on your fortnightly gross salary and the exact calculations can be found on the Australian Taxation Office (ATO) website (https://www.ato.gov.au).

Salary packaging

Public health networks in Australia offer salary packaging allowing hospital staff to spend 'pre-tax' dollars on selected items and services. Pre-tax refers to the money you allocate to salary packaging per pay cycle that is deducted from your gross salary before taxation, thereby decreasing the amount of income tax that will be withheld.

Items and services that are permitted in salary packaging arrangements are known as 'benefits'; they can be fringe benefits, exempt benefits or superannuation contributions. Fringe benefits include items such as loan repayments (including mortgage, personal loans and sometimes credit cards), rent, cars and other personal expenses. In public hospitals, junior doctors are currently permitted to package around $9000 of fringe benefits per Fringe Benefits Tax (FBT) year (March to March, as distinct from the traditional end of financial year). Exempt benefits have no cap, and include items such as portable computers and software.

Another popular benefit scheme is the meals and entertainment packages that permit pre-tax dollars to be used on a specialised card; however, each hospital packaging organisation offers slightly different arrangements. It is therefore best to speak to the salary packaging team at your network directly regarding what can be packaged. Keep in mind that salary packaging is not a free service and administrative costs will be deducted. Recent legislation has capped meals and entertainment salary packaging at $2500 per FBT year.

Some quick tips on salary packaging follow:

- If you work at more than one hospital site you could be eligible to package fringe benefits at any of your rostered sites during the same FBT year.

- If you have a HELP debt it's important to remember that your repayments are calculated by your gross income plus your total value of fringe benefits at the end of the financial year. It's worth checking with payroll that sufficient fortnightly tax is being withheld to ensure you meet your required overall repayment for the financial year.

- You will be required to provide evidence to substantiate your claims, such as loan statements, credit card statements etc.

INCOME TAX AND DEDUCTIONS

At the end of the financial year you will need to submit a tax return. You can complete your tax return or seek accounting advice from a qualified accountant who can help submit on your behalf. At this time you can list items to count as tax deductions. If eligible, the value of these deductions will be subtracted from your total income. Items that are considered valid deductions can be found on the ATO website, but it may not always be apparent whether you are eligible. If you are unsure, then it's always best to seek independent advice. Some general items that can be universally considered as deductions include:

- work-related expenses such as professional association fees (e.g. AHPRA registration, specialist college fees and cost of training-related examinations)

- some education costs such as skills courses, which need to relate to your work in the medical field to count as deductions

- charitable donations

- costs of managing your tax affairs.

Some items are eligible for salary packaging *and* tax deductions; however, you are not permitted to list items as both.

Financial advice can be useful for issues relating to salary packaging, taxation and other general advice, but you must weigh the benefits against any cost for yourself. Some companies give free presentations to medical students and junior doctors at various meetings, outlining their various accounting/financial advice packages, which can give some insight prior to utilising any of their services.

SECTION II
INITIAL ASSESSMENTS

CHAPTER 9

THE EMERGENCY DEPARTMENT

Paul Watson and Joseph M O'Brien

Emergency Departments (EDs) are the initial contact point for most patients admitted to hospital. The structure of the ED is therefore different to that of the ward (see Table 9.1), with an enhanced focus on facilitating patient flow. In the past few years, EDs nationwide have adopted the National Emergency Access Targets (NEAT), which specify that a patient should be assessed and admitted or discharged within 4 hours of presentation. The ultimate goals of the targets are to ease ED overcrowding and its association with increased patient mortality. Patient safety is, however, the core value of any health network; therefore, it's important to ensure that patients are reviewed as clinical priority necessitates.

Emergency departments are dynamic work environments with new models of patient care undergoing constant evaluation. As such, there will be slight differences between departments in separate hospitals. Larger ED departments have specialised areas such as paediatrics.

TRIAGE AND PATIENT FLOW

Table 9.2 lists the triage categories and associated maximum waiting times for review.

There are several clinical factors that influence a patient's triage category. For example, acute chest pain generally attracts at least a category 2, and acute abdominal pain is at least a category 3. Higher category patients requiring monitoring tend to be allocated to general cubicles whereas lower category patients that are ambulant can be reviewed in 'fast track' areas, which use examination chairs. These are not set rules, merely guidelines. A dizzy patient may have an ATS category of 4, but they are not ambulatory so a bed in a general cubicle is required.

Patients are sometimes referred to the ED by primary care physicians such as GPs in the community for evaluation of conditions that require rapid investigation or management. Typically, the GP will include a letter with the presenting complaint, assessment and recent investigations. These assessments can provide an

TABLE 9.1 Categories of ED beds

MAIN ED AREA	DESCRIPTION
General cubicles	The most common type of cubicle, for non-ambulant patients or those who require close monitoring
Resuscitation/trauma cubicles	Larger cubicles with a larger array of equipment and specialised nursing staff to deal with potentially life-threatening illness and injury including chest pain, respiratory distress, circulatory compromise, high speed trauma and patients who require sedation
'Fast track' or 'Rapid treatment'	An area where ambulant patients can be reviewed. Commonly used for musculoskeletal injuries and minor trauma. Each ED has specific guidelines on whether a patient may be suitable for review in this area
Short stay unit	A ward style area where patients can be admitted for a period expected to be less than 24 hours for further treatment

TABLE 9.2 Australasian triage scale (ATS)

TRIAGE SCALE CATEGORY	MAXIMUM WAITING TIME FOR REVIEW
1	Immediate
2	Within 10 minutes
3	Within 30 minutes
4	Within 1 hour
5	Within 2 hours

Adapted from: Australasian College for Emergency Medicine (ACEM), 2013. Policy on the Australasian Triage Scale [Internet]. <www.acem.org.au>.

excellent starting point for history and examination, and the GP will always welcome a phone call for clarification, appreciating the update from the ED on the progress of their patient.

The end points of an ED presentation are inpatient admission, Short Stay Unit (SSU) admission or discharge. Some hospitals use a medical assessment and planning unit (MAPU) as an intermediary between the formal medical wards and the ED, with patients admitted under the inpatient acute assessment team. One of the aims of your initial assessment of a patient should be to determine which end point is likely to apply. Keep the consultant and the nurse in charge updated as this will help with planning for your patient and the department overall. As you gain experience it will become easier to determine which patients are likely to require inpatient admission and which can be discharged with appropriate follow-up.

Chapters 10 and 11 offer a glance at the pathway ED provides for separating patients who require admission from those who require short-term management under observation and those who need to have outpatient review from either their GP or a specialist. By identifying crucial factors of disease and injury presentations (and with plenty of experience!) the initial investigation management and referral process comes more readily to the junior doctor.

SHORT STAY UNIT (SSU)

A variety of terms are used by different health networks to refer to 'short stay' units:

- Short Stay and Observation Unit (SSOU)
- Emergency Department Observation Unit (EDOU/EOU)
- Clinical Decision Unit (CDU).

Short stay admissions follow set 'pathways', developed by the senior ED staff as a means of streamlining patients who will require brief ongoing observation, investigation and management away from the general ED cubicles. These pathways vary among hospitals, but generally include conditions that require short intervention and that do not warrant inpatient admission.

Generally, a consultant is responsible for overseeing the short stay unit and will 'round' on the patients at least once per shift to determine their progress and discharge status. If you have a patient who is potentially suitable for short stay, they must be accepted by this consultant. Patients admitted to SSU will need to have an inpatient drug chart completed.

Each short stay pathway will have a document that outlines the inclusion and exclusion criteria for a patient to be accepted (see Table 9.3). SSU admissions should have clear plans with an established diagnosis. Patients admitted to SSU are expected to be discharged within 24 hours.

JUNIOR DOCTORS IN THE ED

The Australasian College for Emergency Medicine (ACEM) guidelines state that junior doctors should be rostered to ED shifts in a manner that allows close supervision by senior staff. The ED provides a great learning environment allowing the junior doctor to develop their assessment skills, begin to understand the role of investigations and become proactive in initiating management.

Junior doctors, especially interns, are required to discuss all cases with the consultant in charge of their area. This includes reviewing all imaging and investigations such as ECGs, allowing greater supervision and providing an opportunity for teaching. If you become concerned about the progress of your patient at any

TABLE 9.3 Commonly used short stay pathways

NAME OF PATHWAY	INCLUSION CRITERIA
Chest pain	Patient unlikely to have an ischaemic event with a negative initial troponin, for observation and serial troponin
Pyelonephritis	Urinary tract infection, for 24 hours on IV antibiotics, analgesia and observation
Paracetamol overdose	Overdose (including low risk intentional), for serial paracetamol levels to determine if NAC required (Chapter 18)
Simple dehydration	Patients who present with hypovolaemia due to decreased intake, for IV rehydration
Migraine	Patients with established migraine, for analgesia and observation
Renal colic	Patients with established renal calculi, for analgesia and observation; CT KUB typically required
Minor head injury	Low impact head strike, patients admitted with suspected concussion for observation
Discharge planning	Patients discharged from ED who presented from supported accommodation or care facilities awaiting transport home Patients awaiting review from discharge support services such as 'Hospital in the Home' to arrange treatment in the community such as IV antibiotics or wound dressings
Post-sedation	Patients who have undergone conscious sedation for simple treatments of injuries (e.g. fracture/dislocations) who are to be discharged with outpatient follow-up

stage or you are unsure of the diagnosis, you should speak to your consultant – don't be afraid to ask questions. The clinical picture is not always immediately clear and further investigation or opinion from specialist teams may be required to guide management.

The following chapters are aimed at giving you a framework for your assessment of patients with a strong focus on the core foundations of diagnosis: history and examination.

CHAPTER 10

CRITICAL CARE ASSESSMENTS

Paul Watson and Todd Galvin Manning

The Emergency Department provides the junior doctor with good exposure to the implementation of treatment guidelines in patients who present with medical emergencies and severe injuries. The guidelines and recommendations are formulated by review of the scientific literature and the use of expert consensus opinion. Depending on the hospital network there may be slight variations based on the resources or staff available. Some of the specific management points contained in these documents are discussed later throughout the text.

THE PRIMARY SURVEY AND RESUSCITATION

For the junior doctor, the key aspect of any patient presentation is recognising a medical emergency, calling for assistance and initiating a primary survey. Triggering a medical emergency call should lead to the rapid arrival of senior staff to assist; however, the junior doctor should be capable of making an early assessment of the patient's status and initiate resuscitation according to the guidelines.

Primary survey

A rapid assessment of the patient's cardiopulmonary status can be performed using the first part of the mnemonic **ABC**DE (airway, breathing, circulation, disability, exposure):

Airway

- Airway management is required in patients who are unable to maintain a patent airway due to being unconscious or obstructed. Assessment of the airway in the unconscious patient is the first priority, superseding concern about spinal injury.
- The airway should be opened to check for obstruction by using a chin lift.

- An obstructed airway or partially obstructed airway may require suction clearance, removal of foreign body or surgical access in case of total obstruction.

Breathing

- The presence of breathing is established by the look/listen/feel technique:
  - looking and feeling for chest wall movement
  - listening for escaping air from the nose and mouth.
- The presence of breathing does not rule out impending airway obstruction from delayed injury response or further loss of consciousness. An ongoing assessment of breathing should be performed.
- Deep chest wounds may indicate pneumothorax.

Circulation

- A pulse check can confirm the presence of circulation but also provide other vital information such as whether there is tachycardia, bradycardia, a cool periphery or a warm, flushed limb.
- A patient with a palpable radial pulse indicates a systolic blood pressure (SBP) of at least 80 mmHg, and a palpable femoral pulse indicates SBP of at least 70 mmHg.
- Blood pressure monitoring cuffs are normally placed on the patient during the early stages of resuscitation; however, if there is difficulty reading BP, invasive monitoring might be considered.
- Patients who have had major trauma are at risk of major blood loss from open wounds, fractures and undetected bleeding in the chest, abdomen and pelvis.

If the patient does not show signs of cardiopulmonary function, advanced life support protocols should be initiated.

Resuscitation

Resuscitation guidelines in the event of an apparent cardiac arrest follow the Advanced Life Support (ALS) guidelines (see Figure 10.1) as set by the Australian Resuscitation Council (ARC). The key focus is to initiate the pathway as soon as the emergency is identified, known as the 'chain of survival', in order to maintain chances of survival from resuscitation. These steps include:

- early access to the emergency team (medical emergency team [MET] or emergency response team)
- early initiation of resuscitation
- early access and use of defibrillation
- early input of advanced care for post-resuscitation.

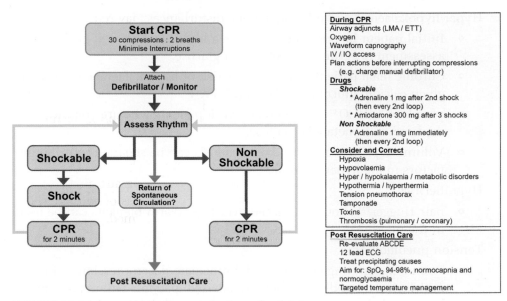

FIGURE 10.1 Advanced Life Support Pathway for Adults.
CPR, cardiopulmonary resuscitation; ETT, endotracheal tube; IV, intravenous; LMA, laryngeal mask airway.

Adapted from: Australian Resuscitation Council and New Zealand Resuscitation Council, 2016. Guideline: Advanced Life Support for Adults.

When a response code is triggered the emergency team is immediately notified, the nursing staff will bring the resuscitation trolley (including the defibrillator) and the intensive care team will automatically be notified, allowing discussion regarding the appropriate post-resuscitation setting.

Large bore IV access should be established and a full set of pathology tubes should be sent for investigations. The chest should be adequately exposed.

During the resuscitation the team members will all have specific roles, including the 'resus team leader' who should consider the reversible causes of cardiac arrest, known commonly as the '4 Hs and Ts'.

Hypoxia

○ All patients undergoing resuscitation receive oxygen therapy to prevent hypoxia. Non-invasive O_2 monitoring such as pulse oximetry is unreliable in patients who have arrested.

Hypovolaemia

○ Shock, due to volume or distributive causes (see below), should be treated with IV fluids to maintain intravascular volume. Hypovolaemia due to volume loss is invariable due to internal haemorrhage in the absence of obvious trauma, and these patients should have surgical input.

Hyper/hypokalaemia and other metabolic disturbances

- Initial patient bloods should include a blood gas that will give rapid assessment of serum potassium and glucose.
- Chronic renal patients are at higher risk of hyperkalaemia and can be given calcium gluconate 10% 10 mL IV.
- 50 mL of $NaHCO^{3-}$ is recommended in patients who are volume depleted with metabolic acidosis.
- Volume depletion and metabolic acidosis can be separate contributing factors to the hyperkalaemia.

Hypothermia

- Bair Hugger™ should be placed over legs. Warm blankets can be used in the interim.

Tension pneumothorax

- From a penetrating chest wound, immediate decompressions with midclavicular needle insertion are advised; patients will require an intercostal chest catheter (ICC).

Tamponade

- Can be due to medical causes (e.g. oncological emergency).
  - Patients may display distended neck veins, tachycardia and hypotension.
  - Pericardiocentesis is indicated in these settings.
- Patients who have tamponade post trauma or cardiac surgery will need rapid surgical input for thoracotomy.

Toxins

- Arrhythmias follow overdose of medications such as cardiac medications and tricyclic antidepressants (see Chapter 19).

Thrombosis

- If from pulmonary embolus or cardiac thrombosis secondary to acute coronary syndrome (ACS) (see Chapter 35), give a fluid bolus and consider anti-clotting agents with expert input.

Once the assessment and management of critical cardiopulmonary pathology has been completed, further steps of the primary survey (ABC**DE**) can be performed, as follows:

Disability

- Involves an ongoing assessment of the patient's mental status as an indicator of neurological function. Decreased neurological alertness can be due to traumatic injury or systemic intoxication or can be an indicator of cerebral perfusion.
- The Glasgow Coma Scale (GCS; see Table 10.1) provides a method of tracking the neurological progression of a patient, with a drop in GCS score used as a guide for escalation of management.

TABLE 10.1 Glasgow coma scale

EYE OPENING		BEST VERBAL		BEST MOTOR	
Response	Score	Response	Score	Response	Score
Closed by local factor	Not testable (NT)	Factor impairing communication	NT	Paralysed or other limiting factor	NT
None	1	None	1	None	1
To pressure	2	Incoherent sounds	2	Extension response	2
To speech	3	Words	3	Abnormal flexion	3
Spontaneous	4	Confused speech	4	Normal flexion (withdrawal)	4
		Normal	5	Localising	5
				Obeys command ('squeeze my hand')	6

Adapted from The Glasgow Coma Scale © Sir Graham Teasdale, 2015.

Exposure
  ○ No emergency assessment is complete without a complete head-to-toe inspection including logrolling the patient to inspect the back, which is critically important in the trauma patient.
  ○ Though a more thorough inspection of the patient is considered part of the secondary survey, the exposure step allows for identification and rapid management of severe injuries hidden under clothing or on the posterior aspect of the patient.

SHOCK

The definition of shock is acute circulatory collapse with evidence of insufficient end organ perfusion. The multiple causes of shock affect the onset and clinical presentation.

Initial management steps remain largely the same:

- primary survey
- large bore IV access × 2; pathology bloods including group and hold
- urinary catheter to measure urine output, allowing for monitoring of renal failure
- in patients with abdominal pain and >50 years, an urgent bedside ultrasound focused assessment with sonography in trauma (US FAST) scan and abdominal aortic aneurysm (AAA) assessment.

Causes of the different categories of shock are discussed in the following sections.

Hypovolaemia shock

- Common causes include haemorrhage and dehydration.
- Haemorrhage can be due to:
  - massive trauma
  - GI bleeding (Chapter 37)
  - ruptured AAA (Chapter 47).
- Dehydration can be due to:
  - external fluid losses such as vomiting, diarrhoea (particularly in elderly patients), burns
  - internal losses such as fluid loss in pancreatitis, bowel obstruction and chronic liver failure (ascites).

Cardiogenic shock

- Due to 'pump failure' loss of cardiac function:
  - acute coronary syndrome, arrhythmia (Chapter 35)
  - valve leaflet rupture.

'Distributive' shock – systemic vasodilatation

- Sepsis
  - Two components are required for clinical diagnosis of sepsis:
    - systemic inflammatory response syndrome (SIRS) – 2 or more of:
      - > heart rate >90 beats/min
      - > temperature <36° or >38°
      - > respiratory rate >20 breaths/min
      - > white cell count >12 × 10^9/L
    - source – confirmed or suspected source of infection.
  - Septic shock is defined as severe sepsis with persistent hypotension despite fluid resuscitation:
    - most commonly due to bacterial infection
    - high mortality, with 50–60% rate in ICU patients.
  - Initial therapy includes aggressive fluid replacement, initiation of empirical antibiotic therapy and potential circulatory support with vasopressor therapy:
    - early ICU input is helpful for management and post-resuscitation planning
    - critical to identify potential surgical causes of infection.
- Spinal shock
  - Neck injury causing disruption to sympathetic tone of peripheral vasculature.

- Anaphylaxis
  - Patients may present with other anaphylactic features such as angio-oedema, urticaria and possibly dyspnoea secondary to laryngeal oedema:
    - impending airway obstruction:
      - > immediate IM adrenalin and IV hydrocortisone
      - > oxygen via facemask
      - > seek urgent expert airway management – **code blue**
    - circulatory compromise:
      - > initially manage with IV crystalloid fluid bolus
      - > if persisting despite IV fluids and IM adrenaline, IV infusion of adrenaline should be considered.
  - Patients will need close monitoring post management of anaphylaxis, looking out for recurrence of symptoms

TRAUMA

Trauma calls are hospital policies for the activation of rapid medical staff review of a patient with confirmed or potentially serious injury. Each hospital has its own specific trauma call relating to which patients constitute a trauma, the staff members who are required to attend and guidelines for management for particular injuries tailored to the resources of that particular institution. Generally, a trauma call includes ED, surgical and, sometimes, anaesthetic staff.

The Royal Australasian College of Surgeons has developed a set of guiding criteria for patients who could be considered at high risk of injury from trauma (see Table 10.2).

There is extensive communication between the hospital and ambulance ser vices to coordinate pre-hospital care and ensure that the hospital is capable of and prepared to receive the patient.

- Upon presentation, a handover is commenced by the pre-hospital staff (usually paramedics, but can be retrieval medical staff if at a major trauma centre).
- Other medical staff conduct the primary survey, including assessing for other injuries during exposure.
- IV access with large bore cannula with full panel of bloods sent for investigation.
- It is common for these patients to undergo routine trauma series imaging:
  - chest X-ray, abdominal X-ray and pelvis X-ray
  - limb X-rays where injury suspected
  - cervical spine (C-spine) X-rays as initial investigation (see below)

TABLE 10.2 General trauma criteria as per the RACS trauma guidelines

GENERAL TRAUMA CALL CRITERIA FOR ADULTS	TRAUMA CRITERIA FOR TRANSFER TO MAJOR TRAUMA CENTRE
Vehicle crash at over 60 km/h	Penetrating injury to head, neck, chest, abdomen, perineum or back
Major deformation of the vehicle, entrapment for >30 minutes	Head injury with coma, a dilated pupil, open head injury or severe facial injury
Fatal injury in the same vehicle, ejection from the vehicle	Chest injury with flail segment or subcutaneous emphysema
Fall of over 3 m	Abdominal injury with distension and/or rigidity
Cyclist or pedestrian hit by vehicle at over 30 km/h, driveway run-over injuries	Spinal injury with weakness and/or sensory loss
Any mechanism causing injuries to multiple body regions	Limb injury involving vascular injury with ischaemia of the limb, amputation, crush injury of the limb or trunk, bilateral fractures of the femur, complex pelvic injury
	Burns, partial or full thickness, more than 20% of body surface area in adults or more than 10% in children

Royal Australasian College of Surgeons (RACS), 2012. Guidelines for a Structured Approach to the Provision of Optimal Trauma Care. Sydney: RACS.

- US FAST
  - ultrasound of abdomen assesses for free fluid in abdomen that may indicate intra-abdominal bleeding; scan conducted around the liver, spleen and bladder
  - used correctly FAST scans can give input into whether a patient requires laparotomy.

Head injury

Patient or collateral history can help establish the risk of intracranial pathology:
- high speed motor vehicle accident
- fall from height >3 m
- falls in affected population groups:
  - elderly patients unable to brace falls
  - patients affected by alcohol
- decreased or fluctuating consciousness.

Examination findings can give insight into the presence and ongoing development of intracranial pathology:

- obvious major facial trauma
- GCS to assess consciousness, track patient's alertness
- cranial nerve exams, particularly of long tract nerves such as the occulomotor nerve; compression of nerve indicates increased intracranial pressure, manifested as:
  - ○ pupil dilatation on the affected side via impingement on parasympathetic nerve fibres
  - ○ ongoing compression that will result in eventual insult to bilateral parasympathetic supply, leading to contralateral pupil dilation
- base of skull fractures that may present as bilateral periorbital collections (Figure 10.2), or mastoid bruising (Battle's sign) in the late setting.

Patients with obvious severe head injury should have rapid computerised tomography (CT) (Chapter 14) to determine the extent of injury and neurosurgical input.

Patients with apparent mild head injury may not lose consciousness and may appear cognitively intact. Mild head injury includes those with a GCS score of

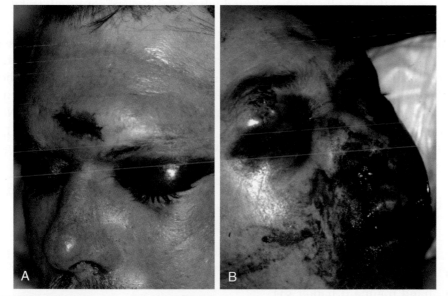

FIGURE 10.2 Two patients with periorbital haematoma collections secondary to base of skull fractures (raccoon eyes).

Reproduced from: Geisler, F.H., Rodriguez, E. & Manson, P.N., 2012. Traumatic skull and facial fractures. In: Ellenbogen, R.G., Abdulrauf, S.I. & Sekhar, L.N., Principles of Neurological Surgery, 3rd ed. Philadelphia: Saunders, Fig. 22.9. Macpherson, D. & Webb, R. 2012. Immediate care (emergency room). In: Ward Booth, P., Eppley, B. & Schmelzeisen, R. Maxillofacial Trauma and Esthetic Facial Reconstruction, 2nd ed. Philadelphia: Saunders, Fig. 3-12, pp. 28-58.

13–15, and patients may experience transient amnesia, confusion and headaches. If there is no other injury presentation, these patients can be monitored in the short stay observation unit as per hospital policy for the recommended period of observation.

Suspected spinal trauma

Patients presenting with potential injuries to the spine should be treated with full precautions until spinal cord function can be properly assessed. Often, the assessment of potential cord injury is made in the pre-hospital setting by paramedic staff and the patient presents to the ED with a hard collar and spinal immobilisation board.

For unconscious patients, these precautions should be kept in place until the patient can undergo complete examination and investigation. These patients should still undergo a full primary survey upon presentation with prioritisation of airway management over all.

Patients who are conscious can undergo clinical examination with a focus on:

- midline tenderness (facilitated by logrolling and inline stabilisation with assistants)
- neurological examination, specific testing of myotomes for muscle power
- supplemented by testing for sensation in each cutaneous dermatome
- noting that results can be affected when patients are confused, agitated or have other distracting injuries.

Patients with inconclusive clinical examination findings with trauma presentations may require imaging to effectively rule out C-spine pathology. A structured approach, such as the 'Canadian C-spine rule' (see Figure 10.3), has been shown to offer superior sensitivity for spinal injury over individual clinician judgement and reduced rates of radiography compared to patients assessed by the Nexus criteria.

Patients with spinal injuries should have ongoing immobilisation until review by the inpatient team responsible for spinal surgery (Chapter 50).

Limb trauma

Limb trauma includes:

- open fractures and closed long bone fractures (discussed in Chapter 46)
- acutely ischaemic limb (Chapter 47)
- hand trauma (Chapter 51).

Severe burns

Severe burns represent a spectrum of thermal, chemical and electrical injuries with the potential to inflict massive soft tissue damage. Though grossly severe burns are obvious, the presentation of a life-threatening injury can be insidious, requiring careful history and examination.

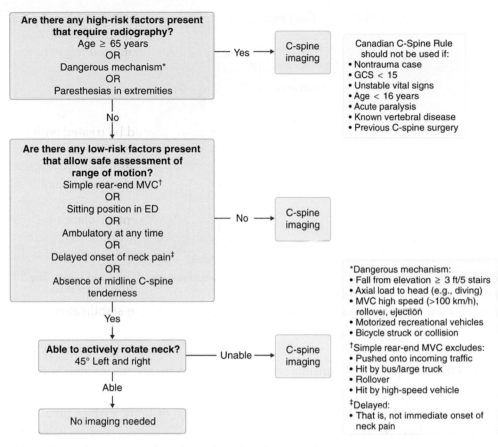

FIGURE 10.3 Implementation of the Canadian C-spine rule.

Ling, G.S.F., 2012. Chapter 406: Traumatic brain injury and spinal cord injury. In: Goldman, L. & Schafer, A.I., Goldman's Cecil Medicine, 24th ed. Philadelphia: Saunders, pp. 2252-2257.

The Australian and New Zealand Burns Association (ANZBA) has developed a structured approach to assist with the early management of severe burns, as follows:

- Primary survey ABCDE as routine for any major trauma:
  - particular attention should be paid to the airway with close examination of the nose and mouth for burns on the mucosa
  - noisy breathing with stridor may indicate laryngeal oedema; rapid progression can occur, requiring proactive management and low threshold for intubation
    - *Note*: inhalation of hot gases can cause lower respiratory tract damage with a combination of inflammatory response and systemic intoxication due to noxious gases such as carbon monoxide (CO):
      - perform a blood gas on arrival to accurately measure levels
      - give O_2 therapy.

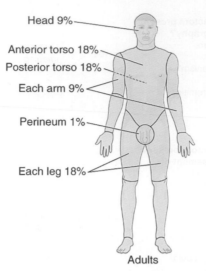

Head 9%
Anterior torso 18%
Posterior torso 18%
Each arm 9%
Perineum 1%
Each leg 18%

Adults

FIGURE 10.4 Rule of 9s for estimating the total body surface area (TBSA) of burns. The palm of the patient's hand roughly correlates to 1%.

Ferri, F., 2014. Practical guide to the care of the medical patient, 9th ed, St. Louis, Elsevier.

- Once the patient is considered stable, the next management step is FATT:
  - fluid resuscitation based on the Parkland formula:
    - 3–4 mL × body weight (kg) × percentage of body surface area burned (refer to Figure 10.4)
    - crystalloid fluid typically used
    - half of the prescribed fluids should be given in the first 8 hours, and the remainder over the next 16 hours; the 24 hours starts from the onset of injury
  - analgesia:
    - burns can be exquisitely painful; generous analgesia may be required
  - tubes:
    - large surface areas burns >20% may require a nasogastric tube (NGT) due to association with decreased GIT motility
    - indwelling catheter (IDC) is essential to measure output for fluid balance chart
  - tests:
    - blood tests and other trauma imaging depending on mechanism of injury (e.g. explosions).

Patients with circumferential burns may require escharotomy to prevent damaged skin causing a compartment syndrome effect on the underlying oedematous soft tissue. Urgent burns surgery input should be sought.

CHAPTER 11

INITIAL ASSESSMENT OF PATIENTS: HISTORY AND EXAMINATION

Joseph M O'Brien and Paul Watson

Modern medicine is focused on patient-centred care. You will meet anywhere between 10 and 50 new patients in a day, whether it be on the wards, in the emergency department or in busy outpatient clinics. You should therefore have a focused approach that you can apply to each situation for your first interaction with a patient you have never encountered before.

Your examination of the patient begins as you enter the room, and will guide the framework you use for the rest of the encounter. For the purposes of this chapter we will assume the patient you are meeting for the first time is either on the wards or in an emergency department cubicle. Take careful note of their overall clinical state – when training for physician exams, people often say you should be able to describe this patient in five terms or so to immediately give your examiner a mental picture (e.g. a thin, pale man, comfortable at rest, but tachycardic and diaphoretic). If the patient is stable you can proceed to history-taking and clinical examination – if they are clearly unwell or even breaching MET criteria, step into action and do what is necessary to stabilise their condition. Do not be hesitant to call for assistance if necessary – no senior clinician should ever lambast you for prematurely calling an emergency code, but they are definitely within rights if you call for help too late.

HISTORY

Begin by introducing yourself to the patient with your name, job title and the purpose of your examination, while gaining consent (e.g. 'Do you mind if we have a quick chat?'). Bedside manner is incredibly important and your first few sentences with a patient can colour the rest of the interaction, so remember to not be an automaton and tailor your style to the patient (e.g. politeness with the old woman in no apparent distress, but more casual and entertaining with a child).

If you don't already have the demographic information, briefly ask about the patient's age, background and where they are from. Ask the patient what they feel their primary issue is – if they are a medical patient, expect there to be multiple active conditions! Use the number of problems to plan your time. Explore their issues one at a time, cycling through the system review questions (see Table 11.1), then move on to past history, family history and social history before progressing to examination.

History of presenting complaint (HOPC)

A good framework for investigating an acute issue (particularly pain) is as follows, denoted as WWQQAA(PB):

- **When** did this symptom first begin? What were they doing at the time?
- **Where** is this symptom (particularly the location of any pain)?
- What **qualities** does the symptom have (e.g. pain could be burning, throbbing etc)?
- Can the patient **quantify** the symptom (e.g. 'What would you rate your pain out of 10?' or 'How many times have you vomited?')?
- Do they have any **associated symptoms** that began at a similar time?
- Are there any **alleviating or aggravating factors** for their symptom (e.g. 'Does anything make it better? Conversely, does anything make it worse?')?
- Has the patient ever experienced this in the **past**?
- What does the patient **believe** the symptom is?

Medical history

When exploring issues for a medical patient, all major disease processes should be probed in the following manner (using the example of type 2 diabetes mellitus):

- When did this condition first get **diagnosed**? How was it diagnosed (e.g. incidental finding, symptomatic disease or late-stage complications)? What were the initial symptoms? What diagnostic testing was performed (e.g. oral glucose tolerance test)? Was any further staging or testing performed (more relevant for malignancies)?
- What was the initial **management** of the condition? What was the response of the disease?
- Have they required any further **treatment** of the disease?
- Have they experienced any **complications** of the disease? Have they experienced any complications of the disease **management**?
- If the disease is one such as asthma or insulin-dependent diabetes, ask if the patient has an **action plan** for sudden deteriorations in their condition.

TABLE 11.1 System review questions

SYSTEM	SYMPTOMS TO CHECK
Cardiovascular	Chest pain (and its nature), palpitations, dyspnoea, orthopnoea, paroxysmal nocturnal dyspnoea, intermittent claudication, syncope (or pre-syncopal symptoms), oedema, pallor, fatigue, baseline effort tolerance (and level of exercise) Risk factors include hypertension, dyslipidaemia, family history, past macrovascular events, diabetes, renal disease, rheumatism, alcohol abuse and erectile dysfunction
Respiratory	Cough (productive? duration? sputum colour? haemoptysis? worse at any time of day?), chest pain, dyspnoea, wheeze, hoarseness of voice, sore throat, sinus pain, atopy, fevers, night sweats, rigors, weight loss, baseline effort tolerance Travel, drug, smoking and occupational history are very important
Gastrointestinal	Anorexia, weight change, fever, lethargy, jaundice, waterbrash, nausea, vomiting (haematemesis), reflux, dysphagia/odynophagia, early satiety, abdominal pain, ascites, change in bowel habit (constipation, diarrhoea, haematochezia, melaena, pale or altered colour stools, tenesmus), anal pain, pruritus, dark urine If PR bleeding is present, ask about the quantity of blood, its colour, presence of mucus, whether the blood is on the paper or mixed with the stool, if it is constant or intermittent, if they can feel rectal lumps and if they have had previous scopes, surgery or inflammatory bowel disease It is important to ask about drug history, alcohol intake, infectious disease risk and travel history
Neurological	Headaches, photophobia, nuchal rigidity, seizures ('fits'), syncope ('faints'), TIAs ('funny turns' or 'mini-strokes'), dizziness or vertigo (clarify which), back pain, disturbances of vision, smell, or hearing, gait disturbance, urinary or faecal incontinence, involuntary movements, tremors, speech disturbance, dysphagia, altered cognition and confusion Neurological risk factors to consider include cardiovascular risk (e.g. HTN), smoking, atrial fibrillation, sepsis, haematological disease and family history

continued

TABLE 11.1 System review questions—cont'd

SYSTEM	SYMPTOMS TO CHECK
Genitourinary	Loin pain, dysuria, pyuria, haematuria, change in colour of urine, polyuria, oliguria/anuria, nocturia, incontinence (determine if urge or stress), oedema, malaise, lethargy, nausea, anorexia, fevers, pruritus, prostatism (difficulty initiating micturition, hesitancy, dribbling, poor stream), urethral discharge, genital rash
	Cardio, menstrual and family history are also important
Endocrine	*General*: anorexia, weight change, sweating, disturbed defecation, change of hair distribution, lethargy, skin changes, pigmentation changes, stature, change in libido, erectile dysfunction, polyuria, goitre
	Hyperthyroidism: preference for colder weather, tremor, weight loss, polyphagia, mood disturbance (irritability or nervousness), diarrhoea, oligomenorrhoea/amenorrhoea, hyperhidrosis, palpitations, proptosis, exertional dyspnoea, tachycardia
	Hypothyroidism: preference for warmer weather, periorbital oedema, lethargy, weight gain, retarded movement, mood disturbance (depression), hoarse voice, constipation, coarse skin, confusion, menorrhagia, bradycardia
	Diabetes: lethargy, polyuria, polydipsia, weight change, visual changes, recurrent infection, altered conscious state
	Primary adrenal insufficiency: pigmentation (bronze), fatigue, weight loss, anorexia, nausea, diarrhoea, mood disturbance, seizures (due to hypoglycaemia or hypotension)
	Acromegaly: fatigue, weakness, hyperhidrosis, weight gain, heat intolerance, enlarged peripheries, enlarged and coarsened facial features, visual changes, voice changes, libido loss, erectile dysfunction
	Cushing's syndrome: truncal obesity, purple striae, moon-like facies, myopathy, bruising buffalo hump
	Male hypogonadism: decreased libido, impotence, reduced body hair, weakness, depression, osteoporosis
	Female hypogonadism: amenorrhoea, hot flushes, vaginal dryness, weakness, depression, osteoporosis
	Polycystic ovary syndrome: hirsutism, oligomenorrhoea, glucose intolerance, obesity, infertility
	Hypopituitary: elements of adrenal insufficiency, hypothyroidism and hypogonadism
	Hyperprolactinaemia: galactorrhoea, hypogonadism

TABLE 11.1 System review questions—cont'd

SYSTEM	SYMPTOMS TO CHECK
	Osteoporosis: calcium intake, sunlight exposure, exercise, age of menarche/menopause, past fractures, height loss, gonadal hormone therapy, corticosteroid use *Paget's disease of the bone*: deformity, bone pain, arthritis, fractures, neurological deficit (deafness), heart failure, sarcoma *Hypercalcaemia* (e.g. hyperparathyroidism): polyuria, nephrolithiasis, weakness, fatigue, confusion, nausea and vomiting *Hypocalcaemia* (e.g. hypoparathyroidism): paraesthesia, muscle spasm, tetany, lethargy, confusion and seizures Take a menstrual history in women, including use of hormone-replacement therapy Family and drug history (especially steroids) are very important
Haematological	*Anaemia*: weakness, tiredness, dyspnoea, fatigue, postural dizziness, bleeding *Coagulopathy*: abnormal bleeding from GI tract, urinary tract, respiratory tract or postoperatively; bleeding into joints, history of protracted immobility, easy bruising, purpura *White cell abnormalities*: recurrent infections, fever, jaundice, neutropenic ulcers, abdominal pain *General*: symptoms of malignancy (lymphadenopathy, weight loss, fevers, rigors, sweats, recurrent infection, fatigue, bone pain) Family history and ethnicity is very important, as is a history of hepatic disease.
Rheumatological	Joint pain, swelling, morning stiffness, stiffness after inactivity, loss of motion or function, instability, weakness, deformity or changes in sensation; dry or red eyes; Raynaud's phenomenon, rash, fever, fatigue, sweats, chills, rigors, weight loss, diarrhoea, mucosal ulceration
Oncological	Diagnosis (symptoms, method and staging), current stage, current therapy, complications of therapy thus far, fevers, rigors, sweats, chills, weight change, anorexia, ± relevant systems review, ± purpose for planned admission, ± advanced care planning Detailed family and social history important

continued

TABLE 11.1 System review questions—cont'd

SYSTEM	SYMPTOMS TO CHECK
Surgical	*General – AMPLE*: **a**llergies, **m**edications, **p**ast history, **l**ast meal, **e**vents leading up to illness/injury *Trauma*: as above, plus mechanism of trauma (incredibly important for evaluating the likelihood of further injury) For motor vehicle accidents – in what position in the car was this person? how many cars were involved? what was the speed of the vehicle before the accident? associated pains? what was the time to extraction? smoke inhalation? other environmental hazards at scene?
Obstetric and gynaecological	Intermenstrual bleeding, post-menopausal bleeding, menorrhagia, dysmenorrhoea (i.e. pain during menstruation), oligomenorrhoea or amenorrhoea, passage of clots, pelvic pain (with relation to cycle), possibility of pregnancy and brief sexual history, anorexia, weight change, post-coital bleeding, dyspareunia (deep or superficial), contraceptive use, discharge (colour, frequency, duration, volume, odour, symptoms in partner), dysuria, loin pain, genital pain or pruritus *Obstetric history*: gravidity parity status (gestation at delivery, dates of delivery, weight and gender of babies and nature of delivery), complications (pregnancy, labour and puerperium), miscarriages and terminations and gestation at which they occurred, postnatal problems (including depression), conception difficulties/infertility, blood group, serology and immune status, congenital disease screening, last pap smear *Menstrual history*: last menstrual period (first day of bleeding, a.k.a. LMP), cycle length and frequency (noted as, e.g., 5/28), flow, clots, intermenstrual bleeding, age of menarche (first period), age of menopause (if relevant) and any post-menopausal bleeding
Paediatric	Relevant system review questions, plus: *Current health*: behaviour (towards family and friends; discipline), elimination (bowel movement frequency/quality, urination, problems toilet training), nutrition (breast milk or formula? quantity? frequency? supplements? problems with sucking or swallowing, reflux?), development (gross motor, fine motor, language, cognition, social/emotional), sleep (quantity, quality, disturbances such as snoring, apnoea, enuresis or restlessness, interventions, waking up refreshed

TABLE 11.1 System review questions—cont'd

SYSTEM	SYMPTOMS TO CHECK
	Development: pregnancy history (adoption status, gravida/parity status of mother, maternal age, duration; exposure to medications, alcohol, tobacco, drugs, infection and radiation; complications of birth; planned pregnancy or not; problems with other pregnancies), labour and delivery (length of labour, rupture of membranes, foetal movement, medications, presentation, assistance with vacuum or forceps, complications, APGAR, immediate breath/cry, oxygen requirement), neonatal (birth weight/height, abnormalities or injuries, length of hospital stay, respiratory distress, anaemia, cyanosis, jaundice, seizures, anomalies or infection, behaviour, maternal concerns) and infancy (temperament, feeding, family reactions to child) *Extended social history*: living conditions, parents' education and occupation, pets, water (city or tank?), lead exposure, smoke exposure, family religion and finances, family dynamics, risk-taking behaviours, school and day care, other caregivers
Geriatric	Relevant systems review Social history is vital, and should include home situation (including home modifications), use of gait aids, effort tolerance, frequency of falls and services in place (e.g. home help, meals on wheels, home nursing, carers) What medications do they take (screen for polypharmacy), and who administers them? Ask if they complete their own cooking, cleaning, financial tasks, driving and self-hygiene. Discuss advanced care planning in detail – would they like to be resuscitated with CPR, intubation, inotropes or transfer to intensive care? Document clearly
Travel	Relevant systems review + destination, length of stay, type of travel, prophylaxis taken, vaccinations received prior to travel, any sick contacts or any exposure to: fresh or untreated water, raw foods, animals, unprotected sexual intercourse, IVDU/tattoos Discuss the timing and pattern of any fevers and/or rashes

APGAR, Apgar score or acronym for **a**ppearance, **p**ulse, **g**rimace, **a**ctivity, **r**espiration.

Adapted from: American College of Surgeons (Trauma Committee), 2012. Advanced Trauma Life Support, 9th ed. Chicago: American College of Surgeons, pp. 14-15. <http://www.fpnotebook.com/er/Trauma/TrmHstry.htm>. Lissauer, T. & Clayden, G., eds, 2007. Illustrated Textbook of Paediatrics, 3rd ed. London: Mosby. Roberton, D.M. & South, M., eds., 2007. Practical Paediatrics, 6th ed. Melbourne: Churchill Livingstone. Talley, N.J. & O'Connor, S., 2014. Clinical Examination: A systematic guide to physical diagnosis, 7th ed. Sydney: Elsevier Australia.

Be aware patients often do not have all of this information. A patient who knows *too* much about their medical history can be a red flag! If experiencing difficulty in gathering history, consider the much simpler 'CCC' approach for each issue – cause, course and complications!

Medication history

Ask the patient about their prescribed medications, as well as over-the-counter (OTC) medications, complementary and alternative medicines and nutritional/ vitamin supplement usage. Common problems experienced include a patient forgetting a medication (or all of them), not knowing the doses, knowing only the brand names or describing the pill and not knowing anything else about it ('You know, the little blue pills!'). If possible, document the generic name of the drug, its dose and its frequency. Ask about recently ceased medications, and what is new. Ask how the patient is coping with their 'pill burden' and how their drugs are managed (e.g. do they take their drugs of their own accord, or do they need a Webster pack or even home nursing?).

Allergies and adverse drug reactions

Enquire about adverse drug reactions and allergies. As you become a more senior doctor, this is a good place in the history to consider the risk of polypharmacy and carry out 'pharmacological debridement'. If the patient does not know their usual medication regimen, you could call their GP or regular pharmacy or, if after hours, use the discharge summary from their most recent previous stay and talk through with the patient to see what has changed since then. If a patient has a Webster pack, don't forget to ask about their non-packed medications (e.g. inhalers and refrigerated drugs).

Preventative medicine

If time allows, ask the patient about how regularly they see their GP, their immunisation status and screening for appropriate diseases (e.g. breast cancer in a woman over 50, cervical cancer in all women, colorectal cancer in people over 50, prostate cancer in men over 50 and skin cancer in almost all Australians).

Past history

For so many conditions, the risk factor with the biggest positive predictive value is past incidence. Patients will often forget about their past history, so some good memory prompts include, 'Have you ever had any serious medical conditions before?', 'Have you ever needed admission before?' and 'Have you ever had any operations before?' Use the framework above to probe any past medical conditions. With surgeries in particular, ask where and when they were performed (as you may need to contact that health service), who performed them and if they were well postoperatively or required additional treatment.

Social history

This part of the history is often neglected by junior doctors, but can be invaluable in both deciding on suitable therapies and planning the discharge of the patient. A full history should cover their present and past occupations (including potential exposures to chemicals, radiation and trauma), marital status and housing arrangements ('Who is at home with you?' is a question that can reveal a lot about a patient's living circumstances), mobility, ability to independently or partially complete their activities of daily living (cooking, cleaning, household chores, driving, managing finances), overseas travel, sick contacts, education, hobbies and adequacy of income. A sexual history would only be necessary if it is related to the presentation (e.g. recent HIV infection). Otherwise, you run the risk of alienating the patient unnecessarily.

During the social history, quantify the patient's use of tobacco, ethanol and illicit substances. A full tobacco history includes the duration of smoking, type of cigarettes smoked, number of cigarettes smoked per day and time since they quit (if they have). This is overall expressed as a patient's number of 'pack years' (i.e. number of years smoked multiplied by cigarette packets smoked per day, with 20 considered one pack).

Similarly, estimate the patient's alcohol consumption by asking what they would drink in an average day, the type of alcohol they drink, if they drink more on weekends, if they ever binge, if they used to drink more heavily in the past and if they have any alcohol-free days. One standard drink contains 10 g of ethanol. You can explore this further by asking the CAGE questions – 'Do you feel you need to **cut down** on your alcohol intake?', 'Do you get **annoyed** when people imply you should drink less?', 'Does your drinking ever cause you **guilt**?' and 'Do you ever need an **eye-opener** (i.e. a drink first thing in the morning)?' These questions are a screening tool for alcohol abuse, with more than two positive responses holding a strong predictive value.

This approach can be used for the screening of abuse of other substances, but has not been extensively validated. It is not necessary to ask every patient about their illicit drug use, but be mindful – the young adults of the 1960s and 1970s are getting on in years and you might be surprised by what you find!

Family history

Enquire about conditions known to 'run in the family'. Ask about the health of their parents, siblings and children. If the patient is old enough that their parents have likely died, delicately ask, 'What did your parents pass away from?' Quantify the patient's risk by asking at what age their relatives were affected by these conditions. Ask specifically about malignancies, and conditions related to the presentation (e.g. for chest pain, ask if there is a family history of ischaemic heart disease, diabetes, arrhythmias, dyslipidaemia or hypertension). For psychiatry patients or genetic diseases, consider a genogram.

EXAMINATION

It is important to have a general approach to examining patients. After introducing yourself, gaining consent, washing your hands and positioning the patient appropriately (including exposure), begin with general appearance. Note the patient's vitals, complexion (e.g. pallor, cyanosis or jaundice), ethnicity, body habitus and any items (medical or otherwise, e.g. Hudson mask) around the patient. Comment on whether they are comfortable at rest or in distress/discomfort. People vary in where they take their examination from here – it is accepted practice to either move onto the peripheries, or to the head and neck. Decide what works for you and stay consistent to reduce errors. It is standard practice to examine from the right side of the bed (it's tradition). Be mindful of the patient's comfort, and cover sensitive areas when not examining them. With each new area, proceed through the principles of **look, palpate, move, listen** and **special tests.** This section is only a brief introduction to clinical examination, and a more appropriate text should be sought for individual system examinations.

Examine the peripheries for signs of systemic disease (e.g. palmar pallor, clubbing, nicotine staining etc). If relevant test for asterixis, and take the patient's pulse. While they assume you are taking their pulse, check their respiratory rate. Move up to the upper arm and take a blood pressure. If relevant, check the axilla for lymphadenopathy.

Examine the head and neck for typical disease facies. Check the eyes for pupillary response, icterus and conjunctival pallor. Consider a brief visual examination. Ask the patient to open their mouth and assess their mucous membranes for hydration status. Note dentition and any oral ulcers, discolouration or thrush. Ask the patient to recline to 45° and measure their jugular venous pressure. If relevant, from behind the patient check for lymphadenopathy in the occipital, pre- and post-auricular, submandibular, deep cervical and supraclavicular nodal regions. Check tracheal deviation.

At the chest, inspect, palpate and measure chest expansion. Feel the apex beat. Percuss the lung fields as necessary. Listen to the chest (at least posteriorly, but preferably also anteriorly) and the heart sounds.

Moving to the abdomen, ask the patient to lie flat. Ensure they are comfortable in this position. Note any surgical scars. Palpate lightly then more firmly, taking note of any masses (especially central and pulsating), sites of tenderness or involuntary guarding. Note any organomegaly and, if time allows, measure the liver span. Consider balloting for renal tenderness. Listen for bowel sounds.

In the lower limbs, check calf tenderness, look for pitting oedema by pressing firmly then sliding your fingers over the depression and feel for peripheral pulses. Note any nail changes or fine hair loss that may represent systemic disease.

When documenting your examination findings, it is acceptable to use shorthand, including symbols. The most common symbols are listed in Figs 11.1 to 11.4. An arrow from bottom-left to top-right through the symbol indicates that there were no abnormalities detected in that area. Abnormalities are denoted by an 'X' and should be described to the right of the symbol.

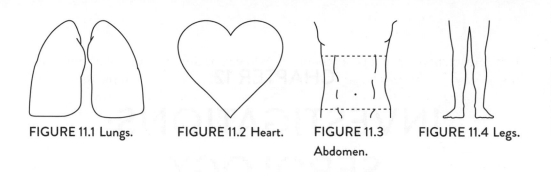

FIGURE 11.1 Lungs.   FIGURE 11.2 Heart.   FIGURE 11.3 Abdomen.   FIGURE 11.4 Legs.

The above framework is for best case scenarios, where you have sufficient time and energy to be unyielding in your approach to clinical history-taking and examination. For example, it is great to have a complete social history but, when you have 20 patients in cubicles waiting to be seen, you don't have the 15 minutes (minimum!) necessary to indulge in a comprehensive social review. Part of the role of the junior doctor is learning to hone time management skills and prioritise the tasks that need to be assessed immediately, while calming your inner perfectionist to let go the tasks that can wait.

CHAPTER 12

INVESTIGATIONS: SEROLOGY

Joseph M O'Brien

Serology is the scientific study or diagnostic examination of blood serum. Ordering bloods is often the role of the junior doctor on a medical or surgical team. Before commencing your internship, you should be familiar with the majority of the investigations discussed in this chapter. A competent intern would be able to identify the indications for these tests; a proficient intern would know when to request them and when they are unnecessary. Over-investigation costs the hospital system millions of dollars annually, with little-to-no gain for the patients. This chapter does not outline normal values (see Appendix II).

Pathology forms differ from service to service, but will all have a few key features such as a box for the tests being requested, as well as the patient details, clinical history, requesting doctor details (with signature), date and collection details. See Fig. 12.1 for an example of a completed request slip. When completing a pathology request form:

- You can use a patient label rather than write out all of their details.

- The minimum requirement for a lab to process your request is your signature (if they have it on file) and the date. If your signature is not recognisable to the lab, you should also print your surname (in fact, some labs insist on this).

- On some forms you are able to have a 'carbon copy' sent to other practitioners. This can be very useful, for example sending a copy of endoscopic biopsy results to their local doctor minimises the chance of a concerning finding being missed.

- If you are sending an important sample (or a sample to a distant lab), consider adding your provider number as well.

- If you took the blood or performed the biopsy yourself, don't forget to put your signature in the correct area as well or the lab may reject the sample. This is a common scenario, as doctors will be called to 'bleed' the most difficult patients – and they are exactly the people you don't want to have to draw more blood from!

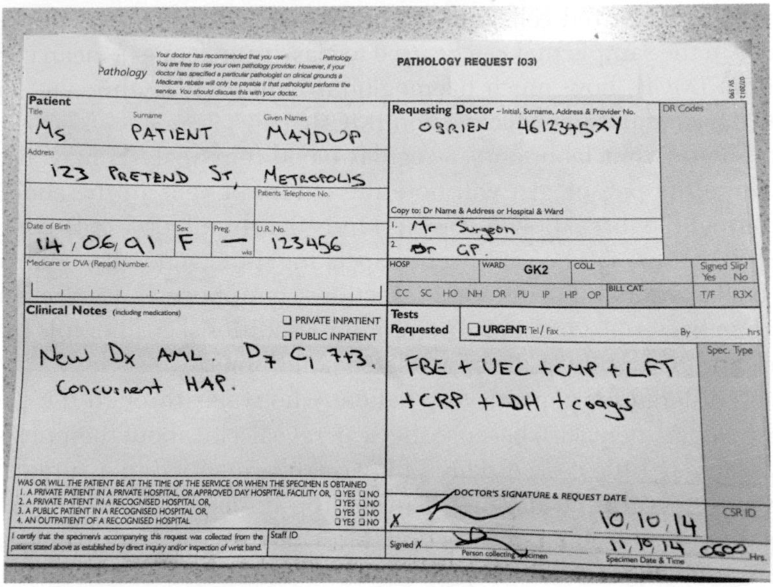

Pathology

Your doctor has recommended that you use Pathology
You are free to use your own pathology provider. However, if your doctor has specified a particular pathologist on clinical grounds a Medicare rebate will only be payable if that pathologist performs the service. You should discuss this with your doctor.

PATHOLOGY REQUEST (03)

Patient
Title: Ms | Surname: PATIENT | Given Names: MAYDUP
Address: 123 PRETEND ST, METROPOLIS
Patients Telephone No.
Date of Birth: 14/06/91 | Sex: F | Preg. — wks | U.R. No. 123456
Medicare or DVA (Repat) Number.

Requesting Doctor – Initial, Surname, Address & Provider No.
OBRIEN 4612345XY
DR Codes
Copy to: Dr Name & Address or Hospital & Ward
1. Mr Surgeon
2. Dr GP.
HOSP | WARD GK2 | COLL | Signed Slip? Yes No
CC SC HO NH DR PU IP HP OP | BILL CAT. | T/F R3X

Clinical Notes (including medications)
❑ PRIVATE INPATIENT
❑ PUBLIC INPATIENT
New Dx AML. D7 C1 7+3.
Concurrent HAP.

Tests Requested ❑ URGENT: Tel / Fax .... By .... hrs
Spec. Type
FBE + UEC + CMP + LFT
+ CRP + LDH + coags

WAS OR WILL THE PATIENT BE AT THE TIME OF THE SERVICE OR WHEN THE SPECIMEN IS OBTAINED
1. A PRIVATE PATIENT IN A PRIVATE HOSPITAL, OR APPROVED DAY HOSPITAL FACILITY OR, ❑ YES ❑ NO
2. A PRIVATE PATIENT IN A RECOGNISED HOSPITAL OR, ❑ YES ❑ NO
3. A PUBLIC PATIENT IN A RECOGNISED HOSPITAL OR, ❑ YES ❑ NO
4. AN OUTPATIENT OF A RECOGNISED HOSPITAL ❑ YES ❑ NO

DOCTOR'S SIGNATURE & REQUEST DATE
X 10/10/14
CSR ID

I certify that the specimen/s accompanying this request was collected from the patient stated above as established by direct inquiry and/or inspection of wrist band. | Staff ID
Signed X .... Person collecting specimen | 11/10/14 Specimen Date & Time 0600 Hrs.

FIGURE 12.1 Example pathology form.

- When completing the clinical history, try and convey to the laboratory technician what you are thinking as thoroughly as time permits. For example, if you forget to put an important investigation on the slip but you have indicated on the history what your presumed diagnosis is, the lab may help you out and have the test running before they call you for 'official' authorisation.
- Sometimes patients require multiple blood tests on discharge (e.g. a patient who has just commenced warfarin who needs serial coagulation studies, or an oncology patient who will need bloods until their next admission). To save the patient multiple visits to their GP (and a lot of bother), you can give them a pathology slip with the phrase, 'Rule 3 exemption', amongst the clinical history. This works an unlimited number of times over 6 months for anticoagulant therapy, and up to six times for patients on dialysis, lithium, clozapine, methotrexate, leflunomide, cyclosporine, vitamin D, bisphosphonate infusions and/or other immunosuppressants and chemotherapy. The frequency of testing must also be specified in the clinical history box.

FULL BLOOD EXAMINATION

The workhouse of serology, a full blood examination or FBE (a.k.a. complete blood count/CBC in the USA) is the most commonly requested investigation in the healthcare system. Often abbreviated to its three most salient components – haemoglobin/white blood cell count/platelets (e.g. 120/4.5/326) – you are also provided with the haematocrit (or packed cell volume, the percentage of whole blood that is made of red cells), mean corpuscular volume (MCV, the volume of the red cells in the sample that can be used to classify anaemias), mean corpuscular haemoglobin (MCH, how much haemoglobin is in each erythrocyte) and mean corpuscular haemoglobin concentration (MCHC).

Depending on your laboratory, a regular blood film analysis may also be conducted, where the pathologist will note the nature of cells in the slide. A white cell differential (i.e. breakdown of what kinds of white blood cells contribute to the white cell count) can be very useful. Speaking quite generally, neutrophils are elevated in bacterial and acute viral infections; lymphocytes in viral infections; monocytes in bacterial, viral and autoimmune conditions; eosinophils in parasitic infections; and basophils in marrow-related conditions.

FBEs are ordered for almost every patient who walks through the door in the Emergency Department (ED) because they can reveal a lot about their physiological state for relatively little cost. A daily FBE would be justified in a surgical patient, especially postoperatively, to monitor for a drop in haemoglobin or neutrophilia that could indicate bleeding or infection. Most medical patients would also need a daily FBE, unless they are very stable, in which case it could be dropped to biweekly. A weekly FBE (or less frequently) would be appropriate for subacute patients.

An FBE is often requested after a transfusion of red blood cells, or after a platelet transfusion (known as a post-transfusion platelet increment, confusingly denoted as PPI). A venous blood gas could be used if a quick haemoglobin check is required. FBEs are taken into the purple ethylene diamine tetra-acetic acid (EDTA) tubes.

UREA, ELECTROLYTES AND CREATININE

If a urea, electrolytes and creatinine (UEC) is requested, you will get a report of the sodium, chloride, potassium, creatinine, urea, bicarbonate and estimated glomerular filtration rate (eGFR). Americans call this a 'basic metabolic panel'. Be mindful that creatinine (and thus lab-determined eGFR) will vary with factors such as age, muscle mass and total surface area and, for highly sensitive drugs such as chemotherapy, a formal creatinine clearance (CrCl) should be obtained with 24-hour urine collection.

Short-hand annotation for UECs varies, but a $Na^+/K^+/creatinine/eGFR$ or $Na^+/K^+/creatinine/urea$ pattern is common. UECs are similarly performed daily on a regular basis. This is justified in any patient who is postoperative or receiving fluids as renal function should be monitored in these situations. Potassium and sodium should be corrected as outlined in Chapter 24, 'Managing fluids and infusions'.

CALCIUM, MAGNESIUM AND PHOSPHATE

Calcium, magnesium and phosphate are ascribed as CMP, and the only reason these electrolytes aren't included in the normal electrolyte panel is cost. Calcium, magnesium and phosphate are three electrolytes with important metabolic roles we won't delve into here (try *Kumar and Clark's Clinical Medicine*). All three have important clinical consequences when outside their normal ranges.

You should consider ordering a CMP on all patients with a cardiac, renal or endocrine complaint, as well as those receiving IV fluids or who have been fasted for a period of time. CMP goes in the same tube as a UEC (containing SST II gel, often gold or white).

Calcium

Calcium is an electrolyte important for the maintenance of sturdy bones (99% of which are calcium phosphate salts), complex cellular pathway signalling, catalysis of enzymatic reactions and the normal contraction of muscles, and as such is tightly regulated by the human body under homeostatic conditions.

The typical assay for a CMP will measure the circulating calcium ions, which can be rather deceptive. Calcium has a high affinity for proteins, and is often bound to proteins in serum (the biggest culprit being albumin). Thus, most labs will also report a 'corrected calcium', which takes into account the serum level of albumin (the most common circulating protein) to give a closer estimate of metabolically active calcium. This formula is: Corrected calcium (mmol/L) = measured calcium (mmol/L) + 0.02(40 − serum albumin in g/L) – don't worry, it's unlikely you'll be expected to memorise that equation until you're sitting your fellowship exams. This is inaccurate in acid–base disturbances as the binding properties of calcium and albumin change at different levels of pH. A neat rule of thumb is to add 0.1 mmol/L to the measured calcium for every 4 g/L albumin is below normal. Additionally, be aware of the patient with malignancy – calcium may appear startling low as their malignancy spews out proteins, binding otherwise free calcium.

The most common cause of hypercalcaemia in hospital inpatients is malignancy – this is due to bone breakdown, output of parathyroid hormone-related protein (PTHrp) by the tumour itself and tumour production of calcitriol (activated vitamin D). Primary hyperparathyroidism will also raise serum calcium, as will less common causes such as hypoalbuminaemia and drugs (check for over-supplementation of calcium and vitamin D to prevent embarrassment).

First-line management is appropriate fluid rehydration, but pamidronate (a bisphosphonate) may also be used if the patient is symptomatic or their serum corrected calcium is headed >3 mmol/L. As 90% of inpatients with hypercalcaemia will have a malignancy or hyperparathyroidism, investigations focus on separating these two causes (and thus request a PTH, PTHrp and malignancy screen).

Hypocalcaemia can be due to hypomagnesaemia, hyperphosphataemia, hyper-albuminaemia, drugs, liver disease, low intake, intravascular overload, sepsis or hypoparathyroidism. Patients with end-stage renal disease will usually have low calcium as 1,25-dihydroxyvitamin D is not produced in adequate volumes and hyperphosphataemia is often present. Calcium (and vitamin D) should be supplemented orally where possible, or by intravenous infusion where necessary.

SECTION II

Magnesium

Magnesium is an electrolyte essential for multiple enzymatic reactions. Its homeostasis is primarily controlled by the kidneys, with the majority excreted in urine. Hypermagnesaemia can be due to over-supplementation, renal insufficiency or, more rarely, DKA, tumour lysis, lithium overdose, milk–alkali syndrome or primary hyperparathyroidism. Treatment for people with intact renal function is simple – don't give them any more magnesium!

For the renally-challenged patient, fluid resuscitation with normal saline and diuresis with frusemide would be indicated. Those with end-stage renal failure may require filtration. As such, never give magnesium to patients with renal impairment without talking to a registrar!

Hypomagnesaemia is more commonly encountered than hypermagnesaemia. It may present as tremor, weakness, delirium or ECG abnormalities, or may be suspected due to other electrolyte abnormalities (hypokalaemia or hypocalcaemia). In patients with a cardiac history (especially atrial fibrillation), we often aim to keep their serum level >1.0 mmol/L (as opposed to the 'normal' upper limit of 0.82 mmol/L).

Phosphate

Phosphate is the electrolyte of the CMP least utilised by junior doctors. It should be monitored and supplemented either orally or intravenously in patients who have fasted for more than 48 hours, as a low phosphate can precipitate refeeding syndrome. Refeeding syndrome is a metabolic disturbance that results in haematological, neurological, respiratory and ultimately cardiac sequelae as magnesium, potassium and phosphate stores are utilised to resume insulin secretion. The most common cause of death in refeeding syndrome is cardiac arrhythmias secondary to potassium metabolism disruption.

Hyperphosphataemia is usually a result of renal impairment or hypoparathyroidism and, due to the high affinity of phosphate for calcium, may result in calcified lesions visible on X-ray. It may also occur with significant tissue necrosis. It is managed with phosphate binders, but these should not be started without consulting a more senior physician.

LIVER FUNCTION TESTS

Liver function tests (LFTs) are a bit of a misnomer. The best true marker of the *function* of the liver is the synthesis of albumin – and, hence, the American term 'liver panel' is perhaps more appropriate. Regardless, LFTs can tell us a lot about the nature of insults to the liver and help us further hone our investigations. LFTs go in the same gold or white SST II gel tube as UECs.

In most laboratories, a request for LFTs will give you a patient's serum bilirubin (BR), alkaline phosphatase ('alk phos' or ALP), gamma-glutamyl transferase (GGT, sometimes γGT), alanine transaminase (ALT), albumin and total protein

(TP). Additional components not included by all services include aspartate aminotransferase (AST), lactate dehydrogenase (LDH) and prothrombin time (PT). You should investigate what your lab offers as a standard, because several of the 'additional' components can be valuable in diagnosis and monitoring of certain conditions.

Bilirubin (BR) is a limited but useful component of the LFTs. A breakdown product of haem, BR circulates in the bloodstream in two forms – unconjugated and conjugated. Unconjugated can be thought of as 'raw' bilirubin produced primarily when haemoglobin in erythrocytes is released after their degradation in the spleen. This newly produced bilirubin binds reversibly to albumin until it reaches the liver, where an enzyme conjugates it with glucuronic acid. Under physiological conditions, the conjugated bilirubin is then excreted as bile or via glomerular filtration. In normal conditions, 95% of circulating bilirubin is unconjugated. Please note that sometimes conjugated bilirubin is denoted as 'direct' bilirubin, and unconjugated as 'indirect'.

In cholestasis or biliary obstruction, the serum concentration of conjugated bilirubin can rise and change the ratio of unconjugated to conjugated bilirubin. At a total serum bilirubin of >35 μmol/L, people will have icteric sclera, and at >40 μmol/L they will be clinically jaundiced. Bilirubin is potentially toxic at high levels and can cause kernicterus, particularly in neonates.

Hyperbilirubinaemia may be due to haemolysis (inherited or acquired), viral hepatitis, drug-induced liver injury, biliary obstruction, ineffective haematopoiesis, hereditary defects of bilirubin metabolism (such as Rotor, Crigler-Najjar, Dubin-Johnson and Gilbert's syndromes), cirrhosis and choledocholithiasis. A mildly elevated bilirubin in the absence of any other abnormality is likely to represent Gilbert's syndrome, a benign, genetic hyperbilirubinaemia due to enzymatic deficiency. Low serum bilirubin is considered normal.

The pattern of changes in the ALT, AST, ALP and GGT – collectively known as the 'liver enzymes' – can help identify the nature of pathology. Increase in serum ALT or AST is most typically associated with intrahepatic disease, with damage directly to the hepatocytes. ALT tends to rise more rapidly than AST in acute illness. The ratio of ALT to AST can also be used in investigating the chronology of chronic liver disease – ALT is initially greater than AST, until the liver becomes cirrhotic and the ratio reverses. It is also said that an AST:ALT ratio >2 suggests alcoholic liver disease (with a ratio <1 suggesting other causes), but with the wide variety of causes of liver disease this rule does not remain true in all circumstances.

In a hospital setting, the most common cause of acute LFT derangement is drug therapy, but outpatient causes include alcoholic liver disease, non-alcoholic steatohepatitis (or fatty liver), viral hepatitis, autoimmune hepatitis, neoplasia, right-sided heart failure, ischaemic hepatitis, portal vein thrombosis, hyperthyroidism, haemochromatosis and metal deposition disease (e.g. Wilson's), hereditary metabolic disorders and coeliac disease.

Elevated ALP (and GGT, to a lesser extent) is often related to biliary tract pathology, and is thus associated with extrahepatic jaundice. Beware the confounding factor of bone-related ALP – if you are suspicious, you can ask the lab to separate skeletal ALP from non-skeletal. ALP is a metabolite-transporting enzyme. Causes of an elevated ALP can be divided into intrahepatic (primary biliary cirrhosis or drug-induced liver injury) and extrahepatic (choledocholithiasis, neoplasia in the head of the pancreas, bile ducts or gall bladder, drug-induced liver injury, cardiac failure, primary biliary cirrhosis and primary sclerosing cholangitis). ALP may also be increased during pregnancy or fractures with no cause for concern, as well as abnormally in the setting of skeletal, haematological, intestinal or renal pathology.

An isolated elevation in GGT – an enzyme found not only in the hepatocytes and cells of the biliary tract but also in the pancreas, renal tubules and intestine – may be secondary to alcohol abuse, cigarette smoking or non-alcoholic steatohepatitis, but it can also be elevated in renal disease and COPD. There are three *common* causes of an *acute* and *severe* derangement of all liver enzymes – hepatic ischaemia, viruses or drugs/toxins.

The serum albumin is also reported with LFTs, in conjunction with the total protein. Albumin production is a good marker of the actual *synthetic* function of the liver as it is produced exclusively by hepatocytes, and its serum level decreases as hepatic disease progresses. This is important as it implies the liver's production of other small proteins – in particular, the coagulation factors I, II, V, VII and X – has also decreased, which may be detectable as a prolonged PT and an elevated international normalised ratio (INR). Be aware that albumin is an acute phase reactant and will be lower than expected in inflammatory states. By comparing the serum albumin with the total protein, you can determine a 'protein gap' – if one is present, further investigation is warranted with a more extensive liver, renal and nutritional screen, serum protein electrophoresis and quantitative immunoglobulins.

LFTs are not necessarily required daily in every patient on either a Medical or Surgical ward. Screening on admission may have some benefits or pick up on underlying disease. Use your clinical discretion – patients with chronic liver disease, gall bladder pathology or infiltrative illnesses, or on known hepatotoxins (e.g. certain chemotherapy, antivirals, antibiotics, anti-lipid agents, anti-epileptics and paracetamol) could benefit from trending LFTs. Most patients would not need this panel repeated more than twice weekly, unless another factor in the clinical picture changes (e.g. new or worsening jaundice, right upper quadrant pain or coagulopathy). As bilirubin is photosensitive, you should try to prevent sample exposure to light.

If a patient has worsening LFTs and the cause is not immediately apparent – e.g. acute cholecystitis demonstrable on ultrasound – then a full 'liver screen' may be necessary. When filling out the request form use your clinical discretion to avoid wasteful over-testing – if the derangement of the LFTs has been acute, it is quite unlikely to be (for example) haemochromatosis or heavy metal accumulation. It might, however, be one of the viral hepatitides, ischaemic hepatitis or drug-induced liver injury! For suggested investigation and management of different patterns of LFT derangement, see Fig. 12.2.

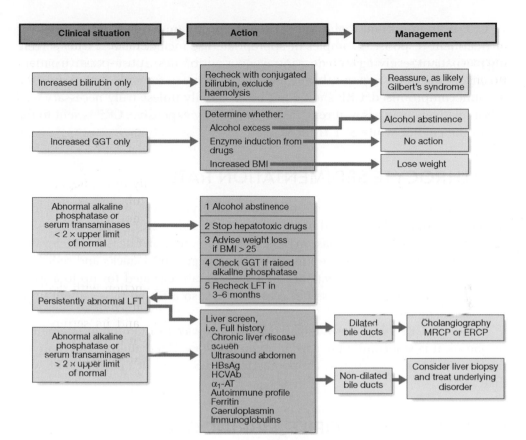

FIGURE 12.2 Suggested management of abnormal LFTs in asymptomatic patients.

Anstee, Q.M. & Jones, D.E.J., 2014. Chapter 23: Liver and biliary tract disease. In: Walker, B.R., Colledge, N.R., Ralston, S.H., et al. Davidson's Principles and Practice of Medicine, 22nd ed. Edinburgh: Churchill Livingstone, pp. 921-988.

C-REACTIVE PROTEIN

C-reactive protein (CRP) is the most commonly used inflammatory marker. CRP is a protein made in the liver during inflammatory states in response to elevated interleukin-6. It binds to the surface of dead cells, dying cells and particular microorganisms to activate the complement system and mark them for phagocytosis. CRP will respond rapidly to systemic insult, becoming elevated within hours. Note, however, that the half-life of CRP is 48 hours, and that CRP will therefore not begin to drop until 2 days after the insult is removed.

CRP levels are less reliable in patients with chronic liver disease as the hepatocytes have a lessened ability to synthesise proteins. CRP is not affected by gender or age and can be performed on aged samples, unlike the erythrocyte sedimentation rate (see below). CRP may remain elevated in chronic inflammatory conditions such as rheumatoid arthritis, inflammatory bowel disease, tuberculosis and malignancy. A low or normal CRP may help exclude organic causes of disease in patients with difficult-to-explain symptoms.

CRP is an important tool as both a screen for inflammation, and as a marker of treatment response. Examples of appropriate use include second-daily screening in a patient receiving high-dose intravenous antibiotics, a postoperative patient (to ensure the trend remains downward) and as a screen for early infection in the immunocompromised. CRP should not be used daily unless truly necessary – as it is a relatively new assay, it remains comparatively expensive. CRP is sent to the lab in the gold or white SST II tubes.

ERYTHROCYTE SEDIMENTATION RATE

A non-specific measurement of inflammation, erythrocyte sedimentation rate (ESR) is the time taken for red blood cells to form sediment in 1 hour, expressed as millimetres/hour. The increase in the serum sedimentation rate is due to elevated fibrinogen (which causes the erythrocytes to aggregate into stacks and sediment faster), and subsequently a patient's ESR will remain elevated for up to a week after the inflammatory process has ceased. It is also affected by a patient's *age* and *biological sex*.

Although CRP has largely replaced ESR as a way to monitor inflammatory responses, it is still commonly used in Rheumatology, Haematology and in investigation of vasculitides such as temporal arteritis. ESR goes in a purple EDTA tube (like FBEs).

COAGULATION PROFILE, FIBRINOGEN, D-DIMER AND ANTI-XA

At its most simple, coagulation is a balance between bleeding and clotting. Coagulation studies or 'coags' are a commonly performed investigation. You will likely see it requested most frequently in the context of warfarin monitoring. Other contexts in which coags would be helpful include suspected or ongoing haemorrhage and diagnosis of coagulopathy (e.g. a thromboembolic event or during use of drugs such as all trans-retinoic acid). Standard laboratories will provide you with a prothrombin time (PT), activated partial thromboplastin time (APTT – sometimes with a lowercase 'a') and an INR.

The PT and APTT are measurements of the time taken for the sample to form a fibrin clot, measured in seconds with detection of the clot by visual, optical or electromechanical methods. The PT is useful for detection of problems with the extrinsic pathway of coagulation, and the APTT the intrinsic.

PT is particularly sensitive to the vitamin K-dependent coagulation factors (in this situation II, VII and X). A prolongation of PT (see Table 12.1) may be due to: anticoagulation; deficiency or inhibition of factors V, VII or X; vitamin K deficiency; liver disease; autoimmune conditions involving antiphospholipid antibodies; or disseminated intravascular coagulation (DIC).

The APTT is measured by re-calcifying the citrate-exposed sample in the presence of both a negatively charged substance and a thromboplastic material.

TABLE 12.1 Causes of prolongation of PT and APTT

PT	APTT	CAUSES
Prolonged	Normal	Factor I, II, V, VII or X inhibition/deficiency, autoimmune conditions, warfarin use
Normal	Prolonged	Factor VIII, IX, XI or XII inhibition/deficiency, heparin, autoimmune conditions, von Willebrand disease (inherited or acquired)
Prolonged	Prolonged	Liver disease, DIC, common pathway coagulopathies, multiple factor deficiencies, vitamin K deficiency, multiple transfusions of red cells, malignancy

SECTION II

Prolonged APTT in a clinical setting is most commonly due to the use of heparin, but the delay may also be due to deficiencies or inhibition of: factors VIII, IX, XI or XII; von Willebrand disease; lupus anticoagulant; liver disease;, autoimmune antibodies; or disseminated intravascular coagulation (DIC).

The INR is a ratio determined by the clotting time for patient plasma, divided by the time for control plasma, multiplied by a correction factor based on the laboratory's local population. As such, it is not measured in any units. A normal INR is 1.0, with the therapeutic range differing dependent on the indication. Typical therapeutic INRs are 2.0–3.0 for deep vein thrombosis, pulmonary embolus or atrial fibrillation; 2.5–3.5 for mechanical heart valves; and 3.0–4.5 for certain highly pro-thrombotic conditions. An elevated INR beyond the target range is referred to as 'supratherapeutic'.

Heparin and its low-molecular-weight variants work by binding to antithrombin III and changing the protein's shape, inhibiting thrombin (i.e. factor II) and the activated form of factor X (denoted as factor Xa). In patients who are pregnant, underweight, obese, renal-impaired or critically ill, it may be necessary to monitor the factor Xa level to measure the pharmacodynamic effect of the low-molecular-weight heparins. It is not deemed necessary for prophylactic dose enoxaparin as it is cost prohibitive. It should be considered in people who have a thromboembolic event on anticoagulation or are on extended therapy. This assay is still not available in many hospitals and may need to be sent to metropolitan labs, delaying results and inhibiting its utility.

Fibrinogen (a.k.a. factor I) is a small glycoprotein assembled in the liver that helps the blood clot by supporting platelet aggregation. It is also elevated as an acute phase reactant. Decreased serum fibrinogen can occur after haemorrhage, haemodilution or sepsis, or via consumption (by thromboembolism or DIC). It can be corrected by the administration of fresh frozen plasma (FFP) and cryoprecipitate (typically 10 units).

D-dimer is a fragment of protein produced during the degradation of fibrin (an essential component of clots). As such it is used to investigate the possibility of deep vein thrombosis (DVT) or pulmonary embolus (PE). It is a good example of a highly sensitive but poorly specific investigation. In a normal physiological state there are no circulating D-dimer fragments – however, the assay used is highly sensitive and will detect even a very small amount of D-dimer. Even a small quantity may be indicative of a large thromboembolic event and requires investigation (often with a ventilation/perfusion scintigraphy scan or CT pulmonary angiogram). In this way D-dimer is very good at *excluding* DVT and PE but, if the test is positive, it does not in any way guarantee the presence of a clot. D-dimer will typically be highly elevated in DIC.

Coags should be drawn into a (usually) blue citrate tube and sent to the lab with reasonable urgency, as it should be processed within 2 hours. It is good practice to have a platelet count within the last 24 hours. The sample should not be drawn from a line that has recently been used to administer fluids or flushed with anticoagulant as this can affect results. It is important that you fill the tube to the line as an under-filled tube contains too much citrate for the sample – if you do not think you will be able to do this, consider drawing the blood into a *paediatric* tube. Ensure you provide the lab with the necessary clinical information (e.g. if the patient is anticoagulated).

Although some people routinely order coagulation studies preoperatively, the Royal College of Pathologists of Australia recommend a screening questionnaire is sufficient for minor procedures unless there are elements of the history that are concerning. Coags (or an INR) should be ordered daily for 3 days when warfarin is either commenced or adjusted, before dropping this down to every 3 days, then weekly, then less frequently as it stabilises. Remember to use the 'rule 3 exemption' when sending a patient home for ongoing monitoring by their local doctor and include it in the discharge summary if you have started an anticoagulant. Patients on a heparin infusion require multiple APTTs – save yourself some time and give the nursing staff a large bundle when starting the infusion! The aim of a heparin infusion is usually to keep APTT within 1.5–2.5 × normal.

BLOOD CULTURES AND SENSITIVITIES

Blood cultures are a vital tool in medicine, often used in conjunction with urine culture, chest X-ray, sputum culture and further serology as part of a septic screen. Although they are more expensive than other forms of serology, cultures should be requested when a patient has had fever, rigors, sweats, rampant inflammatory processes or other signs of sepsis (never forget 'cold sepsis'). 25% of patients with bacteraemia will be afebrile for extended periods, particularly the elderly. If you have a clinical suspicion of either fungal or tuberculosis infection, you should document it in the clinical history section of the slip so that appropriate culture techniques are used. It is also good form to note in this section the patient's temperature, and the site and time of phlebotomy.

Two bottles are sent off simultaneously as a 'set' – one contains medium best for aerobes, and the other anaerobes. An aseptic technique with either chlorhexidine or alcohol must be used to prevent contamination, most commonly indicated by a coagulase negative *Staphylococcus* spp. (such as *S. epidermidis*). To help stop introduction of wayward bugs, consider transferring the blood from the syringe into the bottles by injecting it through an alcohol swab placed on top of each bottle (after removing the plastic shield).

A bare minimum of 5 mL of blood is needed for each bottle, but more than 20 mL is preferred to increase your chance of culturing any circulating bacteria. If you can only withdraw sufficient blood for one bottle, place it in the aerobic container and note this on the pathology request (alternatively, split it between paediatric culture bottles). Label the bottles (without putting stickers over the top of the barcode) and send them to the laboratory urgently. Peel off the miniature barcode and apply to the patient's medical records.

Oncology and Haematology patients often have long-term vascular access such as a central venous catheter (CVC) or port – attempt to send off one set of cultures drawn through this site, and one elsewhere (e.g. a peripheral upper limb vein). The more cultures taken, the higher the yield – supported best by studying cases of infective endocarditis, where a *minimum* of three cultures should be sent.

By the very nature of how they are processed, cultures will take a minimum of 24 hours to return and are processed for up to 3 weeks. Blood cultures should *always* be followed up. Often the Pathology Department will call you to notify you of a positive culture. False positives are not uncommon and you should correlate this information clinically – but regardless, they will need to be repeated. Consider referring to the Infectious Diseases service if there are unusual sensitivities. If bacteraemia is confirmed, blood cultures should be repeated daily until two are negative in a row.

ACUTE PHASE REACTANTS (APR)

This is a term you may hear thrown around on the ward, particularly in the setting of systemic illness (e.g. sepsis). These proteins either increase or decrease in plasma concentration as an inflammatory response. Table 12.2 outlines some of the more common acute phase reactants you should consider when interpreting

TABLE 12.2 Acute phase reactants

MARKER	CHANGE
CRP	Elevated
ESR	Elevated
Albumin	Decreased
Ferritin	Elevated
Haptoglobin	Decreased
Complement	Elevated
Fibrinogen	Elevated
Caeruloplasmin	Elevated
Transferrin	Decreased

your patients' results. While not an exhaustive list, it should cover those you would be likely to encounter on a Medical rotation.

MARKERS OF CARDIAC INJURY – TROPONIN AND CREATININE KINASE

Troponins are three proteins key to muscle contraction. Subtypes troponin-I and -T are both sensitive and specific markers for cardiac injury, leaking into the bloodstream from damaged cardiac myocytes. As such the normal range in a healthy adult is little or no measurable troponin at all. It can be used in combination with dynamic ECG changes and a history of chest pain to assist in the diagnosis of myocardial infarction, although it is not uncommon that one of these elements is absent in a patient's presentation.

It may be elevated without obvious ischaemic cardiac injury in severe left ventricular hypertrophy, cardiomyopathies, renal impairment and heart failure. Coronary vasospasm, rapid ventricular rate, chest-related sepsis, cardiac contusion, PE, aortic dissection and defibrillation may also cause a 'troponin leak' without true ischaemia.

Troponins may not rise until up to 4 hours after the onset of ischaemia – hence the common clinical practice of sending off troponins at the time of pain, and 4 hours post. If troponins are positive and other causes of elevation are not apparent, the patient should be managed as an acute coronary syndrome and serial troponins should be performed until they are trending down consistently.

Creatinine kinase (CK) is an enzyme found in many tissues, notably myocytes. There are three variants, with the MB fraction (CK-MB) being most sensitive to cardiac myocytes. Total serum CK is not specific for cardiac muscle and can be elevated with strenuous exercise, rhabdomyolysis, malignant hyperthermia, muscular dystrophies, seizures, extended rigors and myositis. It may not be elevated in people with a low muscle mass (e.g. the elderly). CK-MB was used historically as a diagnostic marker of myocardial infarction prior to the advent of troponins.

Although troponin is now the preferred biochemical marker of cardiac injury, CK-MB still has a role to play in monitoring for re-infarction. Although more sensitive, troponin can take up to 4 hours to become elevated, and remains elevated for a longer period of time than CK-MB (up to 1 or 2 weeks). If a patient were to have a repeat infarction while their troponin was already elevated, it may be masked biochemically with the use of troponin alone. In contrast, CK-MB rises and falls more rapidly, returning to normal in as few as 3 days. Thus, it can be used to detect re-infarction. See Fig. 12.3 for a visual representation.

LIPID PROFILE

Hyperlipidaemia is an issue affecting over 37% of Australians. Of the five major lipoproteins in human blood – chylomicrons and very low density lipoproteins (VLDL), intermediate density lipoproteins (IDL), low density lipoproteins (LDL)

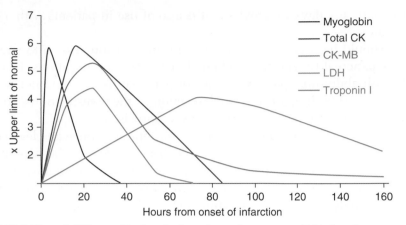

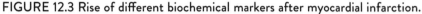

FIGURE 12.3 Rise of different biochemical markers after myocardial infarction.

Sigillum Facultatis Medicae Tertiae Universitatis Carolinae. Pathophysiology of the cardiovascular system. In: Functions of Cells and Human Body [Internet]. <http://fblt.cz/en/skripta/x-srdce-a-obeh -krve/3-zakladni-patofyziologie-kardiovaskularniho-systemu/>.

and high density lipoproteins (HDL) – we routinely measure three: LDL, HDL and VLDL. You will also receive a report of the triglycerides and total serum cholesterol, with some labs providing the total cholesterol-to-HDL ratio.

LDL is often conveyed as the 'bad' cholesterol and HDL as the 'good' (a memory trick – lowlifes are 'bad'). An elevated LDL is the measurement most closely associated with cardiovascular risk, and as such is often the target in monitoring therapy (followed by total cholesterol). VLDL cannot be directly measured yet, and is estimated by taking the total triglyceride level and dividing it by five. This is because VLDL carries the majority of circulating triglycerides.

Serum lipids are measured in a gold or white SST II tube. This investigation should be sent to the lab after a minimum of 9 (optimally 14) hours of fasting. Remember to denote in the clinical history whether they are fasting (always useful) or random (rarely useful). Avoid using a tourniquet for too long when drawing off the sample as it can artificially increase levels.

A lipid profile could be performed opportunistically with some merit in a population >45 years, but all patients with acute coronary syndrome, pre-chemotherapy, newly diagnosed diabetes or a strong family history of sudden cardiac death, should have serum cholesterol and triglycerides performed.

PANCREATIC ENZYMES – LIPASE AND AMYLASE

Both amylase and lipase are enzymes produced by the pancreas for the breakdown of food into more readily available energy. During an episode of pancreatitis they are secreted into the systemic circulation due to a breakdown of the normal synthesis–secretion pathway. Serum lipase is now the diagnostic biochemical marker of choice, having replaced amylase as it has a higher sensitivity and specificity for pancreatitis. Additionally, due to its longer half-life (8–14 days compared with 3–5 days for amylase), it is also of use in patients with a delayed presentation.

Lipase should be used in conjunction with the Ranson criteria to stratify the severity of pancreatitis and the likelihood of further complications. If a patient presents with abdominal pain suspicious of pancreatitis, it would not be unwarranted to send off both lipase and amylase amongst the investigations. Low lipase can be seen in chronic diseases such as cystic fibrosis.

There is *no value* in performing serial serum lipases – once an elevated lipase is detected, the diagnosis of pancreatitis has been made and the patient should be managed as such. The degree of enzymatic elevation does not always correlate with the clinical picture. This is a common question on surgical rounds! Both enzymes are analysed in a gold or white SST II tube.

VITAMIN D

Vitamin D (25-hydroxyvitamin D or 25D) is a lipophilic vitamin necessary for musculoskeletal health. Low vitamin D has been linked with osteoporosis, increased falls and fractures. A severe deficiency once caused rickets and osteomalacia in children and adults with regularity, but this is now rare in developed countries. Subclinical vitamin D appears to be increasing in incidence in Australia and other Western countries, particularly in winter.

Deficiency is considered to be <50 nmol/L, with the elderly, institutionalised and people living in temperate climates at the highest risk. There has been a sharp increase in the number of requests for serum vitamin D in Australia, leading to the Australian Government restricting its use. It is more cost-effective to supplement vitamin D orally if deficiency is suspected. Vitamin D is collected in a gold or white SST II tube.

LACTATE DEHYDROGENASE

Lactate dehydrogenase (LDH) is an enzyme involved in the conversion of glucose to energy, and is present in almost all cell types. It is normally intracellular, with low levels circulating in serum. If elevated, LDH may indicate high cellular turnover, cell death, ischaemia, infection, malignancy, liver disease and haemolytic anaemia. It is a non-specific marker of disease, and is used predominantly in Oncology and Haematology as a loose marker of disease activity. It is measured in an SST II white or gold tube and must be analysed with haste as cell breakdown in the sample can falsely inflate the measurement.

NB: Don't confuse LDH with lactate, outlined below.

LACTATE

Lactate is an ion formed when lactic acid loses a proton from the carboxyl group, such as when dissolved in a solution. Lactic acid is produced during lactic acidosis, when the mitochondria do not have sufficient oxygen to convert glucose into energy (i.e. cellular hypoxia). To compensate, the body shifts towards anaerobic energy production and the primary by-product of this process is lactic acid.

Lactate is a non-specific biochemical marker that can be used to risk-stratify patients with severe sepsis (or in particular used in determining the severity of sepsis in the immunocompromised or elderly who may not be able to mount a full immune response), diabetic ketoacidosis, hypoxia and ischaemia.

Beware if a patient is receiving intravenous CSL – it contains lactate and may affect results. Lactate is typically reported on blood gases. You may see lactate requested when sepsis is suspected, in a patient over 50 years with abdominal pain as a part of the diagnostic work-up for mesenteric ischaemia or on a blood gas in a hypoxic patient. Lactate is no longer recommended as a diagnostic marker for myocardial ischaemia due to the widespread availability and greater sensitivity and specificity of troponins.

AMMONIA

Ammonia is a rarely requested investigation that may be sent off if you suspect hepatic failure or a metabolic encephalopathy in patients with lethargy, tachypnoea or unprovoked seizure activity. It may also be elevated with gastrointestinal bleeding, haematological malignancies (especially myeloma, lymphomas and allograft transplants), certain drug therapies (regular hepatotoxic repeat offenders such as paracetamol, valproate and carbamazepine) and rare genetic conditions with faults in the metabolism of urea and fatty acids. It is usually used in conjunction with neuroimaging (CT or MRI). Ammonia is sent in EDTA tubes that must be delivered to the laboratory *on ice*.

BRAIN NATRIURETIC PEPTIDE (BNP)

BNP is a polypeptide released by the ventricles of the heart when they are dilated – its confusing name comes from the fact it was first identified in the brains of pigs. BNP is secreted by cardiac myocytes when they are stretched, such as in overload. When BNP is cleaved from its prohormone, an inert version (N-terminal pro-BNP or NT-proBNP) is also made, which some labs measure instead of 'direct' BNP. BNP levels are variable in different populations and are affected by age, gender and BMI (with values increased in males, the elderly and the underweight).

BNP first entered clinical use as a diagnostic marker of heart failure – particular diastolic dysfunction – to separate heart failure from pulmonary causes of dyspnoea. Its further use via serial testing to monitor response to therapy in heart failure is still being investigated. However, several studies have also shown BNP and NT-proBNP may be useful as predictors of both hospitalisation for heart failure and all-cause mortality.

Population variance is important, and not all people with high BNP will have heart failure. BNP and NT-proBNP may be elevated in renal failure, pulmonary hypertension, sepsis, valvular disease, atrial fibrillation and acute coronary syndrome. Similarly, a high BNP does not preclude a multifactorial presentation (e.g. pneumonia + heart failure).

HAEMATINICS: IRON STUDIES, FOLATE, VITAMIN B12 AND HAEMOCHROMATOSIS GENES

A haematinic screen may be requested on a patient with anaemia to help elicit the cause, as well as patients with aplastic anaemia, or failure to mobilise after marrow suppression. Iron studies are requested frequently and as a junior doctor you should have a basic understanding of their interpretation.

Iron studies may be requested based on a suspicion of iron overload or anaemia, and you will receive a total serum iron, ferritin, transferrin (or total iron binding capacity, TIBC) and calculated transferrin saturation. Iron replacement therapy is discussed in Chapter 24, 'Managing fluids and infusions'.

- Serum levels of iron do not drop until the body has been depleted for approximately 3 months. Serum iron levels are a weak measure of iron status, as the majority of iron is found within erythrocytes (45%), in muscle and cellular enzymes (15%) and as ferritin or haemosiderin in the liver and reticuloendothelial system (40%), and serum levels fluctuate between meals.
- Ferritin is an iron storage protein that can store up to 4000 iron atoms. A low serum ferritin has a high specificity for iron deficiency anaemia. However, inflammation (and some malignancies) causes a rise in the ferritin levels, believed to be due to the sequestration of iron within the reticuloendothelial system when there are high levels of circulating interleukin-6. In these situations, a low serum ferritin cannot exclude iron deficiency anaemia or be used to diagnose iron overload. Inflammation may cause ferritin to be very highly elevated.
- Transferrin is the combination of a carrier protein (apotransferrin) bound to one or two iron atoms. Transferrin may be low in hepatic disease due to the loss of the liver's synthetic function. Transferrin is also an acute phase reactant and will drop in inflammatory states, and may be falsely normal in situations with low circulating protein. TIBC is an alternate method of expressing the level of serum transferrin.
- Transferrin saturation is determined by serum iron divided by the serum TIBC, and represents the percentage of iron binding sites on the transferrin circulating that are occupied by iron.

Haemochromatosis genetic testing is rarely required, but frequently ordered by the overly keen junior medical registrar. The genetic mutations in question are C282Y and H63D of the HFE gene. They would be justified in a patient with a high serum ferritin and transferrin saturation on two separate occasions.

Haemochromatosis would be suspected in patients with persistently high ferritin and transferrin saturation, or with a first degree relative diagnosed with haemochromatosis. It is unnecessary to test children until late teenage years unless symptomatic. The genetic test report will indicate whether the patient has either a heterozygous or homozygous variation for each of the two mutations tested. Heterozygous patients are less likely to be symptomatic, but are carriers and can pass on the allele to their offspring (and if their partner also has a heterozygous mutation, the children may experience homozygous disease).

Folate and/or vitamin B12 deficiencies can cause a profound, macrocytic anaemia with the possibility of neurological symptoms. The incidence of B12 deficiency in Australians over 65 years is great enough to justify routine screening – these patients may have only a mild (or even no) anaemia. Dietary folate deficiency is rarer. On a peripheral blood film, the erythrocytes will appear larger and ovoid, and may be seen in conjunction with hypersegmented neutrophils. Pancytopenia can be present.

Those most at risk include the elderly, alcoholics and the malnourished (a common exam question is the new vegan with B12 deficiency, as it is mostly found in meat, fish and dairy products). Both folate and B12 can be tested on serum. Folate can be supplemented orally as folic acid, typically 5 mg PO daily for 1 to 4 months. B12 can be given as an intramuscular injection – usually loaded by one 1-mg injection daily for a week, then one injection monthly coordinated by the patient's GP. Before supplementing, the reason for deficiency should be investigated (e.g. insufficient dietary intake).

THYROID FUNCTION TESTS

Thyroid dysfunction affects many people in Australia. Thyroid function tests (TFTs) are comprised of thyroid-stimulating hormone (TSH), total serum thyroxine (T_4) and total serum triiodothyronine (T_3) (see Table 12.3). TSH is produced by the pituitary to stimulate the release of thyroid hormone. The pituitary stops releasing TSH when circulating T_4 is sufficient, and ramps up production when serum T_4 is low (like a thermostat automatically correcting temperature). In hyperthyroidism, TSH may remain high despite treatment for several weeks.

TABLE 12.3 Interpretation of thyroid function tests

TSH	T_3	T_4	MOST LIKELY INTERPRETATION
Undetectable	High	High	Primary thyrotoxicosis
Undetectable	Normal	Raised	Primary T_3 thyrotoxicosis
Undetectable	Normal	Normal	Subclinical thyrotoxicosis
Low	High	Low/normal	Non-thyroidal illness, amiodarone
Normal	Low	Low	Secondary hypothyroidism
Elevated	Low	Low	Primary hypothyroidism
Elevated	Normal	Normal	Subclinical hypothyroidism

Adapted from: Strachan, M.W.J. & Newell-Price, J., 2014. Chapter 20: Endocrine disease. In: Walker, B.R., Colledge, N.R., Ralston, S.H., et al. Davidson's Principles and Practice of Medicine, 22nd ed. Edinburgh: Churchill Livingstone, pp. 733-796.

If a patient has a goitre or symptomatic hyper- or hypothyroidism, you may also send off thyroid antibodies. Three are able to be tested – thyroid peroxidase antibody (TPOAb), thyroglobulin antibody (TgAb) and TSH receptor antibody (TSHRAb). In Hashimoto's thyroiditis, most patients will have a positive TPOAb and TgAb. In Graves' disease, TSHRAb and TPOAb may be positive. Some thyroid cancers are positive for TgAb.

TFTs are not ordered routinely in Australia due to cost – TSH alone is sufficient in detecting thyroid status as it is more sensitive than free T_4. Patients on lithium, amiodarone and thyroid replacement therapy should have regular TSH levels. Note that a high circulating beta-HCG may cause hyperthyroidism, as the alpha-HCG subunit can stimulate pituitary receptors for thyroid hormones. If a patient is hypothyroid during an acute illness (but asymptomatic), the TSH should be repeated in 3–6 months before actively treating. If an abnormal TSH is detected, then assessing the T_3 and T_4 would be warranted. They are drawn into white or gold SST II tubes.

ADRENOCORTICOTROPHIC HORMONE (ACTH) AND SHORT SYNACTHEN TESTS

A relatively common investigation on medical wards is an ACTH stimulation or 'short Synacthen' test (Synacthen® is a trade name for tetracosactide or 'synthetic ACTH'). Typically, a 250-mcg injection of tetracosactide is given intramuscularly at as close to 8 a.m. as possible with serum cortisol and ACTH measured at the time immediately prior to injection, and cortisol alone taken at 30 min post-injection, and (optionally) 1 hour post-injection. The patient should be fasted for a minimum of 8 hours (i.e. midnight the night before).

It is contraindicated in hypersensitivity to Synacthen, psychosis, recent live vaccination, peptic ulcer disease, untreated infection, Cushing's syndrome, heart failure and during pregnancy or lactation. The purpose of an ACTH stimulation test is to identify patients with adrenocortical insufficiency. In normal patients, the administration of Synacthen will stimulate the adrenal glands to produce cortisol. If cortisol remains low despite stimulation by the synthetic ACTH, the results are suggestive of adrenocortical insufficiency or Addison's disease. In Cushingoid patients the serum ACTH is low with elevated plasma cortisol.

DIABETES – ORAL GLUCOSE TOLERANCE TEST, C-PEPTIDE, HbA₁c, SERUM INSULIN AND GAD ANTIBODIES

Diabetes is reaching epidemic proportions in Australia's population with startling speed. A metabolic endocrine disorder caused by either a lack of insulin or lack of sufficient responsiveness to it, there are several investigations you should have a basic understanding of to help diagnose and monitor diabetes.

The gold standard of diagnosing diabetes at this stage remains the oral glucose tolerance test (OGTT). In this test, a patient is fasted for 9–14 hours before being given a 'glucose load' containing 75 g glucose. Serum glucose is measured prior to

TABLE 12.4 Interpretation of oral glucose tolerance tests

CLASSIFICATION	FASTING (mmol/L)	2-HOUR (mmol/L)
Non-diabetic	≥6.0	<7.8
Pre-diabetic	6.1–6.9	7.8–11.0
Diabetic	≥7.0	≥11.1

Reproduced and adapted with permission from The Royal Australian College of General Practitioners from: Phillips PJ. Oral glucose tolerance testing. Aust Fam Physician 2012; 41(6):391-93. Available at <http://www.racgp.org.au/afp/2012/june/oral-glucose-tolerance-testing/>.

the glucose loading, and at 2 hours post-ingestion (see Table 12.4 for interpretation of results). An OGTT should be requested when a random blood sugar level (BSL) is between 5.5 and 11.0 mmol/L or a fasting BSL is between 5.5 and 6.9 mmol/L. An OGTT would be unnecessary if fasting BSL was ≥7.0 mmol/L or random BSL was ≥11.0 mmol/L as these are clearly in the diabetic range. Note that a formal, lab-based BSL should be sent off for any patient with a serum glucose higher than a glucometer can detect, even if asymptomatic.

Equivocal results are sometimes labelled 'pre-diabetes', with a strong correlation with progression to diabetes. These patients have an increased risk of macrovascular events, but there is not yet any evidence they are at increased risk of microvascular incidents. Thus 'pre-diabetics' should have annual OGTTs. Women with polycystic ovarian syndrome should be considered for diabetic screening with an OGTT. Both OGTT and lab-based BSLs are measured in the grey fluoride oxalate tubes.

HbA_{1c} (a.k.a. glycated or glycohaemoglobin) refers to glycosylated haemoglobin, and is gold standard for assessing glycaemic control over a 6- to 8-week period (i.e. the lifespan of the erythrocytes). The HbA_{1c} can help you stratify a patient's risk for microvascular complications – the target for diabetics is ≤7.0% – as well as titrate hypoglycaemic therapy.

The HbA_{1c} may be affected by a change in the turnover of red blood cells (e.g. haemolysis or decreased production due to various deficiencies), abnormal red cell structure, hyperbilirubinaemia, high-dose aspirin, hypertriglyceridaemia, renal disease, chronic opiate use and alcoholism. An HbA_{1c} is a useful measure and, when admitting a patient with diabetes, you should ask if they have had one within 3 months; otherwise it would be a good idea to repeat it.

An HbA_{1c} may be requested on PBS four times yearly and is drawn into a white or gold SST II tube. Online calculators are available that will help you convert HbA_{1c} to average BSL. As of 2015, an HbA_{1c} of >6.5% is considered diagnostic of type 2 diabetes mellitus (T2DM) in Australia and may be used in place of the OGTT for diagnosis. If there are no symptoms of diabetes, the HbA_{1c} should be repeated (with lifestyle recommendations made) before commencing treatment.

Serum insulin has a role in the diagnosis of diabetes, insulinoma (i.e. an insulin-producing tumour) and insulin resistance, or to evaluate the level of endogenous insulin production in a type 2 diabetic patient or determine the success of islet cell transplantation. Insulin is often requested in combination with

C-peptide, a peptide produced by the pancreatic beta cells when proinsulin splits (making one molecule each of C-peptide and insulin). Thus if both are ordered simultaneously in a patient on insulin therapy, it is possible to evaluate how much insulin is being produced endogenously (within the body) and what fraction is being injected subcutaneously (exogenous).

C-peptide is not yet used routinely in diagnosing diabetes, but has several niche uses including in the diagnosis of insulinoma, the prediction of anti-insulin antibodies (as there is high circulating C-peptide by little endogenous insulin), monitoring the activity of beta islet cells and in assessment of response in islet cell transplants. Low C-peptide is associated with low insulin production. Insulin should be drawn into a lithium heparin tube, and C-peptide into a standard gold or white SST II tube. Insulin should be done after a period of fasting and 2 hours post-prandial (i.e. after a meal).

Lastly, glutamic acid decarboxylase auto-antibodies (GAD antibodies) may be used to diagnose type 1 diabetes mellitus or latent autoimmune diabetes of adulthood (LADA). Its most frequent application in clinical practice is in T2DM where the diagnosis is in doubt (e.g. they are not overweight or rapidly progress to insulin dependence). GAD is produced in islet cells and neural tissue, with up to 90% of type 1 diabetic patients having circulating GAD antibodies at diagnosis. They are drawn into a standard gold or white SST II tube.

CROSS-MATCHING AND GROUP AND HOLD

Cross-matching (sometimes written as 'X-match') is performed to ensure a patient is able to receive blood of the same ABO and rhesus (Rh) types. Failure to do so (with administration of incompatible blood) can lead to a transfusion reaction, which can be fatal. As such, the process by which blood is requested is tightly regulated.

When a cross-match is requested by the clinician, the laboratory will perform ABO confirmation and Rh determination of both the recipient's and the donor's erythrocytes, an antibody screen of the recipient's serum and a cross-match of the recipient's serum and donor's red cells. Then they will store the requested number of units of blood product in a refrigerator in the blood bank specifically for the use of the patient on the request form. A cross-match must be performed before administering any blood products – packed red blood cells, granulocytes, buffy coat, platelets, fresh frozen plasma, cryoprecipitate and, depending on the institution policy, even albumins.

Haematology, Oncology and otherwise marrow-suppressed patients will need an existing cross-match at all times during admission, and they are usually performed twice-weekly. Otherwise, you may request a cross-match for a patient who is haemorrhaging, severely anaemic or prior to major surgical procedures.

A group and hold (G&H, or 'group and save') involves ABO and Rh typing and the detection of any red cell antibodies. The Red Cross Blood Bank have a '72 hour rule' in Australia, that is, a cross-match expires at 72 hours and must be repeated before further blood products can be released for the patient. G&H may be performed when bleeding is ongoing or expected (e.g. preoperatively for large surgeries). With a G&H in effect blood can be issued within 10 minutes; without one it will take a minimum of 35 minutes (and that is if the patient does not have atypical antibodies!).

Great care must be taken when requesting a cross-match or group and hold. Urgent transfusions are delayed not infrequently because the doctor did not complete the request properly. All details for a cross-match must be *handwritten* on the tube with a minimum of *three* identifying patient features, the date and time the sample was drawn and the doctor's signature. If any details are absent the sample will be destroyed, no matter how hard it is to bleed the patient or how urgently they require blood! The tubes used are the pink EDTA tubes, which cannot be used for any other investigations. For more on blood products, see Chapter 24, 'Managing fluids and infusions'.

HUMAN LEUCOCYTE ANTIGEN (HLA) TYPING

Sometimes referred to as tissue typing, HLA typing is a very specialist test requested to match organ and tissue transplant recipients with suitable donors by identifying the presence of the major HLA genes and their encoded antigens. They are used most regularly on Transplant and Haematology rotations.

These antigens are proteins present on the surface of all cells in a person's body and help the immune system differentiate 'foreign' and 'self'. Theoretically, the closer the match between the donor and the recipient's HLA antigens, the lower the risk of tissue rejection, the more likely engraftment will be successful and the more likely the overall transplant will succeed.

When preparing a patient for receiving a transplant, their blood samples are sent to your state's Red Cross Blood Service for testing. Take great care when completing the forms, which can be found at www.transfusion.com.au/transplantation_services. One copy is given to the patient, two sent with the samples and one placed in medical records. Be sure to include a brief clinical history in the correct section so that the blood bank knows what the plan is with this patient. If you are also typing a patient's siblings, the form will need to be completed again for each person. It is *highly important* that you fill in the *recipient's details* on the potential donor's forms in the box, or the blood bank cannot match the donor and recipient.

Other reasons to send samples for tissue typing include suspicion of auto-immune diseases such as ankylosing spondylosis (HLA-B27) and idiopathic thrombocytopenia purpura (anti-platelet antibodies) or post-transplant to see if the patient has developed antibodies against the transplanted tissue. Cross-match testing is performed just prior to the transplant (after initial HLA typing) to ensure there is no mismatch.

MARKERS OF MALIGNANCY

'Tumour markers' – as they are so glamorously referred to in the media – are substances (usually proteins) that are either produced directly by cancer, or by the body in response to cancer growth. Junior doctors face a work environment where the number of evidence-based tumour markers is rapidly expanding, but there are several that are already well-documented and in common use.

At this point, routine screening on admission or use in patients presenting with vague symptoms is *not justified*. Tumour markers are of great value when there is a high suspicion of malignancy, in investigation of a cancer of unknown primary or in stratifying prognosis and assessing treatment response. Asymptomatic population-based screening has little merit – even prostate specific antigen (PSA), which shows no mortality benefit. An ideal tumour marker would identify the malignancy with sensitivity and specificity, cheaply, non-invasively and at a stage where intervention is still possible.

In addition to the specific markers listed in Table 12.5, a serum protein electrophoresis (SPEP) is often requested. In this test serum is run through an electrophoresis chamber with charges applied at each end. The different molecules in serum have different sizes and thus different electrical properties and will be separated as such. A 'spike' in one particular protein implies excess production – although this may occur in inflammation, it can also be indicative of malignancy and may even identify the origin.

TABLE 12.5 Tumour markers

MARKER	DISEASE	NOTES
Alpha-fetoprotein (AFP)	Hepatocellular carcinoma, germ cell tumour	Chronic liver disease patients with symptoms of malignancy should always have their AFP checked. Chronic viral hepatitis patients should have an annual AFP. A mild elevation is normal in this population. AFP will be massively deranged in germ cell tumours
Beta-2 microglobulin (B2M)	Multiple myeloma (MM), chronic lymphocytic leukaemia	Also elevated in chronic renal disease and hepatitis, useful for prognosis but not diagnosis of MM
Cancer antigen (CA) 125	Ovarian cancer primarily, but also endometrial, peritoneal, salpingeal disease	Non-specific, it may also be elevated in fibroids, endometriosis, pelvic inflammatory disease, cirrhosis, pregnancy and menstruation
CA 15-3	Breast cancer	Clinical value unclear; often used to assess treatment response

TABLE 12.5 Tumour markers—cont'd

MARKER	DISEASE	NOTES
CA 19-9	Pancreatic cancer, biliary tract malignancies, some colorectal cancers, some gastric cancers	Most commonly used for pancreatic cancers. May also be increased in thyroid disease, rheumatoid arthritis, pancreatitis and inflammatory bowel disease
Calcitonin	Medullary thyroid carcinoma	Produced by parafollicular C cells in the thyroid; can be used to screen family members of patients with medullary thyroid carcinoma
Carcinoembryonic antigen (CEA)	Primarily colorectal, also non-small cell lung cancer, breast, ovarian, bladder and head and neck	Used for prognosis and response, not diagnosis
Chromogranin A (CgA)	Neuroendocrine tumour, phaechromocytoma, small cell lung cancer	Only abnormal in ~33% neuroendocrine tumours. Can be increased by PPI use
Human chorionic gonadotropin (hCG)	Germ cell tumours, choriocarcinoma, gestational trophoblastic disease	An elevated hCG may also cause hyperthyroidism due to cross-reactivity of the protein and TSH receptors
Immunoglobulin (Ig)	Lymphoma, leukaemia, multiple myeloma, Waldenström macroglobulinaemia	May be reported as isolated spikes on SPEP. You can also request serum Ig
Inhibin	Stromal ovarian cancer	
Lactate dehydrogenase (LDH)	High cell turnover, commonly largely elevated in lymphomas and germ cell tumours	As outlined above, quite non-specific and also elevated in non-malignant conditions
Neuron-specific enolase (NSE)	Neuroendocrine secreting tumours, small cell carcinoma of the lung, breast cancer	Useful for disease response in small cell lung cancer

continued

SECTION II

TABLE 12.5 Tumour markers—cont'd

MARKER	DISEASE	NOTES
Prostate-specific antigen (PSA)	Prostate cancer	Often used as a screening test, but this is not routinely recommended. Also elevation in prostatitis, benign prostatic hypertrophy and for 48 hours post-ejaculation. Can be used as a 'trend' and measure of disease response
S-100 protein	Melanoma	Not routinely used yet, but could be used to investigate the possibility of widespread disease in an already-established diagnosis of melanoma
Thyroglobulin (Tg)	Thyroid cancer	Disease response – if used, should check anti-thyroglobulin antibodies at least once

Beng, C., 2006. Tumour markers. In: *IMVS Newsletter* [Internet]. <http://www.imvs.sa.gov.au/wps/wcm/connect/8e862178-7325-4f40-b5b7-69e98d3fbef0/tumour-markers.pdf?MOD=AJPERES>. American Cancer Society. Tumor markers [Internet]. <http://www.cancer.org/treatment/understandingyourdiagnosis/examsandtestdescriptions/tumormarkers/ >.

ASSORTED SEROLOGY PANELS

At times during your internship you may be asked by your registrar to send off one of many 'screens' or 'panels' related to specific conditions. Rather than scramble to your smart phone every time this is requested of you, Table 12.6 is a convenient list of some of the more common panels used on the wards.

TABLE 12.6 Commonly used 'panels'

SCREEN	INVESTIGATIONS
Sepsis	FBE + UEC + LFT + CMP + CRP + ESR + blood cultures (both an aerobic and anaerobic bottle, from 3 sites in total) + urine M/C/S + nasopharyngeal swab + VBG (taking note of lactate) + sputum M/C/S + chest X-ray (CXR) ± faecal M/C/S with CDT ± culture of any other drain or wound
Abdominal pain (or acute abdomen)	FBE + UEC + CMP + LFT + coagulation (in case of need for surgery) + lipase ± amylase ± group and hold (if surgery with significant blood loss is likely)

TABLE 12.6 Commonly used 'panels'—cont'd

SCREEN	INVESTIGATIONS
Haemolysis	FBE + UEC + LFT (mostly for total bilirubin) + haptoglobin + TSH + direct antibody test (DAT) + lactate dehydrogenase (LDH) + unconjugated bilirubin + spherocytes + reticulocyte count + peripheral blood film
Autoimmune	FBE + UEC + CMP + LFT + CRP + ESR + rheumatoid factor (RF) + ANA + ENA + ANCA + anti-dsDNA + C3 + C4 + anti-CCP + anti-cardiolipin + cryoglobulins + immunoglobulins
Neuropathy	FBE + UEC + CMP + LFT + zinc + fasting BSL + HbA1c + TSH + myeloma screen (SPEP + b2M + light chains + LDH + urate + urinary Bence Jones) + B12 + folate + Fe studies + HIV + HCV + HBV + heavy metals + anti-GM1 + cryoglobulins + ESR ± rheumatology screen ± urine immunofixation electrophoresis ± urinary amyloid, porphyrins, and heavy metals + nerve conduction studies ± LP ± nerve biopsy ± gene testing for Charcot-Marie-Tooth disease
Hepatitis	FBE + UEC + CMP + LFT + coagulation + AST + AFP + CK + ANA + ANCA + AMA + ASMA + anti-LKM + copper + caeruloplasmin + vitamin D + folate + iron studies + B12 + coeliac serology + serum IgG + serum protein electrophoresis (SPEP) + alpha-1 antitrypsin + hepatitis A (HAV) IgM + hepatitis B (HBV) core antibody and surface antigen + hepatitis C (HCV) antibodies ± hepatitis D and hepatitis E (if HBV positive) ± haemochromatosis genes (if high ferritin)
Renal	FBE + UEC + CMP + ANA + ENA + anti-GBM + ANCA + anti-LKM + cryoglobulins + serum immunoglobulins + SPEP + urine M/C/S with albumin-to-creatinine ratio, protein-to-creatinine ratio and sodium ± renal tract ultrasound
Rheumatology	FBE + UEC + CMP + LFT + RF + anti-CCP + ENA + ANA + ANCA + uric acid + hlaB27 + ESR + CRP + C3 + C4 + serum immunoglobulins
Myeloma	FBE + UEC + CMP + serum IgG + serum free light chains + SPEP + ESR + LDH + beta-2 microglobulin (b2M) + urate + urine Bence-Jones protein ± skeletal survey and further imaging
Thrombophilia	FBE + UEC + CRP + ESR + factor V Leiden + proteins C and S + antithrombin III + ANA + anti-dsDNA + anti-cardiolipin + anti-b2 glycoprotein 1 + prothrombin gene

continued

SECTION II

TABLE 12.6 Commonly used 'panels'—cont'd

SCREEN	INVESTIGATIONS
Commencing total parenteral nutrition (TPN)	FBE + UEC + CMP + LFT + vitamins A, B12, C, D and E + selenium + chromium + manganese + zinc + folate + iron studies + fasting lipids and glucose
Geriatric	FBE + UEC + CMP + LFT + CRP + vitamin D + folate + B12 + TSH + Fe studies ± fasting lipids and glucose (or HbA1c if diabetic)
Tumour lysis risk	FBE + UEC + CMP + LFT + coags + urate + LDH + CRP
Delirium	FBE + UEC + CMP + LFT + CRP + ESR + TSH + vitamin D + B12 + folate + iron studies ± blood cultures ± drug levels (e.g. anti-epileptic drugs) ± toxins ± ABG + spot BSL ± BAC + urinalysis + MMSE + ECG + CXR ± neuroimaging (CT or MRI) ± EEG ± LP
Diabetes	Fasting BSL + HbA1c + urine AER + opthalmoscopy
Dementia	Delirium screen + rheumatology screen + syphilis + HIV + SPEP ± heavy metals
Fever in returned traveller	FBE + UEC + CMP + LFT + CRP + ESR + HIV + HBV + HCV + HAV + CMV + EBV + VZV + blood cultures + thick and thin films + urine MCS + faecal MCS with ova, cysts and parasites (OCP), *Shigella*, *Salmonella* and *Cryptosporidium* ± further viral serology based on location of origin
Prior to commencing chemotherapy	FBE + peripheral blood film + UEC + CMP + reticulocyte count + coags + B12/folate/iron studies + blood group and hold + direct antibody test + LFT + TSH + glucose + lipids + immunoglobulins + viral serology (VZV + CMV + EBV + HSV + HIV + HBV + HCV + HAV) + blood cultures + CXR + PET/CT studies + TTE or LVEF from a gated blood pool scan + respiratory function tests (RFTs) + ECG + dental review + 24-hour urinary creatinine clearance ± HLA typing

CHAPTER 13

INVESTIGATIONS: OTHER PATHOLOGY

Joseph M O'Brien

Serology samples will not be the only ones you send to the laboratory in your intern year! If the human body produces a fluid, it can be examined under a microscope, cultured and exposed to numerous antibiotics. Investigations other than bloodwork should not be neglected, as identifying causative organisms directly at the source can be an inexpensive and valuable resource.

MICROSCOPY, CULTURE AND SENSITIVITIES

Urine microscopy, culture and sensitivities

One of the most often performed investigations in hospitals, a urine microscopy, culture and sensitivities (urine MCS), can supply a great deal of diagnostic information at a reasonably low cost. It may provide a diagnosis for symptomatic illness, or it may reveal asymptomatic disease. Urinary tract infections (UTIs) are incredibly common, especially in the elderly. It may be performed as part of a septic screen, to investigate urinary symptoms (dysuria, nocturia, loin pain, suprapubic pain, polyuria, oliguria), or to diagnose more serious disease such as diabetes, malignancy or glomerulonephritis. A mid-stream specimen of urine (MSU) is preferred as it is a sample taken after some urine has already left the urethra, and theoretically 'flushed' colonised bacteria that may be at the urethral meatus.

Prior to sending off a 'formal' urine MCS, a patient's urine will often be 'dipsticked'. Urine test strips (a.k.a. 'full ward test' or FWT) can be a good screening test to see if there is value in proceeding to the urine MCS. A FWT will report the acidity (pH), specific gravity (Sp Gr), protein, blood, glucose, ketones, nitrites and presence of leucocytes. The acidity of urine is usually relatively constant, kept between 6.0 and 7.4 by the action of the renal tubules. A drop in acidity can allow a UTI to take hold. The specific gravity refers to the density of the urine, i.e. the ability of the kidney to concentrate (or dilute) the urine produced. A Sp Gr of >1.035 is likely contaminated, or contains excessive glucose and renders the result inaccurate. As the kidneys filter >99.9% of glucose back into the blood, glucosuria is quite closely associated with diabetes. Ketones are an indication of a starvation response, seen they experience a febrile episode. An NPA swab is typically processed for respiratory multiplex polymerase chain reaction (PCR), which is used for the detection of over 30 microorganisms including influenza A and B, parainfluenza strains, metapneumoviruses A and B, *S. aureus*, *Bordatella pertussis*, *Haemophilus influenzae*, cytomegalovirus, *Legionella* species and picornaviruses (including common offenders rhinovirus and enterovirus).

A patient suspected of having an infection transmissible by droplets should be placed in isolation until the PCR results return to prevent the spread of disease to staff and other patients. You should have a low threshold for sending an NPA swab to the lab for immunocompromised patients, but take care not to cause any trauma if the patient is thrombocytopenic.

Faecal microscopy, culture and sensitivities plus *Clostridium difficile* toxin and ova, cysts and parasites

Faecal MCS (a.k.a. stool culture) is an often over-utilised investigation in the inpatient setting. The investigation into diarrhoea should be guided by the duration and severity of symptoms in context with the patient's clinical history. Typically, if a patient is systemically unwell or immunocompromised, has recently returned from overseas travel or has had symptoms for more than 72 hours, a sample should be sent to the laboratory at presentation.

A faecal MCS will provide you with the identification of any bacteria grown as well as their sensitivities. Antibiotic use should be as per the *Therapeutic Guidelines* for your region. The presence of leucocytes and erythrocytes will also be reported. Some of the more common causes of infection include *Campylobacter*, *Shigella* and *Salmonella* species. The travel history should be documented in the clinical history, as it may prompt further investigation into common overseas organisms including *Aeromonas*, *Plesiomonas*, *Yersinia enterocolitica* and *Vibrio* species. The classic causative organism of chronic or sub-acute small bowel diarrhoea is *Giardia*, which is detected on serology just as easily as in the faecal sample.

If a patient has already been on antibiotics (particularly stronger agents), a *Clostridium difficile* toxin (CDT) should also be added. If this is positive, the lab may choose to also perform a *C. difficile* ('C. dif') culture. *C. difficile* is a bacterium that is part of the normal gut flora of the majority of people, which in the presence of antibiotic therapy may become overgrown and pathogenic causing diarrhoea and bowel inflammation. This occurs more commonly in the elderly, postoperative patients, patients with prolonged (or multiple agent) antibiotic exposure and patients on proton pump inhibitors (PPI) and H_2 antagonists. It should be detected as early as possible as it may progress to pseudomembranous colitis.

If the patient has chronic diarrhoea, consider widening the scope of investigation to include investigation for ova, cysts and parasites (OCP). If they are from a residential nursing home or part of an 'outbreak' setting, consider norovirus PCR. Requesting 'viral screen' on a stool sample results only in a search for norovirus (if in an adult). Since rotavirus normally only affects small children, it is not routinely screened for. The sample may be examined for adenovirus if the clinical notes indicate the patient's presentation is part of an outbreak. Although expensive, the cost of these investigations is largely absorbed by the government, since controlling an outbreak of diarrhoea is considered a public health priority. Be aware that several kinds of bacterial diarrhoea are notifiable illnesses – see Chapter 20, 'Notifiable diseases', for more information.

CHAPTER 14

INVESTIGATIONS: IMAGING

Paul Watson

ORDERING IMAGING TESTS

Radiology offers a wide range of diagnostic and therapeutic services. Consequently, the junior doctor can expect to liaise with the Radiology Department on a daily basis organising investigations and procedures and chasing reports from radiologists.

The process of booking radiology tests and procedures varies among hospital networks, but will always involve submitting either a paper-based or online request form. Not all radiology tests can be submitted using the same form, especially requests for nuclear medicine such as PET scans. Timely requests for imaging are essential for efficient discharging of patients (such as orthopaedics), so learn the quickest way to get imaging booked earlier to ensure patients have their tests as soon as possible. During the ward round ensure you inform the nursing staff that imaging has been booked to allow them to liaise with the Radiology Department regarding the booking time.

Ordering simpler imaging such as X-ray or ultrasound does not usually require senior approval; however, CT and MRI scans may need to be discussed with the radiologist or the department registrar before the investigation can be booked. They can also give advice regarding appropriate imaging in cases in which the pathology is unclear or suggestions regarding what modality would be best suited to highlighting a particular pathological process. Radiology Departments receive a high volume of requests for imaging and procedures; therefore, clinical priority will influence how quickly these tests are performed.

Radiologists will usually provide a written report on the same day for any imaging test ordered; however, if there is a critical clinical finding, the radiologist may contact the requesting team directly to discuss the results. Similarly, if the results are likely to influence the management plan of a patient, you may be asked to chase a verbal report from the radiologist.

Online imaging storage allows easy access to images for comparison, transfer to other health networks and compilation for imaging meetings

X-RAYS

Chest X-ray (CXR)

Chest X-rays are one of the most commonly ordered investigations. The image gives a view of the chest of the patient extending from the base of the neck to include the 12th rib and diaphragm inferiorly. The image allows visualisation of a wide variety of bony and soft tissue structures within the thorax and mediastinum and, as such, the chest X-ray has a wide range of uses in the diagnosis and ongoing assessment of cardiac, respiratory and other thoracic disease.

Examination of X-ray films can aid in the diagnosis of both bony and soft tissue pathology. Evaluation of imaging is essential in clinical practice for many specialties, particularly orthopaedics, allowing the possibility of non-operative management for fractures that can be satisfactorily diagnosed on imaging with clinical correlation.

X-ray images are generated by passing radiation energy through the body. The higher the density of the tissue, the less energy passes through to the recorder, and this provides a gradient of white to grey delineating the differing structures in the body.

CXRs can be taken in a number of ways, as follows:

- Posterior-anterior (PA): most fit patients will have standing PA films (see Fig. 14.1). Cardiac silhouette is smaller. In this position the patient places their arms outstretched to rotate the scapula out of view.

- Anterior-posterior (AP): unwell patients who require mobile X-ray have the image taken anteriorly. The head of the bed can be raised to allow the patient to sit up for a portable CXR. In the outpatient setting, elderly patients may be seated for an AP CXR if they are too frail to stand.

- Lateral (LAT): allows appreciation of the posterior mediastinum and lung fields. The lateral X-ray can help place consolidation, collections and foreign bodies in the thorax.

Although the specific pathological findings of chest X-rays are discussed throughout the remainder of this text, it's worthwhile discussing the general approach. The various types of CXR images are illustrated in Figs 14.1 to 14.5.

Abdominal X-ray (AXR)

The AXR is often used as a first-line investigation for the evaluation of potential bowel pathology and urological disease. Although less frequently used than the CXR due to the widespread availability of CT for assessing acute abdominal pathology, AXR can still provide direction regarding:

- bowel obstruction (including volvulus)
- perforation
- constipation (faecal loading)
- ureteric calculi
- foreign bodies.

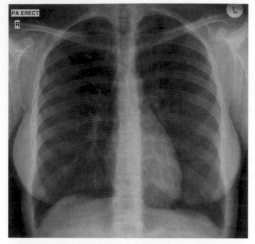

FIGURE 14.1 Normal PA CXR.

Reproduced from: de Lacey, G., Morley, S., Berman, L., 2008a. Chest radiology: the basic basics. In: de Lacey, G., Morley, S., Berman, L., The Chest X-ray: A survival guide. Philadelphia: Saunders, Fig. 1.1.

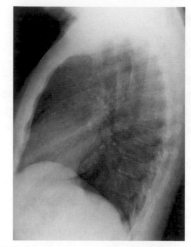

FIGURE 14.2 Normal lateral CXR.

Reproduced from: de Lacey, G., Morley, S., Berman, L., 2008b. The Lateral CXR. In: de Lacey, G., Morley, S., Berman, L., The Chest X-ray: A survival guide. Philadelphia: Saunders, Fig. 2.10.

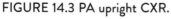

FIGURE 14.3 PA upright CXR.

Reproduced from: Mettler, F.A., 2014. Chest. In: Mettler, F.A., Essentials of Radiology, 3rd ed. Philadelphia: Saunders.

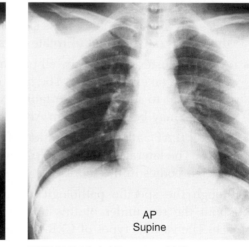

FIGURE 14.4 AP supine CXR.

Reproduced from: Mettler, F.A., 2014. Chest. In: Mettler, F.A., Essentials of Radiology, 3rd ed. Philadelphia: Saunders.

Much like the CXR, there are multiple views available, as follows:

- Supine anterior-posterior (supine AP): is the widespread standard approach with the patient lying on their back.
- Erect AXR: patient is standing, allowing for the observation of air-fluid levels in the bowel (see Fig. 14.8B later).
- Decubitus: patient lying on one side with the beam passing through horizontally, providing an AP view.

Examples of the information afforded by AXRs are given in Figs 14.6 to 14.10.

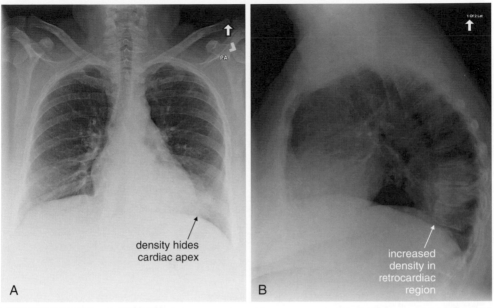

density hides
cardiac apex

increased
density in
retrocardiac
region

A

B

FIGURE 14.5 Lateral CXR (B) demonstrating pulmonary consolidation obscured by the cardiac shadow in the PA view (A).

Reproduced from: Broder, J., 2011. Imaging the chest: the chest radiograph. In: Broder, J., Diagnostic Imaging for the Emergency Physician. Elsevier Expert Consult.

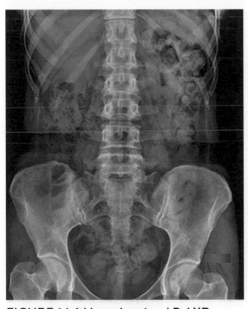

FIGURE 14.6 Normal supine AP AXR.

Reproduced from: Tomei, E., et al., 2011. Plain radiography of the abdomen. In: Tomei, E., et al., Abdominal Imaging. Elsevier Fig. 1-1.

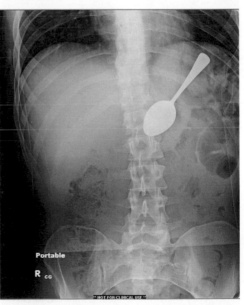

FIGURE 14.7 Intra-abdominal foreign bodies are often obvious.

Reproduced from: Skeik, N., Jabr, F.I., Stark, M., 2013. Unusual case of foreign-body ingestion. Journal of Emergency Medicine 44(3), e307-309.

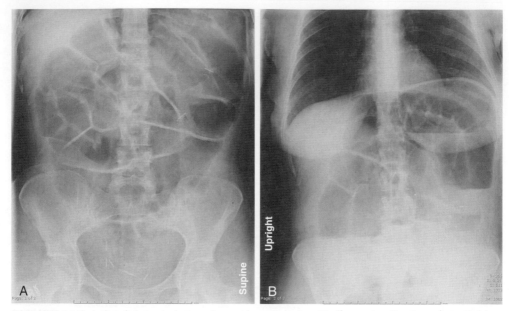

FIGURE 14.8 A Small bowel obstruction – the erect view **B** allows visualisation of air-fluid levels.

Reproduced from: Ferri, F.F., 2015c. Small bowel obstruction. In: Ferri, F.F., Ferri's Clinical Adviser. Philadelphia: Mosby, Fig. 1-866.

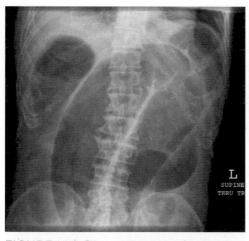

FIGURE 14.9 Obstruction secondary to volvulus.

Reproduced from: Kelly, A.M., 2015. Digestive emergencies. In: Cameron, P., Jelinek, G., Kelly, A.M., Brown, A., Little, M., Textbook of Adult Emergency Medicine, 4th ed. London: Churchill Livingstone, Fig. 7.3.2.

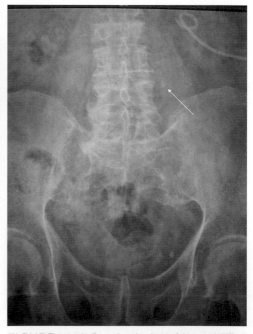

FIGURE 14.10 Renal calculi visible on AXR.

Reproduced from: Linton, K.D., 2013. Obstruction of the upper and lower urinary tract. Surgery (Abingdon: Medicine Group) 31 (7), 346-353, Fig. 1.

Other X-rays

The pelvic X-ray captures the entire bony pelvis, including the articulations with the sacrum and the head of the femur in the acetabulum. Pelvic X-rays are often used to detect pelvic or proximal femoral fractures, particularly of the femoral neck (Chapter 46).

Limb X-ray views are used to evaluate trauma. It's common for wrist and ankle injuries to be screened with imaging and fractures referred to orthopaedic outpatients (Chapter 67).

ULTRASOUND (US)

Ultrasound (sonography) scans provide images by transmitting acoustic signals through the body via a handheld probe. The interaction between the sound and tissue is dependent on the direction of the wave, the position and angle of the tissue relative to the probe, the refraction of the acoustic waves as they hit boundaries between tissues and absorption of sound energy. The reflection of this information back to the probe is used to formulate a visual representation of the tissue. A transducing gel is used to prevent air gaps between the probe and the skin, which causes unwanted reflection of the signal.

Abdominal ultrasound

Ultrasound is a common first-line investigation for intra-abdominal pathology due to the benefits of sparing radiation exposure and excellent imaging of the abdominal organs. It provides useful diagnostic information, as follows:

- Gallbladder:
  - signs of acute cholecystitis (Chapter 45) including gallbladder wall thickness, dilation and presence of gallstones
  - impacted gallstones
- Liver:
  - evaluation of liver masses, including assessing the sizes of cysts and other lesions
  - information regarding the overall structure of the liver architecture such as suggestion of chronic inflammation
- Pancreas:
  - presence of gallstones as the cause of pancreatitis, detecting and draining pseudocysts
- Biliary tree:
  - visualisation of the biliary tree itself for the presence of gallstones and dilatation suggesting obstruction.

Prior to ultrasound of the upper abdomen, patients should be fasted for 8 hours. This allows the gallbladder to dilate and prevents interference from upper bowel gas.

Rapid ultrasound of the abdomen also plays an important role in trauma assessments (Chapter 10) and ruling out abdominal aortic aneurysm in older patients presenting with acute abdominal pain.

Kidney and urinary tract ultrasound

The kidney can be readily visualised using ultrasound, allowing for measurement of kidney size and detection of structural abnormalities. Ultrasound of the kidney/ureters/bladder (KUB) is a common initial investigation for the patient with renal failure, particularly those with suspected post renal obstruction.

- Kidney:
  - dilatation of the renal pelvis (hydronephrosis)
  - cysts and other lesions
  - loss of collecting system suggesting chronic disease.
- Ureters:
  - perhaps difficult to fully visualise due to their course through the abdomen but dilatation can be observed suggesting acute obstruction
- Bladder:
  - bladder calculi
  - bladder wall thickening

Pelvic ultrasound

Pelvic ultrasound has widespread use in women's health for both obstetric and gynaecological issues. Ultrasound of the pelvis can also aid in the diagnosis of appendicitis. Patients undergoing pelvic ultrasound are required to have a full bladder to aid in delineation of the bladder from the hollow viscera.

Peripheral ultrasound

Although most commonly used to assess the peripheral arteries and limbs, ultrasound is also used to:

- assess soft tissue injuries in the hand and forearm such as tendon or ligament disruption
- identify and assist draining of fluid collections
- localise and mark foreign bodies.

Imaging for assessment of deep vein thrombosis (DVT) is universally performed with real-time ultrasound, assessing for complete compressibility of the venous system, screening for intraluminal echogenicity suggestive of thrombus and using the colour Doppler to determine if there is abnormal flow. The Doppler produces a visual representation of flow based on the differences between the frequencies of acoustic reflections of flow moving towards the probe and flow moving away.

These principles and techniques can also be applied to using ultrasound to screen for peripheral artery disease, particularly when examining the carotid vessels. The combination of normal ultrasound and Doppler ultrasound (known as 'Duplex' ultrasound) can be used to detect intramural thickness, thrombus and restriction of flow as a means of measuring stenosis.

The findings of the ultrasound scan are then compiled into a set of images by the sonographer and a technical report with measurements submitted to the radiologist for reporting. Often, the technical report is available much earlier than the radiologist report and can give some useful clinical information for the inpatient team.

Ultrasound of the head and neck

Due to the large amount of soft tissue in the neck ultrasound scans are ideal for assessing neck lumps, particularly in the thyroid. Such lumps can be definitively measured and located for potential fine needle aspiration (FNA). The ultrasound scan can also describe the physical characteristics of the nodule, determining if the shape, size and apparent make-up of the lesion is suspicious for malignancy.

Other uses of ultrasound

Ultrasound also has an important role in the assessment of breast pathology (Chapter 62), the heart (Chapter 35), in the form of transthoracic echocardiography (TTE) and transoesophageal echocardiography (TOE) and the joints (Chapter 46).

Figs 14.11 to 14.16 demonstrate the use of ultrasound in assessing various conditions.

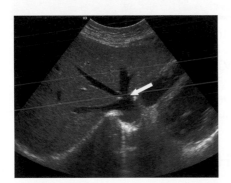

FIGURE 14.11 Transverse view of the venous drainage of the liver.

Reproduced from: Eliot, S., et al. 2011. Liver: anatomy and scanning techniques. In: Allan, P., Baxter, G. & Weston, M., Clinical Ultrasound, 3rd ed. Churchill Livingstone, Fig. 7.4, pp. 93-103.

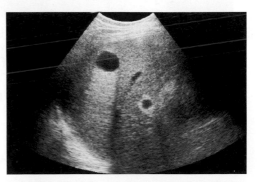

FIGURE 14.12 Simple liver cyst. Note the acoustic shadow as the field extends deeper.

Reproduced from: Farges, O., Vilgrain, V., et al., 2012. Simple cysts and polycystic liver disease: clinical and radiographic features. In: Jarnagin, W.R., ed., Blumgart's Surgery of the Liver, Biliary Tract and Pancreas, 5th ed. Philadelphia: Saunders, Fig. 69.4A, pp. 1052-1065.

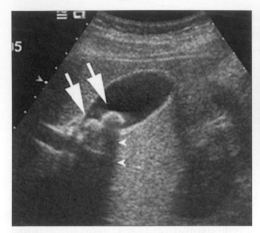

FIGURE 14.13 Two large calculi in the gallbladder.

Reproduced from: Gore, R.M. & Levin, M.S., 2010. Cholelithiasis. In: Gore, R.M. & Levin, M.S., eds., High Yield Imaging: Gastrointestinal. Philadelphia: Saunders, Fig. 1, pp. 512-514.

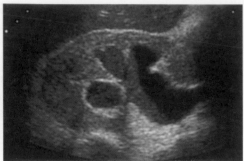

FIGURE 14.14 Kidney ultrasound demonstrating moderate hydronephrosis.

Reproduced from: Middleton, W.D., 2004. Kidney. In: Middleton, W.D., Kurtz, A.B. & Hertzberg, B.S., Ultrasound: The requisites, 2nd ed. Philadelphia: Mosby, Fig. 5-12.

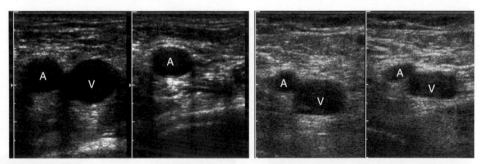

FIGURES 14.15 AND 14.16 Two examples of the transverse view of the femoral vessels; on the right side compression is applied over the vein. In the normal vein (Fig. 14.15) there is complete collapse; however, in the presence of DVT the vessel demonstrates abnormal compression (Fig. 14.16).

Reproduced from: Hertzberg, B.S. & Middleton, W.D., 2016. Extremities. In: Hertzberg, B.S. & Middleton, W.D., Ultrasound: The requisites, 3rd ed. Philadelphia: Mosby, Figs 11-44 and 11-45.

COMPUTERISED TOMOGRAPHY (CT)

CT scans use X-rays to produce slices of images through the body known as 'tomograms'. The use of multiple X-ray detectors and computerised reconstruction of the individual slices allows for accurate depiction of the shape and size of tissue, eliminating the superimposition effect of plain X-rays. Advances in CT have led to improvements in image acquisition, including the following:

- High resolution CT (HRCT) is a process of scanning thinner slices to produce more images, commonly used in the chest. However, the production of thinner slices results in a higher radiation exposure for the patient.

- Spiral or helical CT refers to a dynamic CT machine that rotates the X-ray source with multiple detectors and a mobile patient table. This results in rapid image acquisition in multiple thickness slices and angles. CT software has allowed reconstruction of these images into 3-D representations such as fracture patterns in bones and 'virtual colonoscopies'. With the addition of intravenous contrast, CT scanners can produce angiograms, widely used in medical and surgical specialties.

CT contrast

By using radio-opaque contrast the density of tissue is altered, allowing for greater distinction between the types of tissue. Although CT scans can be performed without contrast, there are a number of scanning requests that require the use of contrast for diagnosis. Junior doctors can liaise with the radiology department to get advice regarding whether a scan will need contrast.

Contrast is most commonly given orally or IV:

- Oral contrast is used for abdominal and pelvic pathology when enhancement of bowel structures aids diagnosis. It's common in non-traumatic causes of abdominal pain where inflammation of the bowel is suspected.

- IV contrast is much more versatile, used to highlight key structure in areas densely packed with soft tissue structure. It's essential for the production of angiograms.

- Rectal contrast is sometimes used to detect recto-sigmoid pathology such as tumours or perforation.

CT contrast media can have potentially adverse effects, particularly in those patients with renal impairment. Contrast containing iodine has a nephrotoxic effect and can lead to acute tubular necrosis in patients with poorer renal perfusion. Therefore, most hospitals have policies in place restricting the use of IV contrast in patients with glomerular filtration rate (eGFR) <30. As with any medication or treatment given to a patient, there is always the potential of allergic reaction. Mild contrast reactions may include erythema, urticaria and tachycardia. These patients should be closely observed as severe reactions can cause bronchospasm and anaphylaxis.

CT of the brain

CT imaging of the brain should be urgently carried out in patients presenting with severe head trauma or those suspected of having a stroke. For patients with head trauma, the scan usually includes the cervical spine and may extend to include the facial bones for complete assessment. CT brains can also provide information relating to chronic changes related to cerebral atrophy, hydrocephalus and evidence of previous cerebral infarction.

For ischaemic stroke, CT scanning may not reveal any imaging changes until hours after the insult; however, haemorrhages can be readily assessed on CT scans (see Figs 14.17 to 14.19).

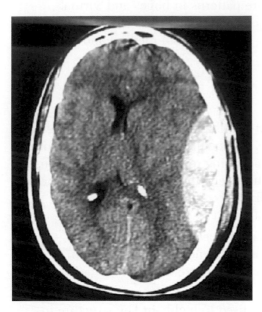

FIGURE 14.17 Epidural haematoma, secondary to blunt force trauma to the side of the head. The haemorrhage is contained between the outer layer of the dura and the skull. Note the size of the haematoma displacing the brain tissue, compressing the ventricular system and pushing tissue across the midline of the brain (so called 'midline shift') This presentation constitutes a neurosurgical emergency (Chapter 50).

Reproduced from: Smith, S.W., Clark, M., Nelson, J., et al., 2010. Emergency department skull trephination for epidural hematoma in patients who are awake but deteriorate rapidly. Journal of Emergency Medicine 39(3), 377-383.

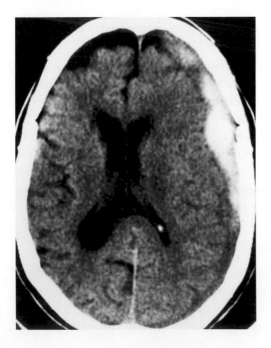

FIGURE 14.18 Subdural haematoma. Typically associated with venous bleeding. the subdural haemorrhage can spread between the dura and brain tissue creating a 'crescent' appearance. Dependent on the effect of the bleed on the surrounding tissue and the patient's clinical status, surgical evacuation is sometimes required. In those bleeds managed conservatively, serial CT scans can be used to determine if there is progression of the haematoma.

Reproduced from: Ferri, F.F., 2009. Subdural hematoma. In: Ferri, F.F., ed., Ferri's Color Atlas and Text of Clinical Medicine, Philadelphia: Saunders, Fig. 37-1.

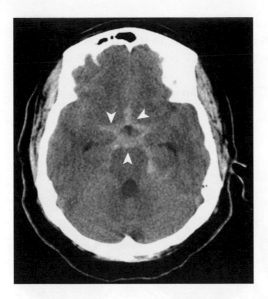

FIGURE 14.19 Subarachnoid haematoma. The arrows indicate a collection of blood in the basal cisterns of a patient who presented with a pathognomonic 'thunderclap headache'. Typically associated with rupture of cerebral aneurysms.

Reproduced from: Rabinstein, A.A. & Resnick, S.J., 2009. Subarachnoid hemorrhage. In: Rabinstein, A.A. & Resnick, S.J., Practical Neuroimaging in Stroke. Philadelphia: Saunders, Fig. 12-8.

CT of the chest

CT scanning of the thorax is performed for:

- evaluation of lung, mediastinal and pleural lesions
- staging for other primary malignancies
- assessment of acute and chronic obstructive and inflammatory lung diseases
- detecting pulmonary embolism (PE).

With the use of contrast, CT chest scans offer excellent localisation of tissue, allowing for masses to be accurately identified despite being in close proximity to other soft tissues. Plain X-ray imaging may indicate thoracic pathology such as hilar lymphadenopathy or pleural thickening with CT allowing accurate surveillance of lesion size and permitting preoperative planning for any potential biopsy. The characteristic appearance of a mediastinal mass on CT can shorten the differential diagnosis, guiding further investigation and management (Chapter 48).

A CT pulmonary angiogram (CTPA) is often used for the investigation of PE following a plain CXR. The indications and criteria for determining the likelihood of PE are described elsewhere, although it's worth noting that the diagnosis can be clinically difficult and, coupled with the potential radiation dose of the scan, the decision to undergo a CTPA becomes a risk vs benefit scenario. Although the ventilation/perfusion (V/Q) scan offers an alternative, it may not be an option out of business hours.

For this procedure the patient will need sufficient IV access to allow proper infusion of the contrast. Typically, an 18-gauge cannula, in the cubital fossa is the recommendation. Ensure the patient has adequate IV access before the scheduled scan to avoid delay.

Examples of the use of contrast in CT chest scans are given in Figs 14.20 to 14.22.

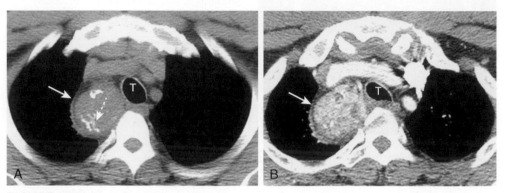

FIGURE 14.20 Use of contrast in the assessment of a retrosternal goitre. The contrast enhanced image demonstrates the classic mottled appearance of contrast uptake in thyroid tissue.

Reproduced from: Herring, W., 2012. Recognizing diseases of the chest. Learning Radiology: Recognizing the basics, 2nd edition. Mosby, Fig. 12-3.

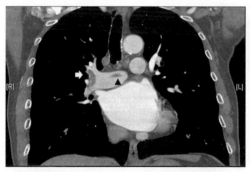

FIGURE 14.21 The coronal view of a CT chest allows appreciation of a saddle embolus.

Reproduced from: Chen, H.Y., 2015. Saddle pulmonary emboli mimicking pulmonary artery dissection. American Journal of Emergency Medicine 33(1), 127.

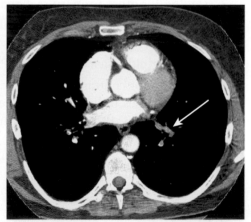

FIGURE 14.22 Loss of contrast in the right pulmonary artery system demonstrates a filling defect (absence of bright contrast), consistent with a PE.

Reproduced from: Reddy, C., 2017. Pulmonary embolism. In: Ferri, F.F., Ferri's Clinical Advisor. Elsevier, Fig. 1P-123.

CT of the abdomen and pelvis (CTAP)

Patients with severe abdominal pain, sepsis and/or haemodynamic instability are likely to have a CT scan to rule out serious pathology; however, some trauma or shocked patients with obvious surgical pathology may undergo rapid plain films or ultrasound assessment before being fast-tracked to theatre. The benefit of CT is the rapid and complete acquisition of images allowing assessment of multiple organs within the one scan.

CT of the abdomen and pelvis can reveal a vast amount of information. Variations on the scanning technique can aid in diagnosis related to the following:

- Liver:
  - masses including cysts, hepatocellular carcinoma and metastatic deposits
  - changes to liver architecture such as inflammation (acute and chronic), steatosis and cirrhosis
  - vascular supply and large intrahepatic ducts
- Biliary tree and gallbladder:
  - CT cholangiograms can demonstrate collections in the biliary system and stone disease that may contribute to biliary sepsis; it has also been shown to be useful in the diagnosis of primary biliary carcinoma
- Pancreas:
  - pancreatitis and necrosis
  - pseudocyst formation
  - pancreatic lesions.

The kidney, ureters and bladder are typically assessed in two ways:

1. a non-contrast CT kidney/ureters/bladder (KUB) for identifying and measuring renal calculi
2. CT intravenous pyelogram protocols provide a plain non-contrast CT image, then images are captured with contrast in the upper and lower urinary tract:
   a. can demonstrate upper tract pathology in the investigation, obstruction and haematuria
   b. used for measuring and staging primary renal tumours and cysts.

CT imaging of the bowel involves the use of oral contrast to highlight the bowel structures, particularly the bowel wall itself. The unwell patient with abdominal pain will typically undergo CT scanning to screen for the following potential surgical issues involving the bowel:

- Bowel obstruction: small and large bowel obstructions can be identified readily on CT including the location of the obstruction and potential causes.

- ○ CT allows for the diagnosis of closed bowel loops in which an entire section is obstructed at both ends, potentially leading to rapid ischaemia.
- Bowel masses: allows for detection of primary lesions or staging following endoscopic detection of primary bowel cancer.
- Bowel ischaemia: includes checking the patency of the vascular supply to the bowel.
- Bowel perforation: can include visualisation of a focus of perforation.

Abdominal CT angiography (CTA) can be used to assess the size and potential rupture of aortic aneurysms. By allowing accurate measurement of the aneurysm, the patient can undergo serial surveillance scans. Observations regarding irregularities in the wall of the vessel and atherosclerotic disease can also give insight regarding the stability of aneurysm. Angiography can also provide information regarding the patency of other major vessels such as the renal arteries.

Examples of CTAP scans are provided in Figs 14.23 to 14.26.

CT of the extremities

CT scans of the extremities assist the diagnosis of fractures and joint disruptions, and assess for vascular injury and patency, discussed in the Orthopaedic and Vascular chapters.

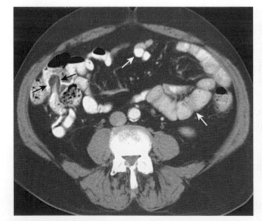

FIGURE 14.23 Normal appearance of the bowel. Note the ileocaecal junction at the black arrow.

Reproduced from: Herring, W., 2012. Computerised tomography: understanding the basics and recognizing normal anatomy. In: Herring, W., Learning Radiology: Recognizing the basics, 2nd ed. Philadelphia: Mosby, Fig. 11-4.

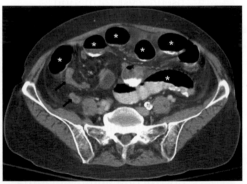

FIGURE 14.24 Small bowel obstruction with dilated loops of bowel indicated.

Reproduced from: Pretorius, E.S., 2011. CT of the acute abdomen and pelvis. In: Pretorius, E.S., Radiology Secrets Plus, 3rd ed. Philadelphia: Mosby, Fig. 20-10.

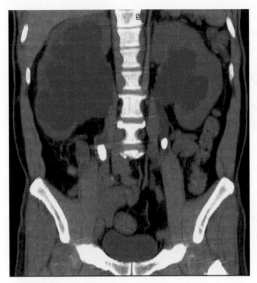

FIGURE 14.25 Plain CT KUB demonstrating bilateral ureteric stones and hydronephrosis.

Reproduced from: Griffin, N. & Grant, L., 2013. Kidneys. In: Grant, L. & Griffin, N., Grainger and Allison's Diagnostic Radiology Essentials. London: Churchill Livingstone.

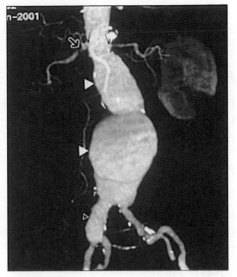

FIGURE 14.26 CTA of an abdominal aortic aneurysm.

Reproduced from: Skow, G., 2011. Abdominal aortic aneurysm. Journal of Men's Health 8(4), 306-312.

MAGNETIC RESONANCE IMAGING (MRI)

MRI scanners produce images by using a superconducting magnet to force the normally randomly spinning magnetic moments of protons in the body to align parallel to the electromagnetic force of the magnet source, using radiofrequency (RF) pulses in bursts. Once the burst has ended, the protons return to their original positions. During this realignment process, RF energy is released and can be detected in signal receivers known as coils.

T_1 and T_2 weightings relate to the different 'relaxation directions' (longitudinal and spin, respectively) of the protons after the RF pulse has ceased. The amount of time for relaxation to occur is different for each direction, and relaxation times also differ depending on the tissue in the body. These differences provide a natural signal contrast between tissues in the body, providing high contrast resolution images. The timing of RF pulses can be altered to change the relative weightings of T_1 and T_2 signals, allowing for ideal tissue contrast in certain areas of the body.

Water has a high T_2 signal intensity; therefore, when looking at an MRI image, a source of water can be used to determine if the image is primarily T_1 or T_2 weighted.

MRI can be used in many of the same settings as CT, including obtaining information from angiography. The advantages of non-ionising radiation are offset against the somewhat limited availability and cost of MRI services and lengthier scan times for patients who are acutely unwell. MRI is useful in the assessment of intra-abdominal masses as it can give indication as to the contents (homogenous vs heterogeneous) based on differences in signal intensity.

MR cholangiopancreatography (MRCP)

By using T_2 weighted imaging (where bile and pancreatic fluid have a high signal), thin slices can demonstrate the presence of stones and duct dilation, offering a dedicated view of the biliary tree.

MRI spine

MRI allows for visualisation of the spinal cord as well as the bony and ligamentous structures surrounding it. Any direct mechanical disruption to the cord can be seen and changes in signal intensity may indicate physiological insult to the cord.

MRI of joints

MRIs are commonly ordered in the outpatient setting for the assessment of soft tissue injuries in and around joints. Where tendon and ligament disorders are suspected, MRI can provide evidence of chronic inflammation, oedema and tears:

- Shoulder: often used in the setting of rotator cuff injuries, chronic bursitis and pain.
- Knee: indicated in suspected ligament injury, can differentiate between partial and complete tears.

MRI safety

All patients must complete a questionnaire prior to undergoing MRI that requires them to list whether they have any metallic implants (especially pacemakers), piercings or previous metallic foreign bodies. Some pacemaker devices are compatible with MRI machines; however, it's important to clarify with the radiology department and obtain the make and model of the pacemaker in question.

Some patients will not tolerate MRI due to claustrophobia. If the patient has an urgent need for an MRI, they may require sedation prior to having their scan, and an anaesthetic team will be required to attend.

Figs 14.27 to 14.31 demonstrate various applications of MRI.

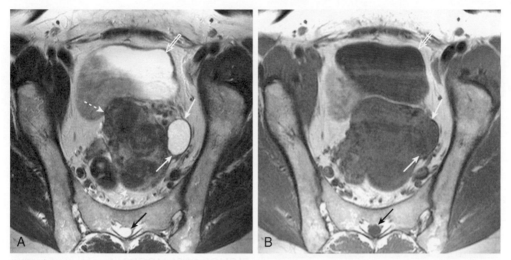

FIGURE 14.27 MRI of left-sided ovarian cyst. T_2 weighted image **A** shows similar signal intensity to that of urine indicated by the arrows. This indicated a simple fluid-filled cyst.

Reproduced from: Kowal, D., 2012. Magnetic resonance imaging. In: Herring, W., Learning Radiology: Recognizing the basics, 2nd ed. Philadelphia: Mosby, Fig. 20-4.

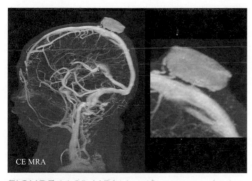

FIGURE 14.28 MRI identifies a mass; high spatial resolution allows for the identification of feeder arteries in preoperative planning.

Reproduced from: Campeau, N., 2012. Vascular disorders – magnetic resonance angiography: brain vessels. Neuroimaging Clinics of North America 22(2), 207-233, Fig. 20.

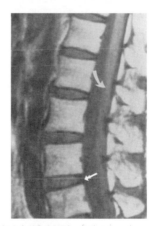

FIGURE 14.29 MRI of the lumbar spine allows for clear identification of soft tissue. Note the intervertebral discs highlighted by the arrow.

Reproduced from: Devlin, V.J., 2012. Magnetic resonance imaging of the spine. In: Devlin, V.J., Spine Secrets Plus, 2nd ed. St Louis, MO: Mosby, Fig. 11-3.

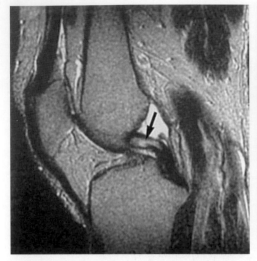

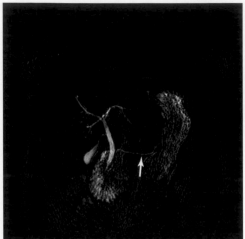

FIGURE 14.30 MRI of the knee. Natural tissue signal contrast allows for excellent distinction between tissue types with a clear view of structures. PCL is pointed out here.

Reproduced from: Witte, D., 2013. Chapter 2: Magnetic resonance imaging in orthopaedics. In: Canale, S.T., Beaty, J.H., Campbell's Operative Orthopaedics, 12th ed. Philadelphia: Mosby, Fig. 2-17, pp. 127-155.

FIGURE 14.31 MRCP indicating the pancreatic duct; the intrahepatic and common bile ducts are also seen.

Reproduced from: Hsu, W., 2011. CT and MRI of the pancreas. In: Pretorius, E.S., Radiology Secrets Plus, 3rd ed. Philadelphia: Mosby.

CHAPTER 15

MAKING REFERRALS

Joseph M O'Brien

Making referrals is a vital role of the junior doctor. It is your job to ensure effective communication between your team and other units, as it is well-documented that when this system breaks down patient care is compromised. As medicine moves further towards sub-specialisation, the ability to make appropriate referrals becomes ever more important. Common scenarios where you may be asked to refer a patient to another team include patients requiring a specialty review, antibiotics approval, procedural interventions or, more rarely, to request another unit take over the care of your patient.

Many hospital networks have a template in place for communicating patient information. One system now popular worldwide is the ISBAR method of handover, developed locally in Australia. ISBAR stands for:

Identify

Situation

Background

Assessment

Request.

It is important to provide structure to your referral, particularly if you find yourself fumbling. ISBAR has been shown in studies to improve the quality of information handed over. It can be used internally among various disciplines and services, or to refer a patient to another hospital. An example would run as in Scenario 15.1.

Before making a referral, consider who is likely to be at the receiving end of your call. In general, consultants prefer to know less detail but have more targeted questions than registrars. Regardless of the recipient, it is important that you familiarise yourself with the patient. It is not always possible to completely understand your patient's situation – especially on very busy units – but it is certainly best practice to know their demographic details, presenting complaint, relevant medical history, clinical findings (particularly vitals) and important investigation results before calling. It is perfectly acceptable not to have memorised all of these details as long as you have the information you expect the recipient will require at hand. For more complex patients this often means sitting

SCENARIO

15.1

'Hi, my name is Joe O'Brien. I am the intern on General Medicine A. Are you the Cardiology registrar on for external referrals today? Do you have time to receive a referral? I have with me Mr John Smith, a 55-year-old gentleman with unstable triple vessel disease that requires transfer for inpatient coronary bypass. He initially presented with severe, central chest pain radiating to his left arm and was diagnosed with an NSTEMI. His ECG shows new ischaemic changes in comparison with a graph from January and he is currently awaiting a transthoracic echo. My consultant is concerned about his welfare if left untreated, and we were hoping to have him transferred to Large Metropolitan Hospital for inpatient bypass. Would you be willing to accept this patient? Do you have a bed available? Thank you for your time – if you need any more information I am holding pager #121.'

---

at a desk with the admission note, observations chart and drug chart, with investigations open on a computer.

Have a targeted, clinical question for the recipient of your referral. Do you want them to review your patient, take over care or simply advise? Think about what will be the most relevant information to the team you are involving in your patient's care and have that information at hand prior to making your call. Table 15.1 outlines some common questions asked by the specialty teams you will most commonly be referring to from either the ward or the emergency department.

Over your junior years you will encounter people who welcome your referrals and others who either reluctantly accept or flat out deny your request. If you are having difficulty making a referral then you should inform your senior colleague, especially if there is concern that patient care will be compromised. Keep in mind there are some consultants who for various reasons will only take referrals from a registrar or above, so discuss this when you review the 'jobs list' with your registrar after ward rounds. It can be of enormous benefit if you know the person whom you are referring to from either cover shifts or socially – another benefit to attending RMO Society events!

Referral etiquette is important. If someone tells you they are too busy to take your referral, accept it and ask when you can call back. If you leave it to the recipient you may not hear back from them. However, if your referral is urgent (life or limb) do not be afraid to stress its importance, keeping in mind they may be attending to an urgent situation themselves.

Where you must page the recipient and await their return call, you are not obligated to sit by the phone for the rest of your shift. A reasonable period of time would be 5 minutes before paging a second time – if there is no response after a further 5 minutes, you have a choice between escalating or trying again

TABLE 15.1 FAQs by referral recipients on specialty teams

SPECIALTY	COMMON QUESTIONS
Cardiology	What does their 12-lead ECG look like? When was their most recent echo? Have they ever had an angiogram? What was their weight on admission and has it changed? Have they had troponins? Has it peaked? Have they had fasting lipids and glucose?
Gastroenterology	Weight loss? Scope history? Family history? Alcohol consumption? If severe vomiting/diarrhoea, what are their UECs? Haemodynamic stability? If IBD – surgical history? If liver disease – outcome of liver screen? If hepatitis – viral load? Genotype?
Renal	UECs? Iron studies? Urinary sodium, albumin to creatinine ratio, protein to creatinine ratio or electrophoresis? Have they had a renal tract ultrasound? Are they making urine? Are they on dialysis, or would they be considered for it?
Surgery	When was their last meal? Are they anticoagulated? Are they bariatric? Surgical history? If they're bleeding, have they been cross-matched? Have you done a PR?
Intensive care	Indication for ICU review? Have they breached MET criteria? Do they have advanced life directives?
Anaesthetics	Have they had an anaesthetic before? Do they have a cardiac condition? Are they bariatric? Do they have dentures? When was their last meal? Are they anticoagulated?

continued

TABLE 15.1 FAQs by referral recipients on specialty teams—cont'd

SPECIALTY	COMMON QUESTIONS
Orthopaedics	As above for surgical referrals, plus: Is the fracture open? Are they neurovascularly intact?
Rehabilitation	What will be their goals? Are they completely stable? What is their follow-up plan with the home team?
Neurology	What are their examination findings (very specific)? What does their imaging show?
Respiratory	Have you done an ABG? What are their saturations? What does their CXR show? Do they have recent spirometry or RFTs? What is their smoking history? Have you done thoracocentesis (if an effusion)? What are their occupational exposures?

later. Prioritise your jobs; some medical teams round until mid afternoon and surgical registrars can be busy with theatre and clinic workloads. Through experience you will learn the best times to contact other teams to make referrals.

Making good referrals is an excellent way to earn a reputation as a competent junior doctor, as you will be interacting with people from all areas of the hospital at various levels of training. You are able to demonstrate in a few minutes that you understand your patients' situations, have the ability to make appropriate judgements about management and recognise your limitations and need for expert input. The best way to improve your referrals is practice, so never give up on an opportunity to put to the test your prowess in this essential workplace skill.

CHAPTER 16

ADMISSIONS

Joseph M O'Brien

A thorough admission is a good start to a patient's inpatient stay. It is well documented in the evidence that patients presenting with common illnesses who have rushed admissions (e.g. on weekends or public holidays) tend to have longer inpatient stays and a moderately higher mortality.

The admission usually begins with a referral to your team – either from your colleagues in the Emergency Department (ED) or from an external doctor. ED staff are under time constraints and will place a lot of pressure on you to review their patient as soon as possible. Not all of your referrals will require admission – sometimes there are alternate outcomes that would better suit the patient's needs, for example sending them home with Hospital in the Home (HITH), back to their nursing home with a residential outreach service or asking them to return to Outpatients Clinic with further investigations completed.

From a junior doctor's perspective, the 'heart' of the admission lies in an organised history-taking and appropriate length examination. A good admission is very similar to a long case, something you may be well versed in – however, in reality there is often a compromise between thoroughness and efficiency as an admitting resident or registrar role is quite busy. It is quite common for senior students and interns to accompany a registrar during an admission, and in many rotations the residents are required to admit without the immediate supervision of a senior clinician. As such, it is a good idea to get a lot of experience with admitting patients as early in your career as possible. As a junior this usually means documenting for the admitting registrar and completing their paperwork for them to speed up the admission (see Fig. 16.1 for an example of a paper admission). While the senior doctor leads the admission, the intern can request imaging, serology and miscellaneous pathology (both for in the emergency department and for the next few days – don't forget to put bloods in for the following morning!), completing the drug chart, writing up fluids and taking note of the GP and other specialists' details to request more information.

HISTORY-TAKING

Being well prepared and having a system for taking a history is covered elsewhere, but remains integral to the task. It is good form to document at the top of the

Example Admission

Patient Details
Mr Joe Blogs
UR 123456
DOB 1/1/1935

Presumed Diagnosis
?Cholecystitis ?Choledocholithiasis

Issues
Mr Blogs is a 79 yo gentleman who was admitted to St Elsewhere on the 29th July with severe RUQ pain, jaundice and intermittent fevers.

?Cholecystitis
- Increasing RUQ pain for two weeks. Associated with intermittent fevers over about a month. Wife did not notice jaundice – was pointed out to patient by his daughter who had not seen him for two weeks.
- Some weight loss – around 5 kg. Patient reports some anorexia.
- Denies chills, rigors, PR bleeding, melaena or reflux.
- Last meal breakfast, cup of tea and toast at 7 am.
- Discussed with surgical registrar on call – to be fasted and prepped for theatre tomorrow. Would like CT-abdo as already booked.

Hypokalaemia
- K^+= 3.3. Patient has a cardiac history, aim >4.0
- Supplemented IV in ED

Acute kidney injury
- Baseline creatinine 120 on bloods from ED one month ago
- Gentle IV hydration, ?dehydration
- Nephrotoxins withheld

Medical Conditions
- NKDA
- Treated hypertension
- Treated hyperlipidaemia
- Osteoarthritis – on NSAIDs, awaiting bilateral TKR by Mr Orthopaedic Surgeon
- Ischaemic heart disease (AMI 1997). No recent TTEs or angiograms as lost to Cardio follow-up.

Past History
- AMI: 1997. Thrombolysed in Regional Hospital.
- MVA: Several long bone fractures, managed at Big City Hospital. No metalwork in place, underwent extensive rehab 1982.

Social History
- Lives with supportive wife, Carol.
- Retired engineer.
- Ex-smoker with 35 pack years (quit 1997). Minimal alcohol consumption.
- Baseline effort tolerance 500 m. Walks without gait aids.
- Drives, cooks, cleans and manages finances independently.

Family History
- Father died of AMI at 54 yo.
- Mother died of stroke at 82 yo.
- Paternal uncle had multiple myeloma.

Medications
- Aspirin 100 mg PO mane
- Perindopril 5 mg PO mane
- Atorvastatin 40 mg PO nocte
- Ibuprofen 400 mg PO TDS

FIGURE 16.1 Example of a paper admission.

Examination
- General: Overweight, severely jaundiced, elderly gentleman in considerable pain despite analgesia. HR 105, BP 140/90, RR 15, SaO$_2$ 97% ORA. Currently afebrile – last recorded fever 38.9°C on presentation to ED at 0900.
- Upper limbs: Pulse regular but tachy. No palmor pallor, asterixis, clubbing or stigmata of chronic liver disease.
- Head and neck: Icteric sclera. No conjunctival pallor. JVP +2 cm. Dry mucous membranes.
- Chest: Chest clear. 2 heart sounds, nil added. Minor gynaecomastia.
  Abdomen: Liver edge palpable 3 cm below costal margin. No palpable splenomegaly. Bowel sounds present. Explicitly tender in RUQ. No venous hum. No masses.
- Lower limbs: Calves soft not tender. Peripheral pulses present. Mild pitting oedema bilaterally at ankles.

Investigations
- LFTs deranged – BR <u>56</u>/ALP <u>127</u>/GGT <u>392</u>/ALT <u>95</u>
- FBE <u>99</u>/11.4/146
- UEC 134/<u>3.3</u>/Cr <u>230</u>/Ur <u>12</u>. Previously documented creatinine 120 one month ago
- CXR NAD
- Abdominal USS: Hypoechoic lines in gallbladder, common bile duct 6 mm thick, gallbladder wall 4 mm
- Awaiting CT-abdo/pelvis on admission

Plan
1. Admit under Gen Surg A (Thompson)
2. Regular medications + VTE prophylaxis while platelets >50
3. HHMN
4. Plan for laparoscopic cholecystectomy
5. Analgesia and anti-emetics as required
6. Morning bloods
7. Gentle IV fluids whilefasting – note AKI, consider med review if does not respond to fluids
8. IV potassium
9. Await CT-abdo/pelvis on ward
10. IV triple antibiotics
11. Withhold nephrotoxins – ACE and ibuprofen ceased

FIGURE 16.1, cont'd

admission a brief summary of the presentation (abbreviations are acceptable for the sake of speed) – for example, '91yo F p/w 3/52 increasing SOBOE on a b/g known CCF and IHD'. Anyone who glances at your admission note will immediately get a sense of why this patient is coming into hospital. This is also important for coding purposes.

From here the logical progression is through the history of the presenting complaint (HOPC), medical history (MHx), past medical and surgical history (PHx), family history (FHx) and social history (SHx). Key facts about the admission may come to light in these latter categories, which are all too often skipped in an effort to save time. They may be brief, but are always worth touching upon.

EXAMINATION

Again, having a system for examination will smooth out this process. A targeted examination may be performed in a busy ED but, for those who are considering the RACP pathway, admissions are an excellent opportunity to practice your long cases. Document well – there's little point in performing a thorough examination and not passing on that information to the other people in the treating team. It is not uncommon to admit patients for other medical teams (e.g. on cover) and you want to convey that you have assessed this patient properly. For patients with a concurrent psychiatric condition (or delirium) it would be prudent to include a brief mental state examination in this section of the admission.

INVESTIGATIONS

Include investigations that have already been completed by the ED or previous treating team. Consider only including those investigations you can personally verify – for example, do not write 'Raised troponins' if you have not seen them on the pathology system yourself. It is good form to write the exact figures if available, but abbreviations are encouraged – for example, 'FBE 135/19.5/563'. Do not forget to include imaging.

IMPRESSION

Alternatively referred to as 'Assessment', here you should consider including a one or two sentence summary of what you think the situation is. For example, 'APO, likely 2° new onset AF. Must exclude infective precipitant'. If the patient's presentation is unclear, this is a good opportunity to document your differential and reasoning.

PLAN

Ultimately, this is the most important part of the admission. What will this patient be doing in hospital? Why is it necessary to admit them? Usually numbered, begin with, '1) Admit under Gen Med Team' and work through your plan stepwise. Do not forget to include medication changes, fluid rates, electrolyte supplementation, non-pharmaceutical components of the plan (such as whether or not venous thromboembolism [VTE] prophylaxis is required), what kind of diet the patient should go on (e.g. nil by mouth for those fasting, diabetic for people with diabetes or low sodium for those with congestive heart failure), the regularity of observations and any altered parameters and future investigations and referrals (including allied health). If any special type of hospital bed is required (e.g. a bariatric bed or an isolation room) specify it here, so that the bed manager can coordinate it.

After the admission is complete, you will often have to liaise with your senior clinician. Remember, they are very busy people who want a rapid overview of the patient you are technically placing under their care. Start with a summary, speed through the *relevant* history and examination findings, report the investigations that have a role in the admission and explain your plan. As always when discussing patient details – never lie!

CHAPTER 17

CLINICAL PROCEDURES

Paul Watson, Joseph M O'Brien, Kerry Jewell,
Kelsey Broom and Lachlan Wight

The key to success with clinical procedures is practice, practice and practice. These basic clinical skills are taught in the early clinical years of medical education; however, extensive reinforcement of the technique is required to become proficient. Some nursing staff are trained and quite skilled at intravenous cannulation and venepuncture; however, it is ultimately the responsibility of the junior doctor to ensure the patient has their procedure in a timely manner.

INTRAVENOUS VENOUS CANNULATION (IVC) AND VENEPUNCTURE

This key skill is the most common clinical procedure performed by medical staff. Peripheral IVCs are indicated for a variety of reasons including:

- antibiotic therapy
- intravenous fluids
- investigations
- pain relief.

When choosing which gauge IVC to use for your patient it's worthwhile considering which indication applies to your patient and whether the gauge will be sufficient (Table 17.1).

Preparation is essential for successful IV cannulation; take the necessary time to identify suitable veins. Where practically possible use a flat immobile surface such as the forearm for IV access as IVCs placed on joints are more likely to kink or be pulled out. Cubital fossa cannulation is suitable for larger gauge cannulation and investigative procedures and, as such, should largely be avoided for routine IV cannulation.

Intravenous cannulation (see Figs 17.1 to 17.8) should be performed using aseptic technique to help prevent catheter-related infection; a sterile set-up is therefore required. Fig. 17.1 demonstrates the required equipment, including:

- sterile surface sheet, gauze, skin antiseptic, clear dressing for IVC (these items typically come in an IVC 'pack')

SECTION II

TABLE 17.1 IVC gauges and indications

IVC GAUGE	INDICATIONS
24-gauge (yellow)	Paediatrics
22-gauge (blue)	Predominantly used in elderly patients with smaller veins. Suitable for slow infusions and IV medications
20-gauge (pink)	Suitable for most infusions including antibiotics. The first choice of cannula for adults
18-gauge (green)	Favored by Radiology for contrast infusions. Ideal cannula for infusion of blood products
16-gauge (grey)	Large bore cannula used for resuscitation purposes
14-gauge (orange)	

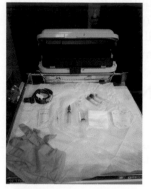

FIGURE 17.1 A standard IV trolley setup.

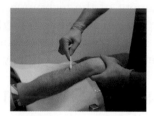

FIGURE 17.2 Apply the tourniquet, palpate the skin for veins. Palpation offers superior assessment of suitable veins over visual inspection.

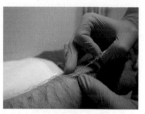

FIGURE 17.3 Approach the selected vein along the path of its course at a 45° angle. Puncture the skin with the bevel facing up. Keep in mind that the vein is superficial – you shouldn't need to advance the needle too far to obtain 'flashback'.

- 10-mL syringe (×2 if taking blood) and 10 mL of normal saline
- tourniquet
- sterile gloves
- IV cannula.

Most hospitals have policies regarding the maintenance and care of IVCs, with some mandating that they be changed every 72 hours to reduce the risk of IVC site infection and thrombophlebitis.

There are several methods of taking bloods from patients. Hospitals have varying equipment including vacuum container needle sets. Basic methods involve using needles and syringes (Figs 17.9 to 17.11).

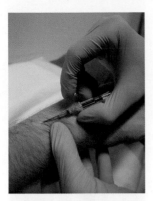

FIGURE 17.4 Once you observe flashback in the needle, flatten the needle and slide the cannula hub towards the skin.

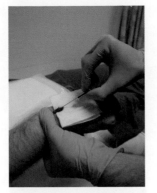

FIGURE 17.5 Withdraw the needle from the cannula hub while applying firm pressure proximally to prevent bleeding.

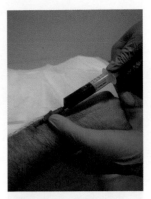

FIGURE 17.6 At this point blood may be taken through the IVC for pathology.

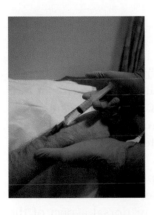

FIGURE 17.7 The IVC must then be 'flushed' with normal saline to clear blood from the cannula tubing and ensure the line is patent.

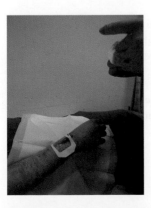

FIGURE 17.8 The IVC is then secured to the skin using a clear adhesive dressing. Consider wrapping the IVC with a protective bandage if it is at risk of knocking into objects such as the bed.

SECTION II

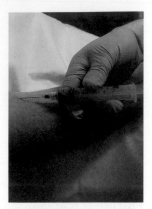

FIGURE 17.9 The 'needle and syringe' method involves piercing the vein with a 21- or 23-gauge needle and withdrawing blood from a syringe.

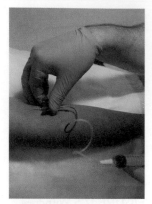

FIGURE 17.10 The butterfly needle offers manoeuvrability in difficult-to-reach positions such as hands or feet; a syringe can withdraw blood through the tubing.

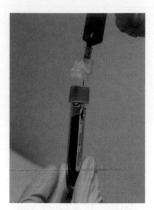

FIGURE 17.11 A needle can be used to empty the syringe into the pathology tube.

PLASTERING

There are a variety of techniques and materials used for immobilisation in limb injuries, the most prevalent of which is plaster-based splints. Although some ED departments and outpatient clinics have staff who specialise in plastering, junior doctors are often required to make the splints themselves. Hand, wrist and ankle trauma are common presentations to EDs and surgical wards that require immobilisation, and the initial treatment is immobilisation with temporary plaster-based splints.

For upper limb trauma, a temporary 'half-cast' plaster splint that facilitates easy removal, especially for hand, finger and wrist injuries, is termed a 'backslab'. This splint can be placed on either the volar (more common) or dorsal aspect of the limb. Modifications can include shaping the plaster to immobilise specific digits. A standard volar-based backslab should extend from at least mid-forearm to the tips of the fingers.

Always use cold water when dipping the plaster and inform the patient that the heat they may feel from the plaster as it sets is entirely normal.

Refer to Figs 17.12 to 17.18 for backslab plastering technique.

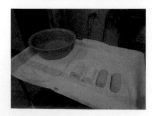

FIGURE 17.12 A typical plaster trolley set-up including cold water, a towel to reduce mess, plaster padding, plaster rolls and crepe bandage.

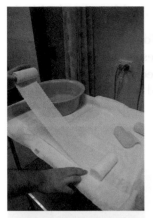

FIGURE 17.13 Use the plaster padding roll to measure the length of the backslab for the patient; this serves as a template for the plaster, which is rolled continuously into 8–10 layers.

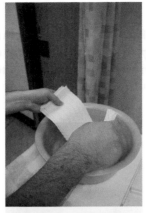

FIGURE 17.14 The plaster layers are then dipped into water. Avoid excessive wringing to prevent loss of the plaster material.

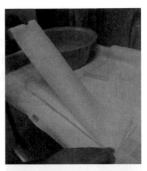

FIGURE 17.15 Place the moistened layer of plaster back over the padding material with several layers of padding rolled over the top; ensure all areas of plaster are covered and will not come into contact with the patient's skin.

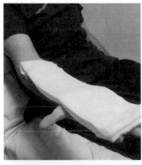

FIGURE 17.16 The plaster can be volar or dorsal. When applying the backslab alone, the patient may tolerate taking the weight of the plaster while the bandage is applied.

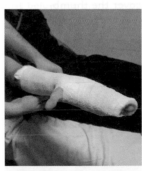

FIGURE 17.17 A crepe bandage is wrapped around the length of the backslab with 50% overlap. A 7.5-cm bandage for the fingers and hand and 10-cm for the forearm can help prevent 'bunching' of the crepe bandage.

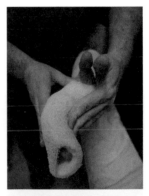

FIGURE 17.18 Before the plaster sets there should be moulding of the backslab to ensure the hand is kept in the 'position of safety' with the MCPJ at 90° and PIPs and DIPJs at full extension.

SECTION II

SUTURING AND WOUND MANAGEMENT

The best opportunity for medical students and junior doctors to practise suturing is in the Emergency Department. Though theatre allows the junior doctor to suture under the supervision of an experienced surgeon, these opportunities can be limited. Suturing of minor traumatic wounds gives great experience in cleaning wounds, administering local anaesthetic and suturing technique.

Preparation of the wound

Initial wound management involves cleaning the surrounding skin around the wound and removing any nearby clothing and jewellery. Irrigation of the wound with normal saline is recommended in traumatic settings to dilute the amount of potential pathogens. Contaminated wounds require local anaesthetic infiltration prior to deep washout and debridement.

Local anaesthetics

These agents are widely used in the Emergency Department for the treatment of pain related to injuries. There are many agents, though three are commonly used (Table 17.2).

Local anaesthetic doses are calculated based on weight, though most small wounds will not need more than 10 mL of short-acting lignocaine. For smaller patients (children and elderly) or those with hepatic impairment, it's essential that you correctly calculate the maximum dose for that patient. This means you'll also need to know the mg/mL. If you can remember that 1% = 10 mg/1 mL, it's fairly simple to work out the dose for any other concentration.

Administer the agent within the open edge of the wound; aspirate as the needle is introduced to avoid intra-arterial injection. Ensure that the infiltration covers the skin where sutures will be introduced.

Suturing

Suturing is a sterile procedure. Most EDs stock disposable packs with tools that should include: needle holder, tissue forceps and suture scissors. Most packs will also contain a drape, sterile gauze and a tray for wash.

TABLE 17.2 Commonly used local anaesthetic agents

AGENT	DURATION	AVAILABLE CONCENTRATIONS	DOSAGE
Lignocaine	Short acting	1%, 2%	3 mg/kg (without adrenaline) 7 mg/kg (with adrenaline)
Bupivacaine (Marcaine®)	Long acting	0.25%, 0.5%	2 mg/kg
Ropivacaine (Naropin®)	Long acting	0.5%, 0.75%, 1%	3 mg/kg

TABLE 17.3 Suture materials

Non-absorbable	
STITCH TYPE	**USES**
Silk	• Secure drain tubes
Nylon (Ethilon®, Dermalon®)	• Skin closure
Polypropylene (Prolene®, Surgipro®)	• Subcuticular wound closure • Vascular anastomosis • Mesh fixation
Absorbable	
STITCH TYPE	**USES**
Gut (Fast, Chromic)	• Skin, particularly skin lacerations in children • Skin grafts
Polyglactin (Vicryl®, Polysorb®)	• Vessel ligation • Subcutaneous wound closure • Rapid degrading versions used for skin closure
Poliglecaprone (Monocryl®)	• Subcutaneous wound closure. Favoured for subcuticular stitches
Polydioxanone (PDS®)	• Abdominal wall closure

Adapted from: Ammirati, C. & Goldman, G., 2012. Wound closure materials and instruments. Dermatology 144, 2353-2363.

Selection of the suture material (Table 17.3) depends on the type of wound. Clean small wounds might be suited to absorbable suture materials that do not require removal. Large, contaminated wounds are generally closed using non-absorbable sutures such as nylon. When in doubt about the best method to close a wound, simple interrupted nylon sutures are a safe option.

Simple interrupted sutures are the most versatile technique and tend to be the default approach to closing a wound as outlined in Figs 17.31 to 17.40.

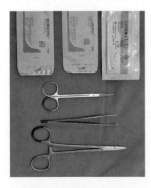

FIGURE 17.31 Basic requirements for suturing including needle holder, tissue forceps, scissors and sutures.

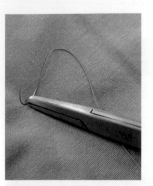

FIGURE 17.32 The ideal position of the suture in the needle holder: two-thirds round from the cutting end, held in the tips.

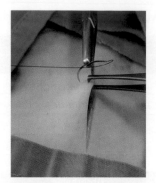

FIGURE 17.33 Using the tissue forceps to evert the skin edge, the needle should enter the skin at 90°.

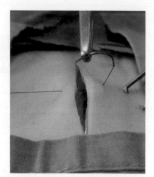

FIGURE 17.34 Use the curve of the needle to your advantage by rotating your wrist, easing the needle through the skin for minimal trauma. Avoid gripping the tip of the needle to prevent blunting.

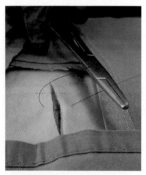

FIGURE 17.35 Tying the suture knot is performed via a series of 'throws' (i.e. looping the suture around the needle holder). Two loops for the first throw, then one for each subsequent throw.

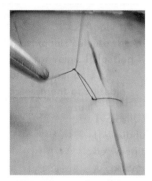

FIGURE 17.36 Correctly performing the throws will result in a non-slip square knot. The tension should slightly evert the skin edges, but not blanche the underlying skin.

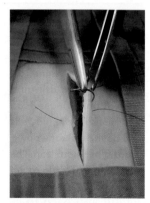

FIGURE 17.37 A backhand throw used in a horizontal mattress suture.

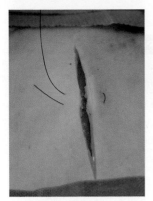

FIGURE 17.38 Ensure the suture is evenly placed.

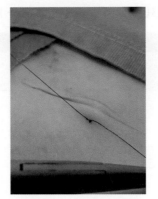

FIGURE 17.39 The horizontal mattress allows for greater eversion of the skin with reduced tension. Useful for rolled-in skin edges.

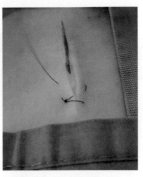

FIGURE 17.40 Most stitch types can be modified into a continuous or running suture.

MALE INDWELLING CATHETER (IDC) INSERTION

Most health networks have policies that allow only medical staff and specially trained nursing staff to perform male catheterisation. Despite obvious anatomical differences, the set-up and method of insertion have a number of similarities.

An IDC 'pack' set-up (Fig. 17.41) includes most of the equipment required to perform the procedure including trays, swabs, gauze, forceps, normal saline, syringe, sterile gloves and a drape. Other required equipment includes:

- lignocaine lubricant gel
- urine drainage bag
- IDC (size dependent on gender and indication).

The exact equipment depends on the indication for insertion of an IDC (Table 17.4).

Sterility is important when inserting an IDC. As such the junior doctor must keep in mind that the genitals are not a 'clean' area, and initial cleaning of the area will involve contamination of the glove. There are two methods of maintaining sterility:

1 double glove – with removal of the top layer of gloves after the area has been cleaned

2 'clean hand/dirty hand' – the non-dominant hand is used to keep the genitals properly positioned and does not make contact with the sterile equipment. A piece of gauze can be used as a sling to hold the penis.

Refer to Figs 17.42 to 17.48 for illustrations of this procedure.

SECTION II

TABLE 17.4 Indications for IDC

INDICATION FOR IDC	SIZE OF IDC	TYPE OF DRAINAGE BAG
Urinary retention	12–16 Fr	Urinary drainage bag Leg urinary drainage bag
Haematuria	22–26 Fr (3-way). May need to obtain from theatre	Large urinary drainage bag, particularly with bladder washouts
Perioperative	12–16 Fr	Urine meter with drainage bag
Immobility	12–16 Fr	Urinary drainage bag Leg urinary drainage bag
Strict fluid balance (i.e. sepsis)	12–16 Fr	Urine meter with drainage bag

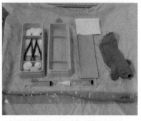

FIGURE 17.41 Typical sterile set up for an IDC.

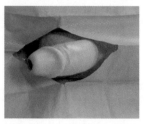

FIGURE 17.42 Cover the area with a sterile drape.

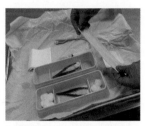

FIGURE 17.43 Fold a gauze for the 'clean hand/ dirty hand' technique.

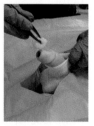

FIGURE 17.44 Cleanse the glans.

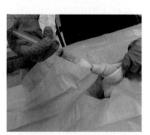

FIGURE 17.45 Administer the lignocaine lubricant jelly.

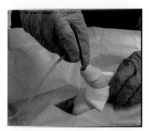

FIGURE 17.46 Lift the penis until vertical and ease the tip of the IDC through the meatus.

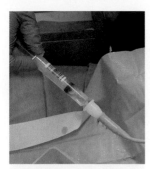

FIGURE 17.47 Once the IDC has been fully advanced, use the empty local syringe to aspirate urine.

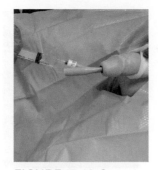

FIGURE 17.48 Once urine is sufficiently draining, inflate the catheter balloon with 10 mL of normal saline and connect the catheter bag.

NASOGASTRIC TUBES (NGTs)

Nasogastric tubes serve two main purposes: to drain excess gastric fluid and allow the passage of food and medications to the stomach. Drainage NGTs are an important part of treating bowel obstructions (Chapter 45); feeding NGTs are indicated in patients with swallowing difficulties or those who are having ongoing sedation.

The insertion of nasogastric tubes is typically done by nursing staff, meaning that some junior doctors have never performed this procedure. As NGTs are a rapid and effective treatment of a patient's symptoms for obstruction, it's essential to know how to perform this procedure (see Figs 17.49 to 17.55) as nursing staff might be otherwise occupied.

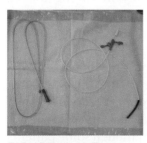

FIGURE 17.49 The two different types of NGTs.

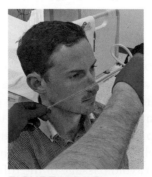

FIGURE 17.50 First measurement: between the bridge of the nose and the earlobe.

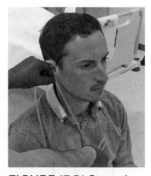

FIGURE 17.51 Second measurement: earlobe to xiphoid process.

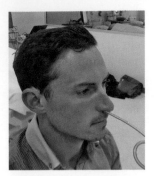

FIGURE 17.52 Position the tip of the drainage NGT within the nostril and introduce by aiming for the back wall of the nasopharynx.

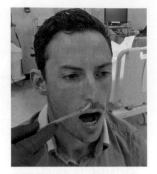

FIGURE 17.53 If there is difficulty feeding the tube, look in the mouth to see if it has become curled.

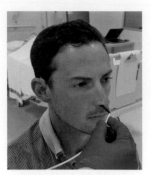

FIGURE 17.54 The nasogastric feeding tube is inserted using the same initial approach.

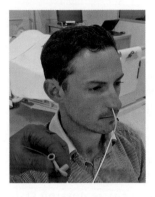

FIGURE 17.55 Remove the stylus at the end of the procedure.

Drainage NGTs are quite firm but flexible enough to allow passage along the back wall of the pharynx and into the oesophagus. Feeding NGTs are thinner and quite flexible; therefore a metal stylet is used to prevent coiling during insertion. During the insertion process, direct the patient to swallow (if able to allow passage through the oropharynx). Suction should be nearby in the case of vomiting.

Position of the NGT can be confirmed by aspiration of gastric contents with a litmus pH test (pH 1–5) or an X-ray. Most hospitals have policies dictating that feeding nasogastric tubes cannot be used until their position has been confirmed by X-ray. Incorrect positioning of an NGT within the trachea and bronchus is typically associated with respiratory irritation (i.e. coughing) though some patients may appear to tolerate it well! The classic contraindication to NGT insertion is a base of skull fracture, so as to avoid passage of the tube into the brain, an alarming and radiologically spectacular complication.

CHAPTER 18

THE PATIENT WITH MENTAL ILLNESS

Paul Watson and Joseph M O'Brien

Although the Emergency Department is the most common setting in which junior doctors are exposed to acute psychiatric presentations, it is important to keep in mind that any patient admitted to the ward with acute medical or surgical issues with an existing mental health condition will require special consideration of their mental and emotional wellbeing.

Psychiatric presentations represent a diverse spectrum of illness including thought, mood and personality disorders. Mental illness has a profound impact on the health of Australians. A 2007 national survey revealed the lifetime incidence of mental disorders in adults (aged 16–85) was around 45%, with 20% of those surveyed revealing an episode within the past 12 months. Refer to Table 18.1 for prevalence data.

There are a large number of affective, mood, thought and personality disorders with a multitude of varied presentations and treatment approaches. Continuing the theme of Section II, this chapter focuses on initial assessment and management. We acknowledge that mental health illnesses require long-term management to achieve optimal outcomes.

INITIAL ASSESSMENT

The goal of an initial assessment is to determine the following:

- Is this a true presentation of mental illness?
  - Is there another cause of mood, thought or behavioural disturbance? Consider:
    - confusion due to infection
    - emotional instability secondary to acute substance intoxication.
- Is this an isolated presentation of mental illness or does the patient demonstrate other features of physical illness?
- Current mental state by performing a mental state examination (MSE) (see the next section) including detailed information about past psychiatric history.

TABLE 18.1 Top three categories of mental illness by prevalence

CATEGORY OF MENTAL DISORDER	PERCENTAGE OF OVERALL PREVALENCE
Anxiety disorders	14.4%
Affective disorders (depression)	6.2%
Substance abuse (alcohol)	5.1%

Adapted from: Australian Institute of Health and Welfare, 2014. Mental Health Services: In brief [Internet]. <http://www.aihw.gov.au>.

- Does this patient present a **risk** to themselves or others? Assessing the risk of violence and suicide should be the first priority for any patient suspected of having a psychiatric presentation. Consider:
  - risk to self requiring constant observation
  - risk to others requiring seclusion and/or restraint.
- Does this patient (satisfying the above assessment criteria) meet the criteria to be admitted as an involuntary patient?

The approach to the patient should be open and honest. Try to set aside any feelings of discomfort and take a thorough history. The act of properly listening to the patient's story, appearing interested and offering an encouraging response to keep talking helps to establish rapport.

Psychiatric history (mental state examination)

General: detailed developmental history – perinatal, infancy and early childhood, middle childhood, adolescence, young adulthood to present. Sexual history. Values. A mental state examination should be performed simultaneously.

Mood: how have you been feeling in yourself? Do you feel 'down' more days than not? Have you lost interest in things that you normally enjoy? Have you experienced any sleep disturbance (identify initial, middle or end insomnia)? Have you had a change in your appetite and/or weight? Do you think about suicide?

Do you sometimes feel 'up' or very energetic? Do you ever have periods where you make rash decisions or spend a lot of money? Do you have any special powers?

Anxiety: have you felt nervy or testy lately? Do you have trouble relaxing? What do you worry about? Have you had any panic attacks? Do they happen with or without triggers? Do you worry about things that most people would not? Do you avoid going out, or avoid situations because you're concerned about a panic attack?

Stress disorders: have you had any problems following (particular incident)? Have you been anxious or worried? Have you had trouble sleeping? Do you have bad memories? Have you been having nightmares? Have you had trouble with your memory? Are you jumpy?

Thought: have you heard people speaking when there is no one else around? Have you heard your thoughts spoken out loud? Do you have any thoughts or beliefs others might find strange? Do you have any special powers? Have you felt people may be against you? Do you ever get any special messages from the TV or radio just for you? Do you feel like someone is spying on you or plotting against you? Do you have any ideas you don't tell others about because you're worried they won't believe you or think there's something wrong with you?

Eating disorders: do you worry about your weight? Do you think you're overweight? Do you diet? Have you ever made yourself sick after a meal? What is your weight today? How often do you weigh yourself? Do you feel the need to exercise a lot after consuming a lot of calories?

Family, past medical and treatment and **substance** histories are all very important when conducting a mental state examination.

RISK ASSESSMENT

Suicide

When patients present to the Emergency Department they may report thoughts of suicide or self-harm. When speaking with the patient, it is important to identify triggers and contributing factors to the patient's state of mind. The junior doctor should not be afraid to ask the seemingly pointed questions regarding whether the patient wants to commit suicide and whether they have made plans. This information allows a determination of level of risk and appropriate management. Scoring systems such as the SADPERSONS (Table 18.2) can be a useful clinical aid.

A score of ≥6 is the cut-off for admission to hospital with a sensitivity of 97%. Patients considered at high risk of suicide within the Emergency Department should:

- be checked for sharps and have access to all sharps removed
- have a nurse or 'psych special' for observation of the patient to prevent self-harm or absconding
- not be physically restrained unless posing a significant and uncontrolled risk of violence to self or others.

Violence

Though a common fear, most violence is not initiated by patients with mental illness but by those with a past history of violence and substance abuse. It has been previously established that patients with schizophrenia have a five-fold increased risk of violence; however, this particular subset of psychotic patients with violent tendencies is strongly associated with substance abuse.

TABLE 18.2 SADPERSONS assessment of suicide risk for non-psychiatric medical staff

RISK FACTOR	SCORE
Sex (male)	1
Age (≤18 or ≥45 years)	1
Depression or hopelessness	2
Previous attempts or psychiatric care	1
Excessive alcohol or drug use	1
Rational thinking loss	2
Separated, divorced or widowed	1
Organised or serious attempt	2
No social supports	1
Stated future intent	2

Adapted from: Hockberger, R.S. & Rothstein, R.J., 1988. Assessment of suicide potential by nonpsychiatrists using the SAD PERSONS score. Journal of Emergency Medicine 6(2), 99-107.

The junior doctor should take precautions when approaching a potentially violent patient and observe for the following key signs:

- Always have an exit from the room or cubicle.
- Note if the patient:
  - becomes flustered or angered with their speech
  - begins to becomes restless, pacing around the room
  - demonstrates gritting of the teeth or clenching of a fist
  - issues verbal abuse and threats.

Attempt to defuse the situation calmly by asking the patient what is concerning them and attempt to identify issues that are distressing the patient. This may be difficult when the patient is under the influence of drugs or alcohol. If the patient becomes violent, a security presence will be required to help manage the patient. Most hospital security guards are well trained in de-escalation of hostile patients and provide fantastic support.

PSYCHOSIS

Psychosis is a disturbance of thought (delusions) and/or perception (hallucinations), which can lead to changes in a patient's mood and behaviour. Psychosis associated with agitation or anxiety is a red flag for unpredictable behaviour. These patients should be seen as quickly as possible to determine the nature of psychosis, establish a cause and initiate prompt treatment to de-escalate the situation. Keep the patient informed at all times about your actions and intended management

TABLE 18.3 Common causes of psychosis

ORGANIC	PSYCHIATRIC
Drug intoxication (prescribed and illicit) Delirium Dementia	Acute/chronic schizophrenia Mood related psychosis: • psychotic depression • manic psychosis

Unless there is an established formal thought disorder such as schizophrenia, it can be challenging to determine if the cause is organic or psychiatric in nature (see Table 18.3).

ANXIETY

Anxiety is a particularly common presentation, accounting for 14% of all mental health disorders. Anxiety refers to an abnormal state of arousal leading to patient distress. Identifying the cause of the patient's anxiety is the key to developing a treatment plan:

- Organic (exogenous):
  - drug intoxication or withdrawal (particularly alcohol withdrawal)
  - metabolic disorders such as hyperthyroidism are also implicated in anxiety.
- Psychiatric (endogenous):
  - primary – anxiety disorder, panic disorder
  - associated – post-traumatic stress disorder mania.

Assessment of these patients is aided by finding a quiet place in the ED or the ward. If the patient has a close family member or friend with them during the review it can help offset the unfamiliarity with their surroundings and the junior doctor.

History should focus on establishing the frequency and pattern of anxiety. It's also helpful to identify potential triggers for episodes of anxiety. Ask about associated physical symptoms: patients with a short burst of intense anxiety (panic attacks) often describe physical symptoms such as chest pain and shortness of breath. Patients with generalised anxiety are more likely to have disruptions to mood such as depression (see Table 18.4). A single one-off event of anxiety related to an extreme stressor does not necessarily constitute an anxiety or panic disorder.

Examination should include taking the patient's vitals, looking for tachycardia or cardiac arrhythmias. Physical symptoms such as diarrhoea and abdominal pain are often brushed aside as somatisation, but can represent metabolic disturbance.

Management

Exclusion of an organic cause is the first step, particularly looking for delirium or substance use. Withdrawal from alcohol is a common emergency presentation

TABLE 18.4 Features of anxiety disorders

ANXIETY DISORDER	FEATURES
Generalised anxiety disorder (GAD)	• Patient describes a constant feeling of unease regarding their own wellbeing and the surrounding world around them • Can have a particular focus such as the patient's health, financial status or loved ones • Somatisation with non-specific physical feelings is common
Post-traumatic stress disorder (PTSD)	• Acute anxiety secondary to a traumatic event • Classic symptoms include hypervigilance, triggering of anxiety when reminded of the trauma and reliving the trauma in the form of nightmares or flashbacks
Panic attacks and disorder	• Sudden onset severe anxiety • A response to patient stress but can sometimes have no triggers • Persistent episodes are termed 'panic' disorders
Phobias	• Exaggerated fear of an object or situation that impedes a patient's ability to lead a normal life • Common pathological phobias include claustrophobia (enclosed spaces) and agoraphobia (outside congested spaces) • 'Social phobia' is considered an archaic term, a diagnosis of 'social anxiety disorder' should be considered

and anxiety is an indication that the patient warrants admission for observation and management with an alcohol withdrawal scale (AWS)

For patients with an acute, severe anxiety a short-acting benzodiazepine can be used for symptomatic management, though this should be considered a last resort. Longer term pharmacological management is dependent on whether the patient has a comorbid mood disorder that might respond to an antidepressant. Specialist psychiatric input should be sought before commencing any of these medications. In the community patients with mild anxiety can respond well to psychotherapy.

DELIBERATE SELF-HARM

The act of intentional self-injury or poisoning is a common ED presentation, responsible for 1 in 200 presentations overall and as high as 1 in 100 for teenagers.

Serious self-harm episodes represent a smaller number of overall presentations, approximately 1.5 in 1000.

The junior doctor is exposed to a wide spectrum of self-harm behaviours. Self-poisoning makes up around two-thirds of self-harm presentations with analgesic medications responsible for 39% of presentations with paracetamol the largest single contributor at 15% overall; antidepressants (15%) and benzo-diazepines (9%) were the next two most common classes. Consider calling the Poisons Hotline (13 11 26) for advice for all patients who have overdosed.

Though sometimes not taken seriously by medical staff due to the superficial nature of their wounds and common associations with personality disorders, it should be noted that over 5% of patients who present with self-harm will commit suicide within 10 years. It is therefore essential to explore all risk factors and put community supports into place to help reduce this risk

Paracetamol overdose

Protocols for managing paracetamol overdoses involve the measurement of serum paracetamol levels and referencing a timeline-based curve (see Fig. 18.1). However, this requires accurate information regarding:

- When was the overdose taken?
- How much was ingested? Was this all at once? Did the patient vomit?

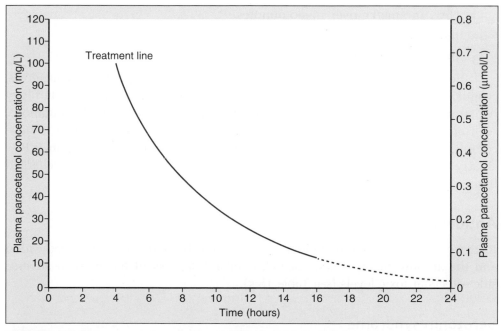

FIGURE 18.1 Plasma paracetamol concentrations and prognosis in paracetamol poisoning: specific treatment is indicated if the concentration is above the treatment line.

Adapted from: Marshall, W.J., Lapsley, M. & Day, A., 2017. Therapeutic drug monitoring and chemical aspects of toxicology. In: Marshall, W.J., Lapsley, M. & Day, A., Clinical Chemistry, 8th ed. Elsevier, Fig. 22-9.

- Have there been repeated ingestions of overdoses?
- Is the patient taking any other medications that interact with paracetamol?

A supratherapeutic dose of paracetamol is classified as >10 g or >200 mg/kg in 24 hours with the lesser amount used to determine a 'toxic dose'. Acute liver injury can occur at times or levels above the line of the normograph curve; this information is used to determine whether N-acetyl cysteine (NAC) therapy is commenced. Therapeutic Guidelines recommend:

- Presentations <4 hours after ingestion have NAC withheld until results for serum levels at the 4-hour mark return.
- Presentations <8 hours after ingestion should have serum levels performed, and NAC commenced if the serum level is above the normograph line.
- Presentations >8 hours after ingestion should have NAC commenced with serum levels sent. If serum levels are below the normograph line, NAC can be ceased.
- If the patient presents at an unknown time after ingestion and has deranged liver function tests, NAC should be commenced.

NAC infusions are given in three steps over a 20- to 21-hour period as an IV infusion:

1 NAC 150 mg/kg over 15–60 minutes
2 then NAC 50 mg/kg over 4 hours
3 then NAC 100 mg/kg IV over 16 hours.

Patients who show signs of liver failure such as encephalopathy, acidosis, coagulopathy and hypoglycaemia should be discussed with the Gastroenterology registrar for guidance. For patients who have ingested slow release formulations, seek advice from Clinical Toxicology or the Poisons Hotline. If patients have completed their course of NAC and have been assessed by the Emergency Psychiatry team as not requiring psychiatric admission, they can be safely discharged home.

Antidepressant overdose

As there are many different antidepressants, identifying the particular medication and the amount taken is key. Each class of antidepressant has its own adverse side effects at toxic levels (see Table 18.5).

Serotonin syndrome

Onset is typically hours after toxic overdose and is classically described as a triad of clinical symptoms:

1 *central nervous system (CNS) effects* including agitation, anxiety and confusion

2 *autonomic effects* including hyperthermia, sweating and tachycardia

3 *neuromuscular excitation,* including hyperreflexia and clonus (inducible or spontaneous).

There are no investigations to confirm the presence of serotonin syndrome, and the varying levels of severity mean that there is often a mix of symptoms. Hunter's Serotonin Toxicity Criteria has a sensitivity of 84% and specificity of 97% in the diagnosis of serotonin syndrome. To fulfil the criteria a patient must have had a serotonergic drug and have at least one of the following:

- spontaneous clonus
- inducible clonus + agitation or diaphoresis
- ocular clonus + agitation or diaphoresis

TABLE 18.5 Summary of antidepressant overdoses

MEDICATION	TOXIC DOSE	SIDE EFFECTS	MANAGEMENT
Serotonin and noradrenaline reuptake inhibitors (SNRIs)[a]			
Desvenlafaxine	Unknown	The noradrenergic effects tend to be more pronounced: hypotension, arrhythmias, hyperthermia and seizures Serotonin toxicity normally only seen when taken with MAO inhibitors	Telemetry, ECG and monitoring delayed seizure activity at toxic dose level Get toxicology input
Duloxetine	8.5 mg/kg		
Reboxetine	~3 mg/kg		
Tramadol	Toxic: >5 mg Seizure activity: >1.5 mg		
Venlafaxine	Seizure activity: >5 mg Cardiac toxicity: >8 mg		
Selective serotonin reuptake inhibitors (SSRIs)[b]			
Citalopram	600 mg	Overdoses rarely cause noticeable side effects, seizures are rare Serotonin toxicity only severe if combined with other serotonergic drug Escitalopram and citalopram can cause QT interval elongation	ECG Observation
Escitalopram	300 mg		
Fluoxetine	Toxic dose not well established		
Paroxetine			
Sertraline			
Fluvoxamine			

continued

TABLE 18.5 Summary of antidepressant overdoses—cont'd

MEDICATION	TOXIC DOSE	SIDE EFFECTS	MANAGEMENT
Tricyclic antidepressants (TCAs)[c]			
Amitriptyline Clomipramine Dothiepin Doxepin Imipramine Nortriptyline Trimipramine	10 mg/kg are potentially toxic 20 mg/kg result in severe toxicity	TCAs are associated with serious risk of cardiovascular effects including QRS widening and ventricular arrhythmias Hypotension, bradycardia and seizures are also potential side effects	ECG Patients will need monitoring of telemetry Activated charcoal if presents within 1 hour QRS widening: bicarbonate therapy in combination with hyperventilation therapy to raise pH

ECG, electrocardiogram; MAO, monoamine oxidase.

[a]Adapted from: Therapeutic Guidelines Limited, 2014. Toxicology: serotonin and noradrenaline reuptake inhibitors [revised Nov 2014]. In: eTG complete [Internet]. Melbourne: Therapeutic Guidelines Limited. <http://online.tg.org.au>.

[b]Adapted from: Therapeutic Guidelines Limited, 2014. Toxicology: selective serotonin reuptake inhibitors [revised Nov 2014]. In: eTG complete [Internet]. Melbourne: Therapeutic Guidelines Limited. <http://online.tg.org.au>.

[c]Adapted from: Therapeutic Guidelines Limited, 2014. Toxicology: tricyclic antidepressants [revised Nov 2014]. In: eTG complete [Internet]. Melbourne: Therapeutic Guidelines Limited. <http://online.tg.org.au>.

- tremor + hyperreflexia
- temperature >38°C + hypertonia, + ocular clonus or inducible clonus.

A CNS infection should be excluded in these patients; therefore, pathology and imaging may be required. Benzodiazepines can be given to ease agitation, while cyproheptadine is the serotonin antagonist used for the reversal of symptoms.

Benzodiazepine overdose

Another common medication used for self-harm, benzodiazepine ingestion causes sedation and CNS depression. The range at which adverse effects may manifest is highly variable among agents.

The major concern is respiratory depression; however, most patients will maintain a patent airway despite profound drowsiness, simply requiring regular observations while lying on their side. Young and healthy patients are unlikely to require intervention to reverse the effects, although elderly patients and those at risk of respiratory compromise due to respiratory disease should be considered for treatment with flumazenil (a benzodiazepine receptor antagonist). The half-life of this medication is much shorter than most benzodiazepines; therefore, sedation is only going to be postponed and multiple doses may be required. Expert opinion should be used in these settings.

Self-injury

Patients also present with instances of cutting, particularly to the limbs. Commonly, the wounds are superficial and may require a dressing or suturing. Dependent on the area of injury there is risk of damage to deeper structures and a full examination is warranted. Some patients will self-harm with burns or by consuming caustic substances that may cause damage to the pharynx and oesophagus, requiring an airway examination and observation.

Patients can present with life-threatening self-harm injuries such as from jumping from a height or hanging. These patients require urgent trauma assessment for serious intracranial, thoracic and spinal injuries. Once they are stable, a psychiatric assessment can be made.

INPATIENT PSYCHIATRIC REFERRALS

Often patients or allied health staff on the ward will report symptoms suggestive of psychological distress such as low mood, hallucinations, delusions and suicidal ideation. Some of these patients will have a longstanding psychiatric history with good out-of-hospital support, and others will have never had any contact with mental health services previously. All symptoms should be given due attention and require exploration with the patient. There are two considerations in the initial phase:

1 Are these symptoms due to an organic cause? Examples include confusion and agitation secondary to delirium, or iatrogenic hallucinations or delusions from medications.

2 Are symptoms of low mood reactionary to poor physical health or recent life events?

In the first instance a delirium screen is beneficial to rule out infection (see Chapter 12, Investigations: serology). It is worth noting that elderly patients with baseline cognitive impairment can develop a delirium merely from change of environment, disruption to sleep–wake cycle or metabolic imbalances secondary to fasting. These factors need to be identified and treated. Patients who are on strong opioid medication require a review of their analgesia requirements, with a careful withdrawal of medication as tolerated by the patient.

Patients with longstanding disease, particularly malignancies, can develop a low mood and agitation while an inpatient. This is especially true if there are complications that further affect physical health. Some specialties (e.g. general surgery) have specialised breast care nurses who are particularly adept at offering psychological support during periods of breast cancer care. Most hospital networks have a psychologist who can speak to the patient and identify issues for outpatient follow-up.

The referral for inpatient psychiatric review should only be made for those patients who require psychiatric diagnosis, medication management and urgent review due to increased risk of harm. The junior doctor should take a full psychiatric history from the patient, including information regarding their social situation, prior to making a referral.

INVOLUNTARY PATIENT STATUS

Patients with acute psychiatric presentations with impaired judgement may be resistant to remaining in the hospital environment for treatment. There are provisions in legislative law, different in every state, to deem a person mentally incompetent to make a medical decision and declare them as an involuntary patient. The decision is made based on certain variables, as follows:

- The patient has a severe physical or mental illness that requires inpatient care.
- This level of care cannot be provided in the community.
- The patient is unable to recognise the consequences of non-treatment.
- The patient is at risk of harm to self or others.

After the patient has been declared involuntary it is mandated that they be reviewed by the inpatient psychiatric team within a set period, typically 24 hours.

It's wise to check the current involuntary admission laws as covered by your state mental health act and properly understand the criteria that a patient must meet to be declared incompetent. These situations can be messy, particularly when there is a presentation including an additional medical or surgical issue that requires urgent attention and the patient refuses treatment.

The decision to 'section' a patient under the mental health act should be done in conjunction with an experienced senior doctor or psychiatric nurse liaison who are familiar with the process and associated paperwork. There is a well-known urban legend of the intern who incorrectly filled out the involuntary patient paperwork, 'sectioning' themselves.

CHAPTER 19

FORENSIC MEDICINE

Joseph M O'Brien

As a medical student or junior doctor, you are unlikely to have frequent involvement in cases with legal implications. Of course, every admission has the *potential* to have legal consequences in the future, which is why everything you and your team do should be thoroughly documented. It is frequently said that when note-taking for your team, you should imagine it being read aloud in a court of law. However, the situations discussed below require particular steps to be taken. Although uncommon, it is not unheard of for a junior doctor's presence to be requested at a criminal case as an 'expert' witness. Please note that this chapter is purely a guideline, and that your institution will likely have its own specific procedures. It should not be substituted for professional, legal advice.

NON-ACCIDENTAL INJURY IN A MINOR

Child abuse, or 'non-accidental injury (NAI) in a minor' is defined in Australia as 'any non-accidental behaviour by parents, caregivers or other adults that is outside the norms of conduct and entails a substantial risk of causing physical or emotional harm to a young person or child' (Price-Robertson R., 2012. What is child abuse and neglect? Australian Institute of Family Studies. <http://www.aifs.gov.au/cfca/pubs/factsheets/a142091/> [accessed 12 September 2014]). It is commonly divided into the five subtypes of: physical abuse, emotional maltreatment, neglect, sexual abuse and/or the witnessing of family violence.

If you suspect a paediatric patient (i.e. less than 18 years old) of yours may be a victim of a non-accidental injury, you should immediately notify the senior clinician on your service as they may reassign the case to either themselves or a registrar. In fact, it is mandatory in many hospitals that all injuries in children under 4 years of age be reviewed and signed off by a consultant prior to discharge. In Australia, it is mandatory to report to your state's government authority if you have belief on reasonable grounds that child abuse may be taking place. Although the exact definitions differ from state to state, universally it is appropriate to report if there is a significant chance of physical or sexual assault, serious psychological harm or serious neglect. All jurisdictions in Australia protect the identity of the reporter. This is certainly not something that would be expected of a junior doctor, and if you are placed in this situation it would be advisable to seek legal counsel before acting.

Comprehensive history-taking, examination and documentation are all essential in this potentially volatile situation. You should take note of consistency between the history given by the patient (if they are able to communicate it), the individual parents, any witnesses to the accident and to the story given to the triage nurse and paramedics. Consider the history you've collected and whether or not it is congruent with the nature of the child's injuries, and whether or not the child's developmental stage would allow for those events to have taken place (e.g. a child who cannot yet run who 'ran into the corner of the table'). With a high degree of suspicion, think about contacting the paediatric registrar on call early for their input.

The Royal Children's Hospital has an excellent guide for dealing with child abuse. The first priority is to diagnose, treat and document the child's injuries; then establish if there is a pattern of injury leading to suspicion of abuse; then notify the appropriate authorities for your state; and, lastly, provide a written report to the police (where consent can be obtained).

Ideally, written consent should be obtained for a physical examination of the child from their primary caregiver. It would not be unwise to request a member of the nursing staff to escort you during the examination as a secondary witness. If consent cannot be obtained, do not proceed unless it is a medical emergency. Examine the patient very carefully, and document all injuries thoroughly.

The past history should be pored over thoroughly – children who have catastrophic NAI that results in permanent disability or death have often presented to a health service multiple times, and 12% have presented to a hospital as their first point of contact. Without appropriate intervention, 35% of cases will be recurrent. Most children's histories are brief – any long histories should prompt further review.

Investigations should be ordered appropriately. Remember, medical conditions may explain the child's presentation and these should never be missed, and even the most suspicious history may be due to miscommunication.

Children often injure themselves and end up with bruises; however, some patterns are more concerning than others (see Fig. 19.1). Accidental bruises are usually over the anterior surface of the body and most commonly over bony prominences, and it is very rare to have accidental bruises on ears, genitals, buttocks or soft surfaces. A forensic investigation of bruising includes bloods (FBE + UEC + LFT for proteins + calcium + coagulation studies ± an extended clotting profile ± autoimmune disease markers). Other causes of abnormal bruising in children include blood leukaemias, haemophilia, post-infectious vasculitis and idiopathic thrombocytopenic purpura.

Fractures in children can also occur accidentally, with the most common being young boys with upper extremity fractures. A bone scan and skeletal survey are recommended together in children less than 3 years to search for occult fractures. In children older than 3, bone scans would only provide additional evidence if healing fractures are suspected. Rib fractures in younger children are consistent with squeezing of a child, and rib fractures in kids less than 3 years old have a

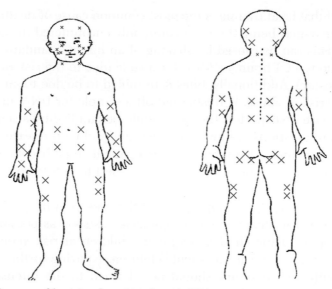

FIGURE 19.1 Pattern of bruising found in abused children.

Maguire S, 2008. Bruising as an indicator of child abuse: when should I be concerned? Paediatrics and Child Health 18(12), 545-549, Fig. 2.

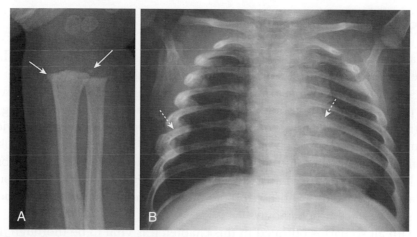

FIGURE 19.2 Radiographic examples of non-accidental injury.
Metaphyseal corner fractures (A) and several healing rib fractures (B) are annotated by the white arrows.

Reproduced from: Herring, W., Chapter 22: Recognising fractures and dislocations. In: Herring, W., Learning Radiology: Recognizing the basics, 2nd ed. Philadelphia: Mosby, Fig. 22.19, p. 234.

95% positive predictor value for NAI. Metaphyseal fractures, particularly in long bones in the absence of trauma, are always suspicious. Children with unusual fractures (see, for example, Fig. 19.2) should also have bloods performed (FBE + UEC + CMP + vitamin D ± TSH ± PTH ± copper ± CRP ± genetic testing for osteogenesis imperfecta). If a child presents with burns or scalds, consider performing a skeletal survey due to the incidence of multiple methods of abuse.

Be mindful that head trauma is the most common cause of death in NAI, with subdural haematomas being the most commonly encountered in the Emergency Department. This can be caused by shaking of an infant. Standard investigation in this scenario is a CT-brain, or MRI if available (due to the risk of unnecessary radiation exposure). Additionally, bites determined to be due to an adult human signify a high risk of abuse. If fresh, send off a sample for DNA analysis.

If sexual abuse is suspected, the case should be handled by a senior clinician. These tragic presentations are incredibly delicate, and require extensive training to conduct appropriately. If you begin to see a patient and it becomes evident that the case may involve a crime of this nature, it is best to excuse yourself and hand it over to a senior.

In addition to notifying the appropriate authorities, your hospital's social work service and paediatrics team should be contacted as soon as possible to provide additional support to the child as required. Children at risk should always be admitted for escalation of care, as should children requiring further medical care. Any infant with a head injury should be admitted to the intensive care unit overnight. Dealing with children who have been abused can be a very stressful situation and, if you feel you need help with strategies, you should contact the AMA, your HMO support unit or a senior member of your team, to put you in touch with appropriate support.

PHYSICAL ASSAULT IN AN ADULT

Physical assault is defined by Singh and Thoburn (in Physical assault, published by Elsevier FirstConsult in 2012) as: 'the intentional infliction of pain or injury by the means of brute force'. In this context, we are referring to people over the age of 18. Examples of intentional injuries include fractures, burns, bruising, other blunt trauma, penetrating wounds and bites. Although intimate partner violence is the most common situation you will encounter, be careful not to overlook elder abuse. Risk factors for domestic violence include increased disability, substance abuse, low socioeconomic status, low level of education, history of child abuse (in the attacker), psychiatric illness (in both attacker and/or victim), pregnancy and precedence of violent behaviour.

As with all scenarios outlined in this chapter, it is vital to be thorough in your history-taking, examination and documentation. As a junior doctor, you may encounter both victims and perpetrators of physical assault. Your primary role as the doctor remains true – regardless of whether your patient is the alleged attacker or victim (remember 'innocent until proven guilty') – you must identify injuries and risks and manage them as such before proceeding. This includes requesting the necessary investigations and making the appropriate referrals, e.g. to the Plastics service for lacerations or Orthopaedics for fractures. Sadly, some patients will be injured so severely they require Trauma input. Throughout your interaction with the patient it is important to remain supportive and sensitive. Occasionally, physical abuse will be more insidious, and dependent on the extent of injuries may not be detected until later in an admission. Beware the patient who presents multiple times with somatic complaints such as headache, functional gastro-intestinal dysfunction or chronic pain, as they can be indicators of a more deep-seated issue.

Documentation can be both written and photographic. Annotate the history from the patient and any witnesses to the alleged crime. Don't forget to take a medical and past history of unrelated conditions. Different departments will have varying procedures, but most will have a proforma for this situation that helps prevent you from missing vital information. Often, these forms have an anatomi-cally correct diagram of a human where you can circle and describe the injuries sustained by the patient. Other hospitals will have a dedicated clinical photogra-pher (if not, and you are asked to take clinical photographs on a hospital camera, you *must* obtain consent prior to taking the images). It is important everything is documented very clearly as, even if the victim chooses not to immediately press charges, they may in the future and the documentation you are completing now could completely change the outcome of their legal endeavours. You are gathering evidence that will be examined in-depth by the legal system and representation for both parties.

As with children, recurrence is frequent. Inquire about previous episodes. Ensure privacy, where possible. Offer to put the patient in touch with the psychia-try service. If the victim is a woman, most regional or metropolitan areas will have crisis centres (for those who do not require admission but need somewhere to go). If it is possible, interview the victim alone – even supportive family members can colour the responses given.

As a junior member of the emergency team it would be advisable to have a more senior member of the team see your patient with you. On examination, inspect for staged injuries of multiple ages, injuries to areas normally well pro-tected (such as eyes, genitals, perineum and buttocks), petechial lesions above the neck, lesions in the shape of objects, cigarette burns, rib fractures and complex skull fractures. If a bite mark is present, try and get a scrape for DNA (however unlikely it is that the perpetrator's DNA would be remaining on the victim's skin).

Investigations are usually limited to radiography of suspected fractures and routine bloods, but can be expanded as clinically indicated. If there is suspicion of an intracranial injury (even low), a CT- or MRI-brain would be warranted. In female trauma patients, a beta-HCG (human chorionic gonadotropin) should also be sent. Do not forget urinalysis (looking for blood, and again in women beta-HCG). If you suspect old, healing fractures, a bone scan could be of use. If there is thoracic trauma, an ECG should be performed in addition to X-ray. If the victim has an altered conscious state, toxicology and blood alcohol should also be sent. The differential diagnoses here include bleeding disorders, central nervous system disturbance, accidental trauma, vasculitis and osteomyelitis.

Your management of these patients should include appropriate analgesia, debridement and cleaning of any wounds (with antibiotics if indicated), booster immunisation for tetanus, definitive management of fractures, management of coexisting medical disorders and strong psychosocial support with referrals to the appropriate agencies in your area. Although difficult in the Emergency

Department, you should ensure the patient has an ongoing medical point of contact with a suitable plan for follow-up – this may involve calling their general practitioner yourself to confirm they have been informed of the situation. There is no mandatory reporting for physical assault of adults in Australia and it is at the discretion of the victim to press charges.

SEXUAL ASSAULT IN AN ADULT

Sexual assault is defined by Blok, O'Hanlon and Nikkanen (2012) as: 'any sex act undertaken by force, threat of bodily injury, or with the inability of the victim to give appropriate consent'. Victims may be male or female and of any age group, race or socioeconomic status. Two-thirds of these crimes are committed by people known to the victim, with 40% committed by intimate partners. It is common for the victim to experience a number of post-traumatic sequelae including depression, anxiety, headaches, sleep disturbance, anorexia, sexual dysfunction, suicidal ideation and somatoform disorder.

As with physical assault, the primary aim of treatment is to manage any life-threatening injuries first but, after the patient is stabilised, forensic examination should be completed before they can wash, defecate, urinate, eat or drink to mini-mise the loss of evidence. This should *never* be completed without consent. Once 72 hours have elapsed, a modified forensic examination of the pubic region should be completed (so that injuries can still be documented). The forensic examination must be completed by a physician with the appropriate training, unless there are extenuating circumstances and this doctor is not able to do so. In those situations, a sexual assault kit (which will be in most Emergency Departments) should be used by a senior doctor to collect evidence and perform the examination with a same-gender chaperone. Samples of all fluids should be collected, and the patient's clothes kept as evidence.

Investigations should include pregnancy and sexually-transmitted infection screening, toxicology (on serum and urinalysis) and imaging if indicated. Treat-ment is multi-pronged, aiming to provide psychosocial support through appropri-ate referrals and avoiding putting the patient back into a dangerous situation, preventing unwanted pregnancy and preventing contagion of infection. Any other injuries, such as lacerations, should also be managed appropriately. Sexually transmitted infection (STI) prophylaxis may be appropriate in adult patients. It is vital that a follow-up plan is devised before the patient leaves, as many of the STIs require repeat screening, the psychological effects of the assault are often delayed and good aftercare is strongly associated with better outcomes.

ROUTINE BLOOD ALCOHOL CONCENTRATION TESTING

Motor vehicle accidents (MVAs) represent a reasonably large proportion of patients seen in Emergency Departments. Although each state's laws surrounding this issue differ slightly, nationwide it is a law that all drivers of vehicles involved in a crash must have their serum blood alcohol concentration (BAC) taken – this includes those riding motorbikes, bicycles, marine vessels and horses(!). If there is doubt about who the driver of the vehicle was, a passenger may also be tested. Great care must be taken with the sample and it must be in the sight of the doctor who withdrew the blood at all times until it is handed over to the police – there is a precedent of clearly intoxicated drivers being found not guilty because the doctor broke the chain of evidence. Only a doctor may take the sample. The patient can refuse the BAC test, but if they do you must document it carefully and notify the police. Similarly, if the patient's behaviour prevents you from safely obtaining a sample, if blood sampling would delay proper care of the patient or if they have presented more than 12 hours after the accident, document this clearly in the notes.

In Victoria, for example, BAC packs are present in the emergency room that contain chlorhexidine skin wipes, blood-taking equipment, three blood tubes, three plastic bags and an information card to give to the patient. Do not use the hospital alcohol swabs to cleanse the area prior to venepuncture (for hopefully obvious reasons). Chlorhexidine swabs are provided in the police BAC pack. You must bleed the patient from a new site, rather than use an existing cannula. After you have filled the three tubes with blood, fill out the police book and use the provided labels for the tubes. Accuracy is vital as these documents are admissible in court. Of the three samples, two are put into a dedicated, locked police box, and the third is given to the patient for independent testing. Place the tubes in the locked box immediately as you can be asked if they were ever out of your sight. Ensure the patient has received their sample and information card, as the police sample is otherwise invalidated. Document clearly that all of the above has happened in the official hospital notes.

SECTION II

TABLE 20.1 Diseases notifiable to the Australian Department of Health—cont'd

	DISEASE	NOTES
Sexually-transmitted infections	Chlamydia	
	Chancroid	
	Gonorrhoea	
	Donovanosis	
	Syphilis (including congenital)	
	Human immunodeficiency virus (HIV)[c]	
Vaccine preventable disease	Diphtheria[a b]	
	Haemophilus influenzae (type b only)[b]	
	Influenza (lab-confirmed)	
	Measles[a b]	
	Mumps	
	Pertussis[c]	
	Pneumococcal disease (invasive)	
	Poliomyelitis[a]	
	Rubella (acquired or congenital)	
	Tetanus[c]	
	Varicella zoster (chickenpox OR shingles)	
Vector-borne illnesses	Arbovirus	
	Barmah Forest virus	
	Chikungunya	*Aedes* mosquito-borne
	Dengue[a b]	
	Japanese encephalitis virus[a]	
	Kunjin virus[a]	
	Malaria	
	Murray Valley encephalitis virus[a]	Notify if detected regardless of whether or not it is causing encephalitis
	Ross River virus	

TABLE 20.1 Diseases notifiable to the Australian Department of Health—cont'd

	DISEASE	NOTES
Zoonoses	Anthrax[a]	
	Australian bat lyssavirus[a]	Even potential exposures
	Brucellosis	
	Hendravirus[a]	
	Leptospirosis	
	Lyssaviruses	
	Ornithosis (a.k.a. psittacosis)	
	Q fever	
	Tularaemia[a]	
Miscellaneous	Legionellosis[a]	
	Leprosy	
	Meningococcal disease (active)[b]	
	Tuberculosis[b]	
	Acute flaccid paralysis[a c]	Has both infective and non-infective causes; report regardless
	Creutzfeldt–Jakob disease (and variant)[b]	
	Lead exposure	Serum lead >10 mcg/dL
	Non-tuberculous mycobacterial infections	
	All adverse reactions to vaccinations	
	Hand, foot and mouth disease	

[a]Requires immediate phone call to the local public health unit.
[b]Requires notification on provisional grounds, even if lab confirmation is pending.
[c]Requires notification once a clinical diagnosis is made.

Adapted from: Department of Health, 2014. Australian national notifiable diseases and case definitions [Internet]. Canberra: Department of Health. <http://www.health.gov.au/casedefinitions#list>.
Queensland Health, 2011. Communicable diseases control manual for clinicians [Internet]. Brisbane: Queensland Health. <http://www.health.qld.gov.au/ph/documents/cdb/19682.pdf>. Department of Health Victoria, 2014. Bluebook – infectious disease epidemiology & surveillance [Internet]. Melbourne: Department of Health Victoria. <http://ideas.health.vic.gov.au/bluebook.asp>.

TABLE 21.1 Examples of inpatient wards

WARD	DESCRIPTION
General ward	Mixture of medical and surgical wards with some wards dedicated to specialty fields Beds can include telemetry (constant cardiac monitoring)
Coronary/cardiac care	For patients considered at risk of serious cardiac events Standard for patients post acute coronary syndrome and cardiac intervention
Intensive care	For unstable patients with need for invasive circulatory monitoring, respiratory support and close observation

(ANUM) supports the NUM in each shift of nursing staff by facilitating the flow of patients through the ward, coordinating discharges of patients and preparing the ward for admissions, transfers and post elective procedure patients.

The junior doctor on the inpatient unit is the primary contact for the ward staff, and is required to coordinate with many hospital services to ensure patient care goals are being met. For example, speaking daily with physiotherapy staff regarding postoperative orthopaedic patients can highlight issues (such as pain control and persistent hypotension) that are preventing postoperative mobilisation and delaying patient progress. Communication on the inpatient ward is the key; make sure you keep yourself and your registrars informed.

Some hospitals use acute medical units (AMUs) or acute general surgical units (AGSUs) as a means to expedite admissions from ED. Typically, these patients are transferred to another inpatient team once a diagnosis and management plan has been determined. Keep the ANUMs informed regarding the transfer of these patients so that there is a clear understanding of which team is currently looking after any particular patient.

An inpatient's contemporary medical record is typically split between two folders:

1 the patient's bedside 'chart' containing the drug chart, observation chart, fluid orders and other specialised charts requested by the medical team (e.g. bowel chart, neurovascular observations chart)

2 the patient's 'notes' folder for medical, nursing and allied health staff to document the patient's progress.

Some health networks keep all patient paper work in the same folder, and some specialised wards such as ICU use different charts to record observations. It's important to remember what differences exist between the wards so that they can be easily identified during the ward round.

Most health networks use scanned medical records with paperwork from previous admissions scanned onto the hospital network, allowing the team to reference previous admissions, investigations and operations.

LIFE ON THE INPATIENT WARD

Prioritising the daily jobs is key to ensuring smooth running of the ward. Ordering investigations, making referrals to other inpatient teams and inpatient discharges are key priority areas during the morning. It can be difficult to predict the workload for the team in any given day due to new admissions and deterioration of current inpatients. As such the junior doctor should endeavour to pre-emptively complete any paperwork, referrals and new drug charts that may be otherwise put off until the next day. After the completion of morning ward tasks and if there are no clinic or theatre sessions, the team should focus on completing:

- discharge prescriptions for patients who are expected discharges in the coming days

- a preliminary discharge summary for all current patients, especially complex patients who have had ICU admissions, multiple procedures or significant complications

- outstanding discharge summaries from previous patients

- updates of weekly or regular audits of meetings on a daily basis to avoid the impact of any particular day becoming too busy to complete the audit (particularly for the work intensive X-ray meeting!).

If the junior doctor is expected to attend a morning clinic, the most essential tasks can be completed after the round. Discharge paperwork can be completed on the ward, then radiology requests handed in on the way to a clinic. Outpatient clinics are outfitted with computers and phones, allowing referrals and further discussion with radiology to be coordinated between clinic patients.

Pagers are widely used across health networks, allowing any staff member to send a short text-based message followed by a phone number for return call. Junior doctors also use the pager system to contact other medical teams in order to make referrals. Some hospital teams have portable hospital phones as opposed to pagers. The junior doctor is allocated a pager at the beginning of a rotation and is responsible for ensuring it remains in working condition. Nursing staff will primarily contact the junior doctor through the paging system with important patient progress updates and tasks.

A good method of keeping track of received pages is to transfer pages related to ward jobs straight to the ward round list. Any pages regarding calling the ward or clinic should be returned as soon as feasibly possible. A quick response to pages to ward staff demonstrates a positive working attitude aimed at resolving clinical problems as they arise. If you're busy, let the person paging you know to avoid duplicate pages. Unreturned pages for issues considered important might result in a call to your registrar or consultant!

COVER SHIFTS

'On-call' or 'cover shifts' are a large part of the junior doctor's roster. This cover shift can be an after-hours addition to your regular in-hours roster or a dedicated after-hours shift. Your 'cover' will likely involve providing medical support across multiple units, during which time you will be responsible for reviewing inpatients as requested, performing any ward tasks handed over from the 'in-hours' teams and admitting patients in conjunction with the on-call registrar or consultant.

If a patient during your cover shift begins to deteriorate (Chapter 25), has multiple MET calls or an emergency code call, you need to inform the senior doctor on call for that team, allowing for earlier input from the home team, especially with complex patients. Remember to document all your activity while on cover shifts, especially for procedures.

It's important to ensure that handover is received from each team. Although it should be the responsibility of the 'home' team to give a handover, it's wise to chase a handover when you're cover to ensure you're aware of any complex or problematic patients. At the conclusion of your cover shift it's equally important to give handover to the next team, particularly with respect to patient reviews or emergency codes.

CHAPTER 22

WARD ROUNDS

Paul Watson and Joseph M O'Brien

PREPARING FOR THE WARD ROUND

Preparation is the key to ensuring the ward round progresses smoothly. Ward rounds are common to both medical and surgical teams. Surgical teams begin their rounds earlier in the morning to accommodate finishing before the morning theatre lists. Despite the variation in how ward rounds are conducted between different units, the principles of effective and efficient ward rounds remain the same.

Every inpatient team will begin the day by 'rounding' on all of all their current inpatients at the bedside. During this time the patient's progress is reviewed and the management plan formulated. Typically, the ward round will consist of the interns, residents and registrars, but can also include:

- consultants and fellows, as either a routine post-admitting round or at a designated weekly time
- nurse unit managers (NUMs) or assistant nurse unit managers (ANUMs)
- allied health
- medical students.

Understanding what your team needs during the ward round is essential for preparation. If you're on a surgical round, new emergency and trauma admissions require consent forms, so ensure you have these pre-filled templates in your folder. Carry around sets of sterile scissors, sterile towels and gloves so dressings can be taken down during the round. If your team commonly performs neurological examinations during the round, keep a tendon hammer nearby. Having these necessary items means that the ward round is not interrupted to find paperwork or equipment.

Medical teams are increasingly using computers on wheels (affectionately referred to as 'COWs'), and you should understand how best to use these prior to your round. Turn on the computer prior to starting the round, and consider opening the relevant browser tabs, including serology, imaging and observations, in advance of being asked for them by your registrar or consultant. One advantage of COWs is the ability to order investigations and send pages from the patient's bedside.

Medical ward teams have post-take rounds where the team will present the previous day's admissions to their consultants. Junior doctors should take the opportunity to present their patients, aided by keeping a photocopy of the admission note and checking the most recent investigations. Being prepared and delivering a full presentation is a valuable opportunity to improve these skills and gain feedback.

Having a backup of required paperwork including inpatient progress is useful, especially if the patient's folder isn't available. The notes can be written on a loose-leaf sheet and added to the file later. Keep in mind that the patient's details should be written on the form to avoid confusion if multiple patients' notes are completed in this manner.

THE WARD LIST

The list contains the details of all current inpatients under the team along with any consult patients from other units (see Fig. 22.1). The list will need to be reviewed daily prior to the round to ensure it contains up-to-date information. Some units use word processor or spreadsheet templates for ward lists, while others use prints from hospital patient tracking software to give a printout of the current inpatients. Due to these variations, it's important that, during the handover for a new rotation, time is spent covering how to generate and modify the list of ward patients. These lists can be time-consuming to generate, particularly for teams with patient turnover. Updating as often as possible avoids the necessity of coming in early every morning to perform a long update.

Make a space on the bottom of the list: it's useful to add jobs for non-inpatients (e.g. organising imaging tests for outpatients). Some teams will have patients who are awaiting surgical procedures in the community (Orthopaedics and Plastics) and it's useful to keep an updated list of those patients with current contact information as they may be called for surgery at short notice (day before or morning of). Some teams will also appreciate a printout of the current bookings for emergency theatre as it allows for the team to check if the unit's patients have been booked, and determine what other priority cases are waiting to be done.

THE ROUND

The round itself should involve a thorough assessment of each patient, with particular focus on new undifferentiated admissions and unwell postoperative patients. Less thorough ward rounds have been associated with delayed diagnosis and preventable postoperative complications. The presence of allied health and nursing staff on modern ward rounds allows for expert, tailored input into a patient's progression. The physiotherapist can advise the team that a patient's mobilisation has been poor and is unlikely to improve without a subacute admission. The timing of the round allows input from the multidisciplinary team to stimulate discussion while the patient is present, promoting mutual goals for discharge planning.

Plastics Ward list 11/4/2014 - Capital City Hospital - If found please return to Front reception. Page #222 or #224

Bed	UR No.	Name	Age	Cons.	Diagnosis + Operations	Investigations	Management	Jobs
7W2B	002232	Reynolds, M	34M	ND	L) Hand Dogbite - 10/4 W/O - BJ/G/C + BS - OT planned 12/4 on PM List. PMHx: Nil	9/4: FBE: 145/11.5/332 UEC: 134/3.4/Cr:87/>90 CRP: 23.4 Wound Swab: Multiple leukocytes 10/4: FBE 140/13.5/288 CRP: 50.6 11/4: FBE: 141/13.2/298 CRP 77.1	Elevate Limb OT Tomorrow Continue IV Tazocin	Fast from EMB on 12/4 Chase Wound swab MCS
7W2D	334223	Washburne, Z	65F	RN	R) Mastectomy + Axil Clearance + DIEP flap 10/4 - Joint with Surg 2 PMHx: R Breast Ca. IDC.	10/4: FBE: 123/15.2/280 CRP: 19.4 11/4: FBE: 109/13.2/276 CRP: 41.0	Flap obs Monitor DT output Gen surg to follow-up Histopath	Physio review
7W5	433553	Serra, I	29F	ORTH (AM)	R) Thigh Haematoma - Evacuation and W/O 8/4 - Drain out 10/4 PMHx: R Femoral IM Nail 6/4 from MVA	9/4: FBE: 145/10.3/332 UEC: 134/3.4/Cr:87/>90 CRP: 23.4 10/4: FBE: 143.9/288 UEC: 135/4.4/Cr105/<90 CRP: 40.3 11/4: FBE: 129/10.2/298 CRP 37.5	Review WED	
4E1A	433455	Cobb, J	45M	RF	L) Shin Wound Breakdown - SSG 9/4. PMHx: HTN, Obesity, T2DM	10/4: FBE 129/7.6/300 UEC: 135/4.2/Cr130/45	2/7 RIB then toilet privileges Dressing down 14/4	Endo
3W14A	555464	Frye, K	67F	RF	R) Index/Middle/Ring detip. from dropsaw - W/O and debridement + Island flap to Index with SSG coverage 10/4		Leave dressing intact until wound clinic appointment	D/C with Wound OP appointment
ED - B6	004340	Tam, R	88F	RF	R Hand skin tear			

FIGURE 22.1 Typical ward list.

When at the bedside the patient's observations should be checked, looking for any particular trends that might warrant further investigation. If there are medical students attached to the unit they can assist in locating the charts and reading out the latest observations while the junior doctor is writing the ward note. Collaboration leads to a more efficient ward round. It's also essential to check progress notes from the the previous 24 hours to determine if the patient has had any urgent reviews/MET calls, input from other medical teams and allied health progress.

The ward round represents the only time during the day that the patient gets to speak directly to the entire medical team and this short window of time may only last several minutes. To the medical team the patient is one on a (potentially) long list to be efficiently checked off in order to attend to other urgent clinical matters such as theatre and clinic. To the patient these few minutes offer what might be the only chance for an update on their progress for the next 24 hours. A rushed and inattentive patient review leads to miscommunication and patient frustration. An extra 5 minutes speaking to a flustered patient saves a much longer conversation later in the day when a lack of information feeds a patient's doubt and unease regarding their clinical situation.

WARD ROUND NOTES

The role of the junior doctor on the ward round is to document in the patient's notes. Although there is no true standardised method of documentation, the ward notes must contain the following information as a minimum:

- date and time
- name of the team and the medical staff present (on consultant ward rounds list every consultant present)
- title of the ward round with the two most senior team members' surnames at the top (e.g. 'Medical CWR – Stark/Rogers et al.')
- patient's responses to direct questions regarding progress
- patient's observations (often kept in a separate bedside chart), including drain outputs, daily weights and abnormal findings
- examination findings
- management plan
  - any discussion regarding treatment plan should be documented, especially when a new treatment option and associated risks are explained to the patient.

Poor patient documentation leads to confusion regarding patient progress, particularly with the timeline of the management plan when making referrals or during emergency calls. When writing ward notes it is important to be mindful that any medical, nursing and allied health staff member who subsequently reviews the file should easily understand them.

The notes in Fig. 22.2 are an example of poor documentation, because there is:

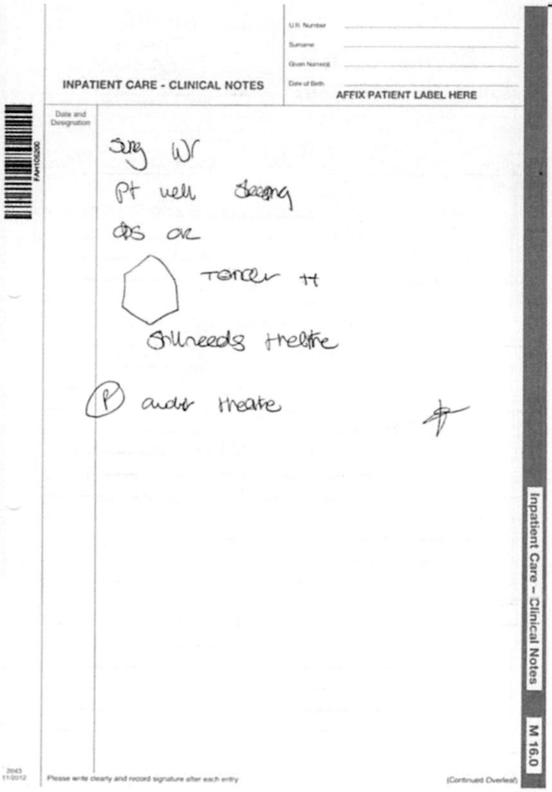
INPATIENT CARE - CLINICAL NOTES

U.R. Number
Surname
Given Name(s)
Date of Birth
AFFIX PATIENT LABEL HERE

Date and Designation

Surg WR
Pt well sleeping
obs ok
Tender ++
Still needs theatre
(P) under theatre

Inpatient Care – Clinical Notes
M 16.0

Please write clearly and record signature after each entry
(Continued Overleaf)

FIGURE 22.2 An example of poor inpatient ward notes.

- no date or time listed
- unclear identification of rounding team and no pager number on signoff.
- disorganised and illegible annotation with an unclear representation of examination findings
- a vague and unspecific plan.

Although there is no 'right way' to document ward round notes, two common methods can help give a consistent structure. This is particularly helpful when reviewing the patient's notes during the discharge summary.

Issue-based documentation

For complex patients with multiple active issues, most medical specialties prefer an issue-based list that separates the patient's progress under individual subheadings. The examination findings and plan are then documented under separate headings.

The notes in Fig. 22.3 outline the current issues and then proceed to discuss examination findings and the management plan in a clear, logical order.

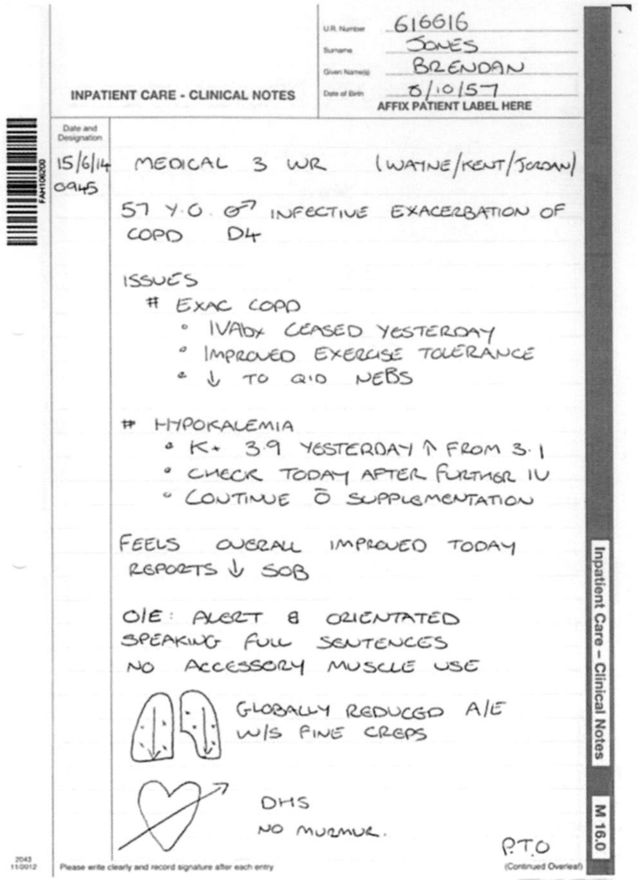
INPATIENT CARE - CLINICAL NOTES

U.R. Number 616616
Surname JONES
Given Name(s) BRENDAN
Date of Birth 6/10/57
AFFIX PATIENT LABEL HERE

Date and Designation

15/6/14 0945 MEDICAL 3 WR (WAYNE/KENT/JORDAN)

57 Y.O. ♂ INFECTIVE EXACERBATION OF COPD D4

ISSUES
EXAC COPD
- IVAbx CEASED YESTERDAY
- IMPROVED EXERCISE TOLERANCE
- ↓ TO QID NEBS

HYPOKALEMIA
- K+ 3.9 YESTERDAY ↑ FROM 3.1
- CHECK TODAY AFTER FURTHER IV
- CONTINUE c̄ SUPPLEMENTATION

FEELS OVERALL IMPROVED TODAY
REPORTS ↓ SOB

O/E: ALERT & ORIENTATED
SPEAKING FULL SENTENCES
NO ACCESSORY MUSCLE USE

GLOBALLY REDUCED A/E
W/S FINE CREPS

DHS
NO MURMUR.

P.T.O
(Continued Overleaf)

Please write clearly and record signature after each entry

Inpatient Care – Clinical Notes M 16.0

FIGURE 22.3 Issue-based ward notes.

'SOAP' notes

This structure mnemonic, '**s**ubjective, **o**bjective, **a**ssessment, **p**lan', is used for shorter, single-issue ward patients:

- *subjective*: patient reported progress (i.e. what the patient tells you – 'feels well'")
- *objective*: examination findings (i.e. what you observe of the patient – 'looks well')
- *assessment*: impression of the patient's clinical progress
- *plan*.

The SOAP notes in Fig. 22.4 are from a consultant ward round, denoted by CWR (note that the C can be substituted with an 'F' for fellow or 'R' for registrar), with the consultant's name underlined. Assessment and management notes clearly document the discharge plan and follow-up for patients. In most hospital networks the nursing staff will liaise with ward clerks to book outpatient appointments.

SECTION III

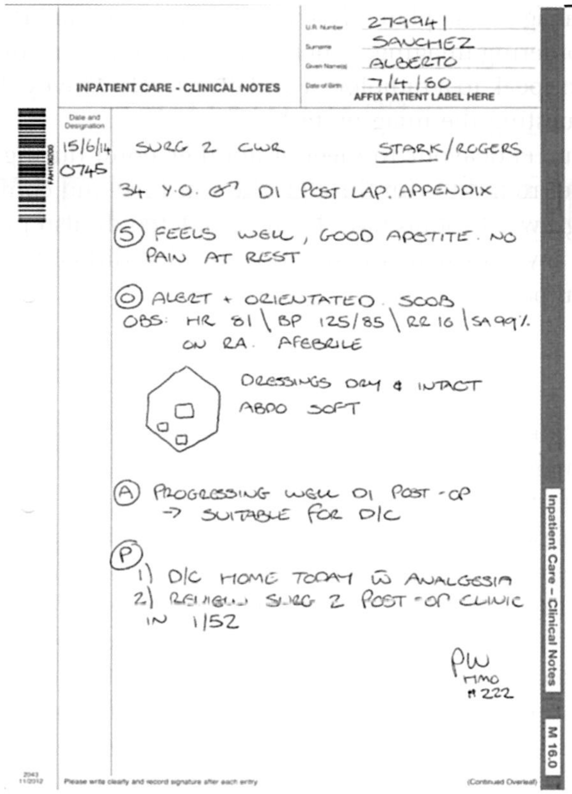

INPATIENT CARE - CLINICAL NOTES

U.R. Number 279941
Surname SANCHEZ
Given Name(s) ALBERTO
Date of Birth 7/4/80
AFFIX PATIENT LABEL HERE

Date and Designation

15/6/14 0745 SURG 2 CWR STARK/ROGERS

34 Y.O. ♂ D1 POST LAP. APPENDIX

(S) FEELS WELL, GOOD APETITE. NO PAIN AT REST

(O) ALERT + ORIENTATED. SCOB
OBS: HR 81 \ BP 125/85 \ RR 16 \ SA 99%
ON RA. AFEBRILE

DRESSINGS DRY & INTACT
ABDO SOFT

(A) PROGRESSING WELL D1 POST-OP
→ SUITABLE FOR D/C

(P)
1) D/C HOME TODAY ω ANALGESIA
2) REVIEW SURG 2 POST-OP CLINIC IN 1/52

PW
HMO
#222

Please write clearly and record signature after each entry

(Continued Overleaf)

Inpatient Care – Clinical Notes

M 16.0

FIGURE 22.4 SOAP ward notes.

At the completion of any documentation, the junior doctor must sign below the notes and provide their pager number for any staff member who may need to clarify the daily management plan with you. It is common for medical students to practice writing in the inpatient notes, but the team is ultimately responsible for ensuring that the information is accurate and therefore supervision and countersigning of the notes by an intern or registrar is essential.

If a NUM or ANUM did not round with the team or if you have completed a round in a ward where the team does not normally have patients, it is advisable to give an update to the nurse in charge regarding the progress and management plan. This gives an opportunity to clarify any specific management points, preventing delay in implementation.

AFTER THE WARD ROUND

During the round the junior doctors should note all the new jobs from the management plan and any task requested of the nursing staff (such as cannulas or paperwork) on their ward list. Following the round, the team should meet to perform a 'paper round' by reading through their list and dividing the jobs between the junior doctors, clarifying any unclear management points. If you're

BOX 23.1 Risk factors for medication-related harm developed by The Society of Hospital Pharmacists of Australia

- Age 65 years and older
- Currently taking five or more regular medications
- Taking more than 12 doses of medication per day
- Significant changes made to medication treatment regimen in the past 3 months
- Medication with a narrow therapeutic index or medications requiring therapeutic monitoring
- Sub-optimal response to treatment with medicines
- Suspected non-compliance or inability to manage medication-related therapeutic devices
- Patients having difficulty managing their own medicines because of literacy or language difficulties, dexterity problems or impaired sight, confusion/dementia or other cognitive difficulties
- Patients attending a number of different doctors, both general practitioners and specialists
- Recent discharge from a facility/hospital (in the past 4 weeks)

Adapted from: The Society of Hospital Pharmacists of Australia, 2015. Risk factors for medication related problems. <https://www.shpa.org.au/sites/default/files/uploaded-content/website-content/Fact-sheets-position-statements/shpa_fact_sheet_risk_factors_for_medication_related_problems_june_2015.pdf>.

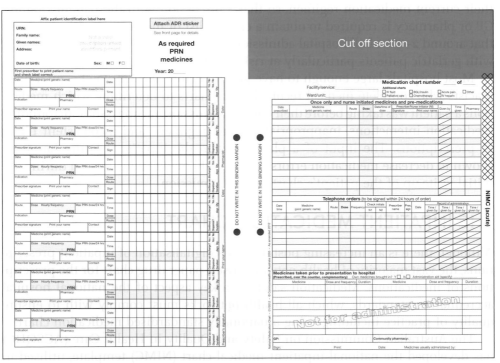

FIGURE 23.1 The cover of the NIMC standardised inpatient drug chart.

Australian Commission on Safety and Quality in Health Care, 2012. National inpatient medication chart [Internet]. Sydney: ACSQHC. <http://www.safetyandquality.gov.au/publications/national-inpatient-medication-chart-2011-for-acute-care/>.

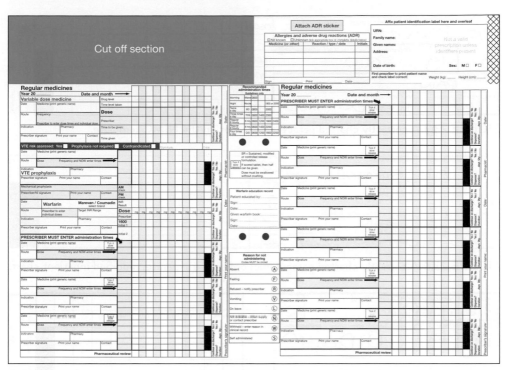

FIGURE 23.2 The inside of the NIMC standardised inpatient drug chart.

Australian Commission on Safety and Quality in Health Care, 2012. National inpatient medication chart [Internet]. Sydney: ACSQHC. <http://www.safetyandquality.gov.au/publications/national-inpatient-medication-chart-2011-for-acute-care/>.

The NIMC is designed to give instructions to prescribers in order to encourage accurate and standardised prescribing. The charts are sometimes modified to include VTE prophylaxis guidelines on the front cover or summarise acceptable usage and notations on the back cover.

The core of the NIMC standardisation lies in the individual order sections. This template is somewhat modified by each health network before being distributed to the inpatient wards; however, the layout of the key aspects of this order does not vary as demonstrated in Figs 23.3 and 23.4.

A correctly filled order clearly states:

- Generic name of medication
- date of commencement
- route of administration
- dose and frequency including administration times
- indication for use to assist the pharmacist and other health practitioners rationalise a patient's medication usage
- legible signature and contact information.

SECTION III

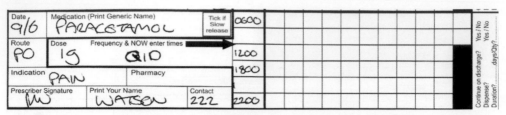

FIGURE 23.3 A correctly charted paracetamol order on the NIMC template.

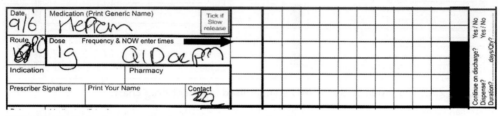

FIGURE 23.4 A correctly charted paracetamol order on a separate, modified inpatient chart.

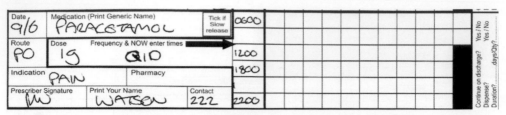

FIGURE 23.5 An incorrectly charted paracetamol order.

Fig. 23.5 shows an incorrectly charted order:

- The order is illegible.
- It refers to a brand name 'Herron' as opposed to the generic term paracetamol.
- This medication section is for strictly regular prescriptions. PRN orders are to be listed in the appropriate section.
- The prescriber has attempted to re-write the route of administration, but has done so clumsily.
- The order is unsigned and the contact details are unclear.

Use of decimal places in orders needs to be particularly clear. As demonstrated in Figs 23.6 and 23.7, the distance between the two numbers should be sufficient to leave an isolated decimal place well clear of the numbers to ensure it is not obscured.

Some medications have a variable dosage course, commonly seen with oral steroid therapy for exacerbation of lung disease (see Fig. 23.8). This section is also useful for medications with a narrow therapeutic window that requires regular monitoring of serum levels, such as gentamicin.

The NIMC also has a separate section for *'pro re nata'* (PRN, Latin for 'as needed') medications that can be requested by the patient and given by the nursing staff within the parameters of the documented order (see Fig. 23.9).

Date 9/6
Medication (Print Generic Name) METOPROLOL
Tick if Slow release
Route PO
Dose 125mg
Frequency & NOW enter times BD
0800
2000
Indication IHD
Pharmacy
Prescriber Signature PW
Print Your Name WATSON
Contact 222
Continue on discharge? Yes / No
Dispense? Yes / No
Duration? ....days/Qty?........

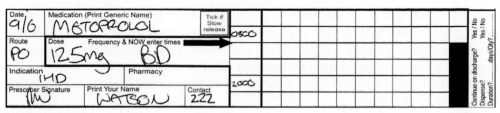

FIGURE 23.6 A metoprolol prescription dose with an unclear decimal place.

Date 9/6
Medication (Print Generic Name) METOPROLOL
Tick if Slow release
Route PO
Dose 12·5mg
Frequency & NOW enter times BD
0800
2000
Indication IHD
Pharmacy
Prescriber Signature PW
Print Your Name WATSON
Contact 222
Continue on discharge? Yes / No
Dispense? Yes / No
Duration? ....days/Qty?........

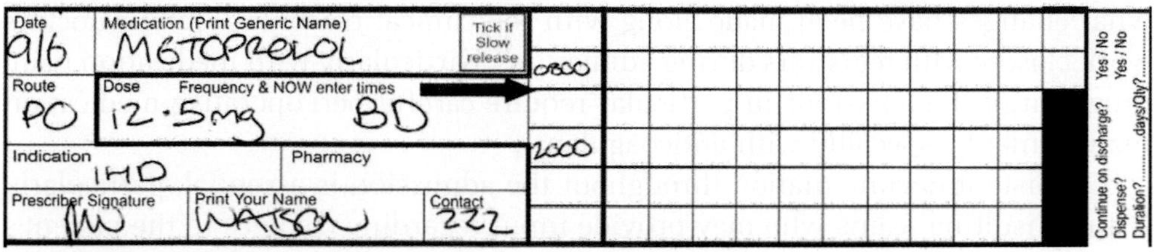

FIGURE 23.7 A metoprolol prescription clearly identifying the decimal point.

REGULAR MEDICATIONS
YEAR 20 15 DATE & MONTH → 9/6 10/6 11/6 12/6 13/6 14/6 15/6
VARIABLE DOSE MEDICATION
Date 9/6
Medication (Print Generic Name) PREDNISOLONE
Route PO
Frequency DAILY
Dr to enter dose times and individual dose
Time of Dose: 0800
Drug level
Time level taken
Dose 25 mg 25 mg 25 mg 12.5 mg 12.5 mg 12.5 mg 10 mg
Prescriber PW PW PW PW PW PW PW
Time given
Nurse
Indication COPD
Pharmacy
Prescriber Signature PW
Print Your Name WATSON
Contact 222
Continue on discharge? Yes / No
Dispense? Yes / No
Duration: ....days Qty:........

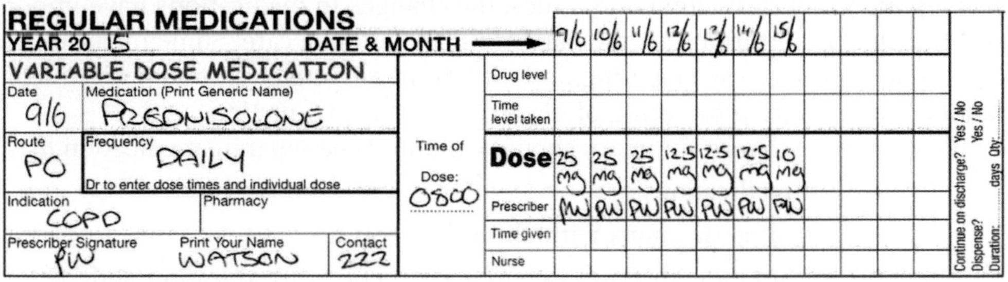

FIGURE 23.8 An example of a prescription for a variable dose medication.

Date 9/6
Medication (Print Generic Name) METOCLOPRAMIDE
Route PO
Dose 10mg
Hourly frequency TDS
PRN
Max dose/24 hrs 30mg
Indication NAUSEA
Pharmacy
Prescriber Signature PW
Print Your Name WATSON
Contact 222
Date
Time
Dose
Route
Sign

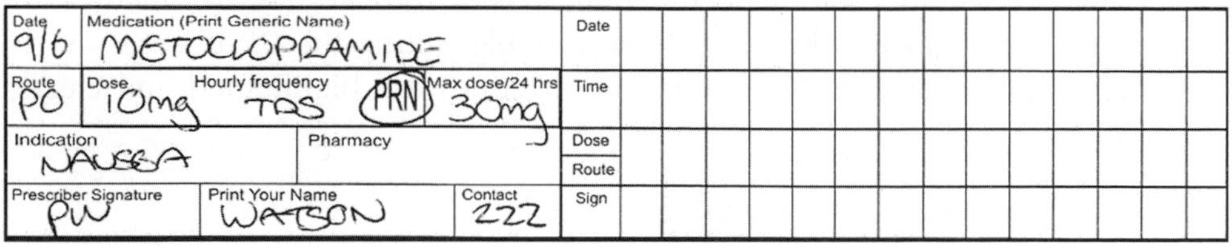

FIGURE 23.9 A PRN order for antiemetic medication.

These medication orders are typically used to treat symptoms such as pain and nausea; however, they can include medications that patients use as required in the community, such as glyceryl trinitrate (GTN) for angina. These orders must specify a maximum dose within a 24-hour period to avoid potential overdose and alert the team that a patient's symptoms (e.g. pain, nausea) have not been sufficiently alleviated by the current regimen and require review.

ADMISSION AND DISCHARGE MEDICATIONS

The admitting team is ultimately responsible for ensuring the patient's regular medications are correctly charted. Patients may present with a current list of their medications, although this is often not the case. If a patient is unsure of the correct dose of a particular drug, clarification should be sought from the patient's primary prescriber (typically their GP) or pharmacy. The inpatient pharmacist will generate a medication summary as part of the admission episode, highlighting potential harmful pharmacological interactions and determining if there are any missing regular medications. Pharmacists also play an important role in checking discharge prescriptions (Chapter 31).

Changes or additions to the patient's medications are an important aspect of the admission paperwork. It must be clear to anyone reading an admission note what changes have been made along with the clinical reasoning. Junior doctors work closely with registrars during admissions, particularly with medication planning. Surgical admissions in particular require careful peri-operative medication management, especially with anticoagulants.

Consistent documentation throughout the admission is essential, particularly with consulting teams who may provide input regarding changes to the patient's pre-admission medications. This documentation forms the basis of generating the patient's discharge summary. Though GPs are interested in gaining an overview of the patient's overall admission issues, the changes to medications have important practical implications for the patient's postoperative care. Some medications such as steroids require a tapering dose or temporary analgesia, and newer medications may require monitoring of electrolytes or liver function.

Ideally, the discharge summary should contain three separate medication lists:

1 admission medications

2 discontinued medications with clinical reasoning

3 new medications with post-discharge instructions for duration and required follow-up.

A clear focus on medication documentation is the best strategy for medication safety. The junior doctor should feel comfortable calling the GP if necessary to ensure that important discharge medication issues are highlighted and clearly understood.

HIGH RISK MEDICATIONS

All medications carry some risk of side effects and interactions; however, several classes of medications have been highlighted as having capacity to do great harm to patients if improperly prescribed. The ACSQHC recommends the identification of the following groups of medications for close review as part of a hospital's adherence to the medication safety standards, APINCH:

A – anti-infectives

P – potassium and other electrolytes (Chapter 24)

I – insulin

N – narcotics (opioids) and other sedatives

C – chemotherapy

H – heparin and other anticoagulants.

These medications have the potential to cause serious adverse drug reactions (ADRs) when inappropriately prescribed. They also form interesting discussion points for this chapter as they represent some of the more commonly prescribed medications for the junior doctor.

Anti-infectives

Anti-infective medications are mostly temporary medications predominantly used for two reasons:

1 prophylactically to reduce the risk of infection
2 active treatment of infection.

Prophylactic use of anti-infectives is more common in the surgical setting, providing coverage from native flora during clean-contaminated procedures. Cephazolin, a common prophylactic agent, for example, is given 15–30 minutes prior to commencement of the case.

The overarching principles of treating an active infection include:

- identification of a patient with an infective illness
- differential diagnosis based on the patient's presenting history and examination plus early investigative tests (samples taken from suspected source(s) of infection)
- empirical treatment based on predicted source(s) of infection
- identification of the pathogenic organism(s)
- narrow, targeted anti-infective treatment(s).

The latter two points require ongoing checking of pending pathological tests by the treating team. For patients with severe systemic infection requiring the use of restricted anti-infectives and ongoing review, a referral to the infectious diseases (ID) team is prudent to provide treatment advice and gain approval numbers for medications.

Some patients will require ongoing oral anti-infective treatment post-discharge for severe or deep tissue infections. Advice from the ID team will guide management; however, the junior doctor of the treating team will have to gain PBS approval for prescription of the medication upon discharge for the patient.

Dosing of anti-infectives typically follows set guidelines based on a number of disease and patient factors. There are a number of medications that require careful monitoring due their narrow therapeutic window, with two common antibiotics in particular worth discussing.

Gentamicin dosing

Gentamicin provides excellent Gram-negative coverage, commonly used in the surgical setting for prophylaxis, and is still considered top-line therapy for patients with suspected Gram-negative sepsis. However, it is a medication with known nephrotoxic (and ototoxic) side effects at excessive dosages. As such, patients on gentamicin will need serum levels performed to monitor for toxicity.

Gentamicin levels are taken twice after the administration of the dose, typically at 5 minutes, then at 6–8 hours. This information is then used by the pharmacy department to determine if the dose lies under the adequate area of concentration curve (AUC) and subsequently determines the next dose. This principle is used for other aminoglycosides, although a pre-dose level is taken for greater than daily dosing.

For use of gentamicin as a targeted therapy most hospital policies require that the patient's case be discussed with the ID team (Chapter 41).

Vancomycin dosing

Vancomycin is widely used in prophylactic, empirical and targeted therapy settings. Notably, it is used in the targeted treatment of multi-resistant *Staphylococcus aureus*. Vancomycin can be given as an intermittent dose or as a continuous 24-hour infusion, with the former being more common on the ward. The initial dosage and timing of serum level checks are dependent on the patient's baseline renal function.

The 'normal range' of trough level ranges as reported by the pathology department may vary among different service providers; however, the therapeutic guidelines recommend a trough level between 15 and 20 mg/kg. Based on these trough levels the dosage can be reviewed and modified as required. The Pharmacy Department can provide assistance in determining the correct dosage.

Insulin and blood glucose levels

Management of a patient's insulin dosages and regimens presents a variety of challenges for the junior doctor. For any patient with diabetes admitted to hospital there is a potential for large fluctuations in their blood glucose levels (BGLs), particularly with respect to those patients who have electrolyte disturbances, infections and changes in diet due to fasting or injury. Some patients are admitted to hospital for issues primarily related to their diabetes and blood glucose level control; those with severe persistent hypo- or hyperglycaemia are prone to neurological, acid–base and fluid status changes that require expert review by the endocrinology team (Chapter 39). The following discussion relates to the management of abnormal BGLs in diabetic patients who are otherwise well.

Insulin formulations are classified by their onset of action (see Fig. 23.10).

Patients with type 1 diabetes have long-acting basal insulin as a minimum, typically in combination with multiple short acting doses around meal times, known as a basal–bolus regimen. The use of intermediate insulin formulations is limited in type 1. Patients with type 2 diabetes require careful consideration before insulin therapy is commenced; as such the individual patient factors are involved in deciding what insulin therapy regimen is used in combination with oral diabetic agents.

Patients with known diabetes undergo regular BGL readings as part of their routine observations. Any abnormal BGL reading will be reported to the junior

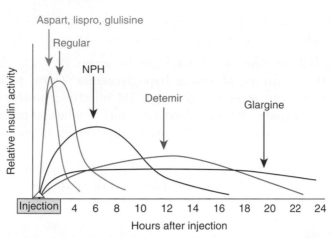

FIGURE 23.10 Onset and duration of action of multiple insulin formulations.

Reproduced from: Meadows, R.Y., 2015. Optimal glycemic control in hospitalized patients. Hospital Medicine Clinics 4(4), 471-488, Fig. 5.

Date 9/6	Medication (Print Generic Name) INSULIN GLARGINE	Tick if Slow release	0800									Continue on discharge? Yes / No Dispense? Yes / No Duration? ....days/Qty?
Route S/C	Dose 28 UNITS	Frequency & NOW enter times MANE										
Indication TZDM		Pharmacy										
Prescriber Signature PW	Print Your Name WATSON	Contact 222										

FIGURE 23.11 An insulin prescription with the dose clearly stated in units.

doctor of the treating team. Initiating or making ongoing alterations to regular insulin regimens in patients with diabetes is best done with advice from a medical or endocrinology registrar.

Predominantly the junior doctor has two tasks related to insulin medications: charting regular insulin therapy and giving temporary insulin orders for patients with elevated BGLs. Any orders for insulin should clearly identify the dose with the word 'UNITS' stated in full. Abbreviating with a 'U' is often confused with a zero (see Fig. 23.11).

Hypoglycaemia

Patients who are conscious, non-confused and able to 'self-treat' (i.e. able to have oral intake) with hypoglycaemia should have oral glucose replacement. Nursing staff will typically initiate these measures in patients, especially for known diabetic patients. Those patients usually are given a combination of high GI and low GI carbohydrates including:

- glucose tablets or paste
- jellybeans
- fruit juice

- fruit
- sandwiches.

Patients unable to have oral intake can be given IV 50% glucose 20 mL, also used in the treatment of severe hypoglycaemia. Those patients who do not have IV access can receive a glucagon IM injection; however, this option requires sufficient hepatic stores of glycogen, which can be compromised in those patients who present with hypoglycaemia in the context of prolonged ethanol intoxication.

When the patient's BGLs have stabilised the underlying cause of the episode will need to be investigated with an exploration of strategies to combat future episodes.

Hyperglycaemia

Hyperglycaemia is a common occurrence on the medical wards, particularly with patients who have recently suffered myocardial infarction and stroke. Persistent hyperglycaemia in these patients is associated with poor outcomes; therefore, these patients require close BGL monitoring and inpatient endocrine input review. It's also imperative that these unstable patients are not put at risk of hypoglycaemic episodes from overuse of supplemental insulin.

For patients who are not critically ill and those with steroid-induced hyperglycaemia, the use of 'sliding scale' insulin is not recommended. Instead, review the patient's current insulin regimen and make appropriate amendments. For patients not currently on insulin, initiation of a basal–bolus combination (provided the patient has sufficient oral intake) has been suggested as a viable treatment option, helping to prevent high-low BGL fluctuations.

'Narcotics' and other analgesia

Opiate-based analgesia is commonly used in the inpatient ward. Although more typically associated with use in the post-procedural acute pain setting, patients can present with complex chronic pain histories, which may include the long-term use of opiate medication.

A detailed history of previous opiate exposure and usage can give an insight into how well a patient's baseline pain levels are controlled and give insight into potential opiate tolerance. In the setting of acute on chronic pain, the primary goal is to provide sufficient analgesic coverage with medication rationalisation once the patient is comfortable, with an aim of preventing withdrawal. Patients with chronic pain admitted to hospital require prudent and accurate charting of their regular analgesia medication. The management of postoperative pain is discussed elsewhere (Chapter 30), including the use of other analgesic medications.

Some of the commonly used opiate medications are listed in Appendix 1. Each medication has the potential for side effects, which commonly include nausea, vomiting and, in ongoing use, constipation. As such every patient charted for opioid analgesia should have anti-emetic and laxative medication charted as PRN. Even so, some patients may not tolerate a particular opiate medication and an alternative should be used.

Short-acting and long-acting opiate medications can be used in combination with one another to achieve effective pain relief. IV preparations of these medications are commonly used in patient controlled analgesia (PCA) infusions. PCAs are initiated with input from the anaesthetic team and reviewed daily by the acute pain team. Hospital policies regarding these infusions include specific instructions regarding escalation of patient review in the event of decreased respiratory effort or increasing sedation (Chapter 30).

When prescribing opiate-based analgesia, it's important to specify:

- the range of dose, frequency and maximum daily dose clearly for PRN orders
- whether the medication is immediate release or a slow release formulation
- the correct setting and appropriate route of administration (PRN IV opiates are not permitted outside of critical care settings in most health networks).

Chemotherapy

Charting new chemotherapy agents is performed by specialist oncology services. Patients who are admitted to hospital may be taking oral chemotherapy agents that will need to be charted with their regular medications.

The most common example is methotrexate. A completed order (see Fig. 23.12):

- clearly indicates a weekly dose including day of week
- blocks out on the recording chart all other days of week to prevent inadvertent administration
- commonly pairs methotrexate with a folic acid regimen given on every day other than the day of methotrexate.

Junior doctors should be aware of potential side effects of methotrexate including nausea, vomiting, cough and shortness of breath.

Venous thromboprophylaxis

Antithrombotic therapies are widely used in all patient settings in a range of acute, chronic and prophylactic contexts. The common practical aspect of prescribing antithrombotic therapies for the junior doctor is venous thromboembolism (VTE) prophylaxis.

VTE refers to both deep vein thrombosis (DVT) and pulmonary embolus (PE). The specific management of these conditions is discussed in Chapter 35; however,

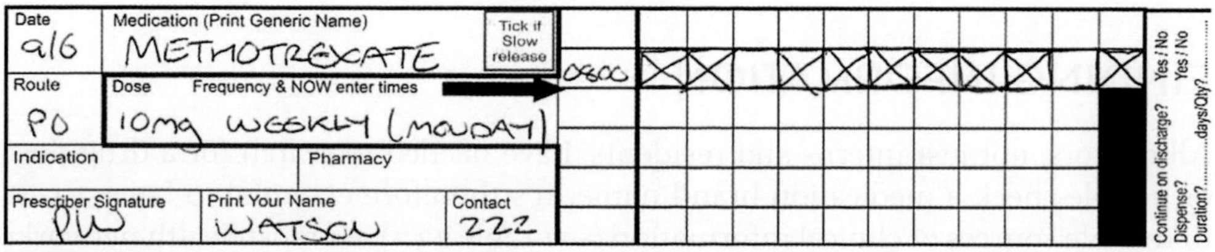
Date
9/6
Medication (Print Generic Name)
METHOTREXATE
Tick if Slow release
Route
PO
Dose Frequency & NOW enter times
10mg WEEKLY (MONDAY)
0800
Indication
Pharmacy
Prescriber Signature
DW
Print Your Name
WATSON
Contact
222
Continue on discharge? Yes / No
Dispense? Yes / No
Duration?........days/Qty?........

FIGURE 23.12 A completed methotrexate order.

it's worth considering at this point that over 30,000 admissions a year are due to VTE, with many considered preventable. There are multiple considerations involved in deciding whether a patient requires VTE prophylaxis, as follows:

- Individual patient risk factors:
  - age
  - obesity
  - smoking history
  - previous VTE
  - family history
  - thrombophilia
- Surgical procedures:
  - lower limb and pelvic surgery
- Disease factors:
  - acute cardiac disease
  - active infection
  - active malignancy.

Hospitals will typically develop their own VTE pathways for the use of prophylaxis. It's worth checking the hospital policy document when using these agents. Surgical teams, orthopaedics in particular, use extended courses of VTE prophylaxis due to the increased risk of VTE following elective arthroplasty. There are two approaches to prophylaxis:

1 pharmacological prophylaxis:
   a most commonly unfractionated heparin (UFH) and low molecular weight heparin (LMWH) such as enoxaparin (requires adjusted prophylactic dose when eGFR is less than 30)
   b in patients who have had intracranial or GI bleeding pharmacological prophylaxis needs to be carefully balanced against the ongoing risk of bleeding; seek expert opinion in this scenario
2 mechanical prophylaxis:
   a graduated compression stockings
   b intermittent pneumatic foot pump devices.

Orders for VTE prophylaxis have a separate order section on the inpatient medical chart (see Fig. 23.13).

FINDING INFORMATION

All doctors, not just interns and residents, have needed to search for a drug dose or double-check a medication brand name. It's therefore essential to have access to reliable sources of clinical information (see Table 23.1). As most health networks

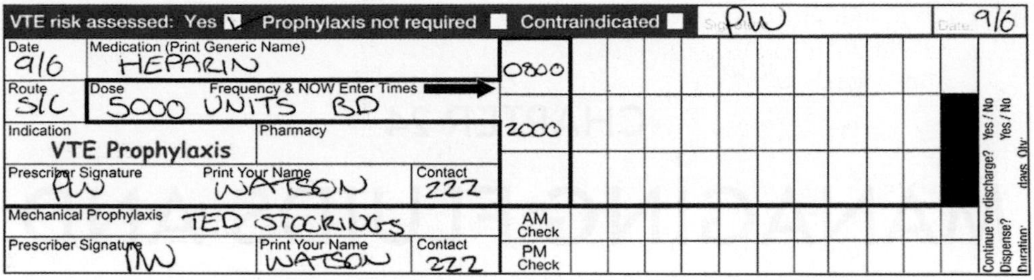
VTE risk assessed: Yes Prophylaxis not required Contraindicated Signature PW Date 9/6
Date 9/6
Medication (Print Generic Name) HEPARIN
Route S/C
Dose 5000 UNITS
Frequency & NOW Enter Times BD
0800
2000
Indication VTE Prophylaxis
Pharmacy
Prescriber Signature PW
Print Your Name WATSON
Contact 222
Mechanical Prophylaxis TED STOCKINGS
Prescriber Signature PW
Print Your Name WATSON
Contact 222
AM Check
PM Check
Continue on discharge? Yes / No
Dispense? Yes / No
Duration: days Qty:

FIGURE 23.13 A completed VTE prophylaxis prescription order.

TABLE 23.1 Sources of clinical information for medication doses and indications

CLINICAL INFORMATION SOURCE	DESCRIPTION
Australian Medicines Handbook (AMH)	Developed with the RACGP, this resource provides evidence-based fact sheets covering medications and therapies
Electronic *Therapeutic Guidelines* (eTG)	This resource compiles therapies across multiple medical specialties to give advice on initial, continuing and second-line therapies
Monthly Index of Medical Specialties (MIMS)	This resource gives information regarding medications including product information and pill identification
Hospital policy documents	All hospitals generate policy documents regarding the approach and management of specific individual clinical scenarios These resources provide guidelines for therapeutic medication options

support specialist training and some level of research there is typically a vast array of applications available designed to assist clinicians and students find clinical information as easily as possible. Individual hospitals also develop policies regarding clinical practice that serve as guidelines for staff based on current literature and input from expert hospital staff.

CHAPTER 24

MANAGING FLUIDS AND INFUSIONS

Joseph M O'Brien

Prescribing fluids will likely be a new task for most junior doctors. As students you are told never to write on the fluid orders – and with good reason. In improperly trained hands, the fluid order can be a licence to kill. Ordering fluids should be done with great care, but it is not something that should necessarily be feared – with a little bit of knowledge and some common sense, fluid management will become one of your most easily handled daily tasks.

PHYSIOLOGY

A commonly spouted fact is that 50–60% of a person's total body weight is fluid, and maintaining or correcting someone's fluid status is an important task that can either hasten or delay recovery from illness. Fluid and electrolytes are both absorbed from the food and liquid we consume, and secreted into the lumen of the intestine. Less than 0.01% of our ingested liquid is excreted as stool – so you can understand why people with poor fluid intake end up constipated!

The recommended fluid intake for a person of average height and weight is ~3.7 L/day for men and 2.7 L/day for women. Keep this in mind when prescribing fluids, taking into account a person's size and body type. The body can be thought of as containing two compartments for fluid – intracellular and extracellular. It is clinically important that the *effective circulating volume* (i.e. the portion of the extracellular fluid within the vascular space that is effectively perfusing tissues) is maintained. Sodium is the most abundant solute and thus drives the retention of water in the extravascular space.

The most common causes of a low circulating volume are gastrointestinal losses (vomiting and diarrhoea), haemorrhage and water loss through endocrine or renal disturbances (e.g. fevers, adrenal insufficiency, diabetes insipidus, syndrome of inappropriate antidiuretic hormone secretion). If a patient continues to be hypovolaemic despite appropriate fluid replacement, consider looking for these causes.

It is estimated that people need 30–40 mL/kg/day of water. Each day, we lose water through urine, faeces and insensible losses that include sweating and respiration. When combined, these losses add up to approximately 1600 mL (500 mL in urine to excrete solutes, 200 mL in faeces and 900 mL of insensible losses).

CATEGORIES OF FLUID

Crystalloids

Crystalloids (see Table 24.1) include normal saline (denoted as isotonic saline, N/S 0.9%, or N/Saline), compound sodium lactate (also known as CSL or Hartmann's solution, and very similar to the American alternative 'Ringer's lactate') and 5% dextrose in water (written as 5% dex or D5W). Crystalloids are your go-to fluids on the wards for volume expansion and replacement for poor oral intake.

Normal saline is typically the most appropriate for all uses, as there are very few drugs that cannot be mixed with it. The danger with too much normal saline (cynically referred to as 'death by saline') is due to hyperchloraemic metabolic acidosis, which may be encountered when more than 3–4 L of 0.9% saline is used in a 24-hour period (especially in patients with renal impairment).

CSL is quite popular and does not cause hyperchloraemic acidosis to the same extent, as it contains some potassium (5 mmol). It can be used as a 'buffer' to correct pH abnormalities. However, there are some medications that it cannot be mixed with (such as piperacillin/tazobactam), it does contain lactate and thus should be used with caution in diabetics due to its gluconeogenic properties, and the potassium may accumulate to dangerous levels.

When you administer 5% dextrose, the majority of the fluid does not remain in the intravascular space (90% is distributed into the cells, which causes cellular swelling). As such, it is not normally used in volume expansion. Due to its dilutional effect use of 5% dextrose may result in electrolyte abnormalities such as

TABLE 24.1 Contents of commonly prescribed crystalloids

SOLUTION	CONTENTS
Normal saline	154 mmol sodium 154 mmol chloride Total osmolarity 308 mosm/L and pH 5.0
Compound sodium lactate	131 mmol sodium 111 mmol chloride 29 mmol lactate 5 mmol potassium 2 mmol calcium Total osmolarity 279 mosm/L and pH 6.5
5% Dextrose	278 mmol dextrose (5 g every 100 mL)

hyponatraemia and hypokalaemia, and pulmonary oedema. Common scenarios in which you may see dextrose given include a type 1 diabetic fasting for surgery, a hypernatraemic patient or a patient fasting for a short period of time (i.e. <48 hours). Use with caution in diabetics and patients with heart failure.

Other solutions you may encounter with more niche uses include 4% dextrose + ⅕ normal saline, 15–20% dextrose for hypoglycaemia and hypertonic saline. Please note that hypertonic saline is *not* the way to manage hyponatraemia (see later in this chapter)!

Colloids

Colloids are an alternative method of volume expansion, but are very rarely used by junior doctors without supervision. Colloids aim to maintain a high oncotic pressure in the intravascular space, as opposed to crystalloids, which dilute the plasma (they also cost more). The three colloids seen most frequently are albumin, gelofusine and hydroxyethyl starch (HES). Albumin is discussed in section 25.7, 'Blood products'.

Gelofusine contains modified fluid gelatine and is used as blood plasma replacement in haemorrhage, trauma or dehydration. The large molecule draws water into the intravascular space by osmosis, mimicking the action of common serum proteins such as albumin. It works over 3–4 hours after administration. The sum of effects include increased circulating volume, venous return, left ventricular end-diastolic pressure and, thus, cardiac output, tissue perfusion and diuresis. It is more commonly used in critical care situations and rarely on the wards. Care should be taken in patients with hypervolaemia, recent myocardial infarction, severe cardiac failure, coagulopathy or severe renal disease.

HES is made from starch, and its most frequent application is in shock (of various aetiologies). Again, caution should be used with renal patients. Patients may also have an allergic reaction to the fluid, and it can cause coagulopathy by halving the available factor VIII (thus prolonging the activated partial thromboplastin time [APTT]).

Colloids come in and out of fashion with intensivists and anaesthetists. If asked to write them up as a junior doctor, you would be well within your rights to ask for assistance from a senior colleague. As a learning experience, it would also be worthwhile to ask why they have chosen that particular fluid.

The evidence base for fluid management is rapidly evolving – for example, some centres are trialling crystalloids that contain ethyl pyruvate as an anti-inflammatory in sepsis and shock! As you practice, you may learn more advanced fluid management techniques. However, the basics remain the same.

PRESCRIBING FLUIDS

Maintenance fluid therapy (for fasting or poor oral intake)

You will regularly encounter fasting patients, whether it be on a surgical rotation or medical rotations such as Cardiology, Gastroenterology or General Medicine. If fasting for more than 8 hours, it is good practice to replace their oral intake with intravenous fluids to prevent the patient from becoming hypovolaemic, and experiencing the discomfort of thirst. Be mindful that many bowel preparations are dehydrating.

If someone is going to be fasting for more than 72 hours, notify the dietitian. If the planned period of fasting is more than 4 or 5 days, consider commencing total parenteral nutrition (TPN). All fasting patients or those on IV fluids should have a UEC performed at least daily, and you should review the fluid chart of every patient on ward rounds. If fasting for multiple days, a daily weight and strict fluid balance are useful.

A standard regimen for a patient who is nil by mouth ('NBM') is three 8-hourly bags of normal saline, ensuring there are enough bags charted to cover their period of fasting. If they are fasting for a period of 24 hours, replace their potassium by adding 30 mmol to two of the bags. An alternative is to use 8-hourly bags of CSL, with the same potassium replacement. This lowers the risk of hyperchloraemic acidosis and more suitably replaces the potassium. Remember to account for all losses – for example, if your patient has a chest tube draining 1000 mL per day, they will need an additional 1000 mL of IV fluids to replace it! Patients with burns, ongoing fevers, drains, diarrhoea or vomiting or tachypnoea will require additional fluid. Conversely, administer less fluid to patients with hypothyroidism, oliguric renal failure, fluid overload and syndrome of inappropriate antidiuretic hormone secretion.

Fluid resuscitation and replacement fluid therapy

Fluid replacement therapy is necessary when either the effective circulating volume is depleted or electrolytes require correction. Hypovolaemia is best estimated by a reduction in body weight, but this method is fraught with inaccuracies (and a baseline weight is often not available). Thus, volume deficit is estimated using clinical examination (as outlined below) and analysis of measurable fluid losses. Hypovolaemia may be due to trauma, burns, haemorrhage, gastrointestinal losses (including bleeding), severe skin conditions (e.g. Stevens–Johnson syndrome or toxic epidermal necrolysis), sepsis, shock or hyperhidrosis (excessive sweating).

The rate with which fluid is replaced is dependent on the severity of hypovolaemia. If the patient is shocked or severely dehydrated, a 'bolus' of normal saline or CSL may be administered (either 1 or 2 L). A bolus or 'stat bag' is a bag of fluid allowed to run through at its natural rate – that is, in about 15 minutes (or measured hourly, 4 L/hour). It can be written up as 'stat' on the fluid chart or as 15/60 (stat is more regularly used).

However, much more regularly, a moderately hypotensive (and thus presumably under-perfused) patient will receive 250 mL as a bolus as a 'fluid challenge' to see if their hypotension is fluid-responsive. If this partially rectifies the issue, a further 250 mL may be given followed by a 4/24 bag of fluid before slowing to an 8- or 10-hourly bag for maintenance.

SECTION III

If the patient is dehydrated or only mildly hypovolaemic, aggressive fluid replacement is not necessary. Instead, fluid should be administered at a slightly slower rate, ensuring that the volume given is greater than their daily requirements and any concurrent losses. A typical regimen for a mildly hypovolaemic person would be a 4-hourly litre of normal saline or CSL, followed by a 6- and then 8-hourly bag to increase their circulating volume back to baseline. A maintenance fluid regimen can then be continued. Use caution in the elderly, and patients with cardiac, renal or hepatic conditions as their ability to receive this volume of fluid is diminished (for example, slow the above rates by 1.5×).

Massive transfusion protocol (MTP)

If the hypovolaemia is caused by bleeding, then packed red blood cells (PRBC) are the fluid replacement of choice. If the volume of haemorrhage is large or it is ongoing, a senior physician can activate the 'massive transfusion protocol'. If a patient requires replacement of more than half of their blood volume in 4 hours or their entire blood volume in 24 hours, has major obstetric, gastrointestinal or surgical bleeding or is experiencing severe thoracic, pelvic or multiple long bone trauma, a series of investigations is sent to the laboratory (FBE [full blood examination], prothrombin time, INR [international normalised ratio], fibrinogen, UEC [urea, electrolytes, creatinine], calcium, arterial blood gas), and the blood bank is notified that the protocol has been activated. The lab will then notify the on-call haematologist, prepare and issue blood components rapidly and minimise test turn-around times.

The clinician and emergency team should optimise the patient's oxygen delivery, cardiac output, perfusion and metabolic state, and the above investigations repeated every 30 minutes (see Table 24.2 for the targets recommended by the

TABLE 24.2 Parameters in massive transfusion investigation and monitoring

PARAMETER	VALUES TO AIM FOR
Temperature	>35°C
Acid–base status	pH ≥7.2; base excess <−6, lactate <4 mmol/L
Ionised calcium	>1.1 mmol/L
Haemoglobin	Should not be used alone as a transfusion trigger; and should be interpreted in context with haemodynamic status, organ and tissue perfusion
Platelets	≥50 × 10^9/L
Prothrombin time	<1.5× normal limit
Fibrinogen	<1.0 g/L

Adapted from: Australian Red Cross Blood Service, 2014. Massive transfusion protocol [Internet]. Table: Parameters in massive transfusion investigation and monitoring. <http://www.transfusion.com.au/disease_therapeutics/transfusion>.

Australian Red Cross Blood Service). Once the bleeding is controlled the lab must again be called to let them know the MTP has been ceased.

A typical regimen of blood product replacement in large-volume haemorrhage is a 1:1:1 ratio of PRBC, fresh frozen plasma and platelets to emulate homeostatic blood components as closely as possible. One bag of platelets is equivalent to four units of PRBC. Additionally, if fibrinogen drops below 1.0 g/L, cryoprecipitate may be given (typically 8 to 10 units, guided by your hospital's policy).

THE FLUID REVIEW

This is an incredibly common task assigned to junior doctors, especially when on a cover or night shift. With so many reasons to give a patient fluid and the lengthy duration of administration of said fluids, it is a regular occurrence that fluid prescribed by the home team will finish running outside business hours. A fluid review is often requested between prescribed fluids (i.e. can this patient continue to receive the fluid written up for them by the home team, or have they became overloaded?). These are not unreasonable requests, as physiological fluid status is dynamic and changes rapidly.

Fluid reviews can be carried out quickly, as long as they are completed accurately. It is mostly guided by your clinical examination skills. Begin by gaining consent, and looking at the patient's observations – particularly their heart rate and blood pressure. Common sense dictates that an intravascularly overloaded patient will have hypertension, and an under-perfused patient will be hypotensive. Tachycardia can occur as the heart attempts to increase venous return with a low circulating volume. If a patient is floridly overloaded, they may be hypoxic and tachypnoeic due to the fluid on their lungs. The observations can be quite sensitive markers of fluid status. While looking at the patient's observations chart, see if they have been having daily weights measured.

As any rapid weight gain or loss is unlikely to be fat or protein, it can be assumed to be fluid. This is a vital part of the fluid review and, if fluid administration is expected to be ongoing, weights should be performed regularly. If the patient is on a fluid restriction, ask if they have been adherent. If the patient is on a fluid balance, check their total input against their total output.

At the peripheries, test capillary refill by pressing on the palmar surface of the finger pads, and skin turgor by *gently* pulling at the patient's skin over the dorsal surface of the hand. Sluggish capillary refill (i.e. >2 seconds) can be a sign of dehydration (or shock). Skin should be elastic, and in a dehydrated state it takes longer to return to normal position after being gently pulled.

Moving on to the head and neck, examine the jugular venous pressure (JVP). This is a feature of clinical examination junior doctors and medical students often struggle with. With the patient at a 45° angle, ask them to turn their head slightly away from you. Measure a hypothetical line horizontally out from the top of where you can see the venous pulsation, then a perpendicular line down at their sternal angle. This vertical distance in centimetres is the JVP (see Fig. 24.1 for a pictorial representation). If you are having trouble visualising the JVP, apply

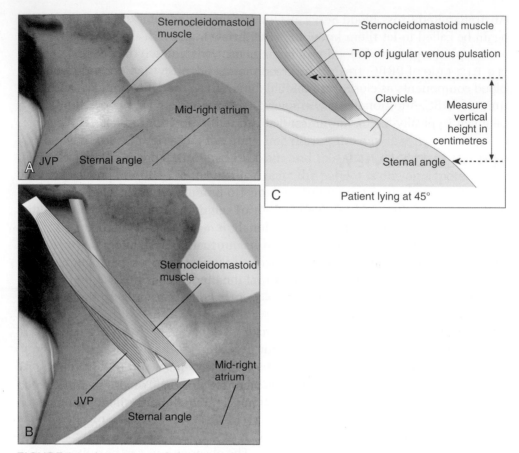

FIGURE 24.1 Assessment of the jugular venous pressure.

Adapted from: Talley, N.J. & Connor, S., 2009. The cardiac examination. In: Talley, N.J. & O'Connor, S., Clinical Examination: A systematic guide to physical diagnosis, 6th ed. Sydney: Elsevier Australia, pp. 57-85.

gentle pressure to the liver to reproduce the hepatojugular reflex. Venous return is increased, transiently elevating the JVP. An elevated JVP is a sign of fluid overload, and a good indicator of venous return to the right atrium. The JVP is considered elevated if >3 cm at 45°, and may be due to overload, right ventricular failure or pericardial disease. If the JVP is not visible (i.e. 0 cm), they may be under-filled.

Open the patient's mouth to see if their mucous membranes are moist and pink. Dehydration may be accompanied by an element of halitosis, so don't get too close. Move on to auscultating the chest. Listen throughout the lung fields for 'crackles' (note that respiratory sounds are usually heard best at the end of inspiration). Note any orthopnoea or dyspnoea. If you are concerned about the degree of crackles you can hear in a patient's chest, consider requesting a chest X-ray and ECG. If they appear to be in respiratory distress (i.e. tachypnoeic or hypoxic), they may require diuresis. Apply oxygen and consider contacting the medical registrar if this is the case.

At the abdomen, note any ascites. Moving to the lower limbs, apply gentle pressure to the skin over the dorsal ankles, shins and sacrum (if the patient has been lying down for a prolonged period of time) to test for pitting oedema. Oedema is considered significant if a depression in the person's skin remains after lifting your finger off the affected area.

If the patient has an indwelling catheter (IDC), check the bag for colour and volume of output. If they do not have an IDC, ask the patient if they are making urine regularly. Normal urine output is 0.5–1 mL/kg/hour, with oliguria being less than this amount and anuria being defined as <100 mL/day.

If the patient's fluid status is still not apparent after your clinical examination, you can check their most recent investigations. A high urine specific gravity, sodium and osmolality are associated with dehydration. Conversely, an overloaded patient will be producing a large quantity of dilute urine. Examine the electrolytes, paying particular attention to sodium, potassium (especially if being diuresed), haematocrit, urea and creatinine. In dehydration the serum sodium, urea and creatinine will be elevated.

Based on your fluid review, you will need to make the clinical decision whether to prescribe additional fluids, withhold already prescribed fluids or to diurese the patient. You may have to correct some electrolyte abnormalities. Regardless of the outcome of your assessment, do not forget to document your findings and plan in the inpatient notes and hand over to the treating team. If you are concerned by a patient's fluid status (either too little or too great), it is perfectly appropriate to escalate your query to a resident or registrar.

ELECTROLYTE ABNORMALITIES

Sodium

An essential salt associated with water homeostasis and action potentials, sodium (Na^+) is vital to maintaining the equilibrium between intra- and extracellular fluid compartments. Hypernatraemia demonstrates a state of hypertonicity – that is, the extracellular component now contains more osmotically active components. Hypernatraemia leads to a reduction in the intracellular space (as the water follows sodium into the vasculature), and the associated cell shrinkage can cause cerebral injury. A 'paired osmolality' (i.e. serum and urine osmolality sampled close together chronologically) could be used to evaluate the cause of hypernatraemia.

If mental state is altered, the patient should be monitored closely with neurological observations. Hypernatraemia is tied very closely to volume state, and causes include vomiting, diarrhoea, diaphoresis (including fevers!) and enthusiastic use of crystalloids as resuscitation fluids. The mainstay of treatment is thus correcting the fluid imbalance. Chronic hypernatraemia or hyponatraemia rarely warrants investigation, making previous bloods very useful.

Hyponatraemia is classified into mild (130–138 mmol/L), moderate (120–130 mmol/L) or severe (<120 mmol/L). Mild and moderate hyponatraemia are able to be slowly brought back to an acceptable range, but severe hyponatraemia requires review as a priority. Hyponatraemia leads to cellular swelling. Sodium levels may be artificially lowered in states of hyperglycaemia (e.g. diabetic ketoacidosis) as the circulating glucose pulls water out of cells and dilutes the serum.

Again, fluid status is vital to assessing the hyponatraemic patient. Hyponatraemia is often considered to be renal or extra-renal. Renal involves excess secretion of sodium (e.g. renal failure or over-diuresis, either endogenously with antidiuretic hormone [ADH] or iatrogenic). Extra-renal causes include congestive heart failure, wounds, gastrointestinal losses, sweating and fevers, burns or fluid resuscitation with fluids that don't contain sodium. Syndrome of inappropriate ADH secretion (SIADH) is another common cause of hyponatraemia, as the hypothalamus secretes extra ADH in an attempt to resolve hypovolaemia.

The mainstay of treatment for hyponatraemia is an appropriate fluid restriction (usually 1.5 L/day) – not salt tablets. If the patient is hypovolaemic and hyponatraemic, crystalloids containing sodium could be used. Hyponatraemia should not be resolved any faster than 10 mmol/L per day, as there is a risk of central pontine demyelination. This is a myelinolytic, life-threatening condition where axons in the pons (in the brainstem) are demyelinated due to the rapid change in tonicity. It is more likely in patients with chronic liver disease, solid organ transplants, severe burns, malnourishment and ongoing gastrointestinal losses.

Potassium

Potassium (K^+) is an element essential for neurotransmission, and the most abundant intracellular cation. It is particularly vital that potassium levels remain in the required range for appropriate conduction of electricity in the heart. Hyper- or hypokalaemia can lead to fatal dysrhythmias.

Hypokalaemia is very frequently seen on the wards, and causes include gastrointestinal losses, diuresis (endogenous or iatrogenic), certain antibiotic use, renal impairment, hypomagnesaemia and malnutrition. Symptoms include palpitations, constipation, paraesthesia and weakness, but patients are rarely symptomatic below 3.0 mmol/L. Although the normal range is 3.5–4.5 mmol/L, when asked to keep a patient at 'cardiac levels' to lessen the chance of arrhythmia you should aim for a serum K^+ of >4.0 mmol/L.

Potassium <2.0 mmol/L is life-threatening and the patient should be moved to ICU for monitoring and replacement. Potassium levels can be brought up either orally or intravenously. If hypokalaemia is mild, oral options include potassium chloride slow release 600 mg oral tablets (marketed as Slow-K) and Chlorvescent®, a mixture of potassium salts. Either of these options can be considered to bring up the serum potassium by ˜0.1 mmol/L but, as the name implies, Slow-K will not raise serum potassium levels for a few hours.

Alternatively, potassium can be given IV. Most commonly used are 'mini-bags' of 100 mL 0.9% normal saline with 10 mmol of potassium chloride added (notated as '+10 mmol KCl') given over 1 hour, expected to raise serum potassium by 0.1–0.2 mmol. Alternatively, 30 mmol could be added to a bag of either normal saline or CSL over 4 hours. When reviewing a patient for a potassium of <3.0 mmol, take an ECG to check for dysrhythmia. Potassium should not be given faster than 10 mmol/hour peripherally as it damages the veins – if potassium supplementation is required at a more rapid rate, an ICU referral would be warranted for electrolyte correction via a central line. If you are having difficulty raising serum potassium, check the magnesium, which may also require supplementation.

Hyperkalaemia can also be a serious condition, and at its highest levels can cause cardiac death. Ensure the specimen is correct, as an overly tight tourniquet can cause haemolysis and artificially inflated potassium. Causes include excess dietary intake, renal impairment, large volume cell lysis (e.g. crush injuries and burns), drugs (e.g. potassium-sparing diuretics) and rigorous exercise. Mild hyperkalaemia (i.e. 4.5–5.5 mmol/L) can be resolved with an oral potassium binder, such as 15 g oral polystyrene sulfonate (Resonium). This works by exchanging sodium or calcium ions in the gastrointestinal tract for potassium ions, and hence the action in lowering potassium is slow.

Moderate hyperkalaemia (5.6–6.0 mmol/L), or patients who have electrocardiographic changes associated with hyperkalaemia (tented T waves, flattened P waves and prolonged PR interval), should be rectified more quickly with 30 g oral polystyrene sulfonate (repeated every 4–6 hours as necessary) and by removing any agents increasing potassium. Notify your registrar.

With severe hyperkalaemia (>6.5 mmol/L) you should urgently contact your registrar for assistance, ask nursing staff for an ECG and consider quickly lowering extracellular potassium with insulin and glucose (a typical starting regimen is 10 units of rapid-acting insulin and 10 mL of 50% dextrose). To stabilise the cardiac membrane administer 10 mL of 10% calcium gluconate. Ask for serial ECGs to review for changes. For more severe hyperkalaemia consider moving to a monitored high dependency unit with cardiac monitoring, and always involve the renal team if the review is for a dialysis patient. Remember that hyperkalaemia is often a *symptom* of an underlying process that should be rectified, and not the end diagnosis.

Calcium

First-line management of hypercalcaemia is appropriate rehydration, usually with normal saline. For more severe cases (e.g. >3.0 mmol/L), consider using a bisphosphonate to lower circulating calcium. You should not initiate this without discussing it with a registrar. It is less effective with malignant hypercalcaemia. A typical dose is 60 mg palmidronate given intravenously. You should continue to monitor the calcium closely, and consider the causes of hypercalcaemia (as outlined in Chapter 12). An Endocrinology referral may be necessitated.

Hypocalcaemia may be supplemented easily as an oral formulation – calcium carbonate 600 mg oral tablets are the most commonly available. Remember to account for high levels of serum protein (see Chapter 12) before acting. If intravenous calcium is required (e.g. for symptomatic hypocalcaemia), 1 g calcium gluconate may be given via a central line (this would be something to call your registrar before doing). Beware bradycardia and hypotension due to peripheral vasodilation.

Magnesium

Primary hypermagnesaemia is rare but, when encountered, will likely be due to renal impairment or over-supplementation. Mild hypermagnesaemia does not require treatment, but consider the trend and repeat the bloods soon. Severe hypermagnesaemia is a life-threatening condition, and may be managed with calcium gluconate in doses similar to those of hypocalcaemia (see above). Frusemide may also expedite excretion of magnesium via the kidneys.

Hypomagnesaemia is far more common, caused principally by dehydration, renal disease, dietary insufficiency or alcoholism. It is often seen in conjunction with low calcium and potassium. 'Cardiac levels' are considered to be >1.0 mmol/L. All patients with a history of dysrhythmia (including atrial fibrillation) and most surgical patients should be kept about this level. Magnesium can be supplemented with oral tablets (usually magnesium aspartate 500 mg tablets) or a 100 mL bag of normal saline with 10 mmol $MgSO_4$ added (both of which can be expected to raise serum magnesium by 0.1 mmol/L).

Phosphate

Hyperphosphataemia is usually a result of renal impairment or hypoparathyroidism. It can be brought down with phosphate-binding agents, but these should not be initiated without speaking to a more senior clinician. Hypophosphataemia is most commonly seen in the hospital setting as refeeding syndrome. To prevent this cascade of electrolyte abnormalities, supplement phosphate orally with phosphate tablets. If hypophosphataemia is more severe, it can be given intravenously as 100 mL of normal saline 0.9% with phosphate added – different facilities will have different mixtures.

Iron

Iron is a mineral essential for the function of living things, with its principal role being the carriage of oxygen to bodily tissues in haem. Iron deficiency is very common and causes include blood loss, growth, pregnancy (due to increased requirements), impaired absorption or dietary insufficiency. The most common pathological cause in men and post-menopausal women is haemorrhage, either overt (e.g. trauma) or subtle (e.g. gastrointestinal loss). It is more common in women of child-bearing age. Certain drugs (e.g. non-steroidal anti-inflammatory agents) increase the risk of GI bleeding.

Iron deficiency may be diagnosed on serology (see Chapter 12 for more on iron studies) or as presentation with fatigue, dyspnoea or bleeding. Iron can be supplemented orally with several different mixtures, which should be taken on an empty stomach. Their absorption can be increased with adequate vitamin C (i.e. ascorbic acid) intake.

If a patient has symptomatic iron deficiency, an iron infusion could be considered. These also come in several combinations, with the most common being 1 g iron polymaltose in 250 mL normal saline 0.9%, or 1 g of iron carboxymaltose in 250 mL normal saline 0.9%. Iron carboxymaltose, while more expensive, causes fewer infusion reactions than iron polymaltose and can be given much more rapidly. If an infusion reaction occurs, cease the infusion immediately, consider giving antihistamines (e.g. hydrocortisone 100 mg IV or cetirizine 10 mg oral) and monitor the patient closely. If a patient has a history of a mild reaction, consider giving them the infusion after some 'premedication' of hydrocortisone and cetirizine (same doses as above). Iron tablets should be stopped for 1 week post-infusion as they won't be absorbed.

Iron overload is most commonly seen in the Western world as haemochromatosis, a genetic condition affecting the storage of iron, or over-supplementation (including transfusion-dependent patients). Presentations are varied but include liver disease, diabetes, cardiovascular dysfunction and renal disease. Haemochromatosis patients often undergo regular phlebotomy to reduce their iron load with monitoring. For transfusion-dependent patients, an iron chelator (e.g. deferasirox) may be given regularly to prevent iron accumulation.

OTHER INFUSIONS

Proton pump inhibitors

A proton pump inhibitor (PPI) infusion is commonly used on the surgical and gastroenterological wards in the management of gastrointestinal bleeding. It works by lowering the acidity of the luminal contents to allow ulcer healing. A standard regimen is 40 mg esomeprazole in 100 mL normal saline 0.9% given over 5 hours (aim for a rate of 8 mg/hour), although some institutions will use omeprazole, pantoprazole or rabeprazole. This should be continued for 72 hours. PPI infusions are used less often, as IV BD PPI is now believed to be non-inferior.

Infliximab

Infliximab is a monoclonal antibody that binds to tumour necrosis factor (TNF)-alpha, an inflammatory cytokine that plays a role in several autoimmune conditions. It is used by neurology, gastroenterology, rheumatology and dermatology services to treat an increasing range of conditions including inflammatory bowel disease, psoriasis and rheumatoid arthritis.

Although you would be very unlikely to prescribe infliximab for the first time, you may be asked to write it up for an outpatient. It is dosed at 5 mg/kg and given as per protocol (APP) in 250 mL of normal saline 0.9%. Doses are typically given at weeks 'zero', 2 and 6, with 8-weekly treatments (if tolerated) thereafter. An infliximab infusion should be rescheduled if a patient is suffering from an infective illness due to its immunosuppressive activity. Before the initial infliximab is commenced, a patient should have had a full infectious disease screen including chest X-ray and viral serology (CMV, EBV, HIV, HSV, hepatitis A, B and C and VZV).

Blood products

Consenting for blood products is a common request for junior doctors, and a task that should not be taken lightly. Inform the patient why they have been prescribed a transfusion, outline the risks and benefits and ask them if they still wish to continue or if they have any questions. Generic risks of blood products include fever, rash, anaphylaxis, incompatibility reaction, infection and fluid overload. Transfusion-dependent patients (e.g. myelodysplastic syndromes) may be consented for 12 months at a time, but the typical duration of consent is the current admission only. These products are supplied by the Red Cross Blood Service in Australia. Prior to receiving blood products a patient's serum must have been cross-matched.

Packed red blood cells

Packed red blood cells (PRBC) are obtained by centrifuging the whole blood collected from donors, and kept mixed with anticoagulant at 2–4°C until ready for use. They are used to treat anaemia. Typical protocol is giving PRBC when the haemoglobin drops below 70 g/L, or is <80 g/L in a symptomatic patient (or in the perioperative period), or <90 g/L in a patient with multiple risk factors (e.g. severe ischaemic heart disease; ongoing blood losses).

One unit of PRBC is thought to raise the haemoglobin by 10 g/L. If a patient has a history of a transfusion reaction but requires blood products, contact your registrar. It may still be possible to give them the product they need with a pre-medication of hydrocortisone 100 mg IV and cetirizine 10 mg oral.

Usually administered over 2 hours, but blood may be given faster in trauma or slowed up to 4 hours in patients with severe renal, liver or cardiac disease. If the patient is overloaded after their transfusion and you have reason to be concerned (e.g. poor cardiac or renal reserve), give a small amount of frusemide (e.g. 20 mg IV).

If a transfusion reaction takes place, immediately cease the infusion. Monitor the patient closely. If necessary, give antihistamines. If anaphylaxis, call a MET call and ask for adrenaline to be drawn up (0.5 mL every 5 minutes as necessary). Correct any electrolyte abnormalities and give fluid if hypotensive. Make a detailed note of the reaction, as it must be reported. There is a requirement for transfusion reactions that involves sending bloods to the lab – ask your hospital for its policy.

Platelets

Platelets are cell components that aggregate to help achieve haemostasis. They are often elevated with inflammation, and fall with marrow suppression, viral illness and liver disease (due to portal hypertension). Normal counts range from 150–400 × 10^{12}/L. Typically, all patients with platelets <10 are given one pool of platelets; those with marrow failure and presence of additional risk factors (e.g. fever, antibiotic use or bleeding) are supplemented below 20; and any patient having a procedure or with ongoing bleeding is supplemented to keep them above 50.

Platelets are usually given either 'stat' or over 30 minutes. A post-platelet increment (confusingly annotated as PPI) is often taken 30–60 minutes after the transfusion, with one pool expected to raise platelets by 10. Patients who may have an allogeneic stem cell transplant should have cytomegalovirus (CMV)-negative platelets. For patients with a poor response to pool platelets, try a single donor bag. If a patient continues to increment poorly, discuss sending off HLA antibodies with your registrar.

Buffy coat transfusions

Rarely given or requested by junior medical staff, buffy coat (the layer of anticoagulated blood between red blood cells and plasma containing leuococytes and platelets) may be given in special circumstances to neutropenic patients. The cells tend to be collected only when needed by a particular patient, usually from family and friends. They are collected from the donor via apheresis. It is administered 'as per protocol'.

Fresh frozen plasma

Fresh frozen plasma (FFP) is the layer of plasma separated from red blood cells and buffy coat when centrifuged. It contains circulating proteins, including coagulation factors. Indications you may encounter include reversing warfarin, treatment of disseminated intravascular coagulation (to replace the consumed coagulation factors), thrombotic thrombocytopenia purpura, during the massive transfusion protocol, chronic liver disease and inherited coagulation defects. It is not necessary to cross-match these patients.

Cryoprecipitate

Cryoprecipitate is the term used for the proteins that precipitate out of fresh frozen plasma when thawed slowly. It contains fibrinogen, factors VIII and XIII, von Willebrand factor (vWF) and fibronectin. It may be given in fibrinogen deficiency (either endogenous or drug-induced), disseminated intravascular coagulation or certain factor deficiencies. It comes in a small quantity and tends to be used in batches of 5 units at a time. It is administered 'as per protocol'.

Albumin

Albumin is a colloid fluid also referred to as concentrated albumin or 'conc alb'. It is administered in either 5% solutions (in 500 mL bottles) or 20% solutions (in 100 mL bottles). Indications include hypovolaemia, particularly in liver disease patients who should not be given normal saline, spontaneous bacterial peritonitis and large volume abdominocentesis). Albumin is not routinely given to supplement low serum levels of albumin! It should be given at no faster than 2 hours per 100 mL bottle of 20% albumin, or 4 hours per 500 mL bottle of 5% albumin, without discussion with a senior clinician.

SECTION III

Intravenous immunoglobulins

Intravenous immunoglobulins (IVIg) is a serum globulin preparation made from donated plasma and used in a range of congenital, acquired and autoimmune conditions including primary hypogammaglobulinaemias, chronic lymphocytic leukaemia, HIV, immune thrombocytopenic purpura, immune haemolysis, some nephropathies, myasthenia gravis and Guillain–Barré syndrome, among many others.

These infusions are commonly given to outpatients of the renal, neurology and rheumatology teams. Ordering IVIg must be done via a special form found on the BloodSTAR website (https://www.criteria.blood.gov.au/). A login will be required the first time you use this website. Several brands and strengths are available including Octagam® and Intragam® (5%) and Kiovig (10%). Although dosage varies with indication, 5% is standard. Premedications may be given if there is a history of adverse reaction. Each bottle is written up to flow 'as per protocol' (denoted APP) as the speed varies during the administration of IVIg. Patient's vaccines should be deferred for 3 months.

SUPPLEMENTAL FEEDING

Enteral feeding – nasogastric tubes, percutaneous endoscopic gastrostomies and percutaneous endoscopic jejunostomies

Malnutrition severely impacts upon patient recovery, and can be somewhat offset with these methods of enteral feeding. It should be considered in patients who are critically ill or have a high risk of malnourishment, and all should be referred to a dietitian for management of their feeds.

Nasogastric tube (NGT) feeds are one method of delivering nutritionally complete feeds to a patient when they cannot tolerate normal feeding (e.g. severe nausea, or postoperatively). A nasogastric tube is passed via the nasal passage directly to the stomach, and may be placed on the wards. Inserting an NGT is outlined in Chapter 17, 'Clinical procedures'.

Alternatively, a percutaneous endoscopic gastrostomy (PEG) or percutaneous endoscopic jejunostomy (PEJ) tube may be placed, bypassing the nasopharynx and oesophagus and delivering nutrients directly to the stomach or jejunum. These are inserted by surgeons or gastroenterologists in an endoscopy suite, and are more suited for long-term use. They may be used in patients with neurological dysphagia (e.g. stroke, motor neuron disease) or oesophageal disease (e.g. malignancy). If they become blocked, trial flushing them with hot water. To prevent this, they should be flushed with saline QID. Monitor these patients for refeeding syndrome. Some drugs will have to be re-written as not all can be crushed and delivered via the various tubes.

Total parental nutrition

Total parenteral nutrition (TPN) is a method of delivering nutritional requirements as a substitute for enteral (i.e. 'by stomach') feeding. It contains lipids, proteins, carbohydrates, trace elements, minerals and vitamins. If necessary, salts (e.g. potassium or sodium) can be added or withdrawn from the solution. There is also partial parental nutrition or PPN, used less frequently as a bridge between forms of nutrition.

TPN is often seen on Surgical, Oncology, Haematology, Intensive Care and Gastroenterology wards in patients who are regularly fasted for prolonged periods (pre- or postoperatively, and those with high output stomae or fistulae, short bowel syndrome, rapid transit syndrome, intractable nausea and vomiting or a prolonged bowel obstruction). TPN should be considered in all patients who must fast for >72 hours and planned with a dietitian. There is a panel of investigations outlined in Chapter 12 that should be sent at baseline, most vital being lipids.

A peripherally inserted central catheter (PICC) is the usual delivery method of choice, as TPN can be quite phlebosclerotic (i.e. damaging to veins). TPN may be charted on a fluids chart or a special form depending on your hospital, with typical rates being between 42 and 84 mL/hour. Special considerations should be taken for patients on a fluid restriction or with renal or liver disease. Weights should be done daily, and blood sugar levels QID. They should have a daily UEC + LFT + CMP (comprehensive metabolic panel), with coagulation studies weekly. Strict fluid balance should be kept with an indwelling catheter.

If a patient has to cease TPN during a cover shift (e.g. dislodged PICC), it can be substituted with 10% dextrose – most hospitals will have a policy to ensure the patient receives adequate nutrition until TPN can be safely recommenced. Like any other line, an infected PICC used to deliver TPN should be removed (after contacting a senior doctor) and cultures sent, including the tip of the PICC line. Although most commonly given in the hospital setting, some patients do go home on TPN.

CHAPTER 25

THE DETERIORATING PATIENT

Joseph M O'Brien

Across your career you will be called upon to assist in the care of deteriorating patients. This type of patient interaction can be difficult, particularly when you do not know the patient well (such as when on cover). Emergency codes – despite their stressful nature – are excellent learning opportunities. When you are more junior you should try and attend as many as possible, and watch how the more senior clinicians handle these situations. Respond as rapidly as possible.

Your role will change as you progress – at first (as a student), simply observe from the sidelines. These scenarios can still be challenging for experienced doctors, and getting in the way is not advised. Start with simple but important roles like documentation, moving things, running urgent bloods and radiology requests and, as you become more confident, IV cannulation and phlebotomy. Always listen to the team leader 'running the code'.

As an intern, you may have the opportunity to perform cardiopulmonary resuscitation (CPR) or even lead an emergency response yourself – remember what you've learned, remain as calm as possible and note that it's okay to ask for help! This chapter is not intended to be an all-encompassing guide to managing deteriorating patients – for that, the authors suggest *On Call: Principles and Protocols* (2nd edition) by Cadogan, Brown and Celenza.

THE MEDICAL EMERGENCY TEAM AND EMERGENCY CALLS

Medical Emergency Teams (tautologically referred to as MET teams, or less frequently as rapid response teams or RRTs) are a Government stipulation in publicly-funded hospitals in Australia. They function as cardiac arrest teams that also respond to significant staff concern, respiratory arrest and serious alterations in urine output, blood pressure, heart rate and respiratory rate. The team's composition will differ depending on the nature and size of the hospital, but will typically include an Intensive Care Unit (ICU) or Emergency Department (ED) registrar, ICU or ED nurse, anaesthetist (consultant, registrar or both), medical registrar and various residents from the anaesthetics, medical and intensive care units. Usually, the most experienced doctor will take on the role of leader, and an anaesthetics team member will manage the airway. In Australia, it was first trialled at Liverpool Hospital (NSW) and Austin Health in the 1990s.

Emergency responses are divided into 'code blues' (i.e. true medical emergencies) and 'MET calls.' MET calls are single-trigger events, called when a patient breaches particular criteria. These aim to respond to patient crises, detect deterioration early and, where possible, prevent cardiac arrest and death. Their introduction has greatly reduced the number of code blues called. If you are ever in a situation where you are seriously concerned about a patient's imminent wellbeing, it is better to call a MET than try and handle the situation without assistance – you will always be scolded for calling too late, but should never be in trouble for asking for help early.

The aim of a MET call is to assess and diagnose a patient's condition, begin treatment and determine whether their level of care requires escalation (e.g. admission to ICU or transfer to a larger hospital). Patients who have multiple MET calls (usually more than three) should be reviewed by a consultant intensivist or physician as soon as possible to make decisions about the direction of their care and whether or not MET calls are appropriate. MET criteria (see Table 25.1) may be altered by the MET team, or the home registrar or consultant. As a resident you may be asked to extend these altered criteria. You cannot institute them yourself without discussing it with a consultant or registrar. Learning the phone number to call a code should be one of the *first* things you do when orienting yourself to a new hospital as it may literally save a life.

Many hospitals have now instituted 'clinical reviews' – these are observations made by the nursing staff that are outside the patient's normal observed range and require review by a junior doctor. They can be considered 'pre-MET calls' and their value in the clinical setting is still being determined. All clinical reviews,

TABLE 25.1 Examples of MET and code blue criteria

PARAMETER	MET CRITERIA	CODE BLUE
Heart rate	<50 bpm or >130 bpm	<40 bpm or >150 bpm
Blood pressure	<90 mmHg or > 180 mmHg	>200 mmHg (some hospitals)
Respiratory rate	<8/min or >24/min	<6/min or >30/min
Oxygen saturation	<90%	<80%
Oxygen requirement	>5 L/min	–
Conscious state	Sudden drop ≥2 GCS	GCS <8/unresponsiveness
Urine output	<0.5 mL/kg/hour lean body mass	–

GCS, Glasgow Coma Scale.

Adapted from: Peter MacCallum Cancer Centre, 2012. Observation and response chart. East Melbourne: Peter MacCallum Cancer Centre.

METs and code blues begin with assessment of the airway, breathing, circulation and disability before progressing to the issue that triggered the call.

HYPERTENSION

Hypertension is a regular ward call. Always compare with older records to determine the 'trend' for the patient's blood pressure (BP) – they may always be hypertensive, or it could be a sudden change. Unless extreme (e.g. systolic BP >180 mmHg), hypertension is usually not an emergency in the acute setting and is of more concern as a cause of end-organ damage long term. Hypertension may be indicative of pain (usually associated with tachycardia), hypervolaemia, cerebrovascular events (i.e. stroke or transient ischaemic attack), renal impairment, endocrine disturbance (e.g. thyroid disease, steroid use or Cushing's syndrome), anxiety or, more rarely, an aortic dissection, acute pulmonary oedema (APO), aortic regurgitation or myocardial infarction (MI). 90% of patients will have 'essential' hypertension where there is no direct cause found.

If the patient is pregnant, consider preeclampsia and call the obstetrics registrar if necessary. If they are a patient with a spinal injury, consider autonomic dysreflexia (a hypertensive response to noxious stimuli) and contact Neurosurgery if concerned. Posterior reversible encephalopathy syndrome (PRES) is a rare constellation of symptoms including hypertension, confusion and sometimes seizures, which may be caused by hypertension or certain drugs (e.g. chemotherapy) and requires careful control of blood pressure.

Assess the patient's regular medications – have any of their usual antihypertensives been withheld and, if so, why? Conversely, are there any agents that might be driving up the blood pressure (e.g. steroids, oral contraceptive pills, MAO inhibitors or other stimulants)? Although rare, you may encounter a patient in hypertensive crisis that can include seizure activity, severe headaches and delirium. In this situation, the BP should be brought down with the assistance of an Emergency or Intensive Care registrar and the patient should have ongoing neurological observations after the MET is stood down.

As with all MET calls, begin with ABC – airway, breathing and circulation. Take a manual BP yourself with the correct size cuff to confirm the findings. If the patient has chest pain (especially 'tearing'), take the BP in both arms and consider an aortic dissection. Perform a fluid assessment – overloaded patients may be hypertensive, and dyspnoea may be suggestive of APO. Consider sending off bloods (FBE + UEC + TSH) and urinary protein, and request an ECG to investigate myocardial infarction. A non-urgent chest X-ray (CXR) could also be done at a later time, or immediately if an intrathoracic pathology is suspected (e.g. APO). If any seizure activity or neurological changes are noted, escalate the patient's care and request a CT-brain to exclude PRES or intracranial haemorrhage.

Treat the underlying cause where detected. If no cause can be elicited and the patient remains severely hypertensive (e.g. >180 mmHg systolic), consider giving 5–10 mg oral amlodipine (in the absence of contraindications for a calcium channel blocker) or applying a glyceryl trinitrate (GTN) 25 mg patch. These should both act quite rapidly – be sure to convey to the nursing staff that the patch should be removed if systolic blood pressure (SBP) drops <160 mmHg. Ask for registrar assistance with hypertensive renal patients. The patient should have observations every 15–30 minutes for 2 hours or until consistently normotensive. Starting any new regular antihypertensives is a decision best left to the home team. Be sure to *document* your review in the patient's notes.

HYPOTENSION

Hypotension, while often benign, can be an early indicator that a patient is deteriorating and is an easily observed component of shock. Similar to hypertension, the concern is the possibility of end organ damage due to hypoperfusion with insufficient blood pressure. A reflex response with hypotension is to fill the patient with fluid (i.e. 'fluid resuscitate' them), but consider the causes of hypotension before doing so. As hypotension may be a sign of more serious illness, all patients with new or worsening hypotension should be reviewed as a priority.

Causes of hypotension include shock (anaphylactic, hypovolaemic from dehydration or third space losses, haemorrhagic from bleeding, cardiogenic from infarction and obstructive from cardiac tamponade, large pulmonary emboli (PE) or a tension pneumothorax), drugs (antihypertensives, alcohol, antidepressants, vasodilators and alpha-blockers), sepsis, autonomic disruption (diabetes, Parkinsonism, vasovagal episode, other primary neurological dysfunction) and hypoadrenalism.

As always, begin with ABC, review the observations chart and the overall trend, and perform a focused clinical examination. Ask if the patient is symptomatic (e.g. dizziness, syncope, headache, confusion). Repeat the BP manually yourself and recline the patient's bed so that their legs are elevated above their heart. If there is any evidence of shock, begin treating without delay by placing a large bore cannula, administering 20 mL/kg normal saline (if no contraindications), applying oxygen by mask and requesting an ECG and bloods (at a minimum, FBE + UEC). If you suspect bleeding request a crossmatch for four units of packed red blood cells (especially relevant in postoperative patients). If anaphylaxis is a possibility ask for adrenaline to be drawn up and consider giving antihistamines (hydrocortisone 100–200 mg IV and/or 10 mg cetirizine orally). Arrange a CXR if there is tachycardia, arrhythmia, chest pain or dyspnoea. If the patient is febrile or infection is otherwise suspected, send off a septic screen and consider commencing empirical antibiotic coverage, especially in immunosuppressed patients.

A person requires a mean arterial pressure (MAP) of >60 mmHg (i.e. ~90–100 mmHg SBP) to perfuse their end-organs, and the patient should receive intravenous crystalloids until their blood pressure reaches this target. A hypotensive patient should have ongoing monitoring and be reviewed by either yourself or another doctor after the MET has been stood down. A patient whose BP continues to drop despite adequate filling and treatment of any underlying cause is a critically unwell patient and transfer to ICU should be considered for vasopressor support. If the patient has any deterioration in neurological status you should have a low threshold for neuroimaging to exclude a watershed infarct (where hypotension leads to infarction in poorly supplied territories of the brain). Monitor LFTs and UECs in the coming days for hepatic ischaemia (global derangement) and acute kidney injury (rising creatinine and urea), respectively.

The aim of your review is to stabilise the patient, determine the cause of hypotension and rectify it, rather than assume it is purely hypovolaemia and refilling the patient. Postoperative surgical patients often have 'third space losses' as fluid sits in the lumen of the bowel as it moves less than usual – these patients do require some extra fluid intravenously, as this fluid is in the extracellular compartment and thus unavailable for use by the body. Note that mild, chronic hypotension is usually not an issue and may be seen in athletic people, chronic liver disease patients, elderly women and younger women of petite build, and may not require action if the patient is well.

TACHYCARDIA

Tachycardia can also be benign or serious and, as a junior doctor asked to review a tachycardic patient, it is your role to stratify the patient's risk. When notified about a patient with tachycardia you should immediately request an ECG as this will guide further management. Keep in mind which arrhythmias are common, which are dangerous and how long a patient can maintain a tachycardia before reaching exhaustion (spoiler: not long in the elderly). Tachycardia with hypotension requires urgent review – although hypotension can in itself cause tachycardia, it could signify systemic inflammatory response syndrome (SIRS), bleeding, shock or anaphylaxis.

Begin with ABC, the observations chart for the trend and their medications (has an antiarrhythmic agent been missed?). An important question is whether or not it is symptomatic (e.g. palpitations, angina, dyspnoea). A focused clinical examination should concentrate on the cardiorespiratory system and attempting to locate any potential signs of infection or bleeding (don't forget to take the pulse yourself). Review the ECG and determine the rhythm – tachyarrhythmias include atrial fibrillation (irregularly irregular), sinus tachycardia (regular but rapid), atrial flutter, supraventricular tachycardia and junctional rhythms (regularly irregular). Look for signs of ischaemia and request a CXR.

If either ventricular tachycardia or ventricular fibrillation is noted immediately escalate to a code blue and commence the advanced life support pathway. Request bloods – FBE + UEC + CMP at a minimum, but also consider troponins, thyroid-stimulating hormone (TSH), blood cultures and inflammatory markers. Haemodynamically unstable patients or those with severe chest pain, altered mental state or dyspnoea should have their care escalated and be moved to a bed with cardiac monitoring. Treat the underlying cause if identifiable. IV access should be obtained and, if hypovolaemic, the patient should be fluid resuscitated appropriately. Document your encounter and consider putting in repeat bloods (especially if you requested troponins).

It is rare for patients to have a chronic resting tachycardia, and thus every attempt should be made to try and diagnose the cause. Causes of sinus tachycardia include hypovolaemia (common in inpatients), hypoxia, left ventricular failure, infection, hyperthyroidism, anaemia, drugs and anxiety.

BRADYCARDIA

Bradyarrhythmias are less commonly encountered, and fortunately have a shorter list of differential diagnoses. If symptomatic (e.g. dizziness, headache, confusion, angina, syncope) review the patient as a priority, but asymptomatic sinus brady-cardia is often benign. Request an ECG upon notification of a bradycardic patient.

Begin with ABC, reviewing the patient's observations chart and completing a medications review. Does the patient appear well? Perform a focused examination. Remember that an inferior myocardial infarction can result in increased vagal tone and, subsequently, bradycardia and even heart block. Review the ECG – bradyarrhythmias include sinus bradycardia, various degrees of atrioventricular (AV) block (a.k.a. heart block), junctional rhythms and slow atrial fibrillation.

Sinus bradycardia is most frequently due to medications (beta blockade, digoxin, calcium-channel blockers, amiodarone, lithium, sedatives, recent anaesthesia) but may also be caused by ischaemia, hypothyroidism and hypothermia. Send off bloodwork – FBE + UEC + CMP ± coagulation studies, troponins, TSH and digoxin level. Consider the need for a CXR. Treat any underlying cause detected. Patients with heart block should be moved to a cardiac-monitored bed (e.g. CCU or ICU) until rectified as pacing may be required. Resting bradycardia (as low as 40 bpm) may be normal in very healthy, athletic people.

HYPOXIA, INCREASED WORK OF BREATHING AND INCREASING OXYGEN REQUIREMENTS

The most common cause of MET calls, hypoxia is often multifactorial in the inpatient population. A truly hypoxic patient (i.e. from a good saturation trace) should be reviewed urgently (recall the saturation curve – haemoglobin saturation drops off rapidly). When called about a hypoxic patient ask the nurse to sit the patient up and increase their oxygen as much as required, noting that any flow rate >6 L/min should be delivered by Hudson mask and not nasal prongs. Keep in mind that anxiety can cause tachypnoea and the sensation of dyspnoea, but never hypoxia.

On arrival, assess ABC, the saturation trend and the medications chart (were their diuretics given? are they on multiple puffers? do they need their regular salbutamol? are they on DVT prophylaxis?). Ask the patient if they are symptomatic (e.g. wheeze, dyspnoea, angina, 'air hunger') – if a patient cannot complete full sentences they are in respiratory distress and you should call for help. Acute respiratory failure is divided into type I (hypoxaemia with normal or low $PaCO_2$) and type II (hypoxaemia with high $PaCO_2$). This is significant as type I is a failure of oxygenation, and thus will normally respond to oxygen therapy, whereas type

II is a failure of ventilation and may require invasive ventilation in an intensive care setting. Important diagnoses to exclude rapidly include MI, pneumothorax, APO, PE, bleeding, sepsis and tamponade and as such your clinical examination should focus on these conditions. Note other signs of respiratory distress such as use of accessory muscles, tracheal tug or diaphoresis.

Bloodwork should be sent marked urgent – FBE + UEC + CMP at a minimum, with inflammatory markers and blood cultures if you suspect infection, and troponins if you suspect MI. An arterial blood gas (ABG) is ideal, but if this is proving too difficult send off a venous blood gas (VBG) to help you determine the $PaCO_2$ – PO_2 <60 mmHg or PCO_2 >50 mmHg is considered respiratory failure and you should call a code blue (if this has not already been done). Compare to old ABGs if available. Call for a mobile CXR and request an ECG. Sudden onset hypoxia, tachypnoea, pleuritic chest pain and signs of right heart strain on an ECG should be sufficient risk factors for you to request a ventilation/perfusion (V/Q) scan or CT-pulmonary angiogram (CTPA) to investigate for PE.

Trial nebulised salbutamol (typically 5 mg) if no contraindications (e.g. hypokalaemia). Continue to up-titrate oxygen therapy as required, but beware the COPD patients who are 'chronic CO_2 retainers' – these patients should have their oxygen slowly increased to prevent an increased PCO_2 and subsequent loss of respiratory drive (and further drop in PO_2). Diurese with frusemide if necessary. Bilevel non-invasive ventilation (NIV) is a method of attempting to decrease PCO_2 but managing bilevel NIV is beyond what would be expected of a junior doctor and this should be done in either ED or ICU. Continue to monitor these patients with serial blood gases and treat any underlying causes noted. If a patient becomes unresponsive, check for circulatory failure and commence the advanced life support pathway. Be sure to document your review.

As mentioned, hypoxia is often multifactorial – patients often present with mixed heart failure and decompensated COPD, but other causes include pneumonia, aspiration, drugs (sedatives, opiates), larger pleural effusions, parenchymal lung disease (e.g. sarcoidosis, pulmonary fibrosis) and neuromuscular disease (e.g. myasthenia gravis, Guillain–Barré syndrome). These patients may require an echocardiogram or respiratory function tests later in their care.

Tachypnoea and bradypnoea may be managed in the manner outlined above. Tachypnoeic patients may have an elevated rate due to pain or anxiety, but always investigate other causes before dismissing it. Causes include sepsis, pain, heart failure, pneumothorax, PE, MI, APO, COPD, metabolic acidosis, pneumonia, hyperthyroidism, drugs (e.g. sympathomimetics, anticholinergics, salicylates) and exertion. Bradypnoea is most commonly due to over-sedation, but can also be caused by MI, heart failure, hypothyroidism, massive electrolyte disturbance or TIA/stroke.

OLIGURIA OR ANURIA

Oliguria is defined as the production of <0.5 mL/kg/hour of urine, an insufficient quantity for unwell patients. It may be of pre-renal, renal or post-renal origin.

TABLE 25.2 Causes of oliguria

PRE-RENAL	RENAL	POST-RENAL
Hypovolaemia (dehydration, third space loss, haemorrhage, GI loss, burns, over-diuresis)	Acute tubular necrosis	Lower urinary tract obstruction (prostatic, cervical carcinoma, calculi, strictures)
Medications (e.g. alpha-blockers, anaesthesia)	Glomerulonephritis	Blocked catheter
Cardiac – MI, CCF, tamponade, PE, constrictive pericarditis	Interstitial nephritis	Upper urinary tract obstruction (calculi, clot, tumours, fibrosis)
Vasodilation 2° shock, sepsis, anaphylaxis, or drugs		
Renal hypoperfusion due to renal vessel occlusion, or aortic dissection		

Adapted from: Cadogan, M., Brown, A.F.T. & Celenza, A., 2011. Urine output: decreased. In: Cadogan, M., Brown, A.F.T. & Celenza, A., Marshall & Ruedy's On Call: Principles & protocols, 2nd ed. Sydney: Elsevier Health Sciences, pp. 293-300.

Common causes are outlined in Table 25.2. Begin with ABC and a medications review (take note of prior diuretic use). Withhold nephrotoxins and renally adjust medications that cannot be immediately ceased until the home team review. A fluid assessment is vital and commence a fluid balance chart, and urinalysis (with MCS, cast analysis and albumin/protein to creatinine ratio) and bloodwork should be sent (FBE + UEC + CMP ± inflammatory markers).

Request a ward bladder scan to see the volume remaining in the patient's bladder. A renal tract ultrasound may be necessary. If the patient is hypovolaemic, commence IV rehydration. If the patient is hypotensive or tachycardic, the issue may be more serious than dehydration and check for signs of infection, bleeding or shock. If the patient is in retention, a digital rectal examination may be necessary to exclude constipation. Continue to observe for late sequelae of acute renal failure, such as hyperkalaemia, metabolic acidosis, hypertension and APO. Document your review. Persistent oliguria may necessitate a renal team review.

ALTERED CONSCIOUS STATE

A change in mental status is the third most common cause of MET calls in Australian hospitals and these patients should be reviewed as a matter of priority. Delirium is an acute confusional state and is a very common scenario in inpatients, particularly the elderly or people with underlying cognitive impairment. It may be multifactorial in origin, with seemingly insignificant features (e.g. mild anaemia) becoming the instigating factor that tips a person into a more serious confusional state. An inpatient delirium is a poor prognostic factor, with a one-year expected mortality of up to 42%.

Start with ABC, review the observations chart for fevers or a change in vital signs and ask the nursing staff or family what this patient's baseline cognition is and if this has happened before. Note their reason for admission. Review their drug chart for medications such as sedatives, antipsychotics, steroids, anti-epileptics or anticholinergics that may explain their change in behaviour. Patients with Parkinson's given anticholinergic medications (e.g. metoclopramide) may experience an oculogyric crisis, with decreased consciousness. Remember the elderly metabolise drugs differently to middle-aged people and 'normal' doses may be within the toxic range for this population. Ask whether or not the patient is on an alcohol withdrawal scale (AWS), as delirium tremens (DTs) may cause seizures. Assess the patient's Glasgow Coma Scale (GCS) and perform a focused clinical examination, targeting the neurological system and possible sources of infection.

If the patient is unresponsive and there are no signs of life call a code blue and commence CPR, continuing the advanced life support pathway. If the GCS is <8, the patient should be considered unable to maintain their airway and you should notify anaesthetics (if they are not already present) as intubation may be required. If the patient is aggressive consider calling a 'code grey' (see 'Code black and code grey' below) and do your best to de-escalate the situation verbally. Send off a full set of bloods and a septic screen, including urine MCS, blood cultures and a CXR. Consider CT-brain if there are any neurological changes, or if the patient is on therapeutic anticoagulants or reports a headache or head trauma. Treat any underlying cause you identify, and continue to monitor the patient with neurological observations.

MEDICAL STAFF CONCERN

If a member of the hospital staff is concerned about a patient but their observations are not breaching any of the above criteria, they may still call a MET response. Common scenarios include prolonged or unexpected seizures, pain crises, ischaemic chest pain, arrhythmias, agitation and delirium, severe electrolyte abnormalities or rigors and febrile episodes.

CODE BLACK AND CODE GREY

These codes vary from hospital to hospital but are called for aggressive patients or visitors when their behaviour is putting other people at risk. Typically, a code grey is called for the hospital's own security to respond, and code black when police are required. The emergency team does not typically attend these codes but, if you hear a code black or grey called on your own patient, you should attend to see if you can give assistance (especially in the case of delirium, where you may be able to help the responders identify a reversible cause).

CHAPTER 26

THE DYING PATIENT

Joseph M O'Brien

Unfortunately, not every patient can be 'saved' and you will regularly encounter patients who are dying. Although you may not be able to prevent their deaths, there is a lot you can do to ensure they die in the manner of their choosing, or achieve a 'good death'. Death is an intensely personal experience, and you must ensure the patient and their family are involved in all palliative care discussions. They become the driving force behind their management, with their medical team acting in a facilitative role.

IDENTIFYING A DYING PATIENT

It is important to detect when a patient is entering the terminal phase of their life, as it allows the patient and their family time to prepare, increases the focus on symptom control, reduces the rate of unnecessary interventions and can prevent unnecessary hospital admissions. Unfortunately, the reality is that many patients die an undignified death, with controllable symptoms. Doctors are poor at predicting prognosis, with the majority of impending inpatient deaths only identified within 4 hours of the event (we are particularly overly optimistic with oncological deaths). Subsequently, the decision to transfer to hospice is often achieved too late to facilitate a 'good death'.

There are several evidence-based indicators that a patient is approaching the end of their life, including decreased activity, multiple comorbidities, cachexia, advanced disease, weight loss greater than 10% of body mass within 6 months and a sentinel event (e.g. serious fall, bereavement or escalation of supportive care). More than one of these criteria should prompt thought about advanced care planning.

ADVANCED CARE PLANS

Having this discussion with both the patient and their family can be very difficult. Most commonly, the thought of declining treatment is overt and confronting. The way you approach this topic is important. Careful wording is necessary so as not to shock or upset the patient, but also to remain clear about the intention of the discussion. For example – 'If time were to run short, and your heart were to stop beating, would you want us to attempt CPR or perform a shock to restart it?' Many patients have a limited understanding of the likely outcomes of these interventions, and assume that emergency treatment such as defibrillation will keep them alive. Practice is key, and so too is observing masterful professionals. As a junior doctor take your opportunities to sit in on family meetings and observe how palliative and intensive care specialists navigate these conversations.

There are several key components you should cover with the patient, at a minimum:

1   Would they like CPR and/or defibrillation to be performed?
2   Would they like to be referred to ICU if they deteriorate?
3   Would they like to be intubated or receive invasive ventilation?
4   Would they like inotrope supports?
5   Would they like emergency calls (i.e. METs and code blues) to be made if they were deteriorating rapidly?

It is possible for a patient to choose any combination of the above treatments, but keep in mind a patient must be in ICU for inotropes or invasive ventilation, and if you do resuscitate a patient who is 'for' CPR and but 'not for' ICU, where would they go? It is quite common for a patient to remain for MET calls for comfort only, and this is usually not unreasonable (especially on nights or weekends where you may need assistance to keep the patient comfortable). This decision is ultimately a medical one and the treating team (or MET responders) can choose not to offer futile treatment.

Patients or their families can make some inappropriate decisions. A misbelief commonly held by the public is that once a patient is 'not for resuscitation' they will no longer receive appropriate care – you should make it very clear that they will still be reviewed regularly and have ongoing supportive care. Be sure to document this discussion *very clearly* – most hospitals will have their own form for discussing resuscitation orders. There is no point having a thoughtful and productive advance care planning discussion if no one can locate the outcome in an emergency.

As a side point, terminology to describe end-of-life care is tricky at best, so here are a few pointers:

• Avoid using 'to palliate' as a verb, instead opt for the noun and advise that a patient is for or receiving 'palliative care'. 'Comfort measures' is another frequently used term many people find helpful.

• A treatment limitation form (or equivalent) is a document initiated by the medical team to clearly outline the limits of management. You do not need a patient's consent to make a patient 'not for CPR' but you should inform the patient and their family as to your decision and rationale to avoid confusion and grief reactions from these parties later.

• Advance care plans are patient-initiated, and not only outline what their preferred ceiling of care is, but also non-medicalised aspects of end-of-life wishes such as who they would like present prior to death, whether they would like to be read last rites and how they would prefer to manage their nutrition.

ROLE OF THE PALLIATIVE CARE TEAM IN AN INPATIENT SETTING

The palliative care team is a valuable resource, not just for end-of-life care but also for assistance in controlling refractory symptoms that are causing distress to a patient. They are most readily required when there is intractable pain or other symptoms unresponsive to standard management, for conscious patients where secretions are an issue or where there is significant stress on the caregivers or family. Analgesia should never be withheld while waiting for a palliative care team review, and you should have started at least the first-line treatment for any symptom you are requesting help with prior to contacting the team.

A useful framework for managing the dying patient is the Liverpool Care Pathway (LCP). Although the LCP has been discussed in the British media recently as a 'euthanasia' pathway, the truth is less controversial. The LCP serves as a series of prompts to ensure no factor of a patient's end-of-life care is forgotten. A patient on the LCP must be reviewed every day (like any other patient) and, although this is uncommon, may improve to the point where they are taken off the LCP at which point the goals of care should be revised.

ARRANGING OUTPATIENT PALLIATIVE CARE

It is recommended a patient who is identified as being in the last 12 months of life should be referred to a palliative care service. If their death is imminent or expected to be within 3 months, it is not unreasonable for their care to be managed at an inpatient palliative care unit (see Table 26.1 for issues and management). However, some people living with terminal illness will survive beyond that window and should be referred to the local palliative care outpatient service. It is quite reasonable for a patient to want to remain in his or her own home.

Outpatient palliative care services are geographically-based (if referring publicly), and you need to contact the service in your patient's distribution area. This may be done by the nursing staff in your hospital network. They are a vital part of end-of-life care, and will devise a plan in consultation with the patient and their family as to what the plan will be at the time of death.

RATIONALISING MEDICATIONS

Once it is confirmed that a patient is dying, their 'pill burden' is minimised by ceasing all non-essential medications such as antihypertensives, electrolyte supplements and anticoagulants. Typically, all that remain are those that provide symptomatic relief, or whose removal would cause withdrawal symptoms (e.g. a rebound hypotension with beta blockade). Analgesia, anti-emetics, anti-reflux medications and drugs that modify respiratory symptoms should always be kept. Aperients should be considered carefully in the context of the patient. Medications should be kept oral until no longer practical.

TABLE 26.1 Common palliative care issues and their management

SYMPTOM	MANAGEMENT	NOTES
Pain	• Paracetamol 1 g PO or IV Q4H PRN • Oxycodone Instant Release 5–10 mg PO Q4H PRN • Oxycodone with naloxone (starting at 10 mg/5 mg PO Q10H PRN) • Fentanyl patches topical changed daily (12–100 mcg/hour, consult registrar) • Morphine 2.5 mg subcut or IV PRN (no limit) • Morphine 10 mg in a syringe driver over 24 hours, with unlimited 2.5 mg subcut or IV breakthrough up-titrated as needed • Ketamine infusion (contact palliative care)	Pain management in the terminal phase of life can be very difficult. Assess the patient's pain regularly and titrate as needed, especially if they are still verbalising that they are in pain. Avoid steroids due to central side effects. Oral medication will eventually need to be stopped and, at this point, a syringe driver can provide good background analgesia. A patient should never have to die in significant pain. Oxycodone with naloxone can be useful in patients with constipation as the naloxone is not absorbed across the gut wall and minimises the localised constipating effect of opioids
Cough and dyspnoea	• Normal saline 5 mL nebs PRN • Salbutamol 5 mg nebs PRN (initially QID, but in end of life can be escalated) • Ipratropium 500 mcg nebs Q4H PRN • Codeine linctus 10 mL PO Q6H PRN • Ordine mixture 10 mg PO Q4H PRN • Morphine (various forms)	Can be difficult to control. Consider non-pharmaceutical methods such as positioning them upright. If very distressed, midazolam may help

TABLE 26.1 Common palliative care issues and their management—cont'd

SYMPTOM	MANAGEMENT	NOTES
Pruritus	• Cirtirizine 10 mg PO daily to BD • Loratadine 10 mg PO daily • Steroids – low dose prednisolone (e.g. 5 mg PO daily), and work up as required • Neuropathic analgesics (e.g. gabapentin) • SSRIs (e.g. mirtazapine) – don't start without speaking with your registrar	Accompanies several terminal illnesses, and can cause great distress to a patient. If not systemic, try topical therapy first. Try keeping the area cool. Make sure there are no medications that may be the cause
Hiccup	• Haloperidol 0.5 mg PO Q6H PRN	Surprisingly effective. Consider starting at a BD PRN dose. Alternatively, consider a prokinetic such as metoclopramide
Terminal agitation	• Haloperidol 0.5–1 mg PO Q12H PRN (consider making a regular order if ongoing restlessness) • Diazepam 5 mg PO Q4H PRN • NB: Midazolam 10 mg or clonazepam 1 mg is often used in a syringe driver with analgesia	Delirium will be fluctuant, and patients may hallucinate, be confused or aggressive and become restless. It is quite common. Review for reversible causes, including medications
Noisy airway or secretions	• Glycopyrrolate 400 mcg subcut as a PRN only	Patients often do not find the 'gurgling' associated with upper airway secretions distressing in their final hours, but the family may. Anticholinergics have significant side effects so only use glycopyrrolate if the family are particularly disturbed by the noises. Often they will understand it is not distressing to their loved one

continued

TABLE 26.1 Common palliative care issues and their management—cont'd

SYMPTOM	MANAGEMENT	NOTES
Nausea and vomiting	• Metoclopramide 10–20 mg PO or IV Q4H (daily maximum of 80 mg) • Ondansetron 4–8 mg PO/IV/subcut Q4H PRN (maximum of 32 mg/day) • Domperidone 10 mg IV/PO Q4H (daily maximum of 40 mg) • Prochlorperazine 12.5 mg IM PRN (daily maximum of 50 mg) • Cyclizine 25–50 mg PO/IV Q6H (with a maximum of 150 mg) • Hyoscine 20 mg PO Q12H PRN • Levomepromazine 6 mg PO PRN or as 25 mg subcut in a syringe driver (avoid in liver disease, Parkinson's and epileptics) • Aprepitant 80 mg PO daily with a 125 mg PO loading dose (rarely used in palliative care, usually oncology)	Generally used in the order listed to the left Metoclopramide is a gut prokinetic, whereas ondansetron will constipate Prochlorperazine can cause abscesses if given subcutaneously Levomepromazine causes significant drowsiness and hypotension Although not always a concern in palliative care, many of these drugs prolong the QT period
Anorexia	If the patient is palliative, a lack of hunger could be tolerated. If the symptom particularly bothers the patient, a dietitian referral may help	Usually multifactorial in origin, but try and find any reversible causes
Fatigue	Non-pharmaceutical. Allow the patient to rest as required. A normal part of the dying process. Often unrelated to energy expenditure	Incredibly common symptom – 70–100% of oncology patients will be fatigued
Xerostomia	Consider starting regular mouth care – gargles of either Peter MacCallum Cancer Centre mouthwash (2.5 mL PO QID) or Biotene® (2.5 mL PO QID)	Alternatively, ice on a stick may be used gently to relieve a dry mouth. Ensure denture care and brushing of teeth continues as long as possible

TABLE 26.1 Common palliative care issues and their management—cont'd

SYMPTOM	MANAGEMENT	NOTES
Sweats	Non-pharmaceutical – cooling with fans, maintaining fluids, changing of bedding, cotton clothing	Affects about 1/8 cancer patients. If it is due to infection or another reversible cause, consider short-term treatment to relieve symptoms
Depression	• Psychiatry referral *first* • Citalopram 10–20 mg PO mane (avoid in CCF, recent MI or prolonged QT)	Common in the dying patient. Treatment, despite brevity, may improve their last weeks of life. There are other SSRIs available if citalopram is contraindicated. Utilise the counselling service or psychiatry team where possible, but not every patient will require their assistance
Constipation	• Docusate with Senna 100/16 mg PO BD • Movicol 1–2 sachets PO Q12H PRN • Lactulose 20 mL PO Q4H PRN • Fleet 1 enema PR daily PRN	Start patients on opiates on an oral aperient. Some patients will become obstructed and, if they are not for surgical management, should have supportive care such as mouth care and anti-emetics
Bleeding	• Tranexamic acid 1 g PO TDS • Sedation	If the patient is dying rapidly from haemorrhage, consider sedation and analgesia. If death is not imminent consider the need for tranexamic acid with your registrar
Spinal cord compression	• High dose steroids (e.g. dexamethasone 8 mg PO BD started immediately) • Emergency radiotherapy • Surgical decompression • Analgesia	MRI is the gold standard investigation. A radiotherapy emergency. Similar to bleeding, consider the patient's context before referring
Dehydration	• Mouth care as outlined above • Normal saline 1 L subcut over 24 hours	Strongly consider the need for rehydration therapy (e.g. causing discomfort)

Source: National Health Service Scotland, 2010. Palliative care guidelines – symptom control. <http://www.palliativecareguidelines.scot.nhs.uk/symptom_control/>.

MANAGING CANCER PAIN

- Opioids should always be charted with a laxative.
- Breakthrough doses are typically 1/6 to 1/10 of the background dose, and should be charted PRN.
- NEVER give opioid dosing a range or a lock-out period in a palliative patient (e.g. oxycodone IR 5 mg PO PRN, not '5–10 mg PO Q4H PRN'). This way it is easy to calculate breakthrough usage and titrate the background analgesia appropriately, and it prevents the patient from being in pain waiting for their next available medication.
- If a patient is experiencing worsening or new pain, avoid the use of extended-release opiates.
- Try and keep the breakthrough opioid the same type as background analgesia.

TABLE 26.2 Preparing a patient for death

Inform the patient and family of their diagnosis or change in prognosis	☐
Chart:	
• Analgesia	☐
• Anti-emetics	☐
• An anxiolytic (e.g. benzodiazepine)	☐
• Antipsychotics for terminal agitation	☐
• Mouth care	☐
• Aperients if needed, and/or	☐
• Glycopyrrolate for secretions	☐
If the patient is not eating, consider a 24-hourly bag of subcutaneous saline for comfort	☐
Rationalise the medications	☐
Refer to a palliative care service	☐
Offer to put the patient and/or family in touch with supportive services (including religious ones if required)	☐
If a pacemaker is in situ, consider contacting Cardiology or the patient's pacemaker company to have the device deactivated	☐
Ask the patient and family who they would like to be present at the time of death	☐
Consider using a syringe driver to administer morphine and midazolam	☐
Move the patient to a single room, if possible, to allow for maximum privacy	☐

CHAPTER 27

THE DECEASED PATIENT

Joseph M O'Brien

It is very unlikely you will make it through your first year of clinical practice without being asked to certify the death of a patient. This can be a confronting task for a number of reasons, particularly when the patient is one you knew personally or the cause of death is traumatic. This is rarely something that has to be done with urgency, particularly overnight, so triage accordingly (it also allows the family, if present, to spend some time alone with their loved one). If you expect a patient to die during a colleague's cover shift, it is strongly encouraged you hand over this information with a few basic details about the patient at a minimum.

THE PROCESS OF CERTIFYING DEATH

Before certifying a patient's death, ask whether or not this was an expected death, whether the family are present or on their way, whether they intended to become a tissue donor, or if an autopsy had been planned. If the patient is already known to you (or the home unit gave you a sufficient handover) you may have these details already. In Australian law, death is defined as, 'The irreversible cessation of circulation of the flow of blood in the body of the person, *or* irreversible cessation of all function of the brain of the person'. In clinical practice, you should satisfy three components:

1 no cardiac output

2 no respiratory function

3 no neurological function.

As such, the examination is guided by demonstrating these three concepts. If the family is present, introduce yourself and state the reason you have come to see their relative. Explain it is a routine part of end-of-life care, and ask if they would like to remain in the room – some people will prefer to temporarily stay outside while you complete the certification. Certifying a death does not have to be a lengthy process, and should only take a few minutes. Systematically assess the patient's response (e.g. 'Mr Smith, can you hear me?') and feel their radial pulse, before moving quickly to pupillary reflex, closing the patient's eyes afterwards (sometimes this is not possible). Auscultate the chest for heart and breath sounds, and optionally assess pain response by sternal rub, trapezius squeeze or

BOX 27.1 Select indications for nomination for a coronial investigation

Unexpected, unnatural or violent death

Patient in care of the state (e.g. a patient with a carer, or under the Mental Health Act of your state)

Patients who are pregnant or have been pregnant in the last 28 days

Patients who have had surgery or a major procedure within 28 days

Road and public transport fatalities

Homicides and suicides

Electrocutions

Animal attacks

Deaths due to fire

Where the patient's identity is unknown

Poisonings and deliberate overdoses

Accidental falls within 28 days of death (including inpatient falls!)

Workplace accidents

Adapted from: Coroner's Court Victoria, 2014. Reportable deaths FAQs. <http://www.coronerscourt.vic.gov.au/find/faqs/reportable+deaths+faqs>.

seniors) are uncertain, give the coroner's court a call. They are an excellent source of advice and the final decision makers in this area.

Don't forget to tell a patient's family you have submitted a referral to the coroner. Explain to the family that a coroner's case does not imply errors have been made, but it is rather part of 'due process' for a large range of circumstances. Inform them the coroner's court will liaise with them directly, and the investigation should not unduly delay their relative's funeral arrangements. Expect the police to attend. Do not remove anything from the patient's body (including cannulas, catheters or other lines). When the police arrive you may be asked to witness the identification of the patient's body by their next of kin, but you are not expected to identify them yourself.

During the coroner's investigation, the patient's medical records may be requested by the court. The purpose of the coronial investigation is to identify the patient, their cause of death and the details necessary to register the death with the state Registry of Births, Deaths and Marriages. If you are ever requested to make a statement about a coronial inquest, speak to the consultant involved and your hospital's legal department for advice.

ORGAN AND TISSUE DONATION

Australia has a national organ and tissue donation program – the Australian Government's Organ and Tissue Authority. Our current organ donation system is 'opt-in', where a person is not assumed to be a donor, and must register their intent in advance. Australia is at the forefront of transplant medicine, with high success rates, but an unfortunately low number of donors. The low number is in part due to the low numbers of people identified as being potential donors due to method of death, and partly because Australian families (who have the final say on their relative's donation) refuse on 40–50% of occasions.

The other way in which a patient may wish to contribute to society posthumously is by donating their body to science. This is done differently state by state, but usually involves a coordinating university that collects, prepares and distributes cadavers and tissue for the purpose of education and teaching in their state's tertiary education centres (e.g. the University of Melbourne, the University of New South Wales, the University of Western Australia, the University of Queensland and the University of Tasmania). Often a patient who requests that their body be 'donated to science' will have contacted the coordinating university already, and it is just a matter of calling the university when the patient dies. However, you may also be asked to provide the contact details to this program if the patient has not planned in advance.

CHAPTER 28

THE PREOPERATIVE PATIENT

Paul Watson

Patients admitted to hospital with acute surgical pathology may require extensive work-up prior to heading to theatre. These patients can be acutely unwell due either to their presenting surgical condition or exacerbation of their medical comorbidities and will require assessment and management during the perioperative period.

The junior doctor is responsible for the ward management of these patients during this period and is often required to liaise with the Anaesthetic and Theatre Departments to ensure operations are correctly booked and the patient will be ready for theatre at the specified time.

PREOPERATIVE WORK-UP

A detailed history and examination should take place during the admission. Previous anaesthetic episodes and a surgical history can give clues to the patient tolerance of an anaesthetic.

Baseline pathology tests are indicated for any patient undergoing an emergency procedure; patients who have presented as non-trauma emergency cases should have an FBE and UEC performed to trend inflammatory markers and renal function. Patients with substantial injury or those likely to have intraoperative blood loss should have a group and hold taken. Patients with respiratory disease should have a chest X-ray.

Patients who have presented with infection and persistent nausea and vomiting are prone to hypovolaemia and acute renal failure. Assessment of fluid status and adequate IV resuscitation are an important aspect of optimising the cardiovascular function of such patients. Even in the absence of severe fluid or blood loss, the anaesthetic agents can create hypotension that will be compounded by a dehydrated patient.

Patients who present with trauma should have appropriate imaging prior to progressing to theatre. Orthopaedic, vascular and neurosurgical patients are likely to require preoperative films to appreciate the full extent of injury and guide the operative approach. Neurosurgical patients, for example, with subdural haematomas will sometimes undergo an initial conservative period of management with serial imaging scans to determine changes in the size of the haematoma. Timely ordering of these scans is imperative.

In the preoperative setting the junior doctor should implement the following checklist:

- Is the patient booked, marked and consented (if applicable) for theatre?
- Is the anaesthetic team aware of the patient and their current clinical condition?
- Have appropriate emergency preoperative investigations been ordered?
- Does this patient require high dependency observation postoperatively and has a referral been made?
- Has the patient's next of kin been updated on the patient's progress?

FASTING AND MANAGEMENT OF REGULAR MEDICATIONS

Adult patients should be fasted from solid food for at least 8 hours prior to the theatre to reduce risk of aspiration during the anaesthetic period. Some hospital protocols dictate that patients should be fasted from free fluids for 4 hours and clear fluids for 2 hours. Where possible patients should continue on their regular medications – this is particularly important for patients taking cardiovascular medications that establish cardiac rate and blood pressure control. Patients who present with trauma and a history of chronic pain or opiate tolerance will need to be prescribed adequate analgesia in the preoperative setting to ease the discomfort postoperatively. The hospital pain service can provide useful advice in patients with complicated pain issues.

Patients with diabetes will need glucose replacement in their IV maintenance therapy (such as dextrose – see Chapter 24) to maintain stable blood sugar levels (BSLs). Patients who have a basal dose of insulin should be prescribed a 50% dose while fasting to prevent large swings in their BSLs. Metformin should be discontinued the night prior to surgery. Regular BSLs during the perioperative period allows for close observation. Patients with diabetes should be higher priority for earlier operating theatre times due to the risk of hypoglycaemia during the fasting period.

Patients who are on long-term steroids may require additional therapy during the perioperative period due to their decreased ability to endogenously produce steroids in response to the physiological stress of major thoracic and abdominal surgery. These patients may benefit from regular hydrocortisone on top of their regular steroid dose during their inpatient stay.

ANAESTHETICS

All patients who are to undergo a procedure requiring an anaesthetic will be reviewed by the anaesthetic team in the preoperative period. When emergency cases are booked the treating medical team is required to discuss the case with the anaesthetic doctor on call.

Much like any other referral this discussion should include information regarding the patient's current clinical status, previous anaesthetics and an overview of the past medical history. For patients who are clinically unwell or have extensive cardiac and respiratory medical history, an earlier anaesthetic review may be required to facilitate any investigations or management plans for medically optimising the patient. In the emergency setting there is limited time to thoroughly work up a patient for theatre; a more comprehensive review and consideration of cardiac risk (see Table 28.1) is taken in the elective setting (Chapter 53). It's important to note that cardiac complications are 2 to 5 times more likely in emergency surgery.

There are multiple methods of anaesthesia available for patients (see Table 28.2 and Fig. 28.1).

Major and head and neck trauma often necessitate an altered anaesthetic approach, as follows:

- Head trauma increases intracranial pressure (ICP); to overcome the increase in pressure and maintain perfusion the patient's systolic blood pressure must be maintained (usually above 90 mmHg systolic).

- Cervical spine fractures present an airway challenge for the anaesthetic team with decreased airway visualisation due to immobilisation of the neck.

- Mandibular and maxillary trauma requires that the patient is intubated via the nasopharynx to obtain necessary access.

- Patients who are shocked from hypovolaemia may develop substantial hypotension from the catecholamine inhibition of IV anaesthetic agents. Severely shocked patients may require progression to intubation with muscle relaxants alone to avoid cardiovascular collapse.

TABLE 28.1 American Society of Anesthesiologists (ASA) physical status classification

CLASS	DESCRIPTION	EXAMPLES	SEDATION RISK
I	Normal and healthy patient	No past medical history	Minimal
II	Mild systemic disease without functional limitations	Mild asthma, controlled diabetes	Low
III	Severe systemic disease with functional limitations	Pneumonia, poorly controlled seizure disorder	Intermediate
IV	Severe systemic disease that is a constant threat to life	Advanced cardiac disease, renal failure, sepsis	High
V	Moribund patient who may not survive without procedure	Septic shock, severe trauma	Extremely high

Adapted from: Fitz-Henry, J., 2011. The ASA classification and peri-operative risk. Annals of the Royal College of Surgeons of England 93, 185-187.

TABLE 28.2 Anaesthetic options for emergency surgery

TYPE OF ANAESTHETIC	INDICATION FOR USE
Local anaesthetic	Minor limb and other localised trauma as tolerated by the patient
Regional anaesthetic	Peripheral nerve blocks for limb surgery
Spinal anaesthetic	Lower limb trauma
Local anaesthetic + sedation	Minor facial trauma or deeper trauma to limbs requiring minor debridement For patients with mild trauma who are not comfortable with local anaesthetic only
General anaesthetic	Major trauma, head trauma, acute abdominal emergencies Extensive soft tissue injuries

McCunn, M., Grissom, T.E. & Dutton, R.P., 2014. Chapter 81: Anaesthesia for trauma. In: Miller, R.D., Eriksson, L.I., Fleisher, L.A., et al., eds. Miller's Anesthesia, 8th ed. Philadelphia: Saunders. pp. 2423-2459. Burbulys, D.B., 2014. Chapter 4: Procedural sedation and analgesia. In: Marx, J., Hockberger, R. & Walls, R., Rosen's Emergency Medicine, 8th ed. Philadelphia: Saunders, pp. 50-60.

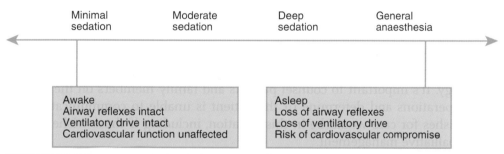

FIGURE 28.1 The spectrum of sedation vs general anaesthesia.

Burbulys, D.B., 2014. Chapter 4: Procedural sedation and analgesia. In: Marx, J., Hockberger, R. & Walls, R., Rosen's Emergency Medicine, 8th ed. Philadelphia: Saunders, pp. 50-60.

PREPARING THE PATIENT FOR URGENT SURGERY

Severely unwell patients may require theatre within minutes to hours of presenting to the emergency department. After initial assessment and diagnosis of the issue, the patient needs to be prepared for theatre. Using the AMPLE mnemonic, the junior doctor can quickly obtain important history for patients who require rapid surgical management:

A – allergies

M – medications (particularly anticoagulants)

P – past medical history (focus on comorbidities and previous surgeries)

L – last meal (solid food, free fluids, clear fluids)

E – events leading to presentation.

CHAPTER 29
THE OPERATING THEATRE

Paul Watson

INTRODUCTION TO THEATRE

The operating theatre is the primary intervention environment for surgical procedures and an ideal environment for the junior doctor for learning and practising of clinical skills under the supervision of senior and experienced clinicians. Even if there's not an opportunity to perform aspects of the case, there's great benefit in observing expert handling of tissue and procedural skill techniques that guide the development of your own skills.

This chapter is a guide to the basics of theatre; each surgical specialty has its own individual approach to setting up and conducting procedures (Section IV). Apart from assisting in theatre, junior doctors are involved in the booking of theatre cases, writing operation notes and liaising with other medical and nursing staff.

Patients who are booked for operations are considered to be in one of two categories:

1   elective – patients who have non-emergency pathology who are booked for surgery under a category-based system of urgency
2   emergency – patients who have conditions that will create a significant impact on mortality and/or morbidity unless there is rapid intervention.

There are different processes for booking emergency and elective patients for theatre. Generally, elective patients are booked as outpatients from clinic, whereas emergency cases present acutely from ED or from inpatient referrals. Emergency theatre time is also used for unplanned interventions for patients with chronic surgical issues, such as debridement of chronic wounds or multiple washouts of a joint due to an infection.

The process for booking emergency cases varies among hospitals; however the basic steps remain the same:

- Patients are assessed and informed consent is obtained.
- Paperwork is lodged to make a booking. In some hospitals this is done via a computer-based system. Any requests for specific equipment should be made at this point.

- The theatre manager or person responsible for booking cases is informed and a discussion takes place regarding potential scheduling. Any further requests for equipment should be made at this point.
- The anaesthetist responsible for the allocated block of theatre time is notified of the booking. It's essential that the Anaesthetics team is provided with the details regarding the specific intervention and the medical comorbidities of the patient as these factors will influence anaesthetic approach. Some patients may require a review by the anaesthetic team before the procedure.

Prior to the commencement of any operating theatre procedure, the patient must undergo a 'timeout'. This process involves all members of the theatre team (Surgical, Anaesthetic and Nursing) checking the identity of the patient and the details of the consent form to ensure the correct procedure is performed on the correct patient. The primary operating surgeon from the surgical team, referring to either the consultant or the registrar, must complete this process.

THE THEATRE

Theatre rooms are designed to facilitate a wide variety of operations. The operating bed lies centrally and can be adjusted to alter the position of the patient. Overhead lights illuminate the surgical field of vision, though some deeper surgery will require the use of headlights worn by the surgeons.

The anaesthetic trolley is typically located at the head of the bed and provides monitoring equipment and induction agents for the anaesthetic team. There will be a number of trolleys for the surgical set-up, depending on the size of the procedure. Familiarise yourself with the positions of the components as this will impact how the theatre equipment is set up around the patient, i.e. suction canisters, diathermy machines, laparoscopy towers.

Other common equipment includes:

- Limb tourniquet – utilised in upper and lower limb surgery to help maintain a bloodless surgical field. The cuff is inflated prior to commencing the procedure. As the cuff creates an ischaemia of the limb to facilitate enhanced visualisation of the field, the tourniquet time is limited to 2 hours to prevent tissue damage.
- Hand table – used for upper limb surgery. The hand must be suspended in the air and prepped before being placed on the table. A scrubbed member of the team's hand holds a prepped section of the limb before it is lowered onto the draped table.
- Stirrups – attached to the theatre bed allowing the legs to be raised and split giving access to the perineum. A common set-up for gynaecological and urological procedures.
- Intraoperative imaging. A portable X-ray machine can be brought into theatre to take intermittent images or provide a continuous screen with radio-opaque dye tests. Examples include:

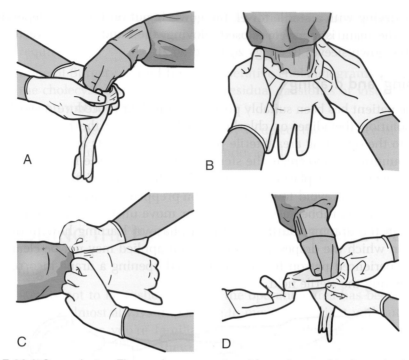

FIGURE 29.2 Open gloving. The scrub nurses assist with putting on the gloves. In this instance the hands are fully pushed through the cuff before applying the glove.

Sullivan, E.M., 2013. Surgery. In: Ballweg, R., Sullivan, E.M., Brown, D., et al., Physician Assistant: A guide to clinical practice, 5th ed. Philadelphia: Saunders, Fig. 25.6.

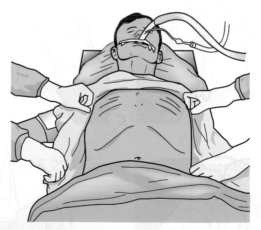

FIGURE 29.3 The bottom and top drapes are applied first, then the side drapes. Drapes can be secured with towel clips.

Sullivan, E.M., 2013. Surgery. In: Ballweg, R., Sullivan, E.M., Brown, D., et al., Physician Assistant: A guide to clinical practice, 5th ed. Philadelphia: Saunders, Fig. 25.11.

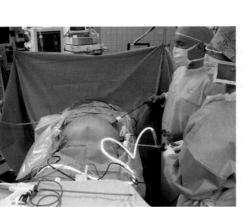

FIGURE 29.4 Intraoperative view of surgeon and camera operator standing on the same side of the patient for adhesiolysis. Patient's arms are abducted and an iodine-impregnated drape covers the abdomen.

Reproduced from: Rosen, M.J., 2014. Laparoscopic ventral hernia repair. In: Cameron, J. & Cameron, A., Current Surgical Therapy, 12th ed. Philadelphia: Saunders, pp. 1497-1501, Fig. 1.

THEATRE EQUIPMENT

The theatre set-up

For each type of operation, the theatre staff create sterile packs that contain the tools that will be used during the case. Each pack can be modified as per the surgeon's preference with extra equipment requested as required. The sterile packs remain the responsibility of the nursing staff and they conduct 'counts' of all the tools and materials used to ensure no unwanted equipment is left behind in the patient. As you might imagine, the scrub nurse may find it hard to keep track of the tools if members of the surgical team 'help themselves', and this may get the junior doctor a stern word from the scrub nurse! It's best practice to request equipment from the nursing staff as this will allow the nursing staff to keep track of the equipment throughout the case.

Suction

Suction canisters are attached into the wall suction, which is then connected to the suction tubing passed off from the surgical team when setting up the case. There are a number of different suction handles, with differing sizes and flows. The canisters allow for the measuring of fluid, which is important for estimating fluid losses (blood) during the case. Often, the suction tools are an 'in case' measure and seldom used. Some surgeons prefer the suction tubing to be clamped or twisted to reduce the noise during the case.

Diathermy

Diathermy or electrocautery is the process of using electrical current to produce surgically desirable tissue damage. The two types of diathermy are monopolar and bipolar, referring to the method of electrical circuit:

TABLE 29.2 Tips for surgical assisting

Laparoscopic surgery: holding the scope (camera)	• Keep the camera centred on the tip of the instrument or the operative field as directed by the surgeon • Don't move the camera to clean the lens unless instructed • Keep in mind that laparoscopes often have an angled view (i.e. 30°)
Retracting	• Most surgeons prefer to place their own retractors, particularly for deeper surgery • Aim to maintain the same position and level of tension when you take over the retractor. Don't remove the retractor until instructed • If the surgeon grabs the retractor to move it, completely relax your hand, allowing them to re-position
Cutting sutures	• Often the surgeon will instruct you to cut the stitches 'long' or 'short' • Remember that non-absorbable sutures will need to be removed when you cut them! • Stabilise your cutting hand with your opposite hand or on the patient to ensure accuracy
Clearing the surgical field	• You may be required to keep the surgical field clear of blood and fluid using suction or packs • Never 'rub' with the pack; dab with pressure then quickly remove the pack from the visual field before any more blood can re-accumulate • Suction should clear the operative field, or can be placed peripherally. Ensure it stays out of the way of the instruments!
Closing wounds	• Junior doctors and medical students have to start somewhere! Usually by closing the skin layer at the end of the case and applying the dressings • Make sure the wounds have been cleaned and dried before applying dressings

- ○ Operation notes may be used by future surgical teams in the case of emergency or revision surgery so it's essential that they accurately reflect the procedure.
- Postoperative plan
  - ○ These instructions should include the short- and long-term management of the patient. If the junior doctor is asked to document this plan, they should consult with the primary operator to determine if there are any special instructions.
  - ○ Consider OPSIDED (Chapter 30) as a template for postoperative issues.

For day cases, the patient will be discharged from the day surgery unit. These patients will need discharge summaries and prescriptions (as required) following the case. Ask the patient prior to the case if they require a medical certificate so you can complete all of the post-op paperwork at the same time.

Patients who will be sent to an inpatient bed postoperatively will need an inpatient drug chart and fluid orders as required. The friendly anaesthetic staff will often chart pain relief, anti-emetics and postoperative fluids; however, the junior doctor will need to chart the patient's regular medications, DVT prophylaxis and antibiotics as required.

MINIMAL ACCESS SURGERY

Widespread use of these approaches exists in general, gynaecological and urological surgery. Minimal access or 'keyhole' surgery aids recovery time and shortens hospital inpatient stays. Junior doctors are often required to assist during these procedures, primarily by holding the camera for the operating surgeon.

Common methods of minimal access surgery include:

- laparoscopic surgery
- arthroscopy
- thorascopy
- robotic-assisted surgery.

Where practically possible, routine emergency general surgery such as appendicectomies and cholecystectomies are performed using this method. The abdomen is pierced centrally with the first 'port' and inflated with an inert (i.e. non-flammable) gas. The camera is then inserted into the abdomen and other port sites are created in the skin through to the cavity under direct vision. See Figs 29.7 and 29.8 for examples of laparoscopic procedures and Fig. 29.9 for a diagram of a 30° scope.

There are a wide variety of procedures performed with minimal access surgery, detailed throughout Section IV.

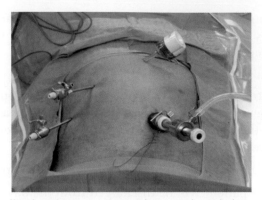

FIGURE 29.7 A centrally placed camera port with two right-sided ports.

Reproduced from: Brunt, M.L., 2014. Laparoscopic cholecystectomy. In: Cameron, J.L. & Cameron, A.M., Current Surgical Therapy, 11th ed. Philadelphia: Saunders.

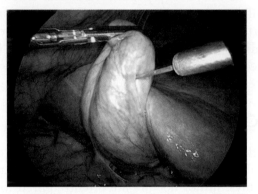

FIGURE 29.8 Technique of needle aspiration of a distended gallbladder. This approach is useful in the setting of a tense, distended gallbladder to avoid perforation from a grasper and spillage of bile and stones.

Reproduced from: Brunt, L.M., 2014. Laparoscopic cholecystectomy. In: Cameron, J.L. & Cameron, A.M., Current Surgical Therapy, 11th ed. Philadelphia: Saunders, pp. 1305-1311, Fig. 4.

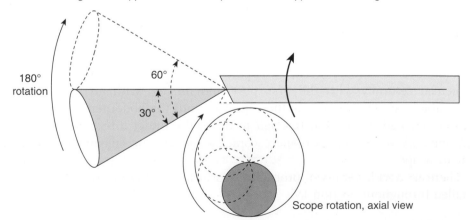

FIGURE 29.9 The use of a 30° scope that can be rotated allows for an increased field of vision.

Reproduced from: Miller, M., 2010. Overview of arthroscopy. In: Miller, M.D., Chhabra, A.B. & Safran, M., Primer of Arthroscopy. Philadelphia: Saunders, pp. 1-11, Fig. 1-10.

CHAPTER 30

THE POSTOPERATIVE PATIENT

Paul Watson

ROUTINE REVIEW OF THE POSTOPERATIVE PATIENT

The postoperative patient is a classic hypothetical clinical scenario for management challenges facing the junior doctor. However, a large number of postoperative patients perform within expected parameters, and are discharged home without incident. The sum of the experience of patients who do well postoperatively should help in the early identification of patients who are progressing slowly, and prudent investigation and management should be initiated to prevent further deterioration.

Some postoperative complications are seen as early as the recovery room or as late as over a week postoperatively. Understanding the natural history of some of the more common postoperative complications can aid in identifying the cause, particularly in the case of postoperative fever. Specific complications of surgery are covered throughout the individual surgical chapters (Section IV).

The postoperative care of the patient begins in the operating theatre. Anaesthetic staff carefully monitor the patient's fluid balance, analgesia and anti-emetics are provided, and drain tubes are regularly observed. Once the patient is considered stable and sufficiently alert after their anaesthetic, the patient is transferred to the ward or an intensive care bed (with the exception of day cases).

The junior doctor should add the patient to the ward list, check the operation note for specific orders (investigations, medications) and be mindful of the patient's likely postoperative progression. The patient may be discharged the next morning so prescriptions and outpatient appointments can be organised.

Provided the patient is well, the entire team may not officially review them until the next day on the ward round. The key focus of the daily round of the postoperative patient is to determine how well the patient is progressing and whether the patient is meeting their goals for discharge. Remember OPSIDED to ensure all postoperative issues are considered (see Box 30.1).

BOX 30.1 OPSIDED mnemonic for routine postoperative review

- **O**bservations: Has the patient been haemodynamically stable? Any fevers?
- **P**ain: Is the patient comfortable? Do they have any IV analgesia (PCA) or regional blocks ongoing? Can this patient have their pain treated by oral medication alone? Does the patient have nausea?
- **S**urgical site: Are there any drain tubes? Dressing intact? Any haematoma, bleeding or infection? Will this patient require ongoing dressings?
- **I**nvestigations: Has the patient had their routine postoperative tests (ie. post-op Hb check)? Chest X-ray post thoracic surgery? Does the patient need electrolyte replacement?
- **D**rugs: Does the patient require antibiotics? Any new regular medication postoperatively? When can regular medications (anticoagulants) be re-commenced? Check DVT prophylaxis.
- **E**ating: Is the patient currently tolerating their prescribed diet (e.g. clear fluids or free fluids post bowel surgery)? Are they suitable for an upgrade?
- **D**ischarge: What is the likely discharge date for this patient? Have they been seen by Allied Health? Will they need rehabilitation? **What is their follow-up plan?**

The documented daily plan should address all relevant issues as per Box 30.1. Clear documentation is essential, particularly with respect to drain tube management. Direct communication with nursing staff during or post-round is key to avoiding misunderstandings and delays relating to the management plan.

PAIN

Pain should be considered a perioperative issue, requiring consideration before and during a procedure. Adequate understanding regarding the likelihood of pain following a procedure can help the junior doctor determine how closely post-operative pain will need to be monitored. Patients who have severe preoperative pain or are particularly anxious during the perioperative period have been shown to be at increased risk of developing postoperative pain syndromes.

In the preoperative setting pain can be controlled by identifying contributing factors. Pain is a physical sensation influenced by a range of mental, emotional and environmental factors. Before and during the procedure steps can be taken to reduce the amount of pain experienced by the patient, including:

- adequate preoperative pain relief for emergency and trauma patients
- accurate estimation of pain levels associated with certain procedures (i.e. procedures involving manipulation of deep soft tissue such as muscle can result in severe pain)
- identification of emergency and elective patients with opioid tolerance

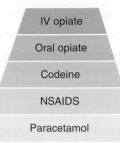

FIGURE 30.1 The 'pain medication pyramid'.

- use of local anaesthetic and regional blocks where possible
- epidural anaesthesia for large abdominal and pelvic procedures where possible.

Non-pharmacological methods of controlling pain include immobilisation and elevation of the affected areas where possible. Having nursing and allied health staff assist the patient in their activities of daily living (ADLs) during the early perioperative period may prevent unnecessarily painful over-exertion.

In the postoperative period patients should have a regular pain regimen charted plus extra PRN medication for breakthrough. Unless contraindicated all patients should be placed on regular simple analgesia

The pain medication ladder (Fig. 30.1) seeks to highlight the role of adequate simple analgesia to help reduce the need for further PRN medications. When patients are in the early postoperative setting and experiencing intermittent pain, they should be encouraged to take their regularly scheduled simple analgesia to provide consistent coverage (Table 30.1). Education regarding the benefits of simple analgesia aids the patient manage their own pain levels when discharged home.

Adequate control of pain is essential for patient progress as patients are unable to have adequate physiotherapy review including mobilisation and achieving independence with ADLs. Adequate relief is also psychologically beneficial as patients are less apprehensive regarding their recovery and discharge.

Acute pain service

Most hospitals offer an Acute Pain Service (APS) that provides perioperative assessment of a patient's pain requirements, particularly with respect to analgesia infusions and patient controlled analgesia.

Continuous epidural analgesia can include long-acting local anaesthetic agents or opiate infusions via the spinal catheter left in postoperatively. These agents require close monitoring by the inpatient and APS teams as these infusions have the capacity to cause respiratory depression and hypotension due to sympathetic blockade. For patients who are stable but demonstrate persistently low blood pressure, high dependency unit (HDU) review and support can be beneficial rather than ceasing the infusion without consulting the anaesthetic or intensive teams first. As these patients have typically had large abdominal and pelvic

SECTION III

TABLE 30.1 Suggested dosing regimens for commonly used perioperative analgesia

SIMPLE ANALGESIA	ORAL	OTHER ROUTES
Paracetamol	1 g 6/24 regularly 1330 mg TDS (controlled release)	Same for IV and PR
NSAIDS		
Ibuprofen	200–400 mg TDS regularly	Same dose PR
Diclofenac	75–150 mg in 2–3 doses (max 200 mg daily)	Same for PR Available in topical 1% gel
Celecoxib	400 mg daily for first daily dose	
Ketorolac	10 mg every 4–6/24 (max 40 mg daily)	IM/IV: 10 mg initially 10–15 mg every 6/24 subsequently (max 60 mg daily) Note: convert to oral as soon as possible
Weak opiates		
Codeine	30–60 mg every 4/24 PRN Most commonly used as a combination medication with paracetamol	
Opiates		
Oxycodone	5–15 mg 4/24 PRN Start with 5 mg in patients >70 years 5–10 mg BD controlled release (CR should not be used standalone in acute pain)	SC: initial dosages • <39 years: 7.5–12.5 mg every 2/24 • 40–59 years: 5–10 mg every 2/24 • 60–69 years: 2.5–7.5 mg every 2/24 • 70–85 years: 2.5–5 mg every 2/24 • >85 years: 2–3 mg every 2/24
Tramadol	50–100 mg 4–6/24 PRN (max 400 mg daily, 300 mg daily if >75)	IV/IM: 50–100 mg 4–6/24 (max 600 mg daily, 300 mg if >75)

TABLE 30.1 Suggested dosing regimens for commonly used perioperative analgesia—cont'd

SIMPLE ANALGESIA	ORAL	OTHER ROUTES
Fentanyl		SC: initial dosages • <39 years: 100–200 mcg every 4/24 • 40–59 years: 75–150 mcg every 4/24 • 60–69 years: 40–100 mcg every 4/24 • 70–85 years: 40–75 mcg every 4/24 • >85 years: 30–50 mcg every 4/24. Patches should not be used in acute pain settings
Morphine		SC/IM: initial dosages • <39 years: 7.5–12.5 mg every 2/24 • 40–59 years: 5–10 mg every 2/24 • 60–69 years: 2.5–7.5 mg every 2/24 • 70–85 years: 2.5–5 mg every 2/24 • >85 years: 2–3 mg every 2/24

Adapted from: Australian Medicines Handbook Pty Ltd, 2015. Articles on: Celecoxib, Codeine, Diclofenac, Fentanyl, Ibuprofen, Ketorolac, Morphine, Oxycodone, Paracetamol, Tramadol. In: Australian Medicines Handbook [Internet]. Adelaide: Australian Medicines Handbook Pty Ltd.

surgeries, ceasing pain relieving measures may create a second management problem that can be avoided if the side effects can be suitably managed in a more supported setting.

Patient controlled analgesia (PCA) is another option of pain relief whereby a patient is placed on a background and/or bolus infusion of analgesia with regulated control over the bolus dose frequency via a delivery button. The device has a lockout period that dictates a maximum amount of bolus analgesia in a specified timeframe. Review of this data by the inpatient team can give insight into the effectiveness of the dosages as the attempts versus delivery of doses highlight how often a patient requires extra analgesia. All PCA orders should be supplemented with regular oral simple analgesia; however, it's best to avoid the combined use of oral and IV opiates to avoid the risk of over sedation and respiratory depression.

The acute pain team will assist in step down of epidural and PCA analgesia to an oral analgesic regimen.

FEVER

Postoperative fever can present a diagnostic challenge to the junior doctor, as there is an exhaustive list of potential causes. This section deals with very general aspects of postoperative fever, as there are specialty specific causes that warrant further discussion later. Some of the more common general causes tend to present in predictable patterns (Fig. 30.2).

Atelectasis

Early postoperative fever with shortness of breath or decreased oxygen saturation is classically associated with atelectasis (see Fig. 30.3). Those patients who have undergone thoracic and abdominal surgery are at particular risk of sputum retention due to restricted chest wall movement and ineffective cough effort.

Adequate pain relief and chest physiotherapy exercises are indicated to improve symptoms. Patients with thick secretions may benefit from nebuliser therapy to aid breaking up the sputum, particularly those patients who smoke or have established chronic airways disease.

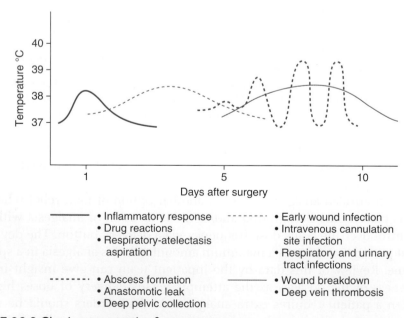

FIGURE 30.2 Classic postoperative fever patterns.

Yii, M., 2010. Postoperative problems. In: Smith, J.A., Fox, J.G., Saunder, A.C., et al., eds. Hunt and Marshall's Clinical Problems in Surgery, 2nd ed. Sydney: Churchill Livingstone Australia, Fig. 11.1.

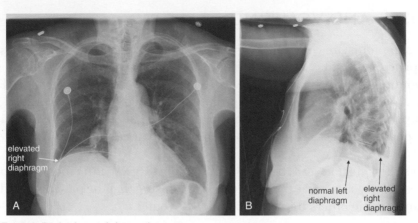

FIGURE 30.3 Right lower lobe atelectasis.

Reproduced from: Raval, D. & Rafeq, S., et al., 2017. Atelectasis. In: Ferri, F.F., Ferri's Clinical Advisor. Philadelphia: Mosby, p. 135, Fig. 1A-139.

Wound infections

During the daily ward round, all patients should have a review of their wound dressings. Some surgical units utilise 'honeycomb' dressings that allow visualisation of the surgical incision through the intact sterile dressing.

Wounds at risk of infection are those contaminated preoperatively such as trauma patients. Despite copious washout intraoperatively, these wounds need to be monitored for the potential risk of infection. Poor wound closure can also leave a portal for infection from the surrounding skin into the wound bed, with dressings used to keep the wound as clean and dry as possible.

If there is gross pus from an infected wound, a swab should be taken for culture. Patients should commence on appropriate empirical antibiotics if they are systemically unwell from wound infection until an organism is identified.

Respiratory tract infections

See the section on hospital acquired pneumonia in Chapter 36.

Deep abdominal infections

Typically associated with 'swinging' fevers and increasing pain, the patient with recent abdominal surgery who becomes febrile after around the 3rd to 4th postoperative day should have prudent investigation for an intraoperative cause of fever.

Deep vein thrombosis and pulmonary embolus

Deep vein thrombosis (DVT) prophylaxis should be instituted for patients at risk of developing DVT. Patients can present with erythematous, swollen limbs that are tender on palpation, requiring investigation and expert opinion for management (Chapter 35).

NAUSEA AND VOMITING

These symptoms are commonly associated as side effects of general anaesthetics and opiate medications as well as manifestations of severe pain. However, nausea and vomiting can be associated with the onset of ileus or mechanical bowel obstruction, which will need to be promptly excluded (Chapter 45).

Current recommendations for prophylaxis in the postoperative setting are based on patient risk factors for postoperative nausea and vomiting (see Table 30.2).

These risk factors can be used as a guide to give anti-emetics to patients postoperatively, as soon as the recovery room. Ensure that the patient has adequate PRN anti-emetic orders for both oral and I/V routes.

HYPOTENSION

There are numerous causes of hypotension in the postoperative setting. The key is to determine the underlying process:

- hypovolaemia
  - intravascular losses (blood loss or bleeding)
  - dehydration (preoperative fasting)
- peripheral vasodilatation
  - systemic inflammatory response, sepsis
  - sympathetic blockade from epidural.

Intravascular losses

Blood loss is an expected aspect of major surgery. Patients are routinely counselled during the preoperative phase regarding the potential for blood loss and possible need for transfusion during or after the operation. Some patients have personal

TABLE 30.2 Risk factors for postoperative nausea and vomiting

Anaesthetic risk factors	• **Intra- and postoperative opioid drugs (primary risk factor)** • Volatile anaesthetic • Nitrous oxide • Inadequate hydration
Patient risk factors (all primary risk factors)	• **Female sex** • **Non-smoking** • **History of postoperative nausea and vomiting**
Surgical risk factors	• Increased length of procedure

Adapted from: Gan, T.J., 2006. Risk factors for postoperative nausea and vomiting. Anesthesia and Analgesia 102(6), 1884-1898. Therapeutic Guidelines Limited, 2014. Post-operative nausea and vomiting in adults. In: eTG complete [Internet]. Melbourne: Therapeutic Guidelines Limited.

objections to receiving blood products, which needs to be discussed with both the surgical and anaesthetic team prior to proceeding to theatre.

During any lengthy procedure or after the observation of a large loss of blood intraoperatively, the patient's haemoglobin (Hb) can be checked and blood products given appropriately. Patients with previous ischaemic heart disease should have particularly close monitoring of their Hb levels to avoid prolonged periods of anaemia (Hb <70). These postoperative patients should have early morning pathology to determine whether there has been loss of blood significant enough to require transfusion. Symptomatic anaemia (dizziness, lethargy, hypotension) can exacerbate underlying medical conditions and delays patient mobilisation postoperatively. The decision to transfuse patients should be made in conjunction with the registrar of the treating team.

An assessment of a patient with active bleeding postoperatively should begin by identifying the likely source of the bleeding. A soaked dressing should be removed and the wound inspected. The distinction needs to be made between skin edge bleeding and deeper bleeding oozing through the wound. Often deeper bleeding will lead to an underlying haematoma surrounding the incision site. Mild oozing from skin edges can be treated with reinforced dressing, while persistent skin edge bleeding, if clearly identified, might be amenable to further suturing on the ward. If there is any suggestion of deeper tissue bleeding the patient should be considered for a return to theatre for exploration.

Fluid balance and electrolyte disturbances

Due to preoperative fasting and intraoperative losses, patients are at risk of dehydration during the postoperative period. Patients who have undergone emergency procedures are particularly at risk as they may have presented with a preoperative fluid deficit that will need to be accounted for in addition to any intraoperative losses and ongoing maintenance fluids.

Patients who have persistent nausea and vomiting postoperatively or a modified diet following GIT surgery will require IV fluids to support them until oral therapy can be safely restarted. For these patients electrolyte replacement will need to be administered via the IV route; keep in mind that oral electrolyte replacement in patients who have just undergone bowel surgery is likely to be ineffective due to poor absorption.

Fluid and electrolyte replacement is a careful balance requiring ongoing assessment of a patient's clinical fluid status to avoid excessive administration of IV products (Chapter 24).

Tachycardia and **low urine output** can be manifestations of hypovolaemia, but other causes will need to be excluded (Chapter 24).

URINARY RETENTION AND CONSTIPATION

Urinary retention in the postoperative setting is associated with an increase in UTIs and prolonged inpatient stays. Patients who develop painful retention or undergo serial bladder scans showing increasing volume with an inability to void may require catheterisation. Encourage the patient to mobilise if possible to encourage voiding.

The causes of urinary retention in a patient with no urological history can sometimes be attributed to lingering effects of anaesthetic and analgesic agents; however, in the older patient, the impact of constipation on the ability of the patient to void should not be underestimated. Surgery around the groin and perineum results in significant local tissue swelling that can contribute to voiding difficulties, particularly in combination with opiate medication.

If a patient has not been able to void, the next question must be about the last time the patient opened their bowels. Any patient on opioid analgesia should be placed on aperient medication to avoid retention and constipation. Patients who require catheterisation for relief of urinary retention should therefore undergo a trial of void once they have opened their bowels.

DELIRIUM

Delirium (Chapter 34) has a variety of potential causes including factors as simple as a change to unfamiliar surroundings and disruption to normal sleep/wake cycle. Elderly patients are most at risk of developing postoperative delirium, and these patients are also susceptible to electrolyte disturbances from poor oral intake. The use of opiate medications leads to further drowsiness and disorientation.

It is prudent to rule out organic causes of confusion such as infection, but equally important is re-orientating the patient by attempting to achieve a normal day–night sleep cycle, reassurance from the nursing staff, proper oral intake as soon as tolerated and avoiding commencing an excessive number of new medications, particularly opiates. Unless the patient poses a constant risk of physical harm to themselves or others, there is no role of physical or chemical restraint.

CHAPTER 31

INPATIENT DISCHARGES

Joseph M O'Brien

DISCHARGE SUMMARIES

Discharge summaries can be the bane of the most junior doctor on a team's life, but they are actually a vital role of interns and residents. They are the main line of communication between the inpatient teams and the primary care doctor who will be coordinating the patient's long-term management and, if a patient is readmitted after a brief discharge, the summary from the prior admission is very useful in ensuring continuous care. It is also worth noting that the words and phrases used in the discharge summary are what allow the coding department to get the hospital funding from the Government for an inpatient stay.

The content that is important in discharge summaries can vary among departments (particularly between medical and surgical rotations), but the principles remain the same. GPs do not have forever to read your seven page essay, and you should emphasise the most important sections (i.e. the medication changes and the plan). Thus, they must be accurate, brief and complete with a clear plan for follow-up.

Discharge summaries should be timely – late paperwork can compromise the quality of patient care. To expedite the discharge process you can and should begin the summary prior to the day of discharge. When writing, keep in mind that the patient and their family are entitled to request a copy of the summary so take care with sensitive issues. Below is a quick guide for what should be in an inpatient discharge summary (see Fig. 31.1 for an example summary).

Introduction

It is good form to start a discharge summary with a one- to two-line recap of why they were in hospital and what their primary diagnosis was. For example, '53-year-old male p/w SOBOE and diagnosed with a NSTEMI who underwent PCI for moderately severe CAD'. This puts a clear picture of the patient's admission in the mind of the reader.

Presentation

How did this patient end up in hospital? Were they sick enough to be brought in by ambulance (BIBA) or did they self-present to ED? Were they referred by their

Example Discharge Summary

Patient Details
Mr Joe Blogs UR 123456
DOB 1/1/1935

Discharge Diagnosis
Diffuse large B cell lymphoma

Complications
Hypokalaemia, hypomagnesaemia, acute kidney impairment

Summary
Mr Blogs is a 79 yo gentleman who was admitted to St Elsewhere on the 29th July with a presumed cholecystitis, ultimately being diagnosed with Stage IV-B DLBCL and underwent two cycles of chemotherapy.

MHx: Treated hypertension, treated hyperlipidaemia, osteoarthritis (on NSAIDs, awaiting bilateral TKR), ischaemic heart disease (AMI 1997, no recent angiograms as lost to follow-up).
PHx: AMI (1997), MVA (several long bone fractures, managed at Big City Hospital, no metalwork in place, 1982).
SHx: Lives with supportive wife, Carol. Retired engineer. Ex-smoker with 35 pack years (quit 1997). Minimal alcohol consumption. Baseline effort tolerance 500 m. Walks without gait aids. Drives, cooks, cleans and manages finances independently.
FHx: Father died of 'heart attack' at 54 yo. Mother died of stroke at 82 yo. Paternal uncle had multiple myeloma.

Cholecystitis
- Admitted under Mr Thompson (General Surgery A) 29th June with severe RUQ pain, jaundice, and intermittent fevers.
- LFTs showed an obstructive picture (attached).
- USS showed multiple hypoechoic lines in gallbladder, suggestive of cholelithiasis.
- Added to emergency list 29th June and underwent laparoscopic cholecystectomy.
- Pathology report suggests chronic cholecystitis, with thickening of the gall bladder wall >5 mm.
- Experienced greater postoperative pain than expected, referred to Acute Pain Service who charted additional analgesia.

AKI
- Renal function decreased postoperatively.
- Baseline creatinine 120 – creatinine peaked at 230, resolved with gentle IV hydration and cessation of nephrotoxins.
  ACE-I can be restarted two weeks post-discharge.

Electrolyte abnormalities
- Hypokalaemia and hypomagnesaemia supplemented PO.

DLBCL
- Postoperatively, no improvement in LFTs or jaundice. RUQ persisted despite review by pain team.
- Could not provide appropriate analgesia, leading to MRCP. No stones.
- Serum LDH noted to be elevated. Malignancy suspected, leading to CT head/neck/chest/abdo/pelvis. No abnormalities detected.
- LFTs continued to worsen. Discussed case with Liver Transplant Team at Large Metropolitan Hospital. Suggested liver biopsy.
- Liver biopsy performed under ultrasound guidance. Tissue sent to Pathology Department of Large Metropolitan Hospital.
- Pathology reported as 'diffuse areas of CD19 and CD20 positive cells with complete obliteration of portal tracts'.
- Referred to Haematology service, who took over care of patient 5th August.
- PET 6th August: High avidity lesions in area of mesenteric chain, left axilla and right inguinal regions. Moderate uptake in spleen. Highly avid, diffuse lesions in liver.
- Bone Marrow Biopsy 6th August: Hypocellular marrow with infiltration of CD19 and CD20 positive cells in a monoclonal capacity.

FIGURE 31.1 Example of a discharge summary.

- Underwent first two cycles of R-CHOP. Experienced some peripheral neuropathy from the vincristine in second cycle. Documented as adverse drug reaction, will receive etoposide in future.
- Discharged with signs of marrow recovery at patient's wishes, will plan readmission for next cycle of R-CHOP in three weeks.

Medication changes
- ACE inhibitor ceased due to renal function.
- NSAID changed to paracetamol due to risk of PUD in >40 yo (risk to liver acceptable as per Gastro).
- Commenced 4 new drugs – valaciclovir (viral prophylaxis), ranitidine (gut cover), fluconazole (gunal prophylaxis) and trimethoprim/sulfamethoxazole (PCP prophylaxis).

Discharge Medications
- Aspirin 100 mg PO mane
- Paracetamol 1 g PO TDS (limit by LFTs)
- Valaciclovir 500 mg PO mane
- Trimethoprim/sulfamethoxazole 160/800 mg PO mane
- Fluconazole 200 mg PO mane
- Ranitidine 150 mg PO BD
- Atorvastatin 40 mg PO nocte

Discharge Plan
1. Follow up in Surg A outpatients, 10 am 12th September.
2. Refer to outpatient Haem clinic anytime patient requires specialist review.
3. Can restart ACE inhibitor in two weeks if eGFR >65.
4. Repeat bone marrow biopsy booked for 12 pm 12th September.
5. Asked patient to see LMO within one week for follow-up UEC (slip given to patient).
6. Patient will receive booking notification for next cycle of R-CHOP.

Distribution
Local GP
Dr Consultant Haematologist
Ms Consultant Surgeon

FIGURE 31.1, cont'd

GP? What were their symptoms? What *relevant* exam findings were present at time of admission? Were any investigations particularly important (e.g. trop rise, CT showing new bleed etc)?

Medical, past and social histories

Not all digital summary programs include these sections but they are all essential. This patient may be going to a new GP or may never have been seen at this hospital before. If you document this in the summary, any future doctor reviewing this patient will easily be able to find out all this information if for some reason the patient is unable to convey it themselves. For medical summaries in particular, document what you can about their past history. For example, if they have COPD – when were their last respiratory function tests, and what did they show? Are they known to a respiratory physician? How do they usually manage this condition? You should separate out each condition as a heading and include this data below it.

Investigations

Only the relevant ones here – we know your patient had an FBE and a UEC every day of their month-long admission but their GP certainly doesn't need to review them. That was your job! Consider attaching the most recent set, but otherwise only include truly investigative bloods (e.g. troponins and CK, haemolytic, renal, liver or malignancy screens, nutritional panel and/or rarely-performed screening bloods like PSA or TSH) and imaging (especially MRIs or CTs). Don't forget special investigations that may not appear in your hospital's pathology system such as Holters, TTEs, stress tests, angiograms, RFTs, scopes, nerve conduction studies and surgical reports (if available). If you don't have the results of these tests, at least convey that they were performed and when the GP will have access to them.

Summary

So your patient presented with haematochezia and a haemoglobin of 65. What did you do about it? Did the patient require any transfusions? Were special precautions required (e.g. negative pressure bed)? Did they need to go to ICU? Did they have any MET calls or code blues called? What medications did you change/cease/commence – and importantly, why? Be sure to include the dates of any surgeries and, if known, the name of the primary operator.

For medical summaries in particular, an issue-based approach is best here. Include the primary issue first – for example, '# CCF.' Then underneath this heading include all relevant information, such as the dry weight, frusemide dose and whether or not fluid restrictions and diets continue post acute care. Continue through all of the issues not forgetting items such as 'hypokalaemia', 'anaemia' and 'fall'. These may not sound important but have large implications for the coding process and therefore funding. If you exclude them you may be hearing from your health information services team asking you to complete the summary again!

Plan

The crux of your summary – where to from here? Include all medications that are due to cease after discharge (e.g. short course antibiotics), follow-up in outpatients, GP review, modified diets (e.g. 'to continue on thick fluids for 2/52'), weight-bearing status and/or investigations yet to be completed. If the plan is complex, it would be good form to contact the GP to discuss the patient's plan with them. Below the plan you should document your name and contact details – a hospital pager number, not your personal mobile!

Also note that a medication summary should be attached. Digital scripts and summaries are usually linked by the hospital's IT system, but if you use digital summaries and paper scripts you must type it out again.

DISCHARGE SCRIPTS

Depending on which hospital you work at, you may be required to write a discharge script for every patient regardless of whether or not any medications have been changed. This is a good habit to develop. Whether your hospital uses digital or paper scripts, you should have them available to your ward pharmacist by 4 p.m. the day prior to planned discharge. Having patients ready for discharge by 10 a.m. is a key performance indicator for Australian hospitals and more strictly enforced at some organisations than others, but having a script prepared the day before allows the pharmacy team to discuss any medication changes or needs with the patient and have their meds ready as early as possible. Conversely, don't try and do scripts too far ahead of time – patients' medications are often changed during their stay and you don't want to accidentally dispense incorrect meds because you were too organised!

Key points to remember when completing a discharge script are as follows:

- Use generic names. Brand names are firmly discouraged. Don't be bamboozled by our corporate overlords!

- Strength refers to the strength of the tablets. For example, a common dose of metoprolol is 25 mg BD, but it doesn't come in any strength under 50 mg. Thus the tablet strength is 50 mg, and the dose is 25 mg (or ½ tab) PO BD.

- Completing the quantity column is not always strictly enforced. If your hospital insists on you writing the quantity, use the PBS website to see what amount of tablets is supplied on the Pharmaceutical Benefits Scheme. Otherwise, writing 'PBS' should suffice, and the PBS quantity can be dispensed (although restricted medications must be written out in words and numbers). You can use this column to put a time course on treatment – for example, dispensing only 10 tablets of Augmentin Duo Forte guarantees a maximum course of 5 days!

- Include your provider number and pager – if there are any issues you can be contacted easily to modify your script with a phone order, rather than starting from scratch.

- Common drugs requiring streamlined authorities include clopidogrel, bisphosphonates and heart failure beta-blockers. If you're on a rotation where you prescribe these regularly, consider jotting them down in your organiser to save time. You can find the list on the PBS website (http://www.pbs.gov.au/browse/streamlined-authority).

- Some drugs require authority scripts, which cannot be streamlined. This includes expensive or potentially harmful drugs (e.g. ciprofloxacin) or drugs with restricted benefits at higher quantities (e.g. oral azithromycin for trachoma). These require a phone call to the 24-hour PBS line on 1800 888 333. Information you should have at hand includes the patient's name and Medicare number (usually on patient labels), the script number (in the top-right corner of the script), your provider number, the name of the required drug and its indication, strength and quantity of tablets required (which can be found on the PBS website). These calls take a bit of practice!

OUTPATIENT FOLLOW-UP

The last consideration on discharge is when the patient will next be seen. Often you will be guided by your registrar but occasionally this falls to you to decide. Take into consideration whether or not this patient requires ongoing specialist care – if so, review in outpatient clinic in 2 to 4 weeks is the standard (unless you have been advised otherwise). All postoperative patients will require at least one appointment for a wound check. If not, ask them to make a booking with their GP in the next week or two. If a patient needs bloods checked between discharge and their outpatient appointment, include this on the summary so their GP is aware.

CHAPTER 32

ALLIED HEALTH AND CLINICAL SUPPORT STAFF

Paul Watson and Todd Galvin Manning

There are a variety of allied health staff positions in inpatient and outpatient settings, each with their own specific skill sets in patient care, providing specialist input separate from medical, nursing and dental.

The junior doctor is the primary liaison between allied health staff and the treating medical team with expectations to make referrals and chase up advice regarding patients. In most inpatient settings, the allied health teams conduct daily reviews of patients, documenting their activities in the patients' notes. It is important that you keep yourself updated on allied health input for all your patients as it has important implications for treatment progression, particularly with respect to discharge planning.

Nursing staff usually make allied health referrals as a matter of routine; however, making referrals to allied health may be the responsibility of the junior doctor depending on the policies of your health network.

ALLIED HEALTH

Physiotherapists

Physiotherapy encompasses a variety of general and specialty practitioners involved in assessing and improving movement and function. The mobility of a patient is a critical component in discharge planning. Patients who come to hospital from home need to be able to effectively move and self care before they can be discharged, especially older patients who live alone. As such, initial assessment of patients should include a detailed history outlining their baseline mobility. Physiotherapists can give input into whether a patient will require further subacute care for further physical rehabilitation once the acute medical treatment goals have been met.

Assessment of function is made in respect to a patient's ability to complete 'activities of daily living' (ADLs), such as personal hygiene tasks. These are important indicators of a patient's ability to care for themselves at home.

Physiotherapists perform a number of specialised roles in disease, too numerous to list. As a junior doctor, some common indications for physiotherapy review to be aware of include the following:

- Chest 'physio' – breathing exercises aimed at improving respiratory effort to prevent sputum retention and atelectasis. Common in pneumonia, rib fractures or a post-surgical setting where thoracic/abdominal pain may limit chest wall movement.

- Mobility assessment and exercises – although typically associated with older patient groups, may also include younger patients with injuries. This assessment will also determine if gait aids are required and state if a patient requires assistance with getting out of bed or a chair. The outcome of these assessments will largely dictate discharge destination. Assessments include walk tests.

- Discharge planning – further to mobility assessments, physiotherapists ensure that patients will be able to safely navigate their home environment including inclines and stairs. If the patient requires further physiotherapy input to reach these goals, they may make a recommendation for a subacute rehabilitation admission.

Occupational therapists

Occupational therapists (OTs) focus on identifying and resolving barriers preventing patients returning to normal activities of daily living with a specific focus on getting patients back to becoming 'job-fit'.

OTs also review patients who have had injuries or acute medical issues (such as stroke) who may require modifications at home such as handrails and ramps to successfully achieve their ADLs. They will continue to monitor the patient's progress in the community to assess whether they need further aids to achieve both work and daily activity goals.

Occupational therapy is widely engaged by surgical services as a means of tracking a patient's progression back to work and identifying short- and long-term limitations. Specialised occupational therapists work closely with surgical units to fast-track the rehabilitation of patients after injury or surgery, including:

- Hand therapists – specialise in hand injuries such as fractures, tendon injuries and scar management. Provide functional assessment and fit splints for patients during their postoperative recovery.

- Orthopaedic occupational therapy – review both trauma patients and elective arthroplasty patients with a focus on aids that may be required to assist discharge from hospital.

Social workers

There are a multitude of personal, cultural, social and economic factors that can influence the physical and mental health of patients. Social workers deal with a variety of issues surrounding a patient's general wellbeing at home, in addition to identifying issues that may impact upon discharge.

Social workers are particularly experienced at working with vulnerable people who have been admitted to hospital, including patients who have:

- longstanding mental illness
- intellectual disabilities
- long-term physical limitations
- no fixed abode
- a low socioeconomic background.

Some of these patients may be unknown to aid services, and a decline in health and subsequent presentation to hospital may reveal areas of concerns regarding a patient's living conditions. Social workers provide patients and their families with information regarding services that can assist patients in the community and help arrange financial support for patients, particularly by filling out paperwork for income support and work-related injury compensation.

Speech pathologists

Speech pathologists (also known as speech therapists) primarily assist patients with communication difficulties. In the inpatient setting, another common indication for speech pathology review is to assess the patient's ability to swallow. This has important implications for feeding and dietary status.

Patients who have had neurological insults, particularly strokes, and those who have had oral surgery would benefit from a speech therapy review to assess their capacity to swallow. The speech therapist will give input on the ability of the patient to swallow thin and thick fluids with a goal to swallow solid food. The primary concern with an inadequate swallow is the risk of coughing and choking and subsequent aspiration.

Dietitians

The overall scope of practice for dietitians is to promote health in patients by optimising their nutritional status. A number of patients are unable to adequately obtain nutrition due to physical injury, surgical procedures or prolonged illness. Dietitians provide input regarding appropriate supplementation and replacement therapies.

Dietitians work closely with patients who have commenced tube-based gastric feeding, guiding which type and the rate of administration of replacement therapy. They also review patients who have a prolonged low oral intake or fasting period who are at particular risk of malnutrition and those patients who are placed on modified diets due to swallowing difficulties.

SECTION III

Diabetes educators

Patients with both newly diagnosed and chronic diabetes can benefit from further education regarding their care. Diabetic educators provide patients with instruction and advice regarding:

- checking blood sugar levels
- dietary habits and lifestyle modification
- medication regimens including advice on insulin dosing and administration.

Ultimately, the diabetic educator seeks to equip the patient with the skills and knowledge to self care, with their diabetes management plan under the supervision of their general practitioner.

The diabetes educator staff are available as both inpatient and outpatient services.

CLINICAL SUPPORT STAFF

Bed manager (or admitting officer [AO])

The bed manager is responsible for coordinating bed allocation throughout the hospital, including overseeing capacity for new admissions based on existing capacity and expected discharge.

The junior doctor is often required to liaise with the bed manager when their inpatient unit is accepting a transfer patient from another hospital network or, in the reverse situation, when they enquire about bed capacity at another hospital. In the latter example, the discussion is aided by first speaking to the accepting registrar at the destination hospital and relaying their contact information to the bed manager to facilitate transfer of patients of high clinical priority. Patients who are to be unexpected admissions directly to the ward from outpatients or day surgery will need to be discussed with the bed manager to ensure there is a bed available.

Post-discharge acute/subacute care

Most health networks offer a number of post-discharge support options to allow clinically well patients to return home while still receiving basic observations and/or treatments that would otherwise necessitate the patient to remain in hospital.

The names of these services vary according to location, but are commonly referred to as 'hospital in the home' (HITH) or early discharge support. An HITH service will conduct daily or twice daily review of patients to administer medications including IV antibiotics and anticoagulants, check VAC dressings and offer drain tube management. An HITH department is generally run by clinical nurses, though a medical registrar can be involved in the referral service screening appropriate patients in some larger health networks.

Other nursing services can offer dressing changes to patients at home, though patients are sometimes required to supply their own dressings. Patients who are suitable for daily dressings of wounds and routine post-discharge graft dressings would benefit from follow-up with these services. Each health network uses different terms to describe these services, which may include:

- post acute care – typically have strict patient criteria for accepting post-discharge care due to funding
- district nursing services – offer a wide range of services dependent on location, more common in regional and rural areas
- cancer support services – are available for post-discharge support of patients with established cancer diagnosis. These services are often linked with outpatient clinics.

These care programs only operate within a geographical area surrounding the health network; for patients from rural and remote areas, a referral is required to the local health network and GP so that the local nursing service has a liaison to discuss and review patients as required.

Clinical support staff vary among hospitals and, as part of a junior doctor's orientation to a new rotation, you should seek to familiarise yourself with staff members who can contribute to smooth discharge planning to ensure this process is put in place at the earliest opportunity.

SECTION III

MULTIDISCIPLINARY MEETINGS (MDMS)

These are formalised meetings allowing for the discussion and formulation of management plans for patients with a cancer diagnosis. The meetings are typically specialised by either region of cancer (e.g. upper GI, HPB, colorectal etc) or by type of cancer (e.g. melanoma). The MDM can occur at any point of the management timeline:

- as a new diagnosis for advice on options for investigation, timing of surgery, role of neo-adjuvant treatment
  - may include a review of images and any available pathology
- post biopsy or surgical intervention for review of pathology and further treatment discussion
- at diagnosis of recurrent or metastatic cancer.

These meetings are typically attended by:

- Radiology
- Pathology
- Medical and Radiation Oncology
- Surgical teams
- Allied Health.

Allied Health staff, such as breast care, prostate care and specialised physiotherapists, attend multidisciplinary and unit meetings to offer input and fast-track referrals. These staff members may suggest changes to the way patients are managed in the outpatient setting in terms of recovery and rehabilitation, as they often become the primary point of contact for patients once they are discharged from the unit.

Depending on the unit, it might be the responsibility of the junior doctor to put patients onto the MDM discussion list – check with the outgoing team during your handover. Each meeting should have a printout of all patients who are to be discussed. Note which patients belong to your team and list any jobs that arise from the discussion (e.g. ordering further imaging, referrals to Oncology).

RADIOLOGY MEETINGS

Some units hold separate radiology meetings to review imaging on current inpatient or interesting outpatient cases. These meetings may vary from an informal sit-down with a consultant radiologist in the reporting room to a scheduled meeting with a fixed agenda.

Orthopaedic Radiology meetings have a specific structure. They involve a review of the imaging for all of the previous week's cases including preoperative and postoperative films in addition to preoperative imaging for upcoming elective cases. The registrar will usually give a brief account of the underlying pathology and the operative approach. Collating the images for this meeting is a time-consuming process that is typically the responsibility of the junior doctor.

Other units such as Cardiology and Vascular Surgery hold meetings referred to as a 'case conference', in which specialised cardiac and vascular studies are reviewed by the unit consultants to discuss a management plan. Often these studies are performed outside the health network and may need to be imported into the hospital imaging system. In some units the junior doctors present these cases so it's important to be familiar with their medical history, previous interventions and current medications (particularly anticoagulants).

SECTION IV

MEDICAL AND

SURGICAL

SPECIALTIES

CHAPTER 34

GENERAL MEDICINE

Joseph M O'Brien

General Medicine (or 'Internal Medicine' if you watch too much American TV) is one of the core rotations completed by interns in Australia, and there is no other rotation quite like it. Does your patient have an unclear diagnosis? Multiple comorbidities? More than one system involved in this presentation? Complex discharge issues? A 'functional' overlay? Or is the specialty registrar simply not interested in your patient? If the answer is yes to any of the above, congratulations – your patient is coming in under 'Gen Med'.

The patients admitted under General Medicine are one of the most heterogeneous groups in the hospital. Expect to care for a lot of elderly patients – the average age of metropolitan Gen Med patients is now in the 80s. Apologies to any current or future geriatricians, but in the interest of space we will cover our aged care issues within this chapter! You might complete Gen Med in a regional or rural setting, where there is less specialty representation. Your case mix here will be especially varied and challenging, as when there are no specialty services General Medicine becomes the default unit.

General physicians (consultants in General Medicine) and Gen Med trainees have a large number of roles in a hospital setting, including managing patients requiring multiple specialty team consults, providing perioperative medical consultations, diagnosing undifferentiated presentations, performing procedures (e.g. lumbar punctures, ascitic taps), responding to emergency codes and educating junior doctors. A career in General Medicine is challenging but enormously rewarding. Most trainees complete 'dual training' with Gen Med and an additional specialty (e.g. Infectious Diseases or Cardiology).

CONGESTIVE CARDIAC FAILURE (CCF)

Congestive cardiac failure (synonymous with congestive heart failure or CHF) is the failure of the heart to meet the metabolic demands of the body's tissues due to either structural or functional cardiac disorders. CCF is highly prevalent, increasing with age. The incidence of CCF is also rapidly increasing, believed to be due in part to the increased survival of patients with CAD.

CCF is under-recognised by junior doctors as an end-stage illness, with a 50% 5-year mortality – higher than several cancers. Patients at a higher risk of CCF are those with existing IHD, hypertension, valvulopathy, cardiomyopathy or diabetes, and men, the elderly and smokers.

Decompensated CCF is an incredibly common cause for admission and thus a condition you should be highly familiar with heading into internship. CCF places significant economic burden on the healthcare system, with up to 18% requiring readmission within 30 days.

Diagnosis

Patients with CCF classically present with increasing exertional dyspnoea, fatigue, rapid weight gain (from fluid retention) and worsening peripheral oedema. The history often includes increased fluid or salt intake (especially in summer!), decreased 'effort tolerance' (previously known as 'exercise tolerance', or the distance a patient can walk before stopping due to dyspnoea or fatigue) or simply being unable to wear their normal shoes.

When taking a history, enquire about other cardiovascular illnesses as there is a large overlap between CCF and other cardiac diseases. Ask if the patient knows their 'dry weight', if they weigh themselves regularly, what their baseline effort tolerance is ('How far can you walk on flat ground before you have to stop because you're short of breath?'), how many flights of stairs they could climb, if they are compliant with salt and/or fluid restrictions, if they have a regular cardiologist and if they have had a recent echo (and if so, where?). Ask about both tobacco and alcohol consumption.

Clinical examination focuses on the cardiorespiratory systems. Examine for clubbing, irregular pulse, nicotine staining, height of the jugular venous pressure (JVP), cyanosis, sternotomy scars, heart sounds, crackles on auscultation and peripheral oedema in the lower limbs (and sacrum/abdomen).

Natural history

Heart failure is now divided into heart failure with reduced ejection fraction (HFREF) and heart failure with preserved ejection fraction (HFPEF). This terminology has replaced the older terms 'systolic' and 'diastolic' failure. An echocardiogram is required to differentiate the two conditions, as their clinical presentations are very similar. Both have a relapsing/remitting course with gradual increase in symptoms and decline in effort tolerance. Depending on the underlying cause, this deterioration can be either rapid or slow.

The most commonly used classification system for heart failure is the New York Heart Association system, outlined in Table 34.1. As effort tolerance decreases, the mortality without proper treatment increases.

Complications of CCF include 'cardiorenal syndrome' (deteriorating renal function; a difficult clinical situation), hepatic congestion, valvulopathies and arrhythmias.

Investigations

A patient admitted with CCF will need baseline bloodwork (FBE + UEC + CMP + CRP), LFTs (for hepatic congestion), thyroid-stimulating hormone (TSH; thyroid

TABLE 34.1 New York Heart Association (NYHA) classification of heart failure

Class I	No limitation with normal physical exercise failing to precipitate dyspnoea, angina or palpitations
Class II	Mild limitation with symptoms during normal physical activity
Class III	Moderate limitation, markedly symptomatic on gentle physical activity
Class IV	Symptomatic heart failure at rest, exacerbated on physical exertion

Adapted from: Ballinger, A., ed., 2012. Chapter 10: Cardiovascular disease. In: Ballinger, A., ed. Essentials of Kumar and Clark's Clinical Medicine, 5th ed. Edinburgh: Saunders, p. 438.

dysfunction can alter cardiac output, contractility and vascular resistance) and brain natriuretic peptide (BNP; used to diagnose and prognosticate heart failure).

If AMI is suspected consider performing troponins, although be wary that troponins may be elevated without ischaemia in severe failure (especially with concomitant renal impairment). A baseline chest X-ray is required to review for cardiomegaly, prominent hilar vessels (i.e. upper lobe diversion), effusions and Kerley B lines. CXR can help differentiate between failure, exacerbation of COPD and pneumonia. Consider a dipstick urinalysis. ECG is essential.

Quite importantly – but often missed – a *baseline weight* should be recorded so an accurate estimate of diuresis can be kept. UECs should be monitored closely as patients are increasingly 'dried out' with diuretics. Despite many units having only limited access to echocardiography, a TTE should be requested. Although this can usually be performed after discharge (aiming for <2 weeks), if a new or worsening murmur is detected its increased urgency should be discussed with the Cardiology registrar.

Although rarely available, cardiac magnetic resonance imaging (MRI) is increasingly employed to definitively assess ventricular volumes, wall motion and structural wall thickness. It may also identify infiltrative disease mimicking failure (e.g. amyloidosis).

Management

When presented with a patient with decompensated failure, begin with ABC – airway, breathing and circulation. Ensure the patient is haemodynamically stable before continuing. If not, escalate appropriately. Once the diagnosis of heart failure is confirmed:

1   Commence diuresis – if the patient is already on loop diuretics (e.g. frusemide), it is standard to double the dose and convert to intravenous administration. For example, if a patient is admitted with a usual dose of 40 mg PO frusemide, it could be escalated to 80 mg IV mane. This can be titrated further as required by the ward team. Frusemide

is *twice* as effective IV when compared with PO administration (e.g. 40 mg IV = 80 mg PO). The aim is to lose *1 kg per day* – you can be confident this is fluid as humans do not lose fat or muscle that quickly!

2   Initiate a fluid restriction (standard = 1.5 L), strict fluid balance and low sodium diet.

3   Request daily weights and UECs.

4   Request an echocardiogram.

5   If there are no contraindications, commence an ACE inhibitor and 'heart failure' beta-blocker (nebivolol, carvedilol, metoprolol extended release and bisoprolol) and slowly up-titrate to the maximum tolerated dose. Be wary of both blood pressure and bradycardia. The beta-blocker should **not** be added until the patient is euvolaemic (or your registrar tells you to!).

6   Continue regular medications and give deep vein thrombosis (DVT) prophylaxis.

7   Consider incidental screening for hyperlipidaemia and diabetes with fasting glucose and lipid profile (much easier to do in hospital than the community).

8   If present in your hospital, refer to a heart failure nurse for patient education.

If the patient is in acute pulmonary oedema (APO) it is a medical emergency and should be escalated immediately. These patients may require non-invasive ventilation (NIV) or inotropic support, performed in the Intensive Care setting. APO is treated with aggressive diuresis ± a GTN infusion, but these should be initiated by more senior doctors only.

Over the first few days of admission, the patient will require ongoing titration of their diuresis. If the patient loses >1 kg, down-titrate and monitor the UECs (a patient who is 'too dry' will underperfuse their kidneys from hypovolaemia). If the patient is losing insufficient weight, increase the diuretics. One useful method is to keep a constant mane dose of frusemide, and put the midi dose in the variable dosing section of the drug chart. This is easier than re-writing the dose of frusemide daily! Don't forget to discuss adjacent diuresis with an aldosterone antagonist or thiazide diuretic if there is loop diuretic tolerance.

Once the patient reaches their dry weight, they will likely be very keen to discharge. CCF patients frequently require readmission, and part of the solution is satisfactory patient education about their dietary and fluid restrictions. Before discharge, have Allied Health review the patient to determine if they should participate in cardiac rehabilitation.

An outpatient appointment should be requested for 2 weeks post-discharge (hopefully with TTE results) for new diagnosis CCF. Patients with preexisting diagnoses can be seen by their GP with a UEC 1 week post-discharge.

Patients with NYHA III–IV heart failure, a QRS >120 ms or LBBB with a left ventricular ejection fraction (LVEF) <30% should be discussed with your registrar for referral to Cardiac case conference for consideration of a biventricular pacemaker for cardiac resynchronisation therapy (CRT) if they have a life expectancy of >1 year.

CHRONIC OBSTRUCTIVE PULMONARY DISEASE (COPD)

COPD is (as the name implies) a chronic, burdensome respiratory illness with airway limitation, progressive symptoms and acute exacerbations. The term COPD incorporates emphysema, chronic bronchitis and irreversible asthma. Although optimally COPD is managed on an outpatient basis (see Chapter 57, 'Respiratory outpatients'), infective exacerbations of COPD (IECOPD) are a frequent cause for hospital admission, especially in winter. Its direct annual costs in Australia are estimated to be >$900 million despite being the 10th most common chronic illness managed by GPs. Risk factors include: tobacco exposure (both primary and passive); asthma; advanced age; occupational exposure to fumes, vapours and dusts; and genetic predisposition (e.g. alpha-1 anti-trypsin deficiency).

The Thoracic Society of Australia and New Zealand have devised the 'COPD-X' plan to improve management of COPD. Its goals are as follows:

1 **C**onfirm diagnosis and assess severity, i.e. regular spirometry and RFTs.
2 **O**ptimise function with bronchodilators (e.g. short-acting beta-2 agonists), combination therapy (with anticholinergics or inhaled corticosteroids), appropriate management of comorbidities, pulmonary rehabilitation and even surgery.
3 **P**revent deterioration with either continuous or intermittent domiciliary (i.e. home) oxygen.
4 **D**evelop a support network and self-management plan.
5 Manage e**X**acerbations, usually in an inpatient setting.

Diagnosis

Diagnosis of COPD is confirmed on spirometry, demonstrating a post-bronchodilator FEV_1/FVC ratio of <0.70. Patients with infective exacerbations of COPD can be very unwell, with many people having a large number of comorbidities. Before admitting the patient, ensure they are stable enough for the medical ward. When taking a history from a COPD patient for admission, be sure to discuss:

- When and how they were diagnosed with COPD, when their most recent RFTs were and who manages their respiratory disease. Do they have home oxygen, and is it continuous or intermittent? How often are they admitted to hospital with COPD?
- What symptoms do they experience and with what frequency? Do they have a chronic cough (what colour is the sputum, and is it ever blood-stained), dyspnoea at baseline or a wheeze? What is their effort tolerance on flat ground at present and at baseline?
- Their full medical history, current list of medications and immunisations.

- Discuss their personal and passive smoking history. Take an occupational history, covering exposure to aerosols, dusts, asbestos and/or other fibres, smoke, or gas and fumes.

- Enquire about exposures at home, including: birds, soil/potting mix and infectious contacts.

- Ask about a family history of respiratory illness and malignancy.

A complete examination of the respiratory system is necessary, inspecting for cyanosis, nicotine staining, signs of respiratory distress, hyper-expanded chest, chest wall deformity (e.g. barrel chest) and proximal muscle wasting (from prolonged steroid use). If possible, a demonstration of inhaler technique is also useful to assess if the patient is receiving adequate therapy at home (or, as with one case study, spraying it on their wrists like perfume).

Investigations

Patients being admitted for COPD should have basic bloods (FBE + UEC + CMP ± LFT) with inflammatory markers (CRP) and blood cultures if febrile. Since this patient population tends to be at risk of nutritional deficit, also consider requesting B12, folate, TSH, vitamin D and iron studies. Either arterial (ABG) or venous blood gases (VBG) should be performed regularly. If the patient is particularly unwell, consider doing this up to Q4H.

Request a sputum sample for M/C/S, if the patient is able to expectorate appropriately. Early morning is best. Consider nasopharyngeal airway swab for respiratory multiplex PCR. RFTs should be updated on discharge if they are older than 12 months.

A CXR is the essential imaging request. A CT-chest is not always required. If an alternate diagnosis is suspected (e.g. interstitial lung disease), consider a high resolution CT-chest (HRCT) as these give better images of the lung parenchyma. Do not order an HRCT if you suspect malignancy, as nodules up to 1 cm in size may be missed by the larger 'slices' taken. A standard resolution CT-chest is preferred for seeking cancer.

Management

Assess the patient's ABC (airway, breathing, circulation) – if the patient appears unwell, move to an appropriate area and escalate. If the patient is stable, a typical plan for admission would include:

1 Admit under General Medicine or Respiratory with regular medications and DVT prophylaxis.

2 Convert regular SABA to nebulised salbutamol (5 mg QID) and tiotropium to ipratropium 500 mcg nebulised QID. Chart a breakthrough reliever and consider charting 5 mL nebulised normal saline PRN for symptomatic relief.

3 If in respiratory failure, consider the need for non-invasive ventilation (NIV) – this is often delivered either on a specialist ward or in high-dependency units (HDU).

4 If the exacerbation is thought to be infective, commence antibiotics as outlined under 'Community- and hospital-acquired pneumonia' in Chapter 36.

5 Chart steroids – depending on the patient's circumstance, either 100 mg IV QID hydrocortisone or 50 mg PO prednisolone. In COPD patients, this is not normally weaned unless used for >1 week.

6 Referral to pulmonary rehabilitation if the FEV_1/FVC ratio is <60% predicted.

7 If a patient has 'failed' pulmonary rehab and has predominantly upper lobe emphysema and a reduced exercise tolerance, they could be referred to Thoracics for consideration of lung reduction surgery.

8 Assistance with smoking cessation, including counselling.

9 Opportunistic vaccination for influenza (Fluvax®) and pneumococcal (PneumoVax®).

If the patient meets criteria, consider referral for domiciliary oxygen. Many patients with COPD exacerbations will require a period of rehabilitation, so make this referral early if your registrar thinks it will be necessary. Patients with COPD should be reviewed as an outpatient 2–4 weeks after discharge – see Chapter 57, 'Respiratory outpatients' for further information.

DELIRIUM

Delirium is almost ubiquitous on General Medical wards – rarely will you have a full patient load without at least one patient experiencing a delirium. 12.5% of patients have delirium during their admission, with this being as high as 20% of General Medical patients. It is defined as a 'heterogeneous and fluctuating syndrome resulting from mostly peripheral conditions that precipitate acute brain dysfunction'[1] or, more digestibly, as an acute confusional state. It is perpetually under-recognised on acute campuses and contributes a significant economic burden.

Diagnosis

The DSM-5[2] criteria for delirium are:

1 rapid onset of symptoms and/or fluctuating sensorium

2 impairment of attention

3 change in cognitive function

4 development of perceptual disturbance.

---

[1]Alasdair, M.J., Anand, A., Davis, D.H.J., et al., 2013. New horizons in the pathogenesis, assessment and management of delirium. Age and Ageing 42(6), 667–674.
[2]American Psychiatric Association, 2013. *Diagnostic and Statistical Manual of Mental Disorders*, 5th ed. (DSM-5). Arlington, VA: American Psychiatric Publishing.

There are a multitude of risk factors for delirium, as any significant disturbance to a person's physiological state can precipitate it. Some of the larger contributing factors include an underlying cognitive impairment, advanced age >65 years, lengthy hospital stays, multiple bed swaps, malnourishment, sensory impairment, polypharmacy, alcohol abuse, recent surgical procedure or immobility.

Natural history

Delirium may be hyperactive (typically rapid onset and fluctuant, with severe confusion and disorientation) or hypoactive (sudden withdrawal from interaction). Hypoactive delirium is less well-recognised by clinicians, perhaps because of a normalisation of somnolence or fatigue in the elderly.

The pathogenesis of delirium is poorly understood and, independent of confounding factors, it has consistently been shown to increase functional decline, institutionalisation and mortality. Delirium can be highly persistent, with a significant number of patients discharged from acute campuses still partially delirious. Patients with delirium tend to stay in hospital twice as long as those without it. Interestingly, the relative risk of diagnosis of a cognitive impairment after delirium is tripled, and a delirium on preexisting dementia doubles a person's 12 month mortality.

Investigations

Due to the large number of precipitating factors, delirium often needs quite extensive investigation (see Table 12.6 for a commonly used delirium panel). Most patients with delirium will require careful history-taking and examination, a full set of serology and a urine culture, CXR, ECG and spot glucose. Consideration should be given to CT-brain in persistent or sudden-onset delirium and, if clinically indicated, also request drug levels, blood cultures, sputum culture, EEG and/or perform a lumbar puncture.

It is controversial, but consider completing some sort of formal cognitive screening (e.g. standardised Mini Mental State Exam [MMSE] or Confusion Assessment Method [CAM]) to objectively monitor the patient's confusion.

Management

The aim when treating delirium is to avoid pharmaceutical management where unnecessary. This may include: using one-on-one nursing; asking family to bring in familiar items, foods and music from home; lowering the patient's bed and minimising falls risk; and orienting the patient where possible (e.g. writing the date on a whiteboard or making a large clock visible).

Additionally, ensure the patient is 'optimised physiologically' (e.g. apply oxygen if hypoxic, rehydrate if hypovolaemic, correct electrolyte abnormalities and treat hyper- or hypoglycaemia). With the registrar you should perform 'pharmacological debridement' – remove any unnecessary medications that may be deliriogenic (including antidepressants, dopaminergics, tramadol and other analgesics, steroids, digoxin and, ironically, antipsychotics).

As a last line, antipsychotics may be used for distress or agitation. Newer generation antipsychotics such as quetiapine or risperidone are commonly employed. Remember to avoid haloperidol in patients with parkinsonism due to the risk of extrapyramidal side effects. Post-discharge follow-up of patients who were delirious as an inpatient is essential, either with their GP or in General Medical Clinic.

COGNITIVE IMPAIRMENT AND DEMENTIA

Cognitive impairments are a variable group of disorders that result in less than normal cognition. A mild cognitive impairment refers to the state of cognition between 'normal' state and dementia, and is usually applied to people with minimal impact upon their ADLs. There has been a recent shift in language used to describe dementia, with some physicians preferring the newer term 'major neurocognitive disorder'. This may be less confronting for patients and their family.

A cognitive impairment may be classified as amnestic (most common) or non-amnestic, and single or multiple domain (e.g. memory complaints, inability to perform ADLs and/or loss of executive functioning, visuospatial skills or language deficits). The amnestic form (associated with short-term memory loss often annotated as 'STML' in notes) is most strongly associated with progression to Alzheimer's disease.

The DSM-5 criteria for dementia include:

- A modest decline in previous cognitive performance is noted in one or more cognitive domains (executive function, complex attention, language, learning and memory, social cognition, perceptual motor) based on the concerns of the individual, a clinician or a relevant informant. The decline is documented by a standardised neuropsychological test or, in its absence, equivalent clinical evaluation.

- The cognitive decline is insufficient to interfere with capacity for independence in daily activities such as paying bills or managing medications. However, greater effort, compensatory strategies or accommodation may be required to maintain independence.

With our rapidly ageing population, Australia is facing an epidemic of people living with major neurocognitive disorders with up to 900 000 people thought to be affected by 2050. This has placed an enormous burden on the aged care system, with a cost of over $4.9 billion in 2010 – a figure expected to double in the next decade.

Diagnosis

There is a common misconception that a diagnosis of major neurocognitive disorder (MCD) requires an assessment by a geriatrician or neuropsychologist. Although these consults are invaluable, they are not necessary and can delay appropriate management. A neuropsychologist review can be useful in determining a person's *legal competence*.

SECTION IV

There are a number of different types of cognitive impairment. Table 34.2 briefly outlines the common characteristics of several pathologies that may present with declining cognition. These features are not always present, but may point you towards a certain diagnosis.

Other commonly examined causes of cognitive decline not outlined in Table 34.2 include alcohol-related dementia, HIV dementia, chronic encephalopathy, Huntington's, trauma and major depressive disorder. Do not forget these in your differential!

TABLE 34.2 Types of cognitive impairment

TYPE OF COGNITIVE IMPAIRMENT	FEATURES
Alzheimer's disease	• Classically presents initially with short-term memory loss. Attention is often preserved. Visuospatial signs may follow • Examination may be normal • Related to burden of amyloid plaques in the brain • May respond to acetylcholinesterase inhibitors (e.g. donepezil) • Further subtypes are now well documented
Frontotemporal dementia	• As above, however the first signs are often a change in behaviour as people become disinhibited. Agitation, personality change, withdrawal and apathy may follow • Examination and pathology the same as Alzheimer's, but with increased frontal atrophy. Frontal signs may be present • No benefit from acetylcholinesterase inhibitors. SSRIs may be of some benefit for frontal behaviours
Vascular dementia	• 'Step-wise presentation' with sudden drops in cognition followed by a plateau, before further acute decline • Symptoms vary depending on the location of the underlying infarction • Examination may reveal other signs of cardiovascular disease or risk factors (e.g. hypertension, CABG scars) • CT- and MRI-brain are very useful • Treatment is aimed at reducing cardiovascular risk factors. Some behavioural symptoms may respond to SSRIs

TABLE 34.2 Types of cognitive impairment—cont'd

TYPE OF COGNITIVE IMPAIRMENT	FEATURES
Dementia with Lewy bodies	• Cognitive decline followed by onset of parkinsonism (e.g. shuffling gait, hypertonicity, sleep disorder, constipation, bradyphrenia etc) • Classic symptom of "Lilliputian" hallucinations, i.e. small people, animals or children. Often do not bother the patient. • Often *highly fluctuating* in their symptoms. • Associated with accumulation of alpha-synuclein deposits (i.e. Lewy bodies) in the brain. • May respond to donepezil.
Parkinson's dementia	• As above, however the motor signs and symptoms present far earlier than the cognitive aspect
Creutzfeldt–Jakob disease	• Rapid onset cognitive decline – people may go from high functioning to completely dependent within 6 months • Examination may reveal personality change, seizures, myoclonus and imbalanced gait • Prion-related illness. Associated with positive 14-3-3 protein on CSF. Cortical ribboning may be seen on MRI brain • Poor prognosis. Average mortality is 12 months
Normal pressure hydrocephaly	• Presents with a classic triad of cognitive decline, incontinence and gait abnormality. May have poor attention • Bradyphrenia and altered gait are common; in the late stages may have upper motor neuron or frontal signs • Ventriculomegaly is seen on CT-brain • A lumbar puncture will show high opening pressure and may relieve symptoms, especially if present <6 months • A shunt may be permanently placed to lower pressure
Mixed dementia	• As it says on the tin – may exhibit characteristics of all of the above. Particularly common is mixed Alzheimer's/vascular dementia

Adapted from: Alzheimer's Association, 2010. Types of dementia. <https://www.alz.org/dementia/types-of-dementia.asp>.

Natural history

The DSM-5 emphasises that neurocognitive disorders exist on a spectrum, from mild to severe. Unfortunately, almost all forms of cognitive impairment tend to worsen with time. Complications include dysphagia, incontinence, constipation, loss of mobility, dysphasia, anorexia, unintentional weight loss and deteriorating behaviour. BPSD, or behavioural and psychological symptoms of dementia, are a particularly difficult set of symptoms for family (and healthcare staff) to manage, as patients may experience disturbed perception, become verbally or physically aggressive, put themselves at risk through impulsive behaviour and/or fluctuate in mood. BPSD can make placement of a patient with cognitive decline very difficult, as only certain aged care facilities are equipped to cope with their behaviour.

The average time between diagnosis and death is highly variable depending on aetiology, with a range of 3–12 years. There is a relation to the age of onset of symptoms with younger patients having an increased life expectancy. The most common cause of death in patients with dementia is pneumonia, followed by AMI and CCF.

Investigations

The Mini-Mental State Examination (MMSE) is a common *screening tool* for cognitive decline, but is not the most comprehensive test. It may be more difficult to track down a template for the Standardised Mini-Mental State Examination (sMMSE), but it provides clearer instructions to examiners to minimise variability in scoring. The Rowland Universal Dementia Assessment Scale (RUDAS, particularly useful for people whose primary language is not English) and the Montreal Cognitive Assessment (MoCA) are also used by clinicians and occupational therapists to assess cognition. A comprehensive neuropsychological assessment may be requested in specialist centres, but is often unavailable in rural sites.

Lab testing should cover a similar panel to those outlined in the 'Delirium' section of this chapter. The utility of lumbar punctures (LPs) is debated and, although markers of certain diseases exist, their routine use is not currently advocated (an exception would be, for example, to look for 14-3-3 protein in suspected Creutzfeldt–Jakob disease or if an intracranial infection were suspected). Non-targeted brain biopsy has a very low pre-test probability and is rarely indicated.

Neuroimaging has always been a part of the assessment of cognitive decline, with at a minimum a CT-brain being required in accordance with the DSM-5. A CT- or MRI-brain may reveal an alternate cause of cognitive decline, including a potentially reversible pathology such as normal pressure hydrocephaly, and is thus essential. Functional neuroimaging with either PET or SPECT is a developing area, but can help in more complicated cases if suggested by a specialist.

Management

Management is dependent on the underlying pathology. If the diagnosis is Alzheimer's, pharmacotherapy with a cholinesterase inhibitor (e.g. donepezil) or memantine (an N-methyl-D-aspartate receptor agonist) may delay the deterioration in ADLs. If the diagnosis is normal pressure hydrocephaly and symptoms have been present less than a year, placement of a ventriculoperitoneal shunt may improve symptoms. SSRIs have modest evidence in the treatment of frontotemporal dementia and frontal variant Alzheimer's disease in improving mood and behaviour. Patients with a vascular component should have their cardiovascular risk profile minimised with blood pressure and lipid-lowering agents.

A multidisciplinary approach to people living with cognitive decline is important. Nutrition should be optimised, alcohol and smoking discouraged and physical activity increased. Future planning is vital and, if the patient is still considered legally competent, an attempt to set up a guardian or enduring power of attorney should be made. Unfortunately, many people with MCD require placement into an aged care facility – a lengthy and emotional process for the patient and their family. This is largely performed from subacute campuses.

FALLS

Falls amongst the elderly remain one of the most common reasons for admission in Australian hospitals, with many patients presenting multiple times. As people age, their risk of being seriously injured with a fall increases. Nearly one-third of people aged over 65 years had a fall in the 12 months preceding admission to General Medical units. Be conscious that this cohort of patients is always one bad ankle away from a neck of femur fracture!

The expression 'mechanical fall' is a controversial one used to describe a slip, trip or stumble without a clear 'medical' precipitant. It is disliked by many physicians, but you may hear it bandied about in ED quite often. Another term you would do well to avoid is 'acopic' to describe a patient admitted due to social stressors. Describing it as a 'social admission' or for 'reversal of functional decline' is more acceptable.

When presented with a fall, the key is to *determine why they fell*. As such, your history should go beyond the immediate consequences of their unplanned meeting with the ground and should determine why they fell in the first place. Ask about physical injury and ongoing pain, *headstrike*, headache, visual change, seizures (including tongue-biting or incontinence), *'funny turns'* (TIA symptoms such as dysphasia or facial palsy), pre-syncope, *loss of consciousness*, dizziness, *vertigo*, lightheadedness, *postural symptoms*, *chest pain*, palpitations, dyspnoea, abdominal pain, *loss of motor function*, imbalance, fever and other localising symptoms of infection (e.g. dysuria or cough). Enquire if they have fallen before, and if they have a 'fear of falling again'.

Ask about the circumstance of their fall – were they wearing their glasses? What footwear did they have on? Were they using gait aids (or should they have been)? Was the area well lit? What were they doing at the time? What surface did they fall on? What was their down time? How did they get up? If memory loss is a concern or there was syncope, collect a collateral history.

A *medication review* is absolutely essential. Antidepressants carry the highest relative risk for falls, followed by neuroleptics and antipsychotics, benzodiazepines, sedatives and hypnotics, antihypertensives and, interestingly, NSAIDs. Be mindful that polypharmacy is itself a risk factor for falling.

NB: It's thought narcotics reduce the relative risk of falls because an antalgic gait (i.e. one in pain) is worse for your stability than the mild sedative effect of opiates.

Examine the patient for signs of physical injury (especially headstrike) and signs of the above causes of falls. A full neurological assessment, especially of the lower limbs, is *compulsory*. Consider a PR exam if neurological compromise is considered. Auscultate the heart for murmurs (e.g. aortic stenosis can cause syncope).

Investigations

Serology and imaging are not always necessary and you should employ that clinical judgement thing consultants keep talking about. If a patient has landed in an awkward way, has persistent pain in an area, significant bruising or tenderness or a cognitive impairment preventing accurate assessment, consider performing plain film X-rays of the affected area. If delirium is present or they have fallen on their chest, request a chest X-ray, but specify in the clinical history for the radiographer that you are looking for rib fractures as this 'view' is different (although clinical examination is often sufficient evidence to treat patients as having a rib fracture).

If lab work is required request an FBE + UEC + CMP + LFT + BSL ± CRP (if infection is considered) + CK if the patient had a prolonged time on the floor to review for rhabdomyolysis. If the patient had chest pain, perform a troponin (being mindful if there was a chest injury it may be slightly elevated and not necessarily indicative of AMI). ECGs *are not optional*. A bilateral carotid Doppler ultrasound could be considered in patients with a high suspicion of severe occlusive disease. If a murmur suspicious for aortic stenosis is present, request a TTE to get the severity of the stenosis graded.

The indications for neuroimaging are less straightforward. A CT-brain should be performed to exclude an intracranial haemorrhage in patients who have a high enough pre-test probability of having a bleed that it must be excluded (e.g. those on therapeutic anticoagulation [not prophylactic doses], multiple antiplatelet agents, headstrike with loss of consciousness, signs of raised intracranial pressure [vomiting, increased confusion, altered conscious state, amnesia]) or a high level of frailty.

Management

There is no routine admission plan for falls, but consider the following (assuming no pathology was identified on admission (e.g. fracture, AMI or stroke):

1 Admission under General Medicine with regular medications and DVT prophylaxis.

2 Postural blood pressures BD for 48 hours.

3 Chase all investigations not yet returned from admission (e.g. cultures).

4 Regular analgesia with PRN breakthroughs charted.

5 Strict bowel chart with new analgesia.

6 If pain in a joint persists, consider escalating imaging from plain films to CT.

7 Physiotherapy, occupational therapy and social work referrals.

8 Minimisation of any risk factors for falling (e.g. polypharmacy, lack of gait aids, poor vision, poor hearing, inappropriate footwear etc).

9 If fracture is being treated conservatively, screen for osteoporosis.

10 If an inpatient fall, the patient should be monitored with neurological observations as per hospital protocol.

Some patients will not need to be admitted following a fall without a precipitant and with no subsequent injury. A portion of these patients will be suitable for transfer to subacute campuses from ED after serious pathology is excluded, but not all services have this option. The remainder will need a short period of monitoring on an acute service before transfer. Many hospitals have a Falls and Balance Clinic patients can be referred to on discharge. They can instruct patients on evidence-based ways to minimise their falls, such as exercise programs, further rationalisation of medications and vitamin D supplementation in deficiency.

POLYPHARMACY

Polypharmacy is when a patient takes >5 (some definitions state >10) regular medications, and is associated with increased falls, hospitalisations, frailty and mortality as well as decreased cognitive performance, nutrition and adherence. On every Medical admission, an attempt should be made to reduce the use of unnecessary medications.

The elderly are particularly susceptible to the negative outcomes of polypharmacy, not only because they are more likely to be prescribed a higher number of medications but because some of the adverse effects can be confused as part of ageing (e.g. tremor, confusion or decline in renal function).

The best management of polypharmacy is to prevent it from occurring. However, this is becoming increasingly difficult. Consider the medications a patient is recommended after an acute coronary event – aspirin, a statin, ACE inhibitor, beta-blocker and possibly diuretics or another antihypertensive or antiplatelet agent. That's five medications already, not to mention their preexisting medications.

Failing prevention, close monitoring and regular review by a GP or physician is essential. Appropriateness should be considered for all regular medications – cease ineffective or short-course medications as required. Criteria such as the Beers criteria may be used to determine the benefit of continuing certain drug classes (e.g. does the 101-year-old really need a statin?). All medication changes should be communicated with the patient very clearly. Consider a Webster pack (a.k.a. dosette box) if they are struggling to administer their own medications.

CONSTIPATION

Constipation is a common complaint amongst the elderly, and is commonly encountered in almost all medical and surgical units. This section was written in reference to inpatients with 'acute' constipation, rather than the chronic constipation experienced by many adults in the community. Patients whose presenting complaint is constipation are often bounced between physicians and surgeons, much like two co-authors trying to decide who will write the section on constipation in a medical textbook.

Diagnosis

Constipation is defined by the Rome III criteria[3] as: 'straining, hard stools, sensation of incomplete evacuation, use of digital manoeuvres, sensation of anorectal obstruction with >25% of bowel movements, and decrease in stool frequency (less than three bowel movements per week)'. Additionally, there should be insufficient signs and symptoms present to classify it as irritable bowel syndrome (see Chapter 37, 'Gastroenterology').

The pathophysiology behind constipation is varied, and may include autonomic neuropathy, pseudo-obstruction, Parkinson's, spinal injury, multiple sclerosis, hypothyroidism, electrolyte disturbance, dehydration, anorexia nervosa, connective tissue disorders, myotonic dystrophy, slow transit, irritable bowel syndrome, medications or dyssynergic defecation. Two serious causes of constipation that should be excluded are obstruction and malignancy.

History-taking and examination should focus on identifying potentially reversible factors (e.g. dehydration) and 'red flag' symptoms (e.g. haematochezia, melaena, unintentional weight loss, anorexia, tenesmus, acute onset of symptoms, refractory constipation, night sweats or fevers), which could signify a malignancy or inflammatory bowel disease.

Ask about incontinence or immobility preventing proper bathroom usage – are they deliberately trying to prevent defecation to avoid social embarrassment? Is there a cognitive impairment preventing proper nutrition and hydration? Are they profoundly depressed? A physical should include abdominal palpation for masses, inspection for inguinal or femoral hernias and a PR examination if there are red flags.

Drugs that can contribute to constipation include opiates, anticholinergics (e.g. oxybutynin, antipsychotics and tricyclics), 5-HT$_3$ antagonists (e.g. ondansetron), calcium, iron and verapamil. Ask about complementary medicines and over-the-counter laxative use.

---

[3]Drossman, D.A., 2006. The functional gastrointestinal disorders and the Rome III process. Gastroenterology 130(5), 1377-1390.

Natural history

Prolonged constipation puts a person at risk of faecal impaction, where the faeces become so dry the peristalsis of the bowel can no longer move it distally. This in turn may cause urinary or faecal 'overflow' incontinence. Elderly patients are at highest risk of this consequence.

When reviewing a patient with constipation, it is essential to consider the differential of a bowel obstruction. This medical emergency is characterised by *total constipation* (often not passing flatus), abdominal distension, nausea and vomiting, abdominal pain (usually cramping) and change in stool calibre. Other symptoms suggestive of obstruction rather than 'simple' constipation include an abrupt onset of symptoms, presence of hernias and a history of diverticulitis.

Investigations

The need for investigation is determined by the severity of symptoms. Without red flags, a patient may simply require the prescription of aperients (i.e. the medical word for laxatives). However, most patients – especially those requiring admission – will have basic bloodwork including FBE, UEC and LFT and urinalysis. If bowel ischaemia is a concern (e.g. an elderly patient with sudden onset abdominal pain), do a VBG to get a lactate.

Imaging to be considered begins with erect and supine plain abdominal X-rays, and escalates to a colon transit study (rarely required), CT-abdomen/pelvis (if red flags for malignancy are present) or a contrast enema.

Management

In the community setting, constipation is primarily managed with non-pharmaceutical interventions such as dietary advice (i.e. meeting daily dietary fibre intake of 25–30 g), appropriate hydration and physical activity (which stimulates intestinal transit). Patients should be encouraged to respond when they encounter the urge to defecate.

In the inpatient setting, the above interventions cannot always be put in place. As such, aperients are often required. Different classes include:

- *Stool softeners* (e.g. docusate; one-half of Coloxyl® + Senna).
- *Osmotic laxatives* (e.g. macrogol [Movicol®] and lactulose). Draw water into the lumen of the bowel, softening and lubricating the faeces. Particularly good for non-ambulant patients. Can work as quickly as 2 hours. Bloating may occur, especially with lactulose. Overuse can result in electrolyte disturbance.
- *Bulk formers* (e.g. psyllium). Not as commonly used, stimulate colonic motility via stretch. Can take >24 hours to work. Not as effective in non-ambulant patients.
- *GI stimulants* (e.g. senna or bisacodyl). As these directly stimulate the bowels, they can cause cramping. Should NOT be used if obstruction is suspected. Usual onset is within 6–12 hours.

- *Prokinetics* (e.g. prucalopride [5-HT$_4$ agonist], erythromycin). Used as short burst therapy of 1–2 weeks.

A typical stepwise approach, as outlined in *Therapeutic Guidelines*, suggests beginning with an osmotic laxative (e.g. Movicol 1–2 sachets PO BD), then adding a stimulant (e.g. docusate/senna 100/16 mg PO BD) and/or a second osmotic laxative (e.g. lactulose). A term you may encounter on the wards is the 'Movibomb' – this refers to up to *eight* Movicol sachets being given simultaneously. This can be understandably messy.

If the patient becomes faecally impacted, an osmotic enema (e.g. Microlax® 1 PR daily) may be used. If this fails to work, consider a fleet enema or oral/PR bowel preparation such as PicoPrep®, but beware fluid and electrolyte disturbance. Consider prescribing an aperient for all elderly patients on opiates, and an 'as needed' option for all inpatients on admission to save yourself or your colleague a page on a cover shift.

CHAPTER 35

CARDIOLOGY

Joseph M O'Brien

Cardiology is one of the most sought after rotations for junior doctors, and a job in Cardiology can be highly rewarding for a physician's exam candidate due to the large crossover with other specialties. They tend to be busy, high turnover units with a patient load that is quite unwell.

As a resident, much of your time will be spent clerking patients for day procedures and '23 hour admissions', bargaining for echocardiograms, chasing external angiogram and echo reports and completing discharge scripts and summaries (include their echo and angio reports!), in addition to your usual ward duties. Particularly when in the Coronary Care Unit (CCU) it pays to listen to the nursing staff, as they are highly skilled. Cardiology is also a great rotation for refining your interpretation of ECGs.

ISCHAEMIC HEART DISEASE

Cardiovascular disease, in particular coronary artery disease (CAD), is the leading cause of adult death in Australia killing one person every 26 minutes (on average). Ischaemic heart disease (IHD) is a result of coronary artery disease and refers to an insufficient supply of oxygen to the cardiac muscle to meet its metabolic demands, resulting in (currently) permanent cardiac myocyte death.

The term IHD covers unstable angina (USA) and acute myocardial infarctions (AMI), which are divided based on electrocardiographic findings into ST elevation myocardial infarctions (STEMI) and non-ST elevation myocardial infarctions (NSTEMI, sometimes pronounced 'non-STEMI'). Acute coronary syndrome (ACS) is another term you may hear, which refers to all symptomatic CAD.

Risk factors for ischaemic heart disease are typically divided into fixed and potentially modifiable. Fixed risk factors include older age, gender (men have a higher incidence than pre-menopausal women, with risk becoming equivalent after menopause) and family history; modifiable risks include obesity, dyslipidaemia, hypertension, diabetes, smoking, alcohol abuse, obstructive sleep apnoea, stress, sedentary lifestyle, chronic inflammatory conditions (e.g. rheumatoid) and previous vascular events (encompassing angina, acute coronary syndrome, transient ischaemic attack [TIA], stroke and peripheral vascular disease).

Diagnosis

The 'classic' history of ischaemic heart disease is central, crushing chest pain although this symptom is not always present during ischaemia. Ischaemic chest pain may radiate to the neck or left arm. Other presentations include sudden onset dyspnoea, palpitations or an 'impending sense of doom'. Some ischaemic episodes are pain-free (known as 'silent' MIs) and are more common in diabetics and pre-menopausal women.

When taking a history from the patient, ask about previous chest pains, exertional chest pain, cardiovascular risk factors (hypertension, hyperlipidaemia, family history), prior vascular disease (AMI/cerebrovascular accident [CVA]/peripheral vascular disease [PVD]) and whether they have a regular cardiologist. Interrogate positive findings further – for example, if they have had an AMI ask where they were managed and if they had any stents inserted or progressed to surgery, and if they have had any subsequent angiograms.

Examination findings may be discrete, but a general inspection will reveal a great deal about a patient with IHD. Note their level of discomfort, diaphoresis (i.e. sweating), skin tone (anaemia may precipitate ischaemia), age, gender and body habitus. Patients may experience dysrhythmia. Assess their fluid status – are they in acute pulmonary oedema (APO)? Listen to their chest and heart sounds. Check for tender calves and peripheral oedema. If the patient appears to be in shock, urgently call a senior clinician to assist you.

Natural history

Patients may initially present with STEMI, having never experienced any symptoms suggestive of unstable angina in the past. However, there is commonly a progression from angina to more significant coronary artery disease. STEMIs are medical emergencies and the aim should be to achieve revascularisation as soon as possible. The 30-day mortality of STEMI is 2.5–10% depending on initial management; and the 30-day mortality of NSTEMI is 3%. Mortality is continuing to decrease as secondary prevention is brought into focus, with more patients on antihypertensives, lipid-lowering agents and antiplatelet agents.

Long-term complications include further IHD, congestive cardiac failure (CCF) and sudden cardiac death (the majority of patients with out-of-hospital cardiac arrest have underlying CAD). These patients are at an elevated risk of stroke and major bleeding.

The Canadian Cardiovascular Society (CCS) uses the grading score outlined in Table 35.1 for the severity of angina pectoris. There is a linear association with mortality due to CAD with grades 1–3, and an increasing all-cause mortality with increasing grades of angina.

Ischaemic heart disease is often seen in conjunction with congestive cardiac failure, hyperlipidaemia, diabetes, hypertension, chronic renal impairment (CRI), stroke and TIAs, dementia and chronic obstructive pulmonary disease (COPD).

TABLE 35.1 CCS grading of angina

SCORE	SYMPTOMS
0	No symptoms of angina
1	Angina on strenuous or prolonged activity only
2	Angina causing slight limitation, on vigorous activity
3	Symptoms while completing activities of daily living
4	Inability to perform any activity without angina; or angina at rest

Campeau, L., 2002. The Canadian Cardiovascular Society grading of angina pectoris revisited 30 years later. Canadian Journal of Cardiology 18(4), 371-379.

TABLE 35.2 ST elevation criteria on ECGs

	LEADS V2 AND V3	ALL OTHER LEADS
Men ≤40 years	2.5 mm	1.0 mm
Men ≥40 years	2.0 mm	
Women	1.5 mm	

Investigations

A full set of basic bloods should be sent including FBE, UEC, CMP, CRP and coagulation studies; however, the most vital and urgent blood test in a patient with suspected ischaemia is troponin. Troponin is a protein 'leaked' from cardiac myocytes during injury. In combination with the history and ECG changes, it is typically used to diagnose cardiac ischaemia (see Chapter 12 for other situations where it may be elevated). Adding a CK may be of value for monitoring for repeat infarction. An urgent chest X-ray (CXR) should be requested, as well as an ECG as soon as possible.

The changes visible on an ECG are how AMIs are differentiated into STEMIs and NSTEMIs. The criteria used to diagnose STEMI are outlined in Table 35.2.

Other changes such as ST segment depression, development of pathological Q-waves or T-wave flattening or inversion can also be useful in diagnosing myocardial infarction, if found in combination with symptoms of ischaemia. The key is to observe serial ECGs (or compare with previous traces).

- *ST depression* may be up- or down-sloping, or even horizontal with the whole ST segment depressed in a flat manner. The current definition requires ST horizontal or down-sloping depression of ≥0.5 mm at the J point (where the QRS complex terminates and ST segment begins) in 2 or more *continuous* leads to be suggestive of ischaemia, with higher mortality and greater specificity associated with greater degree of depression (e.g. 2–3 mm).

- *Q-waves* are a sign that there is abnormal conduction (note the capital 'Q', not lower case q waves, which are a normal part of ECG readings). A significant Q-wave is considered to be one that is ≥0.04 s, or one-third of the height of the following QRS amplitude. These may persist long term after an ischaemic episode.

- *T-wave changes* can be non-specific. T-waves are normally downward in V1 and sometimes V2. An inverted T-wave in a single lead is likely of little significance; however, when ≥1 mm in depth in >2 continuous leads with prominent R-waves they are suggestive of ischaemia.

- *New bundle branch blocks* may also suggest ischaemia and, in the context of symptoms, should be investigated as such. New left bundle branch blocks (LBBB) are always pathological. If there are no ECGs to compare with (e.g. from prior admissions or on digital medical records), a degree of clinical judgement must be used to determine whether or not investigation is required.

  - The *Sgarbossa criteria* are used to diagnose AMI in a patient with a *known LBBB* due to the preexisting drift of the ST segments and T waves, which can be confused with ischaemia. Points are allocated depending on the criterion met, with a score of ≥3 having a 90% specificity for MI:

    - ST elevation >1 mm in leads where the QRS complex is positive (5 points)

    - ST depression >1 mm in leads V1–3 (3 points)

    - ST elevation >5 mm in leads with a negative QRS complex (2 points).

The gold standard of diagnosis for IHD remains the coronary angiogram ('angio'). Angiography retains great value as it is both diagnostic and interventional, allowing a cardiologist to access the coronary vessels via the femoral or radial artery, release a radioisotope to quantify disease severity and perform angioplasty to treat stenosed arteries. Early referral to a Cardiac Catheterisation Lab (CCL) for revascularisation is vital with clear mortality benefit. What is less clear is the benefit of angioplasty in stable angina.

Lastly, if a transthoracic echocardiogram (TTE) were to be performed you may see a regional wall motion abnormality, as the ischaemic tissue no longer moves in sync with the rest of the heart. These are very rarely used in the acute setting due to the much higher sensitivity and specificity of the combination of troponins, ECGs and good history-taking.

Management

When a patient presents with IHD, ensure they are haemodynamically stable. Both STEMI and NSTEMI are medical emergencies where a senior clinician should be involved immediately, as their management is complex requiring the initiation of multiple interventions simultaneously. Once the diagnosis of NSTEMI is confirmed:

1 Manage their ABC and ensure haemodynamic stability. The patient should have ongoing cardiac monitoring for early detection of

dangerous arrhythmias. Apply supplemental oxygen only if the patient is hypoxic or in respiratory distress as there is no benefit in oxygen therapy in a 'normoxic' patient.

2 Administer sublingual nitroglycerine (e.g. 300–600 mcg) if the blood pressure is non-prohibitive.

3 Administer subcutaneous or intravenous morphine to alleviate further pain (e.g. 2.5–5 mg).

4 Administer aspirin 300 mg loading dose orally (or 200 mg if the patient has already had aspirin that day).

5 Discuss adding a second antiplatelet agent with a Cardiology registrar (e.g. clopidogrel 600 mg PO or ticagrelor 180 mg PO), at an appropriate loading dose. Clopidogrel can be used in place of aspirin if there is a reported hypersensitivity reaction to aspirin.

6 Administer treatment dose enoxaparin (1 mg/kg lean body mass subcut BD or 1.5 mg subcut daily, with a maximum of ˜100 mg) for 48 hours, *if* the estimated glomerular filtration rate (eGFR) is >30. Guidelines for renally adjusted doses can be found in the *Australian Medicines Handbook* online.

7 Call the Cardiology Unit on call for referrals, with a view to having the patient assessed in the Cath Lab.

8 Manage any complications of ischaemia, including arrhythmias.

9 Commence a high-dose statin (e.g. atorvastatin 80 mg PO daily).

10 If the NSTEMI appears to be in the inferior leads, discuss giving intravenous fluids with a consultant.

Thrombolysis with anti-fibrin agents should be administered promptly to patients with an acute STEMI, true posterior AMI or a presumed new LBBB as per the American College of Cardiology guidelines. This should never be initiated by a junior doctor and *must* be discussed with a senior. The current guidelines for management of STEMI are similar to the above, with the pathway for thrombolysis or revascularisation shown in Fig. 35.1

Before discharge the patient should have several new medications – a statin, ACE inhibitor or angiotensin II receptor blocker (ARB; promoting cardiac remodelling of the left ventricle), beta-blocker and one or two antiplatelet drugs (dependent on interventions performed and bleeding risk). The beta-blocker should be started within 24 hours if the patient has a non-prohibitive blood pressure and is euvolaemic.

Patients with triple vessel disease, significant left main disease, proximal two-vessel with left anterior descending artery disease or multi-vessel coronary artery disease with significant valvulopathy should be presented by the registrar at a cardiac case conference (a meeting with cardiologists and cardiothoracic surgeons, usually held weekly) for consideration of coronary artery bypass grafts.

The patient should be reviewed in outpatient clinic in 2 to 4 weeks. Long term, the patient should be reviewed by their GP with a view to minimising their

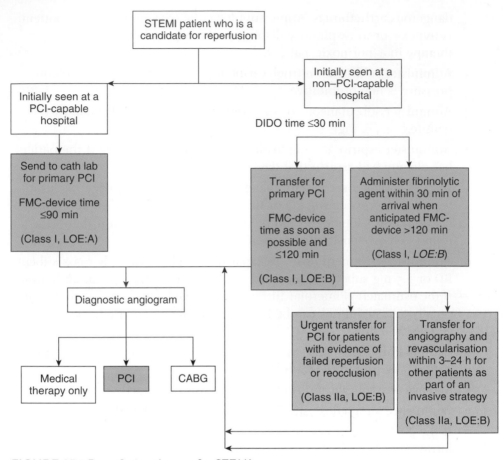

FIGURE 35.1 Reperfusion therapy for STEMI.

O'Gara, P.T., Kushner, F.G., Ascheim, D.D., et al., 2013. 2013 ACCF/AHA guideline for the management of ST-elevation myocardial infarction: a report of the American College of Cardiology Foundation/American Heart Association Task Force on Practice Guidelines. Journal of the American College of Cardiology 61(4), e78-e140, Fig. 2.

risk factors and monitoring for complications or recurrence of ischaemic heart disease.

INFECTIVE ENDOCARDITIS

Infective endocarditis (IE) is an infection of the endocardial surface and/or heart valves, be they native or transplanted. Incidence and prevalence are difficult to determine due to wide variance from region to region; however, overall it remains a relatively uncommon condition. IE is often divided into acute or subacute depending on its presentation.

Risk factors include intravenous drug use (IVDU), congenital heart defects, endovascular hardware (i.e. a permanent pacemaker or mechanical heart valves), recent dental procedures or surgery (especially cardiothoracic) and a past history of rheumatic heart disease. Men and those >60 years are also more likely to experience IE.

The most common causative organisms in Australia are *Staphylococcus aureus*, *Streptococcus* species (especially viridans), the 'HACEK' group (i.e. *Haemophilus* species, *Actinobacillus*, *Cardiobacterium hominis*, *Eikenella* species and *Kingella kingae*) and *Enterococcus* species. More rarely, endocarditis may be caused by *Pseudomonas aeruginosa*, fungi, non-HACEK group Gram-negative bacilli or a polymicrobial source.

Diagnosis

The key to diagnosing IE is a thorough history. In acute endocarditis, patients may report chest pain, fatigue, night sweats, fevers, rigors and anorexia (i.e. loss of appetite). The history of subacute endocarditis is harder to elicit, but may include the above symptoms to a lesser degree (e.g. lower grade fevers).

Examine the cardiorespiratory system. Inspect the hands for the classically taught but rarely seen peripheral stigmata of endocarditis – i.e., Janeway lesions (violaceous, irregular, palmar, painless macular lesions), Osler nodes (red, tender, palmar and lateral digital nodules) and splinter haemorrhages. The key cardiac manifestations of IE are new murmur and signs of CCF.

Patients may also experience a petechial rash or splenomegaly (either from vasculitis or embolic events). Inspect the oral cavity for poor dentition or obvious infection. Consider fundoscopy for embolic events. The Duke's criteria for infective endocarditis are used to predict the possibility of IE in patients with an unclear presentation (see Fig. 35.2).

Natural history

As many symptoms of IE are non-specific, diagnosis is frequently delayed. Some patients present with only embolic signs (e.g. haematuria, joint pain and/or visual changes), further complicating management. Thus IE should always be considered in a febrile patient with no clear focalising signs. Untreated IE has a very high mortality. Even with treatment, mortality remains up to 18%. Long-term complications include embolic damage (e.g. renal impairment, stroke, arthralgias), aortic root abscess, sinus formation and valvular CCF.

Investigations

The cornerstones of diagnosis are positive blood cultures and vegetations identifiable on a TTE. Be mindful that up to 25% of IE will be 'culture-negative', which can result in delayed treatment. If a TTE is negative, discuss with the cardiology registrar whether a transoesophageal echocardiogram (TOE) is warranted.

As described in Chapter 13, 'Investigations: other', cultures should be taken using an aseptic technique and prior to antibiotics, as long as the delay will be <30 minutes. Cultures should be repeated with further fevers. Troponins may also be of use to indicate damage to the myocardium. ECG changes may be present, either demonstrating ischaemia or new onset conduction defects.

Clinical criteria for infective endocarditis require:
• Two major criteria, or
• One major and three minor criteria, or
• Five minor criteria

MAJOR CRITERIA:

• **Positive blood culture for infective endocarditis**
Typical microorganism consistent with IE from two separate blood cultures,
as noted below:
 • viridans streptococci, *Streptococcus bovis*, or HACEK or
 • community-acquired *Staphylococcus aureus* or enteroccoci,
  in the absence of a primary focus

 or

Microorganisms consistent with IE from persistently positive blood cultures defined as:
 • Two positive cultures of blood samples drawn 12 hours apart, or
 • all of three or a majority of four separate cultures of blood (with first and last sample
  drawn 1 hour apart)

• **Evidence of endocardial involvment**
positive echocardiogram for IE defined as
 • Oscillating intercardiac mass on valve or supporting structures, in the
  path of regurgitant jets, or on implanted material in the absence of an
  alternative anatomical explanation, or
 • abscess, or
 • new partial dehiscence of prosthetic valve

 or

New valvular regurgitation (worsening or changing of pre-existing murmur not sufficient)

MINOR CRITERIA:

 • **Predisposition:** predisposing heart condition or intravenous drug use
 • **Fever:** temperature >38.0°C (100.4°F)
 • **Vascular phenomena:** major arterial emboli, septic pulmonary infarcts, mycotic
  aneurysm, intracranial haemorrhage, conjunctival haemorrhages, and Janeway lesions
 • **Immunological phenomena:** glomerulonephritis, Osler nodes,
  Roth's spots and rheumatoid factor
 • **Microbiological evidence:** positive blood culture but does not meet a major criterion
  as noted above or serological evidence of active infection with organism consistent with IE
 • **Echocardiographic findings:** consistent with IE but do not meet a major criterion
  as noted above

FIGURE 35.2 Duke's criteria for infective endocarditis.

Li, J.S., Sexton, D.J., Mick, N., et al., 2000. Proposed modifications to the Duke criteria for the diagnosis of infective endocarditis. Clinical Infectious Diseases 30, 633-638, Fig. 5.7.1.

Management

As always, commence with ABC. If unstable, commence the advanced life support pathway. If stable:

1 Admit with regular medications and DVT prophylaxis.

2 Take blood cultures immediately, from multiple sites if possible. Ideally three cultures will be taken from different sites. Continue daily blood cultures until three consecutive are negative.

3 Start empirical IV antibiotics (Table 35.3) while awaiting culture results.

4 If the patient appears to be in CCF, manage as above.

5 Urgent TTE – should ideally be done <24 hours to identify a culprit valve.

6 Daily bloods, with inflammatory markers second daily.

7 CXR.

8 Urgent surgical referral for consideration of valve replacement if:

  a non-native valves present

  b new NYHA-3 or -4 symptoms

  c valvular abscess

TABLE 35.3 Empirical antibiotics in infective endocarditis

ORGANISM	TREATMENT	NOTES
Empirical for native valves	Gentamicin 4–6 mg/kg IV daily + benzylpenicillin 1.8 g IV Q4H + flucloxacillin 2 g IV Q4H	• Benzylpenicillin is a.k.a. penicillin G • Gentamicin use is controversial, discuss with a registrar first • If hypersensitive to penicillins, gentamicin + vancomycin + cephazolin is used. If the hypersensitivity is immediate, do not use the cephalosporin
Prosthetic valve or pacemaker lead-related	Gentamicin 4–6 mg/kg IV daily + flucloxacillin 2 g IV Q4H + vancomycin IV as per protocol (APP)	• Avoid flucloxacillin in penicillin hypersensitivity, consider cephazolin if the reaction is not immediate hypersensitivity
Viridans streptococci	Benzylpenicillin 1.8 g IV Q4H for 2 weeks + gentamicin 1 mg/kg IV Q8H for 2 weeks OR Benzylpenicillin 1.8 g IV Q4H for 4 weeks	• If non-viridans *Strep*, seek ID review more urgently • Complicated endocarditis (e.g. large vegetations, emboli or secondary sepsis) requires longer treatment • Test the minimum inhibitory concentration (MIC) as some species require longer treatment

continued

TABLE 35.3 Empirical antibiotics in infective endocarditis—cont'd

ORGANISM	TREATMENT	NOTES
Methicillin-sensitive *Staphylococcus aureus*	Flucloxacillin 2 g IV Q4H for 4–6 weeks With penicillin allergy and known to tolerate cephalosporins: ceftriaxone 2 g IV daily With penicillin allergy and unknown tolerance of cephalosporins: vancomycin 1.5 g IV BD then titrated to drug level after third dose	• <u>Minimum</u> of 6 weeks therapy if endovascular hardware • Flucloxacillin is superior to vancomycin for *susceptible* sp. of *Staph*, so use it where possible
Methicillin-resistant *Staphylococcus aureus* **(MRSA)**	Vancomycin 1.5 g IV BD then titrated to drug level after third dose	• ID referral necessary, especially if there is a non-native valve
***Enterococcus* species**	Gentamicin 1 mg/kg IV Q8H for 4–6 weeks PLUS EITHER benzylpenicillin 2.4 g IV Q4H for 4–6 weeks OR amoxy/ampicillin 2 g IV Q4H for 4–6 weeks	• Resistance becoming more problematic, test the MIC for all species isolated • If resistant to penicillin contact ID and consider empirical gentamicin and vancomycin
Pseudomonas aeruginosa	Tobramycin 8 mg/kg IV daily	• Rare, but serious cause of IE
The HACEK group *Haemophilus, Aggregatibacter* spp., *Cardiobacterium* spp., *Eikenella corrodens* and *Kingella* spp.	Ceftriaxone 2 g IV Q24H for 4–6 weeks	• Slow-growing in traditional media, these were former causes of 'culture-negative' IE • Alternative regimens include high dose ampicillin or ciprofloxacin
Fungal	Amphotericin B-containing parenteral azole	• Contact ID immediately • Remove any endovascular hardware surgically

TABLE 35.3 Empirical antibiotics in infective endocarditis—cont'd

ORGANISM	TREATMENT	NOTES
Culture negative	Native valve: ampicillin + gentamicin ± vancomycin Prosthetic valve: vancomycin + gentamicin + cefepime ± rifampicin	• If *Bartonella* infection is considered, contact ID

Adapted from: Therapeutic Guidelines Limited, 2014. Cardiovascular system infections; Treatment of infective endocarditis. In: eTG complete [Internet]. Melbourne: Therapeutic Guidelines Limited. <https://tgldcdp.tg.org.au.acs.hcn.com.au/viewTopic?topicfile=cardiovascular-system-infections#toc_d1e47>.

    d unremitting infection

    e cardiogenic shock

    f severe aortic regurgitation with or without failure

    g cardiac or pericardial fistulae.

  9 If a non-native valve, request operation notes and Cardiology correspondence.

 10 Infectious Diseases referral.

The antibiotic spectrum can be narrowed when a causative organism is detected. If patients develop any neurological signs, a low threshold for neuroimaging should be kept due to the risk of embolic cerebral infarction. Likewise, splenomegaly should be investigated with a CT-abdomen/pelvis. IE patients should have close, ongoing monitoring once well with early review in clinic. They are often discharged with Hospital in the Home (HITH) for continuous antibiotics in the community; however, note that this is not suitable for current IV drug users! Dependent on the responsible organism, the course of treatment may be 4–6 weeks as guided by your consultant or ID team.

ATRIAL FIBRILLATION

Atrial fibrillation (AF) is an incredibly common, irregularly irregular heart rhythm caused by irritable foci in the atria overriding the natural pacing of the heart by the sinoatrial node. Risk factors include progressive age, myocardial infarction, congestive cardiac failure, valvulopathy and hypertension. Atrial fibrillation will be the cause of many clinical reviews you experience as an intern for 'tachycardia' and, as such, a solid understanding of how to manage this condition is important.

Diagnosis

AF may be suspected clinically with an irregular pulse, but is diagnosed on ECG with lack of distinct P-waves and an irregular R-R interval. When taking a history, identify both the duration and frequency of palpitations or symptoms, as well as any underlying causes (e.g. ischaemia or CCF). Take a cardiorespiratory history. Discuss precipitating factors (including exercise, alcohol, emotional state and drugs), presyncopal episodes and signs of CCF. Note the JVP and volume status. Auscultate the heart sounds carefully – they are difficult to discern in AF, but a murmur is likely to be clinically relevant.

Natural history

AF is classified loosely into paroxysmal (pAF; i.e. intermittent and spontaneously terminating), persistent (≥7 days) and chronic or 'permanent' (≥12 months). Patients who are acutely unwell, intoxicated or have undergone a provocative procedure (e.g. one-third of cardiac surgery patients) may have a single episode, which signifies an underlying predisposition but should prompt discussion of future management and monitoring.

AF is also classified based on the rate of conduction to the ventricles. Rapid AF (a.k.a. rAF, atrial fibrillation with rapid ventricular rate, or AF-RVR) is AF with >100 ventricular beats/minute, and 'slow AF' is AF with <60 ventricular beats/minute.

If untreated, the greatest risks are embolic events (such as ischaemic stroke or mesenteric ischaemia) and CCF. Patients with AF have a higher mortality than the general population even when adjusted for their other cardiovascular risk factors.

Investigations

Once confirmed on ECG, first episode or recurrent AF should be investigated with FBE (anaemia or infection can be precipitants) + UEC + CMP (K^+ and Mg^{2+} are particularly important), inflammatory markers, CXR and an ECG. If the patient has not had a TTE in ≥6 months, consider updating it to review for valvular or structural causes of AF. If the patient is anticoagulated, request an INR to ensure they are in the therapeutic range. Any neurological signs should be a strong indication for neuroimaging due to the elevated risk of stroke in AF.

Management

Unstable patients with AF should have their ABC assessed and stabilised. A typical plan for a patient being admitted with AF would include:

1   Admit under General Medicine or Cardiology with regular medications and DVT prophylaxis (if *not* anticoagulated).
2   Daily ECGs and bloods.
3   CXR + TSH + LFT ± BNP (if clinically overloaded).
4   Consideration of troponins with careful interpretation. ACS may cause AF, but a rapid ventricular rate can precipitate a troponin leak.
5   TTE if none <6 months. Tachyarrhythmias may cause cardiomyopathies.
6   **Strong** consideration of anticoagulation with either warfarin or a novel oral anticoagulant (NOAC) such as apixaban, dabigatran or rivaroxaban.

7 Correction of electrolyte imbalances, with targets of K^+ >4.0 and Mg^{2+} >1.0 ('cardiac levels').

8 If the patient appears dehydrated, correction of hypovolaemia.

9 If the blood pressure and heart rate are non-prohibitive (i.e. >120 mmHg systolic and ≥75/min) consider 12.5 mg IV metoprolol. This should be discussed with a registrar before administration. Alternatively, consider amiodarone or digoxin loading depending on the clinical picture.

10 Advise cessation of smoking and alcohol counselling if necessary.

If there is a clear history (e.g. first episode of palpitations), consider direct current reversion (DCR). If the symptoms have been experienced >48 hours or this is not the first episode, the patient must be anticoagulated for 1 month prior to DCR. Patients are typically kept on anticoagulants for 1 month after their DCR and reviewed in clinic prior to stopping them.

The decision of whether or not to anticoagulate the patient will be ultimately the consultant's or registrar's; however, as a general guide the $CHADS_2VASc$ score is used (see Table 35.4). Devised to assess annual stroke risk, it identifies the patients who will most benefit from anticoagulation to prevent stroke. Any patient with a score ≥2 should be anticoagulated (unless strongly contraindicated). An increasingly high $CHADS_2VASC$ score indicates a linear, higher incidence of stroke.

The anticoagulant may be warfarin, but the NOACs are seeing increasing use. If commencing warfarin, the patient should be given low-molecular-weight heparin (LMWH; e.g. enoxaparin) until the INR is therapeutic, as the warfarin has a brief pro-coagulant effect as it affects the vitamin K-dependent coagulation factors, proteins C and S. This can be done with HITH and should not delay

TABLE 35.4 $CHADS_2VASC$ score

FACTOR	SCORE
Congestive cardiac failure	1
Hypertension (including if treated)	1
Age >75 years	1
Diabetes	1
Stroke or TIA	2
Vasculopathy (i.e. AMI or PVD)	1
Age >65 years (i.e. those >75 years get 2 points)	1
Sex **c**ategory (i.e. female gender)	1

Adapted from: Olesen, J. B., Torp-Pedersen, C., Hansen, M. L., et al., 2012. The value of the CHA2DS2-VASc score for refining stroke risk stratification in patients with atrial fibrillation with a CHADS2 score 0–1: a nationwide cohort study. Thrombosis and Haemostasis 107(6), 1172-1179.

SECTION IV

discharge. INR should then be checked at 3 days, 1 week, 2 weeks and, then if stable, monthly.

Patients who are young (e.g. <40 years) and have a re-entry tachycardia, or valvular disease, should be referred to Cardiology Outpatients for further investigation. Certain patient groups benefit from an electrophysiology (EP) study, where an EP cardiologist electrically provokes areas of the atria to identify irritable foci of tissue and ablates them to prevent AF. Patients who have a structural cause of their AF are less likely to respond to ablation. Patients who are anticoagulated should have regular review with their local doctor, and the GP should be notified when they are commenced on anticoagulation.

VENOUS THROMBOEMBOLIC EVENTS: DEEP VEIN THROMBOSIS AND PULMONARY EMBOLUS

Deep vein thrombosis (DVT) and pulmonary emboli (PE) are different presentations of the same underlying pathology, i.e. venous thromboembolic events (VTEs). In VTE, a clot or thrombus has been formed. In a DVT this is located in a deep vein (usually lower limb or pelvis), but in a PE the clot has dislodged from its site of origin and has blocked vessels in the lungs leading to an infarction.

VTEs are common and partially preventable. Every patient in hospital should be on VTE prophylaxis with a LMWH, unless strongly contraindicated (e.g. large surgical procedure within 12 hours, or active and significant bleeding). A standard dose is 40 mg subcutaneous enoxaparin delivered daily, or 20 mg if the patient is ≤50 kg or has an eGFR of ≤30.

Risk factors for VTE include immobility (e.g. hospitalised patients, people on long-haul flights or bus trips), malignancy, obesity, hyperoestrogenic state (including pregnancy, the oral contraceptive pill and hormone replacement therapy [HRT]), trauma, smoking, certain autoimmune conditions (e.g. lupus or antiphospholipid syndrome) and genetic thrombophilias (e.g. protein C or S deficiency, antithrombin III deficiency).

Diagnosis

The classic presentation of a DVT is a patient with a unilateral swollen, erythematous, warm and principally tender lower limb. When taking a history, be sure to cover:

- When did these symptoms set in? Was it gradual or sudden? Have they continued to get worse, or remained stable?
- Have they had an extended period of immobility? Do they have a known malignancy (or do they have symptoms suggestive of undiagnosed cancer)? Have they experienced trauma to the affected area? Have they had any peripheral lines inserted?
- Are they pregnant, on the pill or having HRT?

- Is there a family history of clotting or bleeding disorders?
- Do they smoke cigarettes? If appropriate, do they use intravenous drugs?
- If a PE is suspected:
  - do they have chest pain? dyspnoea? a cough? haemoptysis? palpitations?

Examination of the affected area may demonstrate a limb as described in the paragraph above. Review the peripheral pulses – if they are not present or the leg is dusky, consider an alternate diagnosis of severe peripheral vascular disease and discuss with a senior doctor urgently. Remember to consider differential diagnoses including muscle strains, venous insufficiency, lymphangitis, cellulitis and lymphoedema (usually not tender).

If Radiology is unavailable and a decision about treatment is necessary for a suspected VTE (e.g. on subacute campus or night cover), consider using the Wells score (Table 35.5) to decide whether or not to begin therapeutic anticoagulation. A score of ≥4 suggests a diagnosis of VTE.

Natural history

If left untreated, DVTs can persist for months and the potential for an embolic event is greatly increased. Lymphangitis and venous stasis may also occur. DVTs are often classified based on location. An upper limb DVT is rare, and most often seen in the setting of trauma, malignancy or provocation by a peripheral line insertion.

Lower limb DVTs are split into 'above-knee' and 'below-knee', with more proximal DVTs carrying a higher risk of PE. For treatment, a DVT is classified into either 'provoked' or 'unprovoked'. See Chapter 63, 'Haematology outpatients', for a more detailed discussion on the duration of treatment of DVT/PE. Patients with chronic PE run the risk of developing pulmonary hypertension.

TABLE 35.5 Two-level Wells score for DVT

FEATURE	SCORE
Clinical signs of DVT (e.g. leg swelling, tenderness)	3
Alternative diagnosis less likely than PE	3
Immobilisation >3 days (or surgery within 4 weeks)	1.5
HR >100 bpm	1.5
Previous VTE	1.5
Haemoptysis	1
Malignancy	1

Adapted from: Wells, P.S., Anderson, D.R., Rodger, M., et al., 2000. Derivation of a simple clinical model to categorize patients' probability of pulmonary embolism: increasing the model's utility with the SimpliRED D-dimer. Thrombosis and Haemostasis 83(3), 416-420.

Investigations

Gold standard for diagnosis of DVT is a Doppler ultrasound of the suspected limb. Worth noting is the size of the thrombosis, the amount of flow proximal to the lesion and its anatomical location (consultants will ask these questions!). This ultrasound should be repeated in 6 weeks' time and reviewed by a specialist if the clot has not resolved.

For a PE, the gold standard of diagnosis is a CT pulmonary angiogram (CTPA), a specialised CT scan of the chest. However, this carries a high contrast load and is contraindicated in people who are pregnant, have a contrast allergy or have an eGFR ≤30. In these situations, a nuclear ventilation/perfusion (V/Q) scan might be a suitable alternative. A V/Q scan involves inspiration of an isotope to investigate mismatch of alveoli that are ventilating but not being perfused (or vice versa). Although a mismatch may signify PE, there are other causes (including pneumonia), which could confound results. PE are rarely evident to even well-trained clinicians on CXR.

There are several ECG changes known to occur with PE. The S1Q3T3 pattern refers to large S waves in lead I, Q waves in lead III and inverted T waves in lead III and is quite well known to students and physician's exam candidates alike. Despite its infamy, the S1Q3T3 pattern is relatively rarely seen in PE. The most common ECG finding is a sinus tachycardia, with the second being signs of right heart strain (T-wave inversion in praecordial and occasionally inferior leads).

For either type of VTE basic bloods (FBE + UEC + CMP) and coagulation studies should be requested. With a single VTE, a thrombophilia screen is not necessarily required prior to referral to Haemostasis Clinic. Consider requesting this panel if the patient has no identifiable risk factors, an upper limb DVT, a strong family history of VTE or >1 recurrent episodes. An oft-mentioned test is the D-dimer. D-dimer is a polypeptide resulting from the breakdown of fibrin, and has in the past been used as an indicator of PE. Although it could be used to *exclude* the diagnosis, its high sensitivity but lack of specificity means a positive D-dimer is not useful in confirming a PE and may actually obligate you to expose the patient to a higher radiation dose than necessary. Some consultants like to perform a baseline D-dimer as a measure of response to treatment with anticoagulation.

Management

DVT and PE both require anticoagulation. A PE is a medical emergency, and the patient must be stabilised before progressing any further. An unstable patient with suspected PE will require supplemental oxygen, IV access, analgesia and possibly even inotropic support in an Intensive Care setting. A typical plan for a more stable patient may include:

1   Admit under a Medical unit with regular medications.
2   Commence therapeutic anticoagulation (e.g. warfarin 5 mg PO daily with 1 mg/kg daily subcutaneous enoxaparin) until the INR reaches therapeutic levels.

    a Alternatively, one of the NOACs can now be used for lower limb DVT on PBS.

3 Consider an arterial blood gas (ABG).

4 Consider requesting an inpatient TTE to exclude atrial thrombus.

5 Thrombophilia screen, if indicated, as outlined above.

6 Mane bloods.

7 Ongoing PRN analgesia.

8 Consider telemetry if the patient has been haemodynamically unstable.

9 If DVT, a referral to Haemostasis Clinic in 6 weeks' time with request for repeat ultrasound prior.

Superficial vein thromboses do not require treatment as they rarely embolise; however, if a source of discomfort for the patient anticoagulation could certainly be discussed. The patient should be linked in with their GP so their INR can be monitored. If a patient has an absolute contraindication for anticoagulation, consider referral to Vascular Surgery or Interventional Radiology for an inferior vena cava (IVC) filter. See Chapter 63, 'Haematology outpatients', for further information about the long-term management and follow-up of VTE.

VENTRICULAR TACHYCARDIA AND VENTRICULAR FIBRILLATION

Is your patient unconscious with an ECG that looks like the one in Fig. 35.3? Or like the one in Fig. 35.4?

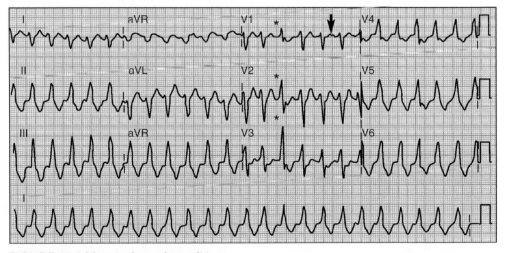

FIGURE 35.3 Ventricular tachycardia.

Young, G.D., Roberts-Thomson, K.C., Stiles, M.K., et al., 2010. Chapter 62: Ventricular tachycardia. In: Crawford, M.H., DiMarco, J.P. & Paulus, W.J., eds. Cardiology, 3rd ed. Philadelphia: Mosby, pp. 847-859, Fig. 62.10.

SECTION IV

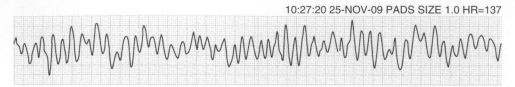

10:27:20 25-NOV-09 PADS SIZE 1.0 HR=137

FIGURE 35.4 Ventricular fibrillation.

Schwartz, J.M., Lee, J.K., Hamrick, J.T., et al., 2017. Chapter 54: Cardiopulmonary resuscitation. In: Davis P.J. & Cladis, F.P., Smith's Anesthesia for Infants and Children, 9th ed. Philadelphia: Mosby, pp. 1236-1281, Fig. 54-18.

If so, put down the book and call a code blue! Ventricular tachycardia (VT) and ventricular fibrillation (VF) are life-threatening tachyarrhythmias and true emergencies. These rhythms are relatively common complications of an STEMI and subsequent cause of death. They are less common but may still occur in the setting of a NSTEMI.

Other causes include severe electrolyte abnormalities, structural heart disease, electrocution, congenital heart disease and end-stage familial channelopathies. The end result is a heart that beats ineffectively, and leads to decreased cardiac output and eventually death if untreated. As they are both shockable rhythms in the advanced life support pathway, they should be rapidly identified and defibrillated with utmost urgency, with compressions commenced in the interim. Both of the above ECGs will ruin your day.

Diagnosis

Diagnosis is based on ECG or telemetry with the above rhythms. VT is a broad complex tachycardia, and is divided into monomorphic (with all QRS complexes being similarly shaped) and polymorphic (differently shaped QRS complexes), pulseless vs conscious and sustained (≥30 seconds) vs non-sustained (NSVT).

VF is a completely disorganised ventricular rhythm, with up to 500 bpm. VT may progress to VF, and either may morph into asystole (i.e. no electrical activity at all and synonymous with cardiac death).

Natural history

This is a medical emergency that will result in death if not immediately treated. Patients may initially present with angina, dyspnoea, fatigue, palpitations or syncope. They may or may not have a prior history of cardiac disease. Long-term complications from survival of an episode of VT or VF may include loss of neurological function (increased with prolonged 'down time'), burns from the pads, rib fractures from compressions, aspiration pneumonia and myocardial injury (leading to CCF).

Investigations

Attaching telemetry or similar devices is incredibly urgent. In hospital, defibrillators will have their own monitors displaying the rhythm and a rhythm check will be performed regularly as part of the ALS pathway. They will print out as required. Urgent bloodwork should be sent, to assess cardiac damage and potential reversible causes. Note that once compressions have begun, troponins and CK will invariably be elevated! Request FBE + UEC + CMP + CRP + LFT + TSH + ABG + troponins + CK ± blood cultures initially. If the patient is stabilised, they should have a CXR.

All of these investigations take the back seat to returning the patient to a safer rhythm. Patients who survive should have a TTE and, if they are eligible, a coronary angiogram to assess for coronary artery disease. Troponins will be elevated post-CPR.

Management

Patients who have pulseless VT or VF should be identified immediately and begun on the ALS pathway. There is a significant correlation between time to compressions and survival.

- Airway.
- Breathing.
- Circulation – commence compressions at a rate of 30 compressions to 2 breaths immediately and continue for 2 minutes, ideally with defibrillator pads being placed simultaneously.
- Rhythm check at 2 minutes and, if shockable, deliver a 120–200 J biphasic or 360 J monophasic shock.
- If non-shockable or no return of spontaneous circulation, continue compressions for a further 2 minutes and repeat the rhythm assessment. Shock again if amenable.
- Give adrenaline 1 mg. Continue compressions. Give further adrenaline after every 2nd shock.
- After 3rd shock, give amiodarone 300 mg IV.
- Attempt to correct any of the 4 Hs (hypoxia, hyper/hypokalaemia and metabolic disorders, hyper/hypothermia and hypovolaemia, as well as tension pneumothorax, toxins, thrombosis and tamponade).
- If the patient has return of spontaneous circulation, continue to monitor very closely. Perform a 12-lead ECG, and treat any underlying causes.
- Therapeutically cool the patient down to 32–34°C for 24 hours (hospital policy-dependent).
- Transfer to Intensive Care Unit or appropriate tertiary centre.
- If the patient reverts to the unstable rhythm, recommence pathway from the beginning.

Patients who survive a cardiac arrest are at greatly increased risk of in-hospital death. They should be stepped down cautiously from ICU to the general medical ward. Angiography should be performed to assess potentially reversible coronary artery disease.

Patients with conscious VT should have their electrolytes optimised, be considered for adenosine (if monomorphic and regular ONLY) and referred to Coronary Care or ICU. IV access should be obtained and they should be monitored carefully. If they are hypotensive, shocked, have an altered mental state or acute heart failure, strongly consider cardioversion.

CHAPTER 36

RESPIRATORY MEDICINE

Joseph M O'Brien

Also known as pulmonology or 'chest medicine', Respiratory Medicine is not a common specialty rotation for junior doctors, being offered at only a few tertiary hospitals scattered throughout the country. It offers quite a variable patient load, with most inpatients experiencing a flare of chronic illness. There is typically a smaller inpatient load, with a large clinic responsibility. You will also usually get some experience with sleep medicine, a growing field. There is unit variation from hospital to hospital – for example, some hospitals also admit chest malignancy under Respiratory (as opposed to Oncology) and others have specialist departments such as The Alfred's Cystic Fibrosis ward.

Practically, your work will also be quite varied. Almost every patient gets a sputum sample (many with acid-fast bacilli). Preparing for Radiology meetings is usually the intern's role. You will work with Oncology, Thoracic surgeons, Cardiology, Intensive Care Units (ICU) and Palliative Care. You will (hopefully) get quite proficient at arterial blood gases (ABGs). Ensure you keep some consent forms in your folder for bronchoscopy + bronchoalveolar lavage ± transbronchial biopsy! There is a reason the 'A' (airway) in ABC comes first, and Respiratory sees some very sick patients with severe asthma, pulmonary embolism and acute respiratory failure. You'll also look after a lot of patients with heart failure, as these patients are often referred to Respiratory with dyspnoea.

COMMUNITY- AND HOSPITAL-ACQUIRED PNEUMONIA

Pneumonia is an acute infection of the parenchymal lung, and is broadly classified based on the patient's location when they contracted the illness due to different pathogens seen in the outpatient setting (known as community-acquired pneumonia or 'CAP') and healthcare institutions (i.e. hospital-acquired pneumonia or 'HAP').

A subtype of HAP known as ventilator-associated pneumonia (VAP) exists with its own unique set of causative organisms, and is seen in patients intubated in ICU. Hospital-acquired pneumonia is defined as pneumonia (not previously incubating) occurring within 48 hours of hospital admission. Aspiration pneumonia may occur as an in- or outpatient, and involves the aspiration of food, saliva or gastric contents into the airways. The term healthcare-associated pneumonia (HCAP) is increasingly being used to describe patients with frequent healthcare contact (e.g. nursing home residents, patients on Hospital in the Home or recent attendance for day chemotherapy or renal dialysis).

In Australia, the most common causative organisms of CAP are *Streptococcus pneumoniae* (i.e. 'pneumococcus'), *Haemophilus influenzae*, *Mycoplasma pneumoniae* and *Chlamydia pneumoniae*. In many cases, the causative organism is not identified. The lower respiratory tract is usually sterile due to innate host defences (e.g. the mucociliary transport system).

Risk factors for CAP include immunocompromise, alcoholism, smoking, seizures, dementia, chronic obstructive pulmonary disease (COPD) and congestive cardiac failure (CCF). Patients who are immunosuppressed are vulnerable to a completely different set of pathogens, including fungi (e.g. *Aspergillus*), *Pneumocystis jirovecii* and *Pseudomonas aeruginosa*.

HAP is second-most frequent nosocomial (i.e. hospital-acquired) infection, closely trailling urinary tract infections. It prolongs hospital admission significantly. The common culprits vary from network to network, but in Australia typically include multiply-resistant *Staphylococcus aureus* (MRSA), *Pseudomonas aeruginosa*, enteric Gram-negatives (*Escherichia coli*, *Proteus*, *Enterobacter*, *Serratia* spp. etc) and *Chlamydia pneumoniae*. Risk factors include hospitalisation for ≥5 days, previous infection with resistant organisms, surgery, pleural effusion, chemotherapy, dialysis, prolonged wound care and residence in a nursing home at baseline.

Diagnosis

A diagnosis of pneumonia should be considered in a patient who presents with a new-onset cough, fevers, rigors, chest discomfort or dyspnoea. Some patients will not present so floridly, and many patient cohorts (e.g. the elderly or immunosuppressed) are unable to mount a sufficient immune response to generate fever. It is also important to try and exclude alternate diagnoses such as CCF or malignancy. Discuss:

- How long have they had the cough? Has the quantity or colour of the sputum changed (e.g. green or yellow is generally thought to indicate bacterial, brown or rust-coloured may signify haemoptysis in the lower airways, clear may be from CCF)? Have they experienced haemoptysis? Have they had fevers, chest discomfort, wheeze or dyspnoea?

- Do they have symptoms suggestive of malignancy (e.g. anorexia, weight loss, pallor, fatigue, rigors, night sweats or common paraneoplastic syndromes)? Note that there is a significant overlap between these symptoms and pneumonia.

- If in hospital – how long have they been admitted, and for what reason? Did they have any symptoms prior to admission?

- Do they have symptoms more suggestive of cardiac failure (e.g. exertional dyspnoea, paroxysmal nocturnal dyspnoea, orthopnoea or peripheral oedema)?

- What is their complete medical history and current medication list? Take particular note of epilepsy, alcohol abuse and dementia as these increase the risk of aspiration pneumonia and change the prospective organisms. Have they ever had surgery (especially thoracic) in the past?
- Quantify their alcohol and tobacco consumption.
- Take an occupational history. Have they been exposed to fumes, asbestos, gases, paints, ionised radiation, guano, sawdust or other aerosols? Were they compliant with personal protective equipment?

Examination is very useful in pneumonia, and is used to guide further investigations. Inspect the respiratory system, and note in particular the breath sounds in the lung fields, the heart sounds, presence of cyanosis (peripheral or central) and the vitals. Fever, tachycardia, tachypnoea and, eventually, hypotension are regularly seen in pneumonia. Note hypoxia at rest and document (if possible) O_2 saturations on room air and a comfortable level of supplemental oxygen. Inspect the sputum sample, if it is by the patient's bedside.

Natural history

Multiple scores of severity for pneumonia exist. Two commonly employed are CURB-65 (Table 36.1) and SMART-COP (Table 36.2).

TABLE 36.1 CURB-65 score for pneumonia severity

VARIABLE	SCORE
Confusion	1
Urea >7 mmol/L	1
Respiratory rate >30/min	1
BP <90 mmHg systolic or ≤60 mmHg diastolic	1
Age >65 years	1

Adapted from text in: Jones, B. E., Jones, J., Bewick, T., et al., 2011. CURB-65 pneumonia severity assessment adapted for electronic decision support. Chest 140(1), 156-163.

Typically, CURB-65 scores of 0–1 are managed safely as outpatients, with a score of ≥2 requiring admission for IV antibiotics and closer monitoring and a score of ≥3 being considered for direct admission to ICU.

The maximum possible SMART-COP score is 11, with patients with a score of ≥7 having a very high likelihood of requiring intensive respiratory or vasopressor support. These guides should be used as an adjunct to your clinical judgement when managing your patient, and not as the sole decision-making tool.

Investigations

The most important investigation for diagnosing pneumonia of any kind remains the chest X-ray (CXR). Be mindful clinical findings can precede radiology changes

TABLE 36.2 SMART-COP tool for assessing the severity of community-acquired pneumonia in adults

CHARACTERISTIC	SCORE
Systolic blood pressure <90 mmHg	2
Multilobar involvement on CXR	1
Albumin <35 g/L	1
Respiratory rate ≥25/min (if <50 years) or ≥30/min (if >50 years)	1
Tachycardia ≥125 bpm	1
Confusion	1
Oxygen low: • PaO_2 <70 mmHg in <50-year-old or <60 mmHg in >50-year-old • Oxygen saturation ≤93% in <50-year-old or ≤90% in >50-year-old • If on O_2 therapy, PaO_2/FiO_2 <333 in <50-year-old or <250 in >50-year-old	2
pH <7.35	1

Adapted from: Charles, P.G., Wolfe, R., Whitby, M., et al., 2008. SMART-COP: a tool for predicting the need for intensive respiratory or vasopressor support in community-acquired pneumonia. Clinical Infectious Diseases 47(3), 375-384.

by a short period. If the CXR is inadequate or a high index of suspicion for another diagnosis remains, a CT-chest may be performed. This is not usually necessary.

Blood work should include an FBE + UEC + CMP + CRP. Some consultants like a second-daily CRP to monitor response to antibiotics. If the patient is unwell, perform serial arterial blood gases (ABGs). Baseline LFTs may be necessary depending on your choice of antimicrobial. Blood cultures should be sent if the patient is febrile >38°C, or if the likely diagnosis is HAP.

If you have a strong suspicion of an atypical cause, consider serum *Mycoplasma* IgM. A sputum sample should be sent for microscopy, culture and sensitivities (M/C/S) + cytology, preferably expectorated (i.e. produced) in the early morning. If clinical suspicion is high, request acid-fast bacilli (AFB). During the winter months, consider a respiratory multiplex PCR on nasopharyngeal swab for particularly unwell patients (not routine). If the patient is very unwell, also consider *Legionella* and *Streptococcus* antigen on a urine M/C/S.

If diagnosis cannot be reached through any of the above investigations and the patient is not improving, a bronchoscopy with bronchoalveolar lavage (BAL) may be warranted. These washings may be sent to the laboratory for M/C/S, cytology, cell count and differential, Gram stain, immunohistochemistry for lymphocyte markers (e.g. CD_4, CD_8) and certain viruses (e.g. CMV), direct fluorescence antibody (DFA) testing for *Legionella* and atypical culture (acid-fast bacilli, fungal, *Legionella* and *Pneumocystis jirovecii*).

Management

Patients with low-risk pneumonia can be given oral amoxicillin 1 g TDS for 5–7 days or, in the presence of penicillin allergy, 250 mg oral clarithromycin BD for the same period. If the patient requires admission, a typical plan may read as follows:

1 Admit under General Medical (or Respiratory) unit with regular medications + deep vein thrombosis (DVT) prophylaxis.

2 Commence IV antibiotics (see below).

3 Fluid resuscitation as required.

4 Early morning sputum sample.

5 Chase investigations sent from Emergency Department (ED) (e.g. blood cultures).

6 ICU referral if high SMART-COP score for consideration of non-invasive ventilation (NIV) and escalation of care.

7 Consideration of an Infectious Disease referral for people with severe pneumonia or multiple antibiotic allergies complicating therapy.

8 Advice on smoking cessation PRN.

9 Allied Health referrals as necessary.

10 Opportunistic vaccinations with influenza and pneumococcal vaccines (Fluvax® and Pneumovax®).

Antibiotic choice is guided by the severity of the pneumonia and underlying risk factors. A standard choice for moderate pneumonia would be benzylpenicillin 1.2 g IV QID until clinical improvement with doxycycline 100 mg PO BD as atypical cover. The typical 'oral tail' for benzylpenicillin is amoxicillin 1 g PO TDS for a total of 7 days (including IV + PO treatment). If an immediate penicillin hypersensitivity is present, consider moxifloxacin 400 mg daily instead of benzylpenicillin (the dose of 'moxi' is the same PO and IV as it has excellent oral bioavailability). Aspiration pneumonia should be treated with amoxicillin, benzylpenicillin or piperacillin/tazobactam for mild, moderate or severe disease, respectively.

In severe pneumonia (e.g. SMART-COP ≥5), ceftriaxone 1 g IV daily would be indicated from admission with azithromycin 500 mg IV daily atypical cover. If Gram-negative organisms are strongly suspected, discuss a stat dose of gentamicin (4–6 mg/kg IV, adjusted in renal impairment) with your registrar. The guidelines for CAP in tropical regions (in Australia this is above 20°S latitude) are slightly different – consider consulting *Therapeutic Guidelines*. There is <5% cross-reactivity between ceftriaxone and patients with a penicillin allergy. If the reaction is a rash, use with caution. Avoid cephalosporins in patients with penicillin anaphylaxis.

In HAP, ceftriaxone is commenced for moderate disease. Consideration is given to piperacillin/tazobactim (i.e. Tazocin®) 4.5 g IV TDS if the patient is immunosuppressed, septic or high-risk for multi-resistant organisms (e.g. has been to ICU or HDU for >5 days), or has grown resistant organisms in the recent past. If the suspected organism is MRSA, add vancomycin at a 1.5 g IV BD loading dose (to be titrated with a trough level after 3 doses). If the patient is allergic to penicillins, consider cefepime 2 g IV TDS ± gentamicin.

After 48 hours, the patient's response should be assessed and switching to oral antibiotics considered. Typically, IV amoxicillin is stepped down to amoxicillin with clavulanic acid (Augmentin® Duo Forte) 875/125 mg PO BD, with any atypical coverage (e.g. azithromycin) converted to doxycycline 100 mg PO BD for 5 days. Ceftriaxone is typically changed to cephalexin 500 mg PO QID. Meropenem or piperacillin/tazobactam is converted to Augmentin Duo Forte.

Unless very unwell, patients do not routinely require specialist outpatient follow-up. They are generally seen by their local doctor within a week of discharge. If symptoms are persistent beyond discharge, they should re-present to their GP. Patients at high risk should continue to get their vaccines regularly (influenza annually, and pneumococcal every 5 years).

ASTHMA

Asthma is an inflammatory, chronic airways disease characterised by recurrent episodes of cough, wheeze, dyspnoea and chest tightness. Obstruction of airflow results from multiple mechanisms, including contraction of smooth muscle in the airway walls, airway oedema and luminal obstruction from mucus.

An acute episode or 'attack' of asthma can be a life-threatening, medical emergency. A very common condition in Australia, asthma is usually managed by GPs with a respiratory physician review in clinic (see Chapter 57, 'Respiratory outpatients'). However, during an acute episode a patient may require inpatient admission.

Diagnosis

Diagnosis is typically made on respiratory function tests (RFTs) with a partially reversible airflow obstruction (i.e. a bronchodilator response). In conjunction with clinical examination and history, an improvement of >12% of the forced expiratory volume in one second (FEV_1) after either inhaled bronchodilators or a 2–3 week course of oral steroids is considered diagnostic. Many patients will report having asthma, without having ever had their diagnosis confirmed in the Respiratory Lab.

Patients may report coughing episodes, 'air hunger', wheeze and chest tightness. Enquire about infective symptoms (e.g. rhinorrhoea, fevers). Ask about their effort tolerance, asthma plan, common triggers (and their methods of avoiding them), regular medications, previous admission to hospital or ICU for asthma and if they measure their peak flow at home.

Discuss whether their asthma has affected their activities of daily living (ADL), caused dyspnoea, kept them awake at night or required breakthrough inhaler use in the past 4 weeks. Obtain full medical, past and family histories. Quantify their tobacco consumption and take an occupational history for respiratory exposures. If they know them, discuss results of their most recent RFTs.

Examination aims to risk-stratify patients, focusing on the respiratory system. Vitals are important – review for tachypnoea, hypoxia, tachycardia (NB: salbutamol can contribute to tachycardia), hypotension and fever. Immediately note interrupted speech, laboured breathing, hypoxia, cyanosis (peripheral on the lips, central on the tongue) and accessory muscle use as these signify respiratory distress and you should escalate patient care immediately.

Inspect for clubbing, nicotine staining, asterixis (for CO_2 retention), sinus tenderness (possible infective trigger) and nasal polyps. Auscultate the chest fields carefully. Wheezing is the most common finding, but reduced wheezing over the course of your examination is unreliable. **Beware** the asthmatic patient who is unable to speak in full sentences and has no breath sounds on chest auscultation – they are **peri-arrest** and should be reviewed by a senior clinician immediately with a view to intubate. One objective measure of this is to ask the patient to count to 20 and see how high they can get before pausing for breath.

Natural history

Asthma is a chronic and incurable illness interjected by acute exacerbations. Patients will need to be reviewed at 2–6 weekly intervals when first starting treatment. An acute asthma episode carries a reasonable risk of in-hospital mortality, increasing with age.

A very common illness in childhood, many patients have fewer and fewer attacks as they age. The aim of asthma management is to reduce the frequency of symptoms, reliance on short-acting beta agonist (SABA) relievers, their impact on the patient's sleep and ADLs, and to optimise the patient's respiratory function.

Long-term complications resulting from asthma include irreversible pulmonary scarring, chronic obstructive pulmonary disease (COPD) and the side effects of steroids, such as cataracts, weight gain, hyperglycaemia, adrenal insufficiency and osteoporosis. Patients reviewed in clinic will be regularly monitored for these side effects.

Investigations

A patient who presents with an asthma attack to the ED should be reviewed as a priority due to their potential to deteriorate quickly. Blood work should include an FBE + UEC + CMP + CRP with serial ABGs to monitor pH, PaO_2 and $PaCO_2$. Ask for an electrocardiogram (ECG) – sinus tachycardia is the most common finding. An urgent CXR should be requested, but should not hamper treatment (a mobile film might be a good alternative). If the patient is stable enough, request serial peak flow measurements and monitor for a change in their volume.

Management

A medical emergency, patients with severe asthma should be seen immediately. Insist on senior supervision. A potential plan may include:

1 Admit under Respiratory or General Medicine with regular medications and DVT prophylaxis.

2 Serial peak flows and ABGs.

3 Apply supplemental oxygen if SaO_2 <95% on room air.

4 Immediate 5 mg nebulised salbutamol, continued as required every 20 min.

   a Alternatively (or if out of hospital), trial 2–6 puffs of 100 mcg salbutamol with a spacer every 20 min and urgently arrange for admission.

5 Continue to reassess severity regularly. If ongoing symptoms, add ipratropium 500 mcg nebulised with the salbutamol every 20 min.

6 Early ICU review if severe.

7 Commence systemic corticosteroids – ideally 37.5–50 mg prednisolone orally for 5–10 days, but if the patient cannot tolerate oral medications consider hydrocortisone 100 mg IV QID.

8 If symptoms continue despite the above therapy, consider ventilation or even intubation.

9 Consideration of 2 g IV $MgSO_4$ in normal saline over 20 min.

10 Consideration of IV salbutamol (consultant-level decision) at 5 mcg/kg/min for 1 hour, reduced as breathing stabilises.

11 Consideration of IV antibiotics, only if indicated.

12 Conversion of inhaled salbutamol to 5 mg nebulised salbutamol QID + PRN.

13 Close and ongoing monitoring in the post-acute phase, watching for the metabolic acidosis that can be caused by salbutamol. Patients should not be de-escalated for at least 1 hour.

14 Chest physiotherapy PRN.

The above therapies are slowly down-titrated in reverse order. Antibiotics should be reviewed at 48 hours and ceased or converted to oral formulations. Steroids do not need to be weaned if used for <2 weeks. If this is the patient's first presentation, they should be linked with a respiratory physician. They should be educated about potential triggers and using a spacer effectively. Before discharge, draft an asthma emergency plan with the patient's input. Their regular medications may need up-titration. For more on the outpatient management of asthma, see Chapter 57, 'Respiratory outpatients'.

PULMONARY HYPERTENSION

In different networks, patients with pulmonary hypertension (PH) may be managed under either a Cardiology or Respiratory bed card. Pulmonary hypertension refers to elevated pressure in the vasculature of the lungs – typically ≥25 mmHg at rest. In adults, it is frequently degenerative and life threatening. It is classified into five groups:

1   pulmonary arterial hypertension, a diagnosis of exclusion

2   PH due to left heart failure (with an elevated left atrial pressure of ≥14 mmHg)

3   PH due to chronic hypoxaemia from lung disease (e.g. COPD or interstitial lung disease)

4   PH due to chronic thromboembolic occlusion

5   idiopathic PH (or PH due to multiple factors).

These groups are worth committing to memory for exams/ward round. There is a genetic component to pulmonary arterial hypertension. Risk factors for and diseases that contribute to PH include congenital heart disease, COPD, interstitial lung disease, CCF, connective tissue disorders, HIV, portal hypertension and valvulopathies. It is not uncommon, and presents in a non-specific manner often delaying diagnosis.

Diagnosis

Gold standard diagnosis is a right heart catheterisation (RHC), but the diagnosis is suspected based on either history or findings on a transthoracic echocardiogram (TTE). History-taking in a patient with known or suspected PH should cover:

- How and when was the diagnosis reached? Did they have an RHC? a TTE? Do they have a cardiologist or respiratory physician?

- Have they experienced a decrease in their effort tolerance, dyspnoea, orthopnoea or paroxysmal nocturnal dyspnoea? Do they have a dry cough, chest pain, unexplained fatigue or syncope? Haemoptysis may rarely occur.

- Have they ever had a DVT or PE?

- What is their complete medical history and current list of medications? Note in particular connective tissue disorders, cardiac disease, respiratory illness, thyroid dysfunction, obstructive sleep apnoea (OSA) and HIV.

- Do they have a family history of cardiac or respiratory disease or malignancy?

- Have they ever had surgery? Were they unwell as a child (possibility of rheumatic heart disease)? Have they ever been hospitalised before?

- What is their occupation, and are there any known exposures? Quantify their exposure to tobacco. Do they use domiciliary oxygen, gait aids or home modifications, or is there a suggestion of need?

Examination aims to review the cardiorespiratory system and try and identify any risk factors or causes for PH. Note in particular the patient's vitals, cyanosis, raised JVP, clubbing, asterixis, heart sounds (particularly a loud P_2, split S_2 or ejection systolic murmur), cool extremities, hepatomegaly, body habitus and signs of right or left ventricular failure.

Natural history

Pulmonary hypertension is typically a disease of slow onset, but continuous progression – particularly if left untreated. It can be fatal if unrecognised. Prognosis differs with the cause of PH, with pulmonary arterial hypertension patients tending to fare the worst with a 5-year survival of 49%.

Investigations

Investigations should include basic blood work (FBE + UEC + CMP) with inflammatory markers (ESR+ CRP), TSH, nutritional panel and, if clinically indicated, an autoimmune screen (particularly rheumatoid factor, ANA and ANCA). If risk factors are present consider HIV testing. If the patient has a productive cough, send a sputum sample to exclude other causes.

A baseline CXR should be ordered. Serial ECGs should be requested. A TTE should be ordered as a semi-urgent scan. If it is suggestive of PH but there is insufficient evidence of left ventricular failure to explain the cause, progress to RFTs (reviewing for a restrictive pattern), a V/Q scan (to look for VTE) and/or overnight oximetry with polysomnography. RHC may be indicated if the diagnosis remains unclear or confirmation is sought, as measuring the pressures in the right heart system remains the gold standard.

Management

Although not necessarily warranting an admission for inpatient work-up, many patients are admitted for investigation of their symptoms resulting in a diagnosis of PH. A complex medical condition, most of the management decisions will be made by a consultant or registrar. A typical plan for someone admitted with the suspicion of PH may include:

1   Admit under Respiratory or Cardiology with regular medications and DVT prophylaxis.

2   Consideration of loop diuresis (e.g. 40 mg oral frusemide mane + midi).

3   Supplemental oxygen if SaO_2 <92% on room air.

4   Optimisation of underlying cause (e.g. COPD or interstitial lung disease)

5   Anticoagulation should be considered in patients with Group 1 or 4 PH.

6   Consideration of digoxin.

7   Consideration of advanced therapy with vasodilators – a consultant level decision based on the class of pulmonary hypertension and its response during a trial of therapy. Agents include calcium channel blockers, prostaglandins and PDE-5 inhibitors (e.g. sildenafil).

8   Referral to pulmonary rehabilitation – exercise can greatly improve a patient's effort tolerance.

9   Consideration of domiciliary oxygen, after a 6-minute walk test (6MWT) or ABG to confirm hypoxaemia.

10   Opportunistic vaccination.

Patients with PH will require ongoing specialist review in outpatient clinics, with regular TTEs as a substitute for multiple right heart catheterisations. They should be reviewed in <4 weeks post-discharge. Patients who are good candidates for a lung transplant (i.e. group 4 on combination vasodilator therapy and with few comorbidities) should be referred early.

PLEURAL EFFUSION

A pleural effusion is an accumulation of fluid in the pleural cavity (i.e. the potential space between the visceral and parietal pleurae). It is classified based on the type of fluid into a hydrothorax (serous), haemothorax (blood), chyle (chylothorax), pus (empyema) or, rarely, urine (urothorax).

Patients tend to present with dyspnoea, hypoxia, tachypnoea and, occasionally, fevers. A small amount of fluid in the pleural space is normal, and likely to be pleural fluid generated by the parietal pleura. An effusion is typically ≥300 mL before producing symptoms and becoming visible on a CXR. Smaller quantities of fluid may be detected on CT scans.

There are many different causes for a pleural effusion, ranging from common (e.g. parapneumonic, CCF) to the rare (e.g. lymphoma). The type of fluid present in the effusion gives a clue as to its origin. The pleural fluid obtained is broadly classified into either transudative (i.e. low protein fluid in the extracellular space as a result of either increased fluid pressure or decreased plasma oncotic pressure) or exudative (i.e. resultant from inflammation). Some of the causes are listed in Table 36.3.

Pleural fluid is sent for biochemical analysis. The modified Light's criteria (common exam fodder) are used to determine whether it is exudative or transudative. It is an exudate if >1 criteria are met:

- pleural-to-serum protein ratio >0.5
- pleural-to-serum LDH ratio >0.6

TABLE 36.3 Transudative and exudative causes of effusions

TRANSUDATIVE	EXUDATIVE
Congestive cardiac failure	Pneumonia ± empyema
Cirrhosis (i.e. hepatic hydrothorax)	Malignancy
Renal disease/dialysis	Drugs
Sarcoidosis	Chylothorax
Pulmonary emboli	Trauma
	Asbestos exposure
	Connective tissue disease
	Pulmonary emboli

Chung, J. & Perrot, M.D., 2010. Pleural effusion and empyema thoracis. In: Bope, E.T., Rakel, R.E. & Kellerman, R.D., eds., Conn's Current Therapy. Philadelphia: Saunders.

SECTION IV

- pleural LDH > $\frac{2}{3}$ the upper limit of normal serum LDH
- pleural protein ≥30 g/L.

Diagnosis

History-taking should aim to help you identify the cause of the effusion, covering not only respiratory symptoms (dyspnoea, cough, chest pain, wheeze, tachypnoea) but symptoms of heart failure, liver disease, malignancy, connective tissue disease and trauma.

Examination should similarly begin with the respiratory system and expand to inspect for signs of more systemic illness. Chest auscultation and percussion is central to the diagnosis of an effusion. Percussion findings over the area of the effusion are classically described as 'stony dull' with decreased breath sounds in the same distribution. Vocal fremitus and resonance, though unreliable findings, may similarly be decreased. Bronchial breath sounds may be heard at the superior edge of the effusion, and a very large effusion may cause tracheal deviation away from the affected side. The chest tends to have a decreased range of movement on the affected side.

Investigations

The CXR is key to confirming a pleural effusion suspected on examination, with a thoracocentesis (a.k.a. thoracic or 'pleural' tap) being instrumental in determining the underlying cause. Patients should have investigations guided by their history and examination findings, as hopefully you will have some appreciation for what may be causing their effusion. Basic blood work would be sent for all patients (FBE + UEC + CMP).

If the source is thought to be infective, a CRP would be sent, and if the patient is febrile blood cultures prior to commencing antibiotics. Consider TSH, LFT, ABG and autoimmune screens as indicated. If a pleural tap is planned, a serum glucose, total protein, pH and LDH should be requested as close as practical to the time of the procedure. If a pleural tap is planned, request urgent coagulation studies as anticoagulation is a contraindication.

An upright CXR may detect 300 mL of fluid, but a lateral or supine film is more sensitive. Look for blunting of the costophrenic angle (where the diaphragm meets the lateral chest wall). CT may be useful for small effusions, but large effusions tend to cloud its utility. CT may be of more use after the majority of the fluid has been drained.

A pleural tap can be both diagnostic and therapeutic, with patients feeling symptomatic relief after large amounts of fluid are drained. The fluid should not be drained too quickly to prevent re-expansion injury – typically, the line will be clamped after every 1–2 L. If the effusion appears loculated (i.e. compartmentalised) on CT, consider requesting an ultrasound-guided tap.

Have the pleural fluid sent for M/C/S, cytology, cell count and differential, Gram stain, pH, glucose, protein and LDH so that the modified Light's criteria may be applied. Fungal culture and viral PCR should be considered if clinically indicated only. Send a small amount of fluid (e.g. 50 mL) when first entering the pleural space, but attempt to collect as much fluid as possible for analysis in the lab.

Management

Management is aimed at the underlying cause of the effusion. Patients admitted with an effusion for investigation should be monitored for signs that may elicit the diagnosis, such as daily weights (CCF) or fevers (pneumonia). Some patients will require their anticoagulation reversed prior to pleural tap.

Recurrent effusions should have consideration of a video-assisted thoracoscopy ± biopsy and pleurodesis. Patients should not be discharged without a clear plan for follow-up of the pleural fluid sent to the laboratory. If malignancy is suspected, patients should be kept in to await the results. The patient should be reviewed in clinic with bloods prior in 2–4 weeks.

CHAPTER 37

GASTROENTEROLOGY

Joseph M O'Brien

Gastroenterology is a fantastic but busy physician's rotation. Gastro registrars will often be called to clinic and endoscopy lists, leaving residents to run the ward. Gastro units at different hospitals will tend towards different sub-specialties – endoscopy, inflammatory bowel diseases (IBD), hepatology and liver transplant – although a basic knowledge of all is required as a resident or intern on these rotations.

Gastro has a high turnover, with many patients presenting with issues that are resolved within 48 hours. As such, keeping current with discharge summaries can be challenging. Any patients with inflammatory bowel disease or viral hepatitis should have their discharge summaries (with endoscopy reports) carbon copied to their primary consultant for continuity of care.

Gastroenterology Departments work very closely with their surgical colleagues, and multidisciplinary meetings with upper GI and colorectal surgeons are common. Specialist units will also have multidisciplinary meetings with transplant teams. Most units will also have weekly meetings with Pathology (to go through biopsies) and Radiology (to discuss potentially management-changing imaging – typically all CTs and MRIs). It is usually a resident's role to complete these lists, accompanied by a brief clinical vignette.

A few general tips:

- Keep plenty of endoscopy referral and consent forms in your resident's folder, as your registrar will regularly require these.
- Most Gastro units have a lot of outpatients under their care receiving ongoing therapy with biological agents (e.g. infliximab) or requiring regular electrolyte infusions. Interns will be paged to write these up in advance or review these patients if there are any issues.
- Stoma nurses are an invaluable resource – utilise them frequently and *always* with patients receiving a stoma for the first time. A stoma can be traumatic and knowing what to expect could just help prevent an adjustment disorder.

INFLAMMATORY BOWEL DISEASE (IBD) – CROHN'S DISEASE AND ULCERATIVE COLITIS

Inflammatory bowel disease is a term that encompasses three conditions – Crohn's disease (CD), ulcerative colitis (UC) and indeterminate colitis (demonstrating features of both Crohn's and UC). IBD is common worldwide, with a higher incidence in the UK, North America and Australia.

Risk factors include positive family history, and being Caucasian or of Ashkenazi Jewish descent. It tends to present in people of a younger age, peaking at 25–30 years. There is also an increased incidence of Crohn's in industrialised areas, leading to speculation diet or environment plays a role in the disease. Smoking has also been associated with Crohn's. Crohn's has been associated with about 30 genes, most significantly NOD2 and XBP1. Poorly controlled IBD can be crippling to live with.

Diagnosis

The typical history for first diagnosis IBD includes weight loss, altered bowel habit (sometimes intermittent constipation, but more regularly diarrhoea) and gastrointestinal bleeding (either melaena or frank blood in the stool, known as haematochezia) with occasional passage of mucus. They may be anaemic if the onset has been insidious.

More rarely, patients with IBD (especially Crohn's) may present with a fistula from bowel to skin (enterocutaneous) or the 'extraintestinal manifestations of IBD' without gastrointestinal (GI) symptoms (see Box 37.1). Although there is a large

BOX 37.1 Extraintestinal manifestations of inflammatory bowel disease

Anaemia

Erythema nodosum

Arthritis – particularly sacroiliitis

Iritis or uveitis

Non-alcoholic steatohepatitis

Corneal ulcers

Calcium oxalate renal calculi

Pyoderma gangrenosum

Hypertrophic osteoarthropathy

Osteoporosis

Aseptic necrosis

Primary sclerosing cholangitis

Delayed growth (in adolescents and children)

Adapted from: Danese, S., Semeraro, S., Papa, A., et al., 2005. Extraintestinal manifestations in inflammatory bowel disease. World Journal of Gastroenterology 11(46), 7227. Talley, N.J. & O'Connor, S., 2014. Examination Medicine: A guide to physician training, 7th ed. Sydney: Elsevier Australia.

SECTION IV

overlap between the presentations of the two conditions, typically UC patients experience:

- less weight loss, fewer fistulae and fevers
- more frank per rectum (PR) bleeding and passage of mucus
- tenesmus (sensation of needing to defecate).

Discuss with the patient the course of their disease so far. When and how were they diagnosed (presumptive vs biopsy, who did the scope)? Do they have a gastroenterologist? What is the main site of their disease (e.g. terminal ileum is most common in Crohn's)? What management have they had in the past, were there any complications and what was the rationale for any recent changes (a sketched timeline may be useful here)? Have they had any prior surgeries? When were their last endoscopies?

On examination, patients may be underweight, febrile and tender in their abdomen with hypermotile bowel sounds. They may also have clubbing (rare), palmar pallor (if anaemic from GI bleeding), arthritis, muscle wasting (from malnourishment), aphthoid ulcers or iritis. Note their volume state. If the patient has known IBD and has been on steroids, look for side effects of long-term steroid use (striae, moon facies, weight gain, thin skin, hypertension, cataracts and proximal myopathy). All patients should have a digital rectal examination (DRE) – the consultant *will* ask you the findings.

Natural history

The natural history of these conditions is a relapsing/remitting pattern. Patients with diagnosed IBD are usually apt at identifying 'flares', manifested in increased frequency of bowel motions, frank haematochezia, melaena, fevers or exacerbation of extraintestinal signs. Patients may experience remissions for years at a time, or may be in and out of hospital monthly.

Long-term complications include malnutrition, fistulae, anaemia (from malabsorption and GI loss), abscesses and anorexia. Ulcerative colitis in particular is associated with toxic megacolon (dilated colon with fever and shock) and dysplasia-associated mass or lesions (DALM), and as such screening colonoscopies should be scheduled regularly.

Many conditions have an increased incidence with IBD, including primary sclerosing cholangitis, psoriasis, ankylosing spondylitis, thromboembolic events, osteoporosis (from steroid-based treatment and poor nutrition), renal calculi, interstitial lung diseases and secondary amyloidosis.

Investigations

When admitting a patient with a flare of inflammatory bowel disease, request an FBE, UEC, CMP, LFT, ESR/CRP (for baseline, can be second-daily), B12, folate, iron studies, vitamin D, TSH and coagulation studies on bloods. As guided by history, order a beta-HCG, lipase and amylase to exclude other causes of abdominal pain. If febrile, request blood cultures. If the patient is actively bleeding (or expected to go to theatre), ask for a group and hold (G&H).

Send a stool specimen for M/C/S, *Clostridium difficile* toxin (CDT) if exposed to antibiotics recently, and a faecal calprotectin (a neutrophil-derived protein found at increased levels in faeces during flares of IBD). A screening urine M/C/S would also be indicated if the patient reports any urinary symptoms.

An erect and supine abdominal X-ray (AXR) is typically ordered to exclude perforation or megacolon, and quantify faecal loading. A CT-abdomen and pelvis is rarely indicated but, if performed, may demonstrate thickened bowel walls in affected areas. If a colonoscopy is absolutely contraindicated, a CT-colonography with contrast (bowel preparation is still necessary, but less strict) could be ordered as a subpar substitute. The gold standard of imaging remains magnetic resonance imaging (MRI) enterography, that is, a targeted MRI of the affected bowel, which can identify areas of chronic and acute disease and any abscesses or large fistulae. Ultimately, many patients will need repeat endoscopy.

If the patient is being considered for a biological therapy (e.g. infliximab), they will need a full infectious disease panel including human immunodeficiency virus (HIV, hepatitis A (HAV), hepatitis B core antibody and surface antigen, hepatitis C (HCV), Epstein–Barr virus (EBV), cytomegalovirus (CMV), herpes simplex virus (HSV), varicella zoster (VZV) and QuantiFeron™ Gold (QFG) with a CXR to screen for latent tuberculosis (TB). Biological therapy can cause reactivation of any of these diseases.

Management

Patients presenting with a flare of inflammatory bowel disease can be very unwell. They may present with sepsis, unrelated infections, haemorrhage, decompensated anaemia or any multitude of complications from their complex disease. A basic admission plan for a patient with an IBD flare should cover:

1 Admission under a Gastroenterology (or Gen Med) unit with their regular medications.

2 Venous thromboembolic event (VTE) prophylaxis – patients with IBD are at high risk of deep vein thrombosis (DVT) and pulmonary emboli (PE).

3 Escalated steroid dose (e.g. 100 mg IV hydrocortisone QID). Withhold any regular oral steroids in the interim.

4 Strict bowel chart, reviewed regularly for melaena and haematochezia.

5 IV antibiotics (covering common enteric organisms), if indicated.

6 Appropriation IV hydration and blood product consent and transfusion if necessary.

7 Consent for endoscopy if indicated, and chart any required bowel preparation.

8 Fast from midnight (FFMN) prior to endoscopy.

9 If there is bright red haematochezia, make a Colorectal or General Surgical referral.

10 If iron deficient, chart an iron infusion.

11 If the patient has UC and is at high risk of toxic megacolon, consider *daily* AXR for 3 days.

12 Request a dietitian (and other Allied Health [e.g. social work, physiotherapy or occupational therapy]) review as required.

Aim to wean the steroids over a long period – for example, 50 mg PO prednisolone daily for 5 days, then 37.5 mg, then 25 mg, then 20 mg, then 15 mg, then 10 mg, then 5 mg. This ensures the patient will still be on steroids when they are reviewed in clinic. Long-term steroids are not ideal, and a more suitable alternative regimen should be sought.

There are many options for treating inflammatory bowel diseases, including oral 5-aminosalicylates (e.g. sulfasalazine and mesalamine), glucocorticoids (e.g. prednisolone, budesonide), immunomodulators (including azathioprine and 6-mercaptopurine) and, lastly, the biological agents (e.g. infliximab and adalimumab). Each has its own advantages and disadvantages (covered briefly below in Table 37.1) and their selection is a consultant-level decision.

As an outpatient, refer for capsule endoscopy ('pill cam') if requested by your consultant. For this to be rebated by Medicare, the patient must have had a negative colonoscopy and gastroscopy within 12 months. Consider referral for outpatient bone densitometry (if <2 years). Ensure they have follow-up either with IBD

TABLE 37.1 Common drugs in inflammatory bowel disease

DRUG	DOSING	COMMENTS
Sulfasalazine	1 g PO BD, up-titrated	<ul><li>A 5-aminosalicylate (5-ASA).</li><li>Common first-line treatment. Inhibits formation of prostaglandins</li><li>Can be up-titrated to 4 g/day</li><li>Can also be given in the same dose as a suppository</li><li>Side effects include GI upset, hepatitis, reversible male infertility, pneumonitis and Stevens–Johnson syndrome</li></ul>
Mesalazine	Mezavant® 1.2 g PO daily or BD Pentasa® 1 g PO or PR daily or BD Salofalk® 500 mg–1 g PO daily to BD	<ul><li>Mesalazine comes in many forms. It is another 5-ASA. Common first-line</li><li>Side effects include GI upset, worsening colitis, blood dycrasia, methaemoglobinaemia and pneumonitis</li></ul>

TABLE 37.1 Common drugs in inflammatory bowel disease—cont'd

DRUG	DOSING	COMMENTS
Prednisolone (PNL)	50 mg PO daily, then weaned slowly (e.g. 5 days each 37.5 mg/day, 25 mg/day, 20 mg/day, 15 mg/day, 12.5 mg/day, 10 mg/day, 5 mg/day, 1 mg/day)	• Side effects include hyperglycaemia, agitation, proximal myopathy, cataracts • Provide patients with a 'weaning pred dose' on their script
Prednisolone enema (PredSol)	20 mg PR mane	• Useful in disease limited to the distal colon • An enema is inserted and quickly passed
Prednisolone suppositories (PredSol)	5 mg PR nocte	• The suppository form is kept in the rectum as long as possible, hence nocte administration
Hydrocortisone	100 mg IV QID	• Typical dose for an acute flare • Do not cease suddenly
Azathioprine (AZA, sold as Imuran®)	50 mg PO mane start, titrated up to 1.5 mg/kg PO daily	• An immunosuppressant and pro-drug of 6-MP that interferes with DNA synthesis • Comes in 50-mg tablets • One serious side effect is myelosuppression, more likely in patients deficient in an enzyme called TPMT. Patients should be tested for TPMT levels prior to starting, and FBEs should be watched cautiously • When a patient goes home on AZA initially, send them with a slip for repeat FBEs weekly for 1 month
6-Mercaptopurine (6-MP)	1.5 mg/kg PO daily	• If brave, you can trial 6-MP in someone who had an adverse reaction to AZA

continued

TABLE 37.1 Common drugs in inflammatory bowel disease—cont'd

DRUG	DOSING	COMMENTS
Infliximab (sold as Remicade®)	5 mg/kg in 150 mL normal saline as per protocol	• Currently on PBS for CD, not UC • Registrar must complete application form for PBS • Must have infectious screen before commencing • Cannot be given if the patient has concurrent infective illness • Given with 100 mg IV hydrocortisone and 10 mg PO cetirizine premedication
Methotrexate (MTX)	12.5–25 mg PO weekly	• An anti-folate drug not often used in IBD • Give 0.5 mg PO folic acid every day except the day of MTX

Adapted from: Ballinger, A., 2012. Chapter 3: Gastroenterology. In: Ballinger, A., ed. Essentials of Kumar and Clark's Clinical Medicine, 5th ed. Edinburgh: Saunders.

Clinic, or their private gastroenterologist. Patients should have an outpatient review in 2–4 weeks. They should also be aware that, if their symptoms recur, they should re-present to ED. If bleeding has been a serious issue, consider sending them with a slip for a repeat FBE + UEC to be checked by their GP in 1 week.

COELIAC DISEASE

Coeliac disease is a chronic, immune-mediated enteropathy resulting from abnormal sensitivity to gluten proteins. Due to this reaction, the villous projections of the small bowel become flattened and atrophied, resulting in malabsorption and nutritional deficiency. It may present as abdominal pain, bloating, weight loss, diarrhoea, fatigue or increased flatulence. Extra-intestinal manifestations are rare.

Coeliac is common in Australia, with 1 in 70 Australians affected. There is a genetic component to the disease, with the genes HLA-DQ2 and -DQ8 associated with the illness. The incidence of coeliac is highest among whites of European descent.

Diagnosis

At this stage, genotyping for mutations in HLA-DQ2 and HLA-DQ8 remains an expensive and usually unnecessary investigation. As such, diagnosis is based on the history, serology and small bowel biopsy. When taking a history from a patient with coeliac, discuss:

- When were they diagnosed with coeliac? Was it based on diet modification (i.e. excluding gluten), serology or biopsy? Has removing gluten from their diet improved symptoms? What happens when they eat gluten?
- What were their symptoms? Did they experience abdominal pain, diarrhoea, bloating, weight change, anorexia or flatulence? Are there any symptoms suggestive of an alternative diagnosis (e.g. haematochezia, fevers or lymphadenopathy)?
- Have they seen a dietitian or had dietary counselling? Do they feel they sufficiently understand which foods they can and cannot eat? Is their weight now stable? Have they been investigated for any vitamin or mineral deficiency in the past, or are they taking any supplements?
- Is there a family history of coeliac disease or GI malignancy?
- Does their coeliac disease affect their work or social life?
- Do they smoke? Offer cessation advice if necessary.

Examination of a patient with early coeliac disease may be without pathological findings. Patients who have lived with coeliac for longer may show signs of malnourishment, specific mineral deficiencies, hypermotile bowel sounds or abdominal bloating.

Diagnosis currently requires ≥4 of the following features:

1 symptoms suggestive of coeliac
2 HLA-DQ8 or HLA-DQ2 genotype
3 coeliac IgA class auto-antibodies positive on serology
4 coeliac enteropathy confirmed by biopsy of small bowel
5 improvement of symptoms with a gluten-free diet.

Natural history

The symptoms of coeliac continue to worsen if it remains untreated, eventually resulting in cachexia, fatigue and weakness. The villi of the small bowel continue to atrophy with time, resulting in worsening absorption issues and potential deficiencies in calcium, vitamins D and B12, folate, iron and magnesium.

If people are compliant with the advised gluten-free diet, the majority of patients remain in 'remission'. A small percentage of people are 'non-responders' to a gluten-free diet, and must have other diagnoses (e.g. IBD, malignancy) excluded, their compliance assessed and consideration of ongoing, low-dose steroid therapy.

Coeliac disease is associated with osteopenia and osteoporosis, hyposplenism, pancreatic insufficiency and a number of skin disorders (most commonly dermatitis herpetiformis). There is controversy regarding the risk of GI malignancy in these patients, with some citing coeliac as a risk factor. There is currently insufficient evidence to support screening endoscopy. Coeliac is quite strongly associated with thyroid dysfunction and diabetes, and older patients should be screened for both.

Investigations

A patient presenting with symptoms suggestive of coeliac disease should have an FBE (review for anaemia), UEC, CMP, LFT (coeliac can cause hepatitis), nutritional screening (vitamin B12, folate, iron studies and vitamin D) and 'coeliac serology', i.e. IgA anti-tissue transglutaminase (anti-tTG) ± IgA anti-endomysial antibodies (anti-EMA). PCR testing for HLA-DQ2 and HLA-DQ8 is not routine.

Radiology is not usually required. Endoscopy is preferred, with a view to obtain small bowel biopsies (gold standard for diagnosis). Bone mineral density (BMD) should be performed at diagnosis (as an outpatient).

Management

It is rare that a person with coeliac disease would be unwell enough to warrant admission; however, you may encounter patients with undiagnosed coeliac who have been admitted for investigation of their symptoms. A typical admission plan may include:

1 Admission under Gastroenterology with regular medications and DVT prophylaxis.
2 Nutritional screening.
3 Screening for diabetes and thyroid dysfunction with HbA_{1c} and TSH.
4 Endoscopy with the aim of obtaining a small bowel biopsy (if space on the Endoscopy list).
5 Fluids if fasting for endoscopy.
6 PRN analgesia.
7 Dietitian review as an inpatient, if possible.

Preferably, a patient will still be on a diet containing gluten when having their diagnostic biopsy. As required, correct any vitamin or mineral deficiencies with oral or IV supplementation. Non-pharmaceutical management for coeliac is a lifelong, gluten-free diet. If the patient is refractory to this change after several *compliant* months, discuss with your registrar or consultant a course of moderate-dose steroids. The mucosal inflammation resolves relatively quickly, but the damage done to the mucosa can take 6–24 months to completely heal. Anti-gliadin on serum can be used to confirm adherence to the restricted diet. Consider family screening, especially if first-degree relatives are symptomatic.

IRRITABLE BOWEL SYNDROME

Irritable bowel syndrome (IBS) is a constellation of symptoms including chronic abdominal pain, altered bowel habit and bloating in the absence of a detectable organic cause. Despite extensive research the pathogenesis of IBS remains unknown, with hypotheses including gastrointestinal hypermotility, visceral hypersensitivity or altered gut flora.

People are often able to identify 'triggers' for their disease, including foods (e.g. lactose), decreased fibre consumption, alcohol, caffeine, infection, medications, menstruation and stress. IBS is common in Australia, with 20% of people experiencing symptoms at some stage of their lives. It can be highly disruptive to a person's life, causing immense discomfort and affecting their ability to complete their activities of daily living (ADLs) at work and home.

Diagnosis

The ROME-III criteria for diagnosis of IBS includes recurrent abdominal pain of ≥3 days/week for ≥3 months, with two of the following features: pain with relief on defecation; onset of pain associated with altered bowel habits; and onset associated with a change in stool formation or appearance. Symptoms should have been present for a total of ≥6 months.

The remainder of the history should focus on excluding other organic causes of the patient's symptoms, including IBD (UC and Crohn's), malignancy, coeliac disease, hyperthyroidism and CMV colitis. Symptoms suggestive of an alternative diagnosis include moderate-to-severe haematochezia, weight loss, iron deficiency anaemia, nocturnal symptoms and a family history of the aforementioned GI illnesses.

Examination focuses on the gastrointestinal system. Note weight change, palmar or conjunctival pallor, cachexia, abdominal tenderness or bloating. When palpating the abdomen, note tenderness or masses. Perform a DRE with consent.

Natural history

IBS is a relapsing/remitting condition, with patients often experiencing flares of their disease. Some people recognise triggers, but they are not always identifiable. There is no association with bowel cancer, but please remember people with IBS are still at the same risk of cancer as the general population and alarm symptoms should be followed up. IBS is associated with fibromyalgia, chronic headaches, multiple allergies and dysmenorrhoea.

Investigations

Investigations for IBS should begin broad, and narrow in as severe diagnoses are excluded. Perform an FBE, UEC, CMP, LFT, CRP, TSH and nutritional screen (as above) on serology. A urine culture may be of use if abdominal pain is present. Consider sending a stool sample for culture, occult blood and calprotectin. If the patient also has chronic diarrhoea, add an ova/cysts/parasites to the stool sample request slip.

Imaging should include an AXR. Due to the high dose of radiation associated with its use, consider the clinical need for CT-abdomen. Endoscopy should be performed (if nothing else, to exclude IBD) with gastroscopy and colonoscopy.

Management

Patients are not usually admitted with IBS. However, an undiagnosed patient with IBS may be admitted for inpatient work-up. A typical plan would include:

1 Admission under Gastroenterology with their regular medications and DVT prophylaxis.

2 Inpatient endoscopy, IV fluids while fasting for the procedure.

3 Bloodwork with nutritional screening.

4 Imaging as outlined above.

5 Dietitian review and advice, ± review by social work, physiotherapy and OT

6 Commencing a high-fibre, low 'FODMAP' (fermentable oligosaccharides, disaccharides, monosaccharides and polyols) diet post-endoscopy.

Once other organic causes are excluded, a patient with newly-diagnosed IBS should go onto a low FODMAP, high-fibre diet low in foods that produce gas. A dietitian review for patient education is strongly advised. This may initially increase bloating, which should resolve in 2–3 weeks.

Diarrhoea should be managed with agents such as loperamide. Anti-spasmodic agents such as hyoscine butylbromide (Buscopan® 20 mg orally) may also provide relief. Patients with IBS frequently have an anxiety component to their illness, which responds well to selective serotonin reuptake inhibitors. Patients with IBS do not necessarily need ongoing specialist review. Most GPs are quite happy to manage these patients' care.

GASTROENTERITIS

Gastroenteritis ('gastro') is a broad term applied to multiple pathological states of the gastrointestinal system, most frequently manifesting as diarrhoeal illness presumed to be of infectious origin. It is typically classified by its duration, with <14 days being 'acute' and >30 days becoming 'chronic.' Globally gastroenteritis is one the five leading causes of death, and even in the Western world remains a common cause of morbidity and mortality.

Gastroenteritis may be caused by viruses (e.g. norovirus, rotavirus, enteric adenovirus), bacteria (e.g. *Salmonella, Shigella, Campylobacter, Clostridium difficile* and *Escherichia* species) and protozoa (e.g. *Cryptosporidium*, giardia, entamoeba). The majority of cases are viral, with low rates of bacterial growth on stool culture.

Risk factors include consumption of contaminated food and water, sick contacts (especially in an institutionalised setting, e.g. nursing homes or hospitals), prolonged recent antibiotic use, immunocompromise and malnutrition. Patients with gastroenteritis do not always require an inpatient admission, unless they appear very unwell.

Diagnosis

Diagnosis is based on the symptoms of diarrhoea and abdominal pain, but anorexia, nausea, vomiting, waterbrash, cramping and bloating may also be present. Discuss:

- When did symptoms begin? How often have they opened their bowels? Can they describe their bowel motions (e.g. watery, poorly formed, hard to flush)? Has there been any bleeding or melaena? Short duration of symptoms (i.e. <24–40 hours) is suggestive of a viral aetiology.

- Do they have nausea, vomiting, anorexia, bloating, cramping or abdominal pain? Have they had any fevers, chills, sweats, fatigue or rigors?
- Have they had any respiratory symptoms (e.g. cough, rhinorrhoea, pharyngitis)?
- Have they recently been on antibiotics? Do they have any sick contacts?
- Food history – what has the patient eaten in the last 24 hours? How long after consumption did the symptoms set in?
- Take a travel history.

Typical examination findings include a mild, diffusely tender abdomen. Patients may be tachycardic or febrile. Note their volume state – severe dehydration warrants admission. If bleeding is reported, perform a DRE. Be thorough in your examination of the gastrointestinal system, as this patient may be presenting for the first time with IBD or malignancy.

Natural history

In the developed world, most people recover quickly from viral or bacterial gastroenteritis. The median time to recovery is reported as 2 days for norovirus, 3 to 8 days for rotavirus and 2 to 7 days for *Campylobacter* and *Salmonella*.

Investigations

Usually, no investigations are required. However, if the patient appears unstable or severely dehydrated, or has GI bleeding, a fever >38°C, abdominal pain or persistent nausea, they should have an FBE + UEC with consideration of LFT + lipase + CRP. Stool samples can be sent for M/C/S and occult blood, and a PCR can be performed for both norovirus and rotavirus. If in an outbreak scenario, also consider adenovirus PCR.

If the patient is immunocompromised or has travelled in a developing country recently, add a request for ova/cysts/parasites. If a patient has recently been on antibiotics, also request a *Clostridium difficile* toxin. Clinical history will guide the pathologist, so if there is an exposure or risk factor for *Shigella, Salmonella,* giardia or cryptosporidium indicate this as some microorganisms require special culture media. A negative stool culture does not exclude an infective cause of diarrhoea.

Consider performing a CT-abdomen/pelvis in older people with severe abdominal pain to exclude other causes (e.g. AAA). An erect + supine abdominal X-ray series may suffice in a patient suspected of having an obstruction, perforation or toxic megacolon.

Management

Acute gastroenteritis will not usually be admitted. The course of illness tends to be brief, and in developed countries is rarely life threatening. If the patient appears unwell enough to launch investigations, it may be prudent to admit the patient to a Short Stay Unit to rehydrate them with IV fluids and await the return of the investigations requested.

Stool cultures will take a minimum of 24 hours to return (although they can take up to 72 hours). Monitor a patient's electrolytes closely and supplement in the IV fluids as necessary (in particular, patients tend to lose K^+ and Mg^{2+}). Oral rehydration therapy remains the preferred first-line therapy. Loperamide (2–4 mg PO PRN) may assist with symptoms.

If the clinical suspicion of a bacterial cause of an inflammatory gastroenteritis is high, consider empirical antibiotic therapy. These patients tend to have either bloody diarrhoea, high fevers, >8 stools/day, immunosuppression or severe dehydration. Once the pathogen is identified, the spectrum of antibiotic coverage can be narrowed. If a patient is admitted to the wards with a suspected infective cause of diarrhoea, they should be isolated.

Patients with gastroenteritis do not require specialist gastroenterologist follow-up unless there was a suspicion of IBD. If a patient was particularly unwell, they may benefit from an appointment with their GP 1 week after discharge with bloods (FBE + UEC) beforehand. You do not need to repeat stool cultures to confirm clearance of the microorganism unless symptoms persist.

UPPER GASTROINTESTINAL BLEEDING

Upper gastrointestinal bleeding (UGIB) – strictly defined as bleeding proximal to the suspensory ligament of the duodenum (i.e. the ligament of Treitz) – is a common cause of admission under Gastroenterology. Depending on severity, UGIB can be a life-threatening condition and carries a high morbidity.

Five 'red flags' on history include: age >60 years, haemodynamic instability, syncope/collapse, haemoglobin (Hb) <90 and/or therapeutic anticoagulation. The most common cause is peptic ulcer disease (PUD), but other causes include oesophageal varices, severe gastritis, Mallory–Weiss tears, angiodysplasia (e.g. arteriovenous malformations or AVMs; GAVE or gastric antral vascular ectasia) and mass lesions.

Risk factors for UGIB include liver disease (through formation of varices), advanced age, chronic renal impairment, NSAID use, multiple vomits, *Helicobacter pylori* infection, aortic valve stenosis, prolonged ICU admission ('stress' ulcers), therapeutic anticoagulation, past oesophageal/gastric surgery and neoplasia of the GI tract.

Diagnosis

Diagnosis is straightforward, with most patients reporting either melaena (jet-black, malodorous, sticky stool), bright-red haematemesis or providing a history of 'coffee-ground' vomiting. You may see this pattern of haematemesis and melaena described as 'H&M'. The history can give a clue as to the location or cause of the bleed:

- Bright-red bleeds tend to be proximal.
- Coffee-ground vomits may be from the stomach or proximal duodenum.
- A patient who reports a series of vomits that do not contain blood, followed by moderate-to-large volume bright-red haematemesis, may have a Mallory–Weiss tear.
- A history of liver disease suggests a source in either oesophageal varices or portal hypertensive gastropathy.
- A history of aortic surgery suggests the possibility of an aortoenteric fistula (very high mortality).
- Oesophageal ulcers may have a history of odynophagia (pain on swallowing) or dysphagia (difficulty swallowing).
- Epigastric or right upper quadrant pain may signify gastric ulceration.
- Gastric cancer tends to have smaller, self-limiting and sporadic bleeds and may also present with fatigue, weight loss and/or early satiety.

Discuss also:

- How many times have they vomited? How many times did it contain blood (or was it like coffee grounds)?
- Have they had abdominal pain? Do they feel dizzy or light-headed? Have they lost consciousness or had palpitations, dyspnoea or chest pain?
- Have they also passed melaena or bright-red blood per rectum? Do they have otherwise altered bowel habit?
- When did they last eat? Do they have any allergies?
- What is their complete medical history? Do they have liver disease, cardiovascular disease or a non-native heart valve? What medications are they taking? Are they on antiplatelet agents, warfarin or other oral anticoagulants? Are they on NSAIDs or bisphosphonates and, if so, what dose?
- Do they have a family history of GI bleeding, IBD or malignancy?
- Quantify their alcohol consumption in grams/day and their tobacco history in pack-years.

The most important part of examination is the patient's vitals, including a postural blood pressure. Signs of a particularly unwell patient include tachycardia, hypotension or a large postural blood pressure drop. A rigid abdomen with hypomotile bowel sounds and rebound tenderness may represent a perforated viscus (e.g. from an ulcer).

A digital rectal examination (DRE) is also *essential* to inspect for melaena or bright-red blood. Note cachexia, palmar/conjunctival/general pallor, fatigue, heart murmurs (especially aortic mechanical valves), surgical scars and signs of liver disease (e.g. ascites, organomegaly, jaundice, hepatic flap, clubbing, caput medusae, spider naevi).

Natural history

UGIB should be swiftly managed, as left untreated it can result in anaemia, hypovol-aemic shock, renal impairment, confusion and ultimately death. Variceal bleeding in particular can be torrential. Some patients do not present with overt bleeding, but instead have an iron deficiency anaemia detected on routine bloodwork.

The Rockall score (see Table 37.2) is used to objectively prognosticate risk. A convenient acronym to remember the variables is ABCDE (A = age, B = 'BP drop', C = comorbidities, D = diagnosis and E = evidence of bleeding). A score <3 has a good prognosis, but a score ≥8 carries a particularly high risk of mortality.

Investigations

Bloodwork should be marked urgent, and include an FBE, UEC (elevated urea suggests an UGIB), CMP (hypercalcaemia may suggest malignancy), LFTs, CRP, coagulation studies and a group and hold (G&H). Consider iron studies and nutritional screening (B12, folate, vitamin D, TSH). If a patient is at high risk of myocardial infarction, consider troponins.

Imaging may include abdominal ultrasound (? portal hypertension), a red cell scan (where the patient is transfused technetium-tagged erythrocytes and scanned to examine their migration into the lumen), CT-abdomen/pelvis or a CT-angiogram of the abdomen. Patients may be referred to Interventional Radiology for a potentially therapeutic and diagnostic CT-angiogram for bleeds not visible on endoscopy.

The gold standard of diagnosis is upper GI endoscopy ± biopsy. Most ulcers iden-tified will have a CLO test performed, i.e. a rapid urease test used on biopsy samples to identify *Helicobacter pylori*. Endoscopy is both diagnostic and therapeutic, with

TABLE 37.2 The Rockall score for upper gastrointestinal bleeding

VARIABLE	0 POINTS	1 POINT	2 POINTS	3 POINTS
Age (years)	<60	60–79	80+	–
Shock	No evidence	HR >100 bpm SBP >100 mmHg	SBP <100 mmHg	–
Comorbidities	Nil major	–	CCF, IHD, other major comorbidities	CRF, CLD, metastatic cancer
Diagnosis	Mallory–Weiss	All other diagnoses	GI malignancy	–
Evidence of bleeding	None	–	Blood, spurting vessels, adherent clot	–

CCF = congestive cardiac failure; CLD = chronic liver disease; CRF = chronic renal failure; IHD = ischaemic heart disease.

Reproduced from: Rockall, T. A., Logan, R. F., Devlin, H. B., et al., 1996. Risk assessment after acute upper gastrointestinal haemorrhage. Gut 38(3), 316–321.

the operator able to use tools to perform argon plasma coagulation (APC), balloon tamponade, clipping of arterial bleeds or variceal banding if necessary.

Management

Patients with UGIB should be admitted under Gastroenterology, Upper GI or General Surgical unit (depending on your hospital's policy). Bright-red rectal bleeding is usually admitted under Surgical units. A typical plan for a patient admitted with UGIB may include:

1 Admit under Gastroenterology with regular medications and DVT prophylaxis (withhold if actively bleeding). Consider ICU referral if the patient remains unstable despite adequate resuscitation.

2 Place two large-bore IV cannulas (preferably 18G+).

3 Send urgent bloods including G&H. Consent for blood products.

4 Make the patient nil by mouth (NBM) until able to go to theatre, and consent them for endoscopy (gastroscopy ± biopsy ± argon plasma coagulation ± variceal banding).

   a Consent forms should cover the possible complications, including further bleeding, infection, anaesthetic complications, perforation (from air sufflation), lack of diagnosis, failure of therapy and damage to other structures.

5 Resuscitate with IV fluid.

6 Some units consider use of a prokinetic agent (e.g. 10 mg IV metoclopramide or 200 mg IV erythromycin) to promote gastric emptying.

7 If the diagnosis is strongly suspected of being varices, chart 200 mcg IV octreotide in 250 mL normal saline 0.9%. This synthetic somatostatin lowers portal venous pressure.

8 If the diagnosis is thought to be PUD, chart a proton pump inhibitor (PPI) IV twice daily (e.g. pantoprazole 40 mg IV BD).

9 If the patient's Hb is <80, arrange a blood transfusion of ≥2 units of packed red blood cells (PRBC) as quickly as is safe for the patient. If the bleed is high volume, activate the Massive Transfusion Protocol (see Chapter 24, 'Managing fluids and electrolytes') and transfuse fresh frozen plasma (FFP) and pools of platelets in a 1:1:1 ratio.

10 Withhold anticoagulants and antiplatelet agents.

11 Cease NSAIDs.

12 Consider reversing therapeutic anticoagulation (registrar-level decision).

   a Warfarin may be reversed with vitamin K (10 mg IV stat with repeat INR in 2 hours), FFP or Prothrombinex® (a cocktail of factors II, IX and X). Vitamin K will cause disruption to anticoagulation for a few weeks. The preferred method of reversing warfarin is FFP. In an emergency situation Prothrombinex (despite its high expense) can be used.

SECTION IV

b Novel oral anticoagulants currently have no antidotes (although dabigatran can be eliminated more rapidly with haemodialysis). If bleeding is life threatening, consider giving Prothrombinex (currently unsupported by evidence), dialysis or tranexamic acid 15–30 mg/kg IV in addition to appropriate fluid resuscitation and transfusion.

c Patients with a strong need to be therapeutically anticoagulated (e.g. mechanical heart valve, phospholipid syndrome) should receive bridging low-molecular-weight heparin withheld for 6 hours prior to endoscopy (for biopsy).

13 If the patient is seen to be iron deficient, chart an iron infusion of 1 g iron polymaltose in 250 mL normal saline 0.9% (or, alternatively, 1 g of iron carboxymaltose in 100 mL normal saline 0.9%).

14 Postural blood pressures BD.

15 If the source of bleeding is thought to be varices, chart the patient for 10 mg PO propranolol BD and up-titrate as tolerated to lower the portal venous pressures.

In some cases, bleeding from ulcers is so severe it requires open, emergency surgery for arterial ligation. Patients should have their PPI given IV for at least 72 hours, then changed to oral. At 1 month this can be dropped to 40 mg/day. Life-long dosages should be considered for patients at the highest risk of recurrence.

The biopsy results should be presented at your Gastro unit's Pathology meeting, as a small amount will be determined to be malignant. Due to the high rate of infection, all patients with duodenal ulcers are treated with *Helicobacter pylori* eradication 'triple therapy' of ampicillin 1 g PO BD, clarithromycin 500 mg PO daily and a PPI (e.g. 40 mg PO daily esomeprazole). If a patient is considered high risk (e.g. high Rockall score) do not discharge them until the stool returns to brown. Patients with gastric ulcers should be booked for repeat gastroscopy in 6–8 weeks to ensure ulcer healing.

OESOPHAGEAL MOTILITY DISORDERS

Oesophageal dysmotility refers to an abnormality of the movement of the oesophagus more than two standard deviations from the median. Classified into primary (e.g. achalasia, hypertensive peristalsis, lower oesophageal sphincter issues) or secondary disorders (e.g. scleroderma, diabetes, chronic GORD). Oesophageal manometry can then be used to further divide the patient cohort into hyper-, hypo- or discoordinated motility.

Oesophageal motility disorders affect 1 in 10,000 people in developed countries, and can be a significant source of discomfort. Patients may present with dysphagia, odynophagia or globus sensation (i.e. feeling of a mass in one's throat). Risk factors include advanced age, diabetes, scleroderma and psychiatric conditions. Some of the different causes of dysmotility include:

1 *Achalasia* – failure of smooth muscle relaxation in the oesophageal sphincter. Possibly antibody-mediated following viral infection, leading to a generalised neuropathy of the oesophageal body.

2   *Diffuse oesophageal spasm (DOS)* – in this disease, the muscles of the oesophagus are able to contract, but do so in a disorganised fashion. Believed to be due to impaired inhibitory innervation. Some cases of DOS develop into achalasia, and there is significant overlap between the two conditions.

3   *Hypertensive peristalsis* – a.k.a. 'nutcracker oesophagus'. The muscles contract *too well*, with an increased amount of force. Patients present primarily with chest pain.

4   *Hypertensive lower oesophageal sphincter* – also due to over-excitation of the nerves innervating the smooth muscles, but located primarily at the lower oesophageal sphincter. Often presents with chest pain and dysphagia.

Diagnosis

Patients usually report dysphagia, but they may also present with globus sensation, reflux, odynophagia (rare), chest pain, regurgitation, nausea or chronic cough. It is important in the history to also ask about symptoms suggestive of malignancy (fevers, rigors, sweats, chills, weight loss, anorexia and early satiety). Ask about whether the patient's symptoms are brought on by solids, semi-solids and/or liquids.

Discuss the patient's full medical history, as some conditions (e.g. scleroderma, diabetes) may cause secondary oesophageal dysmotility. Quantify their alcohol consumption, which may contribute. Enquire about family history and past surgical history. Examination findings may be normal. Some patients will show signs of weight loss due to prolonged difficulty swallowing.

Investigations

Basic bloodwork including FBE + UEC + CMP + LFT + CRP should be sent. If the chest pain sounds cardiac in origin (and has occurred recently) consider troponins and an ECG. If patients show clinical signs of systemic disease that may cause oesophageal dysmotility (e.g. diabetes or scleroderma) consider the relevant serology.

Imaging should begin with a barium swallow ± barium meal. Patients swallow radiopaque barium and a series of plain film X-rays are performed as they swallow and the barium mixture reaches their stomach. The radiographic finding most closely associated with achalasia is the 'bird beak' deformity (see Fig. 37.1). A 'corkscrew' pattern is described with DOS.

Upper GI endoscopy should be performed to exclude structural oesophageal pathology. Gold standard of diagnosis remains oesophageal manometry, whereby a tube is passed via the nasopharynx just through the lower oesophageal sphincter (placed like an NGT). It then measures the pressure while swallowing and at rest. Standard findings are summarised in Table 37.3. 24-hour pH monitoring is only indicated if the patient is reporting significant reflux symptoms.

SECTION IV

SECTION IV

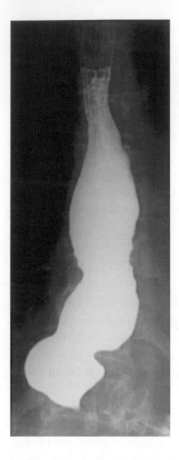

FIGURE 37.1 Oesophagram of a patient with idiopathic achalasia.

Reproduced from: Goldman, L. & Ausiello, D., 2008. In: Goldman, L. & Ausiello, D., eds., Goldman's Cecil Textbook of Medicine, 23rd ed. Philadelphia: Saunders, Fig. 140.7.

TABLE 37.3 Findings on oesophageal manometry with various motility disorders

DIAGNOSIS	FINDINGS
Achalasia	High lower sphincter pressure on contraction. Failure of the sphincter to relax at rest. Lack of coordinated lower oesophageal contractions during peristalsis
Diffuse oesophageal spasm	Simultaneous movement in the proximal and distal smooth muscle of the oesophagus. Intermittently normal peristalsis. Normal intensity. Normal sphincter tone
Hypertensive peristalsis (nutcracker oesophagus)	High-pressure contractions (i.e. >180 mmHg) ± swallow duration ≥6 s. Contraction amplitude must be ≥2 standard deviations greater than normal
Hypertensive lower oesophageal sphincter	Normal peristaltic wave. High residual pressures, with lower sphincter pressure >45 mmHg

Adapted from: Sciortino, C.M. & Yang, S.C., 2014. Disorders of esophageal motility. In: Cameron, J.L. & Cameron, A.M., Current Surgical Therapy, 11th ed. Philadelphia: Saunders.

Management

Management for dysmotility of the oesophagus begins with reassurance, once structural and sinister causes have been excluded. Patients are typically started on a PPI. Calcium channel blockers (± nitrates for hypertensive lower oesophageal sphincter) may be trialled for DOS and nutcracker oesophagus. If these measures fail, patients may progress to endoscopic dilatation of the oesophagus, intrasphincteric injection of botulinum toxin or even surgical long oesophageal myotomy (i.e. incision of the affected muscles to relieve excess propulsion).

Patients are typically only managed as inpatients if they have oesophageal dilatation or intrasphincteric injection of botulinum toxin, where they may be kept as 23-hour cases. Titration of their medications can take place in outpatients. Advise smoking cessation and reduction in alcohol consumption. If weight loss is an issue for the patient, consider a dietitian referral. If other diagnoses were detected during the patient's work-up (e.g. diabetes or autoimmune disease), make the appropriate specialist referrals to their outpatient clinics.

GASTRO-OESOPHAGEAL REFLUX DISEASE

Gastro-oesophageal reflux disease (GORD; or GERD in American English) is a motility disorder characterised by reflux of stomach contents into the lower oesophagus with pathological frequency due to an incompetent lower oesophageal sphincter, resulting in dyspepsia (i.e. heartburn). It is extremely prevalent, with 1 in 5 Australians experiencing weekly symptoms. Although not a 'dangerous' disease, it can impact on a person's psychosocial wellbeing and over time cause transformation (i.e. metaplasia) of the lower oesophagus into a pre-malignant state.

Risk factors for GORD include male gender, obesity, heavy alcohol consumption, hiatus hernias, use of certain medications (including calcium channel blockers, nitrates, alpha-adrenergic antagonists and anticholinergics), tobacco use and a positive family history. Symptoms also occur more regularly during pregnancy.

Diagnosis

A diagnosis of GORD can be made on the classic symptoms alone, with response to a therapeutic trial of a PPI being sufficient confirmation. A typical history should cover the symptoms of GORD, GI malignancies and other similar diagnoses that should be excluded (e.g. peptic ulcer disease or unstable angina). Discuss:

- When did their symptoms begin? How frequently do they occur? Do they note any triggers (e.g. spicy food, chocolate, alcohol, tobacco, activities or stress)?

- Do they experience heartburn, regurgitation (gastric contents re-entering the oesophagus), waterbrash (over-stimulation of saliva from oesophageal acidification) or chest pain? Do they have a chronic cough, or has their asthma worsened? Do they have dysphagia, odynophagia or haematemesis?

- ○ Haematemesis, melaena, odynophagia or dysphagia are considered 'alarm' symptoms and should be investigated more rigorously.
- Have they had signs of malignancy?
- What is their full medical history? What medications do they take?
- Have they ever had a gastroscopy, surgery (especially upper GI) or oesophageal manometry?

Examination findings are very likely to be normal. Note obesity, signs of alcohol abuse or chronic liver disease and general, palmar or conjunctival pallor. Inspect the supraclavicular nodes for Virchow's node (a sign of gastric cancer).

Natural history

GORD is typically intermittent but chronic, with symptoms varying in intensity from mild irritation to debilitating. As such, compliance (even when asymptomatic) must be stressed with patients. 10–40% of patients will have symptoms refractory to PPIs – consider an alternative diagnosis in this group.

If GORD is allowed to continue for a long period of time, the lower oesophageal cellular make-up can begin to change due to the prolonged exposure to a higher pH. The normal, stratified squamous epithelium of the oesophagus becomes columnar, in a condition known as Barrett's oesophagus.

Barrett's is considered a premalignant condition and is associated with the development of oesophageal adenocarcinoma, which carries a high mortality. It is not currently possible to predict which patients will go on to develop Barrett's, and thus patients at highest risk are screened with endoscopy with four-quadrant biopsy at every 2 cm of identifiable altered mucosa. If low-grade dysplasia is found, repeat endoscopy is recommended in 6 months. If two are negative in 12 months, the patient can be reviewed again in 1 year until two subsequent scopes are also negative. High-grade dysplasia, if not surgically managed, should be monitored every 3 months.

Investigations

In some cases (e.g. clear history without alarm symptoms), no investigations are required and a therapeutic trial of a PPI can be commenced. However, if the diagnosis remains unclear or any alarm symptoms (as outlined above) are present, consider doing basic bloodwork (FBE + UEC + CMP + LFT + CRP + coagulation studies) and booking the patient in for either a barium swallow (if dysphagia or odynophagia are present) or upper GI endoscopy.

24-hour ambulatory pH monitoring with oesophageal manometry can also be used to confirm the diagnosis of GORD but, due to impracticality, is rarely performed. It may be done for surgical planning. Biopsies performed at endoscopy can screen for metaplasia and Barrett's oesophagus.

Management

The cornerstone of treatment remains a PPI (e.g. esomeprazole 40 mg PO daily). Alternatively, H_2 antagonists (e.g. ranitidine 150 mg PO BD) may be used. Non-pharmaceutical measures should also be taken, with tobacco, caffeine and alcohol consumption reduced, BMI decreased and avoidance of triggers. Side effects of PPIs include initial interaction with warfarin, increased risk of bacterial gastroenteritis and interstitial nephritis.

Fundoplication can reverse the symptoms of GORD in those who fail medical therapy. If Barrett's oesophagus is found on endoscopy, it should undergo endoscopic resection and surveillance as outlined above. GORD is typically managed by GPs in the community, with only those being monitored for malignancy, or people with severe or refractory cases, being reviewed continuously in a specialist outpatient clinic.

ACUTE LIVER FAILURE

Hepatitis, in its truest definition, means inflammation of the liver (not just the viruses that come to mind!). This may be reflected biochemically with deranged LFTs indicative of damage to the liver or biliary tree, or coagulopathy demonstrating a loss of the synthetic function of the liver. Abnormal LFTs are commonly detected incidentally, but may not indicate true hepatitis in the absence of other symptoms (see Chapter 12, 'Investigations: serology').

Acute liver failure refers to development of severe hepatic injury in <6 months with an element of hepatic encephalopathy. Hepatocellular damage and loss of synthetic function are able to be demonstrated on serology. Risk factors include intravenous drug use (IVDU), alcohol abuse and hepatotoxic medications. Acute liver failure can be severe enough to cause significant morbidity, need for transplant or even death in a relatively short period of time.

In previously well patients, the three causes of massively deranged LFTs (transaminases >1000) are drugs (paracetamol toxicity and/or alcohol are common), hepatic ischaemia and viral hepatitis (hepatitis A, B, C, D and E, as well as HIV, HSV, VZV, CMV and EBV). Drug-induced liver injury may be dose-dependent, such as paracetamol, or idiosyncratic (i.e. different people react to different doses).

Hepatic ischaemia most frequently occurs after systemic hypotension (e.g. during shock), but may also be a consequence of certain drugs (e.g. cocaine) and hepatic vein thrombosis. Hepatitis A is the most likely viral cause. Other, rare causes include autoimmune disease, malignant infiltration, metabolic disorders, sepsis, toxin/heavy metal exposure or acute fatty liver.

Diagnosis

Diagnosis is based on the clinical finding of encephalopathy in combination with deranged LFTs and coagulopathy. History should cover:

CLD signifies progressive damage to liver parenchyma with attempted regeneration, ultimately producing irreversibly scarred tissue known as cirrhosis. It is the eighth leading cause of death in the developed world. Risk factors include advanced age, male gender, alcohol consumption, tattoos, obesity, intravenous drug use, blood transfusions, risky sexual behaviours, polypharmacy, travel, tobacco use and rapid weight loss.

Diagnosis

Patients will often be aware that they have CLD, and can usually tell you the origin of their disease. However, occasionally you will encounter a person experiencing decompensated liver disease who has had little or no prior contact with healthcare services. In this situation, you must take a broad history covering many of the risk factors outlined above. Discuss:

- When were they diagnosed with liver disease? Are they aware of the cause? Do they have a gastroenterologist?
- Have they ever presented to hospital confused (i.e. hepatic encephalopathy), bleeding (i.e. varices) or with a swollen abdomen (ascites) requiring drainage? If so, how recently and on how many occasions?
- If known, when was their last endoscopy for variceal monitoring? Do they get regular blood tests (AFP) and scans (ultrasound) to monitor for liver cancer?

On examination, inspect for jaundice, cachexia, asterixis (a.k.a. hepatic flap, >3 beats/min), palmar erythema (alcohol), clubbing, tattoos and track marks, muscle wasting, icteric sclera, volume state, hepatic fetor, spider naevi, gynaecomastia, ascites (test for shifting dullness), organomegaly, caput medusae, umbilical hernias and peripheral oedema.. Look for infective foci that may have caused the patient's deterioration. A digital rectal examination is *compulsory* to quantify the risk of bleeding (look for melaena or bright-red blood).

Natural history

Chronic liver disease is typically a progressive and long-term illness, with acute decompensation usually requiring admission. Complications of CLD include encephalopathy, portal hypertension, variceal bleeding, ascites, spontaneous bacterial peritonitis (i.e. infection of ascitic fluid), portal hypertensive gastropathy, cirrhotic cardiomyopathy, hepatomegaly, splenomegaly (and secondary thrombocytopenia), anaemia, bone marrow failure, hepatic hydrothorax (i.e. ascitic fluid in the pleural space due to diaphragmatic defects) and hepatorenal syndrome (i.e. liver disease + acute kidney injury; with high mortality).

There are two scoring systems used to objectively stratify the severity and mortality of chronic liver disease – the Child–Pugh system and the MELD (model for end-stage liver disease) score. Child–Pugh (Table 37.4) is more frequently used on the wards due to its simplicity, whereas MELD is employed by gastroenterologists and surgeons when discussing a patient's potential for transjugular

TABLE 37.4 Child–Pugh scoring system

VARIABLE	1 POINT	2 POINTS	3 POINTS
Total bilirubin (μmol/L)	<34	34–50	>50
Serum albumin (g/L)	>35	28–35	<28
INR	<1.7	1.71–2.30	>2.30
Ascites	None	Mild	Moderate to severe
Hepatic encephalopathy	None	Grade 1–2, or requiring medication	Grade 3–4 or refractory

Child, C. G. & Turcotte, J. G., 1964. Surgery and portal hypertension. Major Problems in Clinical Surgery 1, 1.

BOX 37.2 Model for end-stage liver disease (MELD) scoring system

MELD = 3.78 × ln[serum bilirubin (mg/dL)] + 11.2 × ln[INR] + 9.57 × ln[serum creatinine (mg/dL)] + 6.43 × aetiology (0 for cholestatic or alcoholic, 1 otherwise)

　　NB #1: If the patient is dialysed within 7 days, serum creatinine should be 4.0.

　　NB #2: Any value <1 is rounded up to 1.0 to prevent negative scores due to the logarithms used.

Adapted from: Wiesner, R., Edwards, E., Freeman, R., et al. and the United Network for Organ Sharing Liver Disease Severity Score Committee, 2003. Model for end-stage liver disease (MELD) and allocation of donor livers. Gastroenterology 124(1), 91–96.

intrahepatic portosystemic shunt (TIPS) or transplant. MELD is seeing increasing use in research and criteria for other treatment due to its greater reproducibility.

Patients are classified as either Child–Pugh A, B or C depending on points accumulated (5–6, 7–9 and 10+, respectively). These allow estimates of one-year survival – 100% for Child–Pugh A, 81% for Child–Pugh B and 45% for Child–Pugh C. The MELD score is determined by the calculation in Box 37.2.

Understandably, this is slightly harder to determine (and impossible without a calculator). MELD may also be used to determine mortality with a MELD of >40 having a 3-month mortality of over 70%.

Investigations

Investigations aim to quantify the degree of liver damage, identify the trigger for deterioration and, if unknown, recognise the cause of liver insult. The patient's presentation will guide the investigations requested. For example:

- All patients will need an FBE + UEC + CMP + LFT + TSH + coagulation studies (looking for auto-anticoagulation) + AFP (hepatocellular carcinoma screening) + nutritional panel (folate, iron studies and vitamins B12, D and consideration of K, A and E).
- Request fasting lipids and glucose for the following day.

CHAPTER 38

RENAL MEDICINE

Joseph M O'Brien

Renal Medicine (or nephrology) is yet another excellent learning rotation for a junior doctor interested in physician's training, or wanting to become more comfortable with complex and often unwell patients. Patients known to the renal team – especially those approaching or currently on dialysis – have unique needs and are very frequently admitted under Renal even when the primary issue is not renal tract-related. Most Emergency Departments (EDs) will streamline these patients directly to your care. As such, you will work closely with many other treating teams and hopefully get quite proficient at referrals by the end of your rotation!

As a junior doctor, the majority of your work will involve managing renal patients on the ward and troubleshooting issues with dialysis patients. Larger Renal Units will have outpatients come for iron infusions, planned transfusions, renal biopsies, line insertion/removal and other procedures that you will be expected to complete paperwork for. You will likely be expected to attend multiple clinics, and Radiology and Pathology meetings (e.g. to discuss biopsy results) are common.

When completing Renal admissions, document clearly the patient's volume status, weight, baseline renal function (UEC), haemoglobin (Hb), parathyroid hormone (PTH), calcium, magnesium and phosphate (CMP) and iron studies, advance care planning and, if relevant, their dialysis information (i.e. cause of renal failure, method and frequency of dialysis, baseline weight, usual weight removed, site of dialysis and access sites). All Renal patients should be admitted with a fluid balance chart with daily weighs. Consider determining the creatinine clearance (CrCl) using one of the calculators available online, as this has implications for the patient's medical management.

Planning the care of renal inpatients often means coordinating procedures and imaging around their dialysis sessions, so include these on request slips. Avoid cannulation or taking blood pressure on the arm with their fistula (or arm planned for fistula formation). Remember your patient's renal function when ordering imaging that requires contrast (although patients regularly on dialysis can have it dialysed out). Lastly, do not be afraid to discuss concerns with your registrar – they understand the complexity of your patient load and are there to help.

URINARY TRACT INFECTIONS AND UROSEPSIS

Urinary tract infection (UTI) is a broad, encompassing term that refers to a positive urinary culture with an inflammatory response in the urinary endothelium. Although they are a group of conditions that affect people of all ages, UTIs are a very common cause of hospitalisation in the elderly. They are usually managed by General Medicine.

They are most commonly caused by bacteria endemic to the bowel, such as Gram-negative bacteria (e.g. *Escherichia coli*, *Klebsiella* spp., *Enterococcus*), but special populations of patients (such as the hospitalised or immunocompromised) may be infected by *Pseudomonas*, fungi or rare microorganisms. Note that multiply-resistant *Staphylococcus aureus* does not normally cause UTIs and, if grown in urine, should be investigated with blood cultures and potentially a transthoracic echocardiogram (TTE).

Bacteriuria refers to the presence of bacteria in urine (known as pyuria if pus is present), and does not necessarily require treatment. Cystitis describes symptomatic infection of the lower urinary tract (i.e. bladder), and pyelonephritis refers to an infection of the actual renal tissues. If a bacterial infection of a urinary source spreads into the bloodstream, the infection is colloquially referred to as 'urosepsis'. Commonly caused by Gram-negative bacteria, urosepsis carries a high mortality and morbidity, particularly in the elderly. A recurrent UTI is one that recurs after *complete resolution* of symptoms.

Risk factors for UTIs include female gender (males have longer urethras), advanced age, diabetes, structural abnormalities of the urinary tract, immunocompromise, pregnancy, increased sexual activity, prostatism, prolonged inpatient admission, being post-menopausal (as oestrogen drops), urinary tract obstruction and using an 'in-and-out' catheter. The likelihood of a UTI progressing to urosepsis increases with age, renal calculi, immunocompromise, diabetes and indwelling catheter (IDC) use. Infections of the urinary tract are estimated to cost the USA healthcare system over $2 billion annually.

Diagnosis

UTIs may be diagnosed clinically, with a history of dysuria (pain on urination), urinary frequency and nocturia (need for urination overnight). Fever, chills, haematuria, nausea and vomiting and loin pain suggest severe UTI, pyelonephritis or renal calculi. It is very rare for flank pain to be absent in pyelonephritis. Severe UTI may result in delirium, particularly in the elderly. As many of the other symptoms may be absent in the elderly, delirium may be the only sign of a UTI.

When discussing a UTI with a patient, discuss the presence of the above symptoms, their existing medical conditions, any past urinary issues (e.g. structural abnormalities or regular issues as a child), any use of urinary catheters, their family history and, if relevant, a brief sexual history (including method of contraception, possibility of pregnancy and frequency of intercourse).

There may be very little to find on examination. Suprapubic or costovertebral angle tenderness may be present. The patient's observations are important, and note

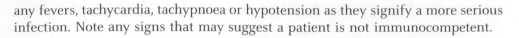

any fevers, tachycardia, tachypnoea or hypotension as they signify a more serious infection. Note any signs that may suggest a patient is not immunocompetent.

Natural history

UTIs are usually self-limiting, especially in younger patients. The risk of recurrence is high despite antibiotic management. Bacteriuria does not always progress to a urinary tract infection and, if asymptomatic, should be left untreated. Sepsis due to Gram-negative organisms carries a high morbidity and mortality and can cause lengthy hospital admissions.

Investigations

In a young person with clear symptoms, no investigations may be necessary and the patient can begin empirical treatment. However, most clinicians will at least request a 'dipstick' urine or full ward test (FWT) to inspect for nitrites (produced by bacteria as they reduce nitrates in urine), leucocyte esterase (indicative of the presence of white blood cells), erythrocytes and an altered pH. If the FWT is positive, request a formal urine microscopy/culture/sensitivities (M/C/S) to identify the organism and review for leucocyte and erythrocyte count. A 'rule of thumb' is that >100 × 10⁶/L leucocytes on urine M/C/S is suggestive of an infection.

　　If the patient is elderly or unwell with their infection, request serology. Blood work should include a full blood examination (FBE, for white blood cell count), urea, electrolytes and creatinine (UEC, for renal function), calcium, magnesium and phosphate (CMP), liver function tests (LFTs) and C-reactive protein (CRP). Blood cultures should be requested if the patient is febrile.

　　Although not always necessary, consider a chest X-ray (CXR). A renal tract ultrasound could be considered if there is a suspicion of structural abnormality. Consider a sexually transmitted infection (STI) screen in younger people with risk factors (including gonorrhoea and chlamydia PCR on urine). If urinary tract malignancy is suspected, a CT-kidney/ureters/bladder (CT-KUB) is often requested.

Management

Asymptomatic bacteriuria should **not** be treated unless the patient is pregnant. If the patient is young, strongly consider outpatient management. The elderly patient with signs of systemic illness should be admitted for treatment and monitoring. A typical plan may read:

- Admission under a General Medical or Renal unit (if known to Renal) with regular medications and deep vein thrombosis (DVT) prophylaxis.
- Empirical antibiotic therapy for 3–7 days.
  - A lower urinary tract infection may be treated with trimethoprim, typically 300 mg PO nocte (given at night so it sits in the bladder and urinary tract longer):
    - if the patient is pregnant, substitute trimethoprim with cephalexin 500 mg PO QID

- – if the patient has recently had a course of trimethoprim without resolution of symptoms, consider amoxicillin/clavulanic acid (Augmentin® Duo Forte) 875/125 mg PO BD
  - – if there is proven resistance, another potential antibiotic is norfloxacin 400 mg PO BD.
  - o In pyelonephritis or complicated infection (e.g. immunocompromise, structural abnormalities, presence of calculi), consider ceftriaxone 1 g IV daily for 2–3 days with an oral antibiotic tail to take the total duration of treatment to 10–14 days.
  - o Urosepsis is most often managed with ceftriaxone 1 g IV daily, or with haemodynamic compromise, consideration of cefepime 1 g IV TDS. With penicillin allergy, consider aztreonam 1 g IV TDS or contact Infectious Diseases (ID).
  - o Urinary tract infection with an extended spectrum beta lactamase (ESBL) organism will require a carbapenem (e.g. meropenem 1 g IV TDS). While the patient has their inpatient IV therapy, the culture should be tested for sensitivity to oral antibiotics to determine the agent used for the oral tail. ID should be notified.
- Intravenous (IV) fluid resuscitation if necessary.
- If the patient is delirious, consider the need for a 'special' to supervise them on the ward. Avoid using physical restraints, and try non-pharmaceutical management before using sedative or antipsychotic medications.
- Regular analgesia and PRN antiemetics. Consider PRN urine alkalisers (e.g. Ural sachets [1 sachet PO up to TDS PRN]).

Provide patient education regarding prevention of UTIs, including maintaining their oral intake, wiping after defecation from anterior to posterior, urinating after sexual intercourse and considering drinking cranberry juice. There is little evidence to support use of hexamine hippurate (Hiprex™) although some patients report it gives them relief of symptoms.

Follow-up is not necessary in outpatient clinics, but people who were particularly unwell could follow-up with their GP 7–10 days post-discharge. A repeat urine M/C/S to confirm bacterial eradication is not necessary.

ACUTE KIDNEY INJURY

Acute kidney injury (AKI) refers to the rapid deterioration in renal function with subsequent retention of renally-excreted substances and alteration of acid–base homeostasis over a period of <48 hours. AKI is covered in detail in Chapter 59, 'Renal outpatients'. This section aims purely to outline the management of inpatients with acute kidney injury.

AKI is common in the inpatient setting, with 5–7% of inpatients experiencing a deterioration in renal function that satisfies its definition (15–40% in the

SECTION IV

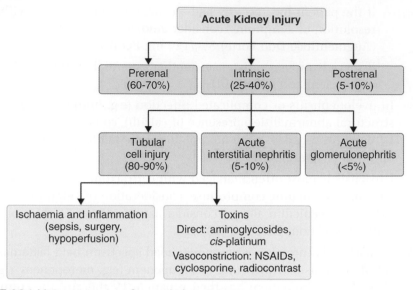

FIGURE 38.1 Main categories of acute kidney injury.

Goldman, L. & Ausiello, D., 2008. Chapter 122: Acute kidney injury. In: Goldman, L. & Ausiello, D., eds., Goldman's Cecil Textbook of Medicine, 23rd ed., Philadelphia: Saunders, Fig. 122.1.

Intensive Care Unit). Diagnosis is based on serology, as the creatinine rises and the estimated glomerular filtration rate (eGFR) drops. Multiple classification systems for defining and categorising AKI exist, as outlined in Chapter 59. Many patients also experience significant electrolyte abnormality, with hyperkalaemia and acidosis being common.

AKI is typically asymptomatic, but the symptoms experienced by the patient may provide clues as to the aetiology of the renal insult. Conceptually, many clinicians think of AKI as being either pre-renal, intrinsically renal or post-renal in origin. Fig. 38.1 outlines the main categories of kidney injury. It is important to note whether or not the patient is continuing to make urine.

Investigations should be requested to exclude chronic renal impairment, that is parathyroid hormone (elevated after months), renal tract ultrasound (kidneys atrophy with chronic impairment), FBE (chronic renal disease leads to anaemia) and CMP (hyperphosphataemia occurs after >1 week).

Management

Managing AKI firstly assumes early identification and an attempt to elicit the underlying cause. Any reversible factors should be rectified (e.g. ceasing nephrotoxins and not adding renal insults such as contrast), and the patient should aim to be euvolaemic and electrolyte replete. A typical plan could include:
- Investigation of the AKI with monitoring of renal function (UEC + CMP), a urinary protein-to-creatinine ratio (PCR), urine M/C/S (to screen for infection).

- Blood cultures if febrile.
- Administer intravenous fluid at a slow rate (e.g. 1 L of normal saline 0.9% over 8–12 hours) to maintain fluid status.
- Correct any electrolyte abnormalities.
- Withhold nephrotoxins, with the exception of frusemide, when a patient is in AKI but also fluid overloaded.
- Commence a fluid balance chart with consideration of daily weighs.
- A renal tract ultrasound to exclude post-renal obstruction.
- Flushing of the indwelling catheter, if one is in situ, to ensure it is still draining.
- If severe, consideration of filtration in a High Dependency Unit (HDU) setting (see Box 38.1 for indications for filtration).
- Consideration of insertion of an IDC for monitoring urine output accurately (patient-dependent).
- Treatment of the underlying cause (e.g. hypovolaemia, sepsis etc).

Pre-renal AKI patients perform best, with a mortality of <10%. Unfortunately, the mortality of patients with intrinsic AKI remains between 30 and 80%, with risk factors for higher mortality including advanced age, medical comorbidities, congestive cardiac failure, diabetes and prolonged ICU admission.

Patients who recover from acute kidney injury should be monitored closely. Once an obstruction is relieved, a large volume diuresis may occur. Necessary nephrotoxins should be slowly reintroduced by their primary physician. There should be an aim to prevent recurrence, by optimising risk factors such as diabetes, maintaining the patient's oral intake, avoiding unnecessary nephrotoxic agents (e.g. NSAIDs), minimising the utilisation of imaging with IV contrast and monitoring and correcting the patient's electrolytes. If the renal impairment becomes chronic, they should be referred to a renal service as a priority.

BOX 38.1 Indications for filtration in acute kidney injury

Fluid overload or pulmonary oedema refractory to diuresis

Hyperkalaemia >6.5 mmol/L refractory to therapy

Severe, refractory metabolic acidosis

Rapidly climbing creatinine or urea

Symptomatic uraemia (especially encephalopathy or pericarditis)

Oliguric/anuric renal failure

Toxicity with drugs amenable to filtration

Adapted from: Goldman, L. & Ausiello, D., 2008. Chapter 122: Acute kidney injury. In: Goldman, L. & Ausiello, D., eds., Goldman's Cecil Textbook of Medicine, 23rd ed., Philadelphia: Saunders. Gibney, N., Hoste, E., Burdmann, E.A., et al., 2008. Timing of initiation and discontinuation of renal replacement therapy in AKI: unanswered key questions. Clinical Journal of the American Society of Nephrology 3(3), 876-880.

CHRONIC RENAL IMPAIRMENT AND DIALYSIS-DEPENDENT PATIENTS

Chronic renal impairment (CRI, a.k.a. chronic kidney disease or CKD) is a progressive reduction in renal function, as measured by the eGFR and proteinuria. There is a subsequent build-up of waste products in the bloodstream, with long-term complications including renal atrophy, anaemia (due to decreased production of erythropoietin and vitamin and iron deficiencies), electrolyte abnormalities, immunocompromise (due to leakage of immunoglobulins via the basement membrane), malnutrition, neurological manifestations of uraemia, multifactorial growth retardation, hypertension, insulin resistance and hyperlipidaemia (as the body tries to increase the intravascular oncotic pressure with lipids).

CRI is outlined extensively in Chapter 59, 'Renal outpatients', including its classification system, history-taking, examination findings and management. The primary aim of management with CRI is to prevent acute deterioration by optimising the patient's risk factors, preserving their existing renal function and preparing them for dialysis early.

When admitting a patient with 'acute on chronic renal impairment' (AoCRI), manage them as per the outline for acute kidney injury above. Patients with diabetes, hypertension, acute kidney injury, cardiovascular disease, structural urinary tract abnormalities, a family history of renal disease, autoimmune illnesses and incidentally-detected haematuria should be screened for CRI.

Principles of renal replacement therapy

Renal replacement therapy (RRT) refers to a number of interventions that supplant the role of the kidney in excreting waste and managing the balance of electrolytes, including haemodialysis (HD), peritoneal dialysis (PD), haemofiltration and, ultimately, renal transplantation. Many people incorrectly use RRT to refer solely to methods of dialysis. They are all considered to be life-prolonging procedures. In general:

- The decision to initiate dialysis is one made between the patient and their nephrologist. There is no specific guideline as to at what serum creatinine or eGFR dialysis should be commenced; however symptomatic uraemia, pericarditis, pleuritis, coagulopathy, fluid overload, refractory hypertension, malnourishment, persistent hyperkalaemia or persistent gastrointestinal upset may hasten the transition to dialysis.

- The patient must be deemed to participate sufficiently in their medical care. Dialysis is a full-time commitment, with frequent medical appointments, lengthy dialysis sessions and many potential complications. On a similar note, all Renal patients should have their advanced care planning updated regularly.

- o People are prepared for dialysis in advance, so that a sudden deterioration in renal function does not become an emergency. Early referral should be made to Interventional Radiology or Vascular Surgery for creation of a fistula.
- o You may be called to review a patient on dialysis for any number of issues. Manage the typical ward calls (tachycardia, chest pain etc) as you would any other patient. Table 38.1 outlines a few specific conditions experienced by patients on dialysis and briefly how to manage them.

TABLE 38.1 Dialysis troubleshooting

ISSUE	MANAGEMENT	NOTES
Blocked fistula	• Urgent blood work, especially noting K^+ and volume status • Request a fistulogram • Vascular surgical referral	• If at a smaller dialysis centre, may require urgent transfer to a hospital with a vascular service
Poor flow through fistula	• Request an ultrasound – if stenosis is identified, request a fistulogram • A fistuloplasty, where a balloon is passed through the fistula and expanded, may be performed by vascular surgeons or interventional radiologists for vascular stenosis	• If no stenosis is identified, discuss with your registrar
Fever during dialysis	• Full septic screen with bloods, CXR and cultures as appropriate • Careful examination, particularly noting the site of access	• Work up exactly like any other patient with fever • Continue dialysis if content there is no line infection • Always notify your registrar – antibiotic treatment will likely be recommended
Vascular access infections	• Swab any discharge • Send basic blood work • Commence antibiotics empirically with skin and Gram-negative cover • Do NOT pull the line without discussing with a registrar	• Notify the registrar – ideally, the site should not be used for dialysis but the patient's options may be severely limited. It may be possible to treat with the line in situ

continued

TABLE 38.1 Dialysis troubleshooting—cont'd

ISSUE	MANAGEMENT	NOTES
Hypotension	• Manually repeat BP • Check weight – was too much fluid removed? • Review for signs of ischaemia, sepsis or other causes of low BP • Place patient in Trendelenburg position • Withhold antihypertensives until SBP >110 mmHg • Request an ECG – cardiac disease is very common in CKD	• Very common, seen in almost half of HD patients • If a regularly-occurring phenomenon with your patient, discuss midodrine with your registrar
Air embolus	• Supportive management (requires early identification) with vasopressors, fluid resuscitation and mechanical ventilation as required • Roll the patient into the left, lateral, decubitus position to potentially move the air 'bubble' • Apply supplemental O$_2$ • Consideration of removal with right heart catheterisation • If the patient arrests, commence the Advanced Life Support pathway with CPR • Consideration of anticoagulation	• Often presents with tachypnoea, tachycardia, dyspnoea and chest pain similar to a pulmonary embolism (PE) • An emergency situation • Remember to exclude other similarly-presenting conditions such as infarction, shock and PE • Notify registrar immediately

Adapted from: Goldman, L. & Ausiello, D., 2008. Chapter 133: Treatment of irreversible renal failure. In: Goldman, L. & Ausiello, D., eds., Goldman's Cecil Textbook of Medicine, 23rd ed. Philadelphia: Saunders, pp. 818-826. Nassar, G. M. & Ayus, J. C., 2001. Infectious complications of the hemodialysis access. Kidney International 60(1), 1-13. Yeun, J.Y., Ornt, D.B. & Depner, T.A., 2012. Chapter 64: Hemodialysis. In: Taal, M.W., Chertow, G.M., Marsden, P.A., et al., Brenner and Rector's The Kidney, 9th ed. Philadelphia: Saunders, pp. 2294-2346. Shaikh, N. & Ummunisa, F., 2009. Acute management of vascular air embolism. Journal of Emergencies, Trauma and Shock 2(3), 180. Perazella, M.A., 2009. Renal vulnerability to drug toxicity. Clinical Journal of the American Society of Nephrology 4(7), 1275-1283.

DRUG-RELATED NEPHROTOXICITY

The medications used in modern medicine are a very common cause of renal injury. There are various mechanisms through which a drug can cause kidney injury, including reducing perfusion (e.g. many cardiovascular drugs, IV contrast), a direct tubular effect or causing interstitial nephritis. The incidence of drug-induced kidney injury is increased when patients have an underlying renal pathology or risk factors such as diabetes, polypharmacy or advanced age.

When taking a history from a patient suspected with acute kidney injury, do not forget to cover their consumption of complementary and alternative medicines as several of these are also nephrotoxic. Table 38.2 covers some of the more common drugs known to cause nephrotoxicity in predisposed patients.

TABLE 38.2 Nephrotoxic agents

MECHANISM OF KIDNEY INJURY	DRUG
Hypoperfusion	IV contrast ACE inhibitors Angiotension-II receptor blockers Allopurinol Cyclosporine Tacrolimus Diuretics (e.g. frusemide)
Direct tubular effect	Aminoglycoside antibiotics Amphotericin B Chemotherapy (e.g. cisplatin, methotrexate) IV contrast Antivirals Osmotic diuretics (e.g. mannitol) Non-steroidal anti-inflammatory drugs
Interstitial nephritis	Proton pump inhibitors (e.g. pantoprazole) Lithium Selective serotonin reuptake inhibitors Beta-lactam antibiotics (e.g. penicillins, cephems, carbapenems, monobactams) Glycopeptide antibiotics (e.g. vancomycin) Ciprofloxacin Rifampicin Sulfonamides Non-steroidal anti-inflammatory drugs H_2 antagonists (e.g. ranitidine) Cimetidine Diuretics – frusemide, thiazides Antiepileptics (e.g. phenytoin, topiramate)

Adapted from: Perazella, M.A., 2009. Renal vulnerability to drug toxicity. Clinical Journal of the American Society of Nephrology 4(7), 1275-1283.

SECTION IV

CHAPTER 39

ENDOCRINOLOGY

Joseph M O'Brien

Endocrinology ('Endo') is a rotation with minimal inpatients, often functioning even in larger hospitals as a predominantly consult-based rotation. Subsequently, residents on Endocrinology are often shared with other specialties, which requires appropriate organisation and prioritising skills. Endocrinology is an excellent rotation to prepare for the physician's examination.

Common referrals for your team will involve labile blood sugar levels (BSLs; a.k.a. blood glucose levels or BGLs), abnormalities in thyroid function tests (TFTs) ordered as 'screening' by General Medical teams, severe electrolyte abnormalities and, in centres with Neurosurgery, diabetes insipidus, pituitary tumours and syndrome of inappropriate antidiuretic hormone secretion (SIADH).

You will be quite busy in clinics on Endocrinology, and you will get to know your hospital's diabetes educator very well. You will hopefully become very comfortable titrating insulin and commencing patients on insulin infusions (with guidance), making you a very useful resident regardless of your future career!

HYPERGLYCAEMIC CRISES: DIABETIC KETOACIDOSIS AND HYPEROSMOLAR HYPERGLYCAEMIC STATE

Diabetic ketoacidosis (DKA) is a common emergency condition seen predominantly in type 1 diabetics, resulting from either absolute insulin deficiency or insulin resistance with relative insulin deficiency, and characterised by the presence of serum ketones, metabolic acidosis with a high anion gap and profound hyperglycaemia.

Hyperosmolar hyperglycaemic state (HHS, previously known as hyperosmolar non-ketoacidosis or 'HONK') is a similar complication seen in type 2 diabetics (particularly the elderly), with hyperglycaemia due to impaired insulin action often precipitated by dehydration. In HHS, hyperglycaemia is accompanied by increased osmolality and the absence of ketones in serum.

Both DKA and HHS represent poor underlying control of a person's diabetes. The incidence of DKA peaks in the teenage years. DKA leads to many inpatient admissions, contributing to a high economic burden on the hospital system. Hyperglycaemic states may be precipitated by trauma, infection (especially sepsis), intercurrent illness, psychological stress, pregnancy, stroke, myocardial infarction and poor compliance. Certain medications may also predispose a patient to a hyperglycaemic state, including antipsychotics, steroids, thiazides and sympathomimetics (including cocaine). Sometimes, DKA is the first presentation of a person's diabetes.

In both DKA and HHS, a lack of insulin activity leads to hyperglycaemia. This induces an osmotic diuresis (bringing fluid into the intravascular space), resulting in loss of electrolytes (particularly sodium and potassium). As the body's metabolism switches from sugar consumption to free fatty acids, ketones are produced, which in turn generate a metabolic acidosis.

In an attempt to correct the acidosis, hydrogen ions (H^+) are forced into cells, pushing potassium out into the extracellular compartment and leading to an overall potassium-deplete state. Further potassium is lost via the gastrointestinal (GI) tract from vomiting. The large-scale diuresis leads to hypovolaemic shock. The absence of ketones in HHS is thought to be due to the presence of a small amount of circulating insulin.

Diagnosis

The cardinal signs and symptoms of hyperglycaemic states include dehydration, polyuria (i.e. excess urination), polydipsia (i.e. excess thirst), polyphagia (i.e. excess hunger), nausea ± vomiting and abdominal pain. Symptoms that occasionally present include altered mental state, Kussmaul breathing (i.e. deep and laboured breathing, not to be confused with Kussmaul's sign, which is increasing JVP on inspiration!) and acetone (fruity) breath. Patients with severe DKA may present confused or even comatose.

The vitals and fluid state are the most important aspect of the clinical examination. Note body habitus and signs of dehydration such as decreased skin turgor, sunken eyes, dry mucous membranes, tachycardia, poor capillary refill and, at later stages, hypotension and decreased conscious state. Inspect for acetone breath, air hunger and signs of a precipitating event such as infection, trauma or vascular episode.

Natural history

Although not a 'hard-and-fast' rule, DKA tends to be quite acute in <24 hours with HHS having a slower, more insidious onset over several days. Both hyperglycaemic states are often associated with a 'pseudo-hyponatraemia' due to the osmotic effect of high serum glucose. Calculators are available online to help you determine the serum sodium.

Due to increased awareness, mortality of DKA is now <1%. Unfortunately, mortality of HHS remains as high as 20% in observational studies. Complications of hyperglycaemic states are rare, but include hypokalaemia, relapse after withdrawal of the insulin infusion, hyperchloraemic acidosis (after excessive use of normal saline), coma, aspiration, cerebral oedema, venous thromboembolic events (VTEs) and rhabdomyolysis that can lead to acute kidney injury.

SECTION IV

Investigations

Diagnosis of DKA is confirmed with a BSL >15 mmol/L, pH <7.15, HCO_3^- <15 mmol/L and elevated ketones on urine or serum. In HHS, the BSL is often very high (e.g. >28 mmol/L), with a pH >7.3, HCO_3^- >15, low ketones (if present) and osmolality >320 mosmol/L.

Venous blood gases (VBGs) are your best friend in DKA and HHS. They are easy to obtain, fast to turn around results and report the major electrolytes, pH and serum glucose. Spot glucometers should report the level of ketones. VBGs should be ordered hourly with formal electrolytes every 2 hours initially.

On presentation, basic bloodwork should be requested including: full blood examination (FBE; review for leukophilia); urea and electrolytes (UEC; review renal function, sodium and potassium); calcium, magnesium and phosphate (CMP); inflammatory markers (CRP); liver function tests (LFTs); and HbA_{1c}. If myalgia is present, request a creatine kinase (CK). Request troponins with angina. Request a urine microscopy, culture and sensitivities (M/C/S) with an albumin-to-creatinine ratio (ACR).

Consider a chest X-Ray (CXR) to exclude pneumonia as a precipitant. Once stabilised consider screening for concomitant autoimmune disease with thyroid-stimulating hormone (TSH) and coeliac serology. A screening ECG should be requested.

Management

The first step in managing DKA and HHS should not be commencing an insulin infusion, but rather beginning urgent fluid resuscitation. If the patient is unstable, resuscitation with ABC (airway, breathing, circulation) should commence. Consider admission to an intensive care unit (ICU) or high dependency unit (HDU) if the patient is haemodynamically unstable, unable to maintain their airway due to lowered conscious state, obtunded or requiring an insulin infusion. A typical plan for a patient admitted with a hyperglycaemic state may include the following:

1 Admission under a General Medical or Endocrine unit with regular medications and deep vein thrombosis (DVT) prophylaxis.

2 Aggressive fluid resuscitation, limited only if the patient has cardiac, hepatic or renal disease. Fluid deficit of up to 5 to 10 L is not uncommon:

   a an example regimen might be 2000 mL of normal saline 0.9% over the first hour with 500–1000 mL over the next 2–4 hours and reassessment

   b patients may require placement of a central line.

3 Commence strict fluid balance with consideration of indwelling catheter (IDC) only if necessary.

4 Close monitoring of sugars and ketones as above. The target BSL is 5–12 mmol/L and the aim is to reduce ketones by 0.5 mmol/L/hour.

5 Slow correction of electrolyte abnormalities as required, aiming for a potassium >4 mmol/L and a magnesium of >1 mmol/L:

a potassium should be given after the first hour if hyperkalaemia is excluded. People with a potassium between 4 and 5 mmol/L should be given 20 mmol of KCl in normal saline; those with a potassium of 3–4 should receive 30–40 mmol KCl replacement; and those with potassium <3 mmol/L should receive 40–60 mmol KCl with consideration of delivery via a central line in a HDU setting (discuss with the registrar).

6 Commence fixed rate insulin infusion (FRII) if necessary. A typical starting solution would be 50 units fast-acting insulin (e.g. Actrapid) in 50 mL normal saline 0.9% via a syringe, run at a fixed rate of 0.1 unit/kg/hour. Your hospital should have a policy for insulin infusions to assist in titrating the rate:

a boluses are no longer given

b the patient continues their long-acting or mixed insulin therapies

c delay insulin therapy in hypokalaemia

d beware insulin naïve HHS patients, who may respond vigorously

e if the patient has an insulin pump, consider disconnecting it while running the insulin infusion

f down-titrate as hyperglycaemia and ketonaemia resolve

g hypoglycaemia should be corrected with a small bolus of 10% dextrose (5 mL/kg).

7 Complete screening for precipitants and treat any detected (e.g. empirical antibiotics for sepsis).

8 Ongoing neurological observations.

9 If the patient is pregnant, notify Obstetrics & Gynaecology.

10 If the patient is a new diagnosis type 1 diabetic, a dose of 0.25 units/kg subcutaneous long-acting insulin should be given once daily to prevent rebound ketosis when the FRII is ceased.

11 Convert the patient to subcutaneous insulin when biochemically stable, i.e. ketones <0.6 mmol/L and pH >7.3. This is ideally commenced by a specialist endocrine unit. Alternatively, if the patient is on an insulin pump this could be restarted with close monitoring.

12 Refer to a diabetes educator and dietitian as an inpatient.

Bicarbonate administration is not generally recommended, unless the pH is <6.9 or arrhythmias are present (either way, this is a registrar or even consultant level decision). Early reintroduction of diet is advocated. A patient with DKA will often recover quickly, especially if young.

First diagnosis diabetics should be linked with an endocrinologist, or if <18 years old, a paediatrician. They should be reviewed in the outpatient clinic a few weeks after discharge where they will be referred to an optometrist and podiatrist if necessary. Patients should undergo extensive education regarding management of their BSLs, and be asked to monitor them and their insulin dose prior to their next review.

HYPERTHYROIDISM

Hyperthyroidism refers to either clinical or biochemical overactivation of the thyroid gland. Thyrotoxicosis is the hypermetabolic state resultant from excess thyroid hormone release. Hyperthyroidism does not always require admission to work up, unless the patient is particularly unwell (see thyrotoxic crisis under 'Natural history' below). It may be detected incidentally in the inpatient population, and is hence a common referral for endocrine units.

Hyperthyroidism has multiple aetiologies, the most common including Graves' disease (a.k.a. diffuse toxic goitre), multinodular goitre, toxic adenoma, thyroiditis and excess iodine intake. Graves' disease is due to antibodies stimulating thyroid hormone release. Goitres or adenomas (cancers of glandular tissue) may spontaneously release excess thyroid hormone.

Hyperthyroidism is very common, affecting up to 1.5% of Australians. Risk factors include female gender, advanced age, exposure to ionised radiation, excess iodine intake (e.g. overconsumption of seafood), family history and medications such as amiodarone and lithium. Thyroid dysfunction often presents itself during pregnancy.

DIAGNOSIS

The history of hyperthyroidism is variable, but inevitably involves 'overactivation' of bodily systems. Classic symptoms include heat intolerance, polyphagia, weight loss (although increased hunger sometimes leads to paradoxical weight gain), goitre, exophthalmos (i.e. eye protrusion), tachycardia (sometimes with palpitations), tremors, labile mood and anxiety, insomnia, xeroderma (i.e. dry skin), diarrhoea and myasthenia (i.e. muscle weakness).

Examination should be thorough, due to the many potential clinical manifestations of hyperthyroidism. Review the vitals for fever, tachycardia, tachypnoea and hypertension. Inspect for onycholysis (loosening of the nail bed), pruritus, vitiligo, alopecia, hyperhidrosis (sweating), hyperreflexia, goitre, exophthalmos, lid lag (i.e. immobility or sluggish movement of the upper eyelid on downward rotation of the eye), flow murmur (due to increased output), dyspnoea, cachexia, mood lability and cognitive impairment.

When examining the thyroid, inspect the patient from behind and remember to palpate the head and neck lymph node chains. When inspecting, get them to swallow some water to see if there is any abnormal movement of the thyroid. Note tenderness or bruit. Percuss the chest for retrosternal extension. In the elderly, consider a mini-mental state examination (MMSE) and note that signs may be more subtle.

Natural history

'Thyroid storm' (a great name for a rock band) or, more appropriately, a thyrotoxic crisis, is a life-threatening but thankfully rare complication of hyperthyroidism characterised by fever, tachycardia (often with atrial fibrillation), nausea, vomiting and agitation. It most frequently occurs in known hyperthyroid patients with an intercurrent illness or who have recently stopped treatment.

Thyroid dysfunction often exists on an axis with other autoimmune conditions, particularly diabetes, pernicious anaemia, Addison's disease and coeliac disease. Anticoagulation in patients with atrial fibrillation associated with hyperthyroidism is a controversial issue, with the majority of clinicians tending to anticoagulate despite inconclusive evidence.

Investigations

Patients with decreased TSH require further investigation. Typically with hyperthyroidism, TSH is appropriately suppressed with increased T4 and T3 (see Chapter 12, 'Investigations: serology' for more detail). If they are normal, the patient may have subclinical hyperthyroidism, non thyroidal illness or central hypothyroidism or may be recovering from hyperthyroidism or an acute dose of glucocorticoids.

If thyroid hormones are elevated, a radionuclide thyroid scan may be indicated to determine the cause. Homogeneous uptake is suggestive of Graves', and heterogeneous uptake suggests either a toxic, multinodular goitre or toxic adenoma. If uptake is absent or near-absent, examination provides further information. A tender, 'cold' thyroid is likely to be subacute thyroiditis. A painless, 'cold' thyroid may be sporadic or drug-induced thyroiditis.

Thyroglobulin may be used as a tumour marker in hyperthyroidism from malignancy, or to monitor effectiveness of treatment for Graves' disease. Antibodies may provide further clues as to the aetiology of the disease. Thyroid peroxidase antibody (TPO Ab) is positive in Graves' and Hashimoto thyroiditis. Thyroglobulin antibody (Tg Ab) is requested when Hashimoto thyroiditis or malignancy is suspected. Lastly, the TSH-receptor antibody (TSHR Ab) or thyroid-stimulating immunoglobulin (TSI) are requested when Graves' is suspected and a thyroid uptake scan cannot be performed (e.g. due to pregnancy or lactation).

Patients with hyperthyroidism should also have basic bloods (FBE + UEC + CMP + LFT) with consideration of screening for concomitant diseases such as pernicious anaemia, coeliac, dyslipidaemia and diabetes. Occasionally, ultrasonography is requested to measure thyroidal blood flow, but does not usually aid in diagnosis.

Management

Management is dependent on the cause of the hyperthyroidism. Beta-blockers may be used prior to beginning antithyroid therapy to relieve adrenergic symptoms (e.g. propranolol 20–40 mg PO TDS). Anticoagulation should be discussed with a consultant for patients in atrial fibrillation (AF).

SECTION IV

The treatment options for Graves', the most common cause of hyperthyroidism in Australia, are antithyroid drugs, radioactive iodine and surgical thyroidectomy. Typically, patients are trialled on oral medications (e.g. carbimazole 10–30 mg PO daily in 2–3 divided doses initially, slowly tapered after 4 weeks to a maintenance of 2.5–10 mg PO daily), and monitored for side effects until ceased at 12–18 months.

Steroids may be used for autoimmune causes of hyperthyroidism, as directed by a consultant. If the patient relapses, radioactive iodine (RAI) could be considered. Patients should be counselled about cessation of smoking, as it carries much higher risk of orbitopathy in Graves' disease.

Thyroidectomy is covered in Chapter 49, 'Ear, nose and throat and head and neck surgery', and is indicated in obstructive goitre, patients unsuitable for radioactive iodine and severely symptomatic pregnant patients. Ideally, patients are close to euthyroid preoperatively. Side effects include hypothyroidism, hypoparathyroidism and, rarely, vocal cord paralysis (from injury to the recurrent laryngeal nerve). Patients may also require referral to a surgeon for consideration of orbital decompression if they experience severe exophthalmos.

Thyroiditis is managed symptomatically with beta-blockers, non-steroidal anti-inflammatory drugs (NSAIDs) and steroids. In lithium-induced thyroid disease the lithium should ideally be switched to another agent. Definitive treatment of a toxic, multinodular goitre involves treatment with antithyroid agents followed by RAI.

For more information about the ongoing monitoring of hyperthyroidism, please refer to Chapter 60, 'Endocrinology outpatients'.

HYPOTHYROIDISM

Conversely, hypothyroidism is underactivity of the thyroid gland resulting in decreased circulating, active thyroid hormones. It is quite common in the community and, due to the non-specificity of symptoms, is most often diagnosed with an elevated TSH on serology. Subclinical hypothyroidism is abnormal biochemistry in the absence of symptoms. Risk factors include pregnancy, female gender, intercurrent autoimmune disease, advanced age, family history, ionised radiation exposure and previous thyroidectomy.

Primary hypothyroidism is by far the predominant cause of hypothyroidism, with Hashimoto's thyroiditis being the most common aetiology in people >8 years old. Other causes include treatment of hyperthyroidism with RAI or surgery, subacute thyroiditis, iodine imbalance, congenital and prolonged iodide treatment.

Secondary hypothyroidism may occur with pituitary dysfunction, neoplasia or infiltrative disease; and tertiary hypothyroidism may result from disease in the hypothalamus (e.g. granulomas or neoplasia). Congenital hypothyroidism is endemic in areas where the soil does not naturally contain iodine, which has led to the iodinisation of salt in many developed countries.

Diagnosis

The presentation of hypothyroidism is highly variable and quite non-specific, with differential diagnoses including depression, cognitive decline and systemic diseases causing specific symptoms (e.g. congestive cardiac failure). Common symptoms include lethargy, weight gain (paradoxically with anorexia), cold intolerance, hyperphonia (hoarseness of voice), constipation, myasthenia, arthralgias, xeroderma, peripheral paraesthesia, alopecia and, in women, amenorrhoea or menstrual abnormalities. People with hypothyroidism often note a depressed mood with blunted affect and limited motivation to participate socially. In the elderly in particular, cognitive decline may be noted.

Similar to hyperthyroidism, examination should be broad. Review the vitals for hypothermia (rare), bradycardia, diastolic hypertension and bradypnoea. Altered conscious state may be present. Note disorientation, and consider an MMSE. Bradykinesia (slow movement) and delayed responsiveness may be obvious. Inspect for obesity, nail changes, skin changes, scalp alopecia, periorbital oedema, thinning of the lateral third of the eyebrows, quietened heart sounds, hyporeflexia and peripheral, non-pitting oedema. Thyroid examination may demonstrate scars suggestive of past surgery, abnormal anatomy of the thyroid gland, tenderness or altered texture.

Natural history

In comparison with hyperthyroidism, hypothyroidism is often more insidious in its onset with slow development of symptoms. Associated conditions include anaemia, pericardial effusion, pernicious anaemia, ascites, carpal tunnel syndrome, gout, coeliac disease, dyslipidaemia, reduced blood sugar and sodium and elevated prolactin and homocysteine.

Long-term sequelae include goitre, dyslipidaemia leading to increased incidence of ischaemic heart disease, depression, peripheral neuropathy, partially reversible infertility, birth defects (if the mother is persistently hypothyroid throughout the pregnancy) and myxoedema.

Investigations

First-line investigations into hypothyroidism include TSH (elevated), with thyroid function tests (with T3 and T4 expected to be low), FBE (for anaemia), UEC, CMP, LFT and fasting lipids and glucose. If GI symptoms are present consider screening for coeliac. As primary hypothyroidism is so common, further testing may not be necessary and, in the absence of intercurrent illness, treatment with thyroxine could be considered. If confirmation of the diagnosis of autoimmune hypothyroidism is necessary request antithyroid peroxidase antibodies. Imaging is not usually necessary; however an MRI-brain may be required if there is a clinical suspicion of pituitary mass.

Management

Patients with hypothyroidism do not require admission for management; however, as in hyperthyroidism, many diagnoses are made incidentally during inpatient stays. The cornerstone of treatment is supplementation of the suppressed thyroid hormone with thyroxine, often started at 25–50 mcg PO daily and up-titrated with TSH every 4–6 weeks as necessary. Young patients may be able to begin on a higher

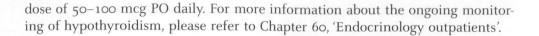

dose of 50–100 mcg PO daily. For more information about the ongoing monitoring of hypothyroidism, please refer to Chapter 60, 'Endocrinology outpatients'.

ADRENAL INSUFFICIENCY

Adrenal insufficiency is a disorder of the adrenal glands resulting in inadequate secretion of corticosteroids. The most common aetiology of primary adrenal insufficiency is autoimmune destruction of the adrenal glands (Addison's or autoimmune adrenitis; contributing to 80% of cases), with other causes including neoplasia, infarction, tuberculosis and rare causes such as AIDS, granulomatous disease, infiltrative disease (e.g. amyloid) and fungal infection. Causes of secondary adrenal insufficiency include decreased stimulation via the hypothalamic–pituitary axis.

The onset of adrenal insufficiency may be acute or chronic, with the latter being quite difficult to diagnose in the absence of clinical suspicion. In some cases, people present with an adrenal (or 'Addisonian') crisis, an emergency often precipitated by infection, trauma or sudden cessation of steroid therapy. Due to the non-specific presentation of adrenal insufficiency, there are a large number of differential diagnoses including sepsis, hypovolaemia, hyperthyroidism and perforated abdominal viscus. Addison's disease is a chronic form of adrenal insufficiency from bilateral loss of the adrenal cortices.

Adrenal insufficiency is relatively rare, with an incidence in the UK of 1 in 10,000 people. Risk factors include concomitant autoimmune disease, family history, retroperitoneal trauma, chemotherapy, vasculopathy and infiltrative diseases.

Diagnosis

Diagnosis can be difficult to elicit. If presenting acutely, patients may report nausea, vomiting, abdominal pain, anorexia, salt craving, muscle cramps, arthralgias and altered bowel habit (either constipation or diarrhoea). Patients with a chronic presentation may report postural hypotension and presyncope, weight loss, fatigue, weakness, mood change and loss of secondary sexual characteristics (seen as loss of pubic and axillary hair in women). Ask about any recent medications or illnesses and, in particular, use and cessation of steroids.

When taking a history from a patient with known adrenal insufficiency, ask them about their current endocrinologist, their usual dose of steroids, if they have been recently unwell or injured, if there is the possibility of pregnancy, if they have needed to up- or down-titrate their steroids, if they have ever had any complications of their therapy in the past and if they have had an adrenal crisis previously and what was done to manage it (e.g. did they require admission to Intensive Care?). Consider screening for common co-related illnesses as outlined below in 'Natural history'.

Patients with an adrenal crisis can present with vasodilatory shock with profound hypotension, bradycardia, hypoglycaemia, anorexia, nausea and vomiting, abdominal pain, weakness, pyrexia and, in later stages, confusion and even coma.

Examination findings will vary dependent on the acuity of the presentation. On general inspection, note body habitus, fluid state, blood pressure, heart rate and temperature in particular. Inspect for vitiligo (i.e. patchy loss of skin pigmentation). If the patient has identifiable risk factors, review for signs of infection with tuberculosis (TB). If they are already on steroid therapy, look for complications of steroids such weight gain, striae, thin skin, proximal weakness and Cushingoid appearance.

Natural history

Many people who go onto steroid therapy for adrenal insufficiency do experience relapse of their illness, usually during times of physiological stress. Adrenal insufficiency of autoimmune origin is associated with many other autoimmune illnesses including thyroid dysfunction, polycystic ovarian syndrome, hypoparathyroidism, myasthenia gravis, pernicious anaemia, type 1 diabetes and adrenoleukodystrophy.

Investigations

Bloodwork should be carried out marked 'urgent' and should include FBE (anaemia or leukophilia may be present), UEC (hyponatraemia and hyperkalaemia are common), CMP (for hypercalcaemia), glucose (often low), LFTs (transaminases may be elevated), CRP (for precipitant) and TSH, HbA_{1c}, coeliac serology and fasting lipids (as screening). If anaemia is present request B12, folate and iron studies and, if B12 is low, consider intrinsic factor and antiparietal cell antibodies. Consider Quantiferon Gold (QFG) in patients with risk factors for TB.

To interrogate the adrenal glands further, request serum adrenal autoantibodies, and renin and aldosterone levels. These should be drawn close in time to serum cortisol, with high renin and low aldosterone seen classically with Addison's. Serum adrenocorticotropic hormone (ACTH) should be measured and is expected to be raised in primary and low or normal in secondary adrenal insufficiency.

The key to diagnosis is a serum cortisol, a 'stress hormone' with levels that vary over the course of the day. As such it is critical to order it between 8 a.m. and 9 a.m. An ACTH stimulation (i.e. 'short Synacthen') test could be considered, as outlined in Chapter 12, 'Investigations: serology'. A normal response is a rise in cortisol after administration of synthetic ACTH.

Imaging should be discussed with your registrar. A CXR and abdominal X-ray to exclude infection, lung mass, signs of latent TB and adrenal calcification would be standard. If autoantibodies were negative a CT-abdomen/pelvis could be considered. If secondary adrenal insufficiency was suspected, consider an MRI-brain to look for structural changes in the pituitary and hypothalamus.

Management

As always, begin with an 'ABC' assessment of the patient and escalate their care if necessary. If the patient is haemodynamically compromised, they will need admission to ICU. Patients with an adrenal crisis may need vasopressor support to maintain their blood pressure. Treatment should never be withheld to aid diagnosis as adrenal insufficiency can be a life-threatening condition. A typical plan may include the following steps:

1 Admission under an Endocrinology or General Medical unit with regular medications and DVT prophylaxis.

2 If in adrenal crisis:

   a urgent assessment and commencement of intravenous fluids

   b correction of electrolyte abnormalities with close monitoring with VBGs

   c intravenous steroid (e.g. dexamethasone 4 mg IV bolus – preferred as it does not interfere with diagnostic evaluation), as soon as possible

   d consideration of admission to HDU or ICU for vasopressor support if hypotension not responsive to steroids and fluid.

3 Steroid therapy should be changed to oral when tolerated, and weaned very slowly. Patients should receive replacement for both mineralocorticoid and glucocorticoid steroids with fludrocortisone and prednisolone, respectively. Prednisolone is slowly weaned down. Fludrocortisone is started at between 50 and 300 mcg PO daily.

4 Postural blood pressures BD for 48 hours.

5 PRN anti-emetics and analgesia.

Prior to discharge, a patient with new diagnosis adrenal insufficiency should be referred to a specialist endocrinologist for ongoing monitoring. The patient will require extensive education regarding management of their steroid supplementation, including an explanation of how to up-titrate during periods of illness. Suggest a medical alert bracelet, which can be purchased from pharmacies, and link them with support groups if necessary. Patients going for surgery will need perioperative review and IV steroids.

Patient response to therapy is measured via BP (including postural changes) and normalisation of sodium and potassium. Patients should be reviewed by their GP after discharge with serum electrolytes prior to all their doctor's appointments. Patients should be monitored for osteoporosis while on steroid therapy with bone mineral density (BMD) scans 2-yearly. When reviewing patients with adrenal insufficiency, screening for mental health issues and sexual dysfunction is advised (low libido is common).

CUSHING'S SYNDROME

Cushing's syndrome refers to a constellation of signs and symptoms secondary to prolonged exposure to excess cortisol, including hypertension, central obesity with limb wasting, striae, 'moon' facies (i.e. rounded face), buffalo hump (i.e. a fat lump between the scapulae), myasthenia, osteoporosis and thin skin. Mood disturbance, headaches and fatigue are also common.

Cushing's *disease* is a specific subtype of Cushing's syndrome caused by pituitary ACTH excess. Pseudo-Cushing's refers to a syndrome with similar signs and symptoms explained by either metabolic obesity, alcohol abuse or depression.

The most common cause is iatrogenic, that is excessive use of glucocorticoid therapy, but other aetiologies include excess pituitary ACTH production, adrenal neoplasia and ectopic production of ACTH (e.g. as part of a paraneoplastic syndrome with lung, renal cell, thyroid, thymus or pancreatic cancers). A rare cause is multiple endocrine neoplasia-1 (MEN-1) syndrome.

Cushing's syndrome is relatively common, although it is difficult to study epidemiologically due to the under-reporting of iatrogenic (i.e. doctor-induced) patients. Peak incidence is at 15–40 years of age, with paraneoplastic causes being more common in the elderly or those with a history of tobacco consumption.

Diagnosis

Cushing's syndrome is most commonly detected by a treating physician who sees a patient intermittently, as the signs and symptoms develop gradually. The issue most commonly presented by patients is weight gain, fatigue or mood disturbance. Take a menstrual history from female patients, discuss impotence with men and enquire about decreased libido in both genders. If the patient is on exogenous (i.e. administered from outside their body) steroid ask about the indication behind the prescription and expected duration of therapy.

On examination, take note of the patient's vitals, body habitus, skin tone and mental state. Inspect for striae, moon facies, facial acne, hirsutism, alopecia, buffalo hump, thin skin, peripheral oedema and demonstrable weakness. Consider examining the thyroid, and reviewing for signs of diabetes, as chronic hyperglycaemia is common with excess cortisol. Palpate for bony tenderness along the vertebral column. Note any signs of chronic liver disease, which may suggest an alternative diagnosis.

Natural history

The natural history of Cushing's syndrome is dependent on the underlying aetiology. With removal of iatrogenic steroids, most patients with Cushing's syndrome perform well. Endogenous Cushing's syndrome (i.e. excess cortisol is produced by their body) can be thought of as ACTH-dependent or ACTH-independent. ACTH-dependent causes include pituitary adenomas (80% of ACTH-dependent cases) and ectopic production of ACTH (i.e. paraneoplastic syndromes from endocrine, small-cell lung or bronchial carcinoid tumours). The ACTH-independent causes include a unilateral tumour of the adrenal gland or, very rarely, adrenal hyperplasia. The majority of cases have a chronic course with periodic exacerbations.

Complications of Cushing's syndrome include metabolic syndrome (hypertension, dyslipidaemia, obesity, diabetes), osteopaenia and osteoporosis, coagulopathy (thrombophilia) and panhypopituitarism if resection of the pituitary is necessary. Patients with Cushing's syndrome have a fivefold increase in mortality, with common causes of death including cardiovascular disease, uncontrolled diabetes and infections.

Investigations

Investigations should first aim to confirm the presence of Cushing's syndrome and rule out any preexisting complications. Basic bloodwork including FBE (leukophilia is common), UEC (hypokalaemia and metabolic acidosis), CMP, LFT, TSH, CRP and fasting glucose and lipids should be requested at baseline.

The key pathology for diagnosis is a 24-hour urine free cortisol, plasma ACTH and an overnight 1 mg dexamethasone suppression test. Gold standard for diagnosis would be three separately measured samples, with creatinine clearance measured simultaneously, that demonstrate a cortisol >3× the upper limit of normal (ULN).

Plasma ACTH varies over the day, and should be measured at 8 a.m. If ACTH is low and cortisol is high, this suggests an ACTH-independent cause (i.e. the ACTH is appropriately suppressed but the adrenal glands are continuing to produce cortisol). If ACTH and cortisol are both high, an ACTH-dependent cause is suggested (e.g. pituitary adenoma).

The low-dose dexamethasone suppression test can be used as a substitute if, for whatever reason, a patient is either unable or unwilling to perform a 24-hour urinary free cortisol measurement. Dexamethasone 1 mg PO is administered 'stat' between 11 p.m. and 1 a.m. with a serum cortisol requested for 8 a.m. **strict** the following morning. A normal response to dexamethasone would be low cortisol. The 2-day suppression test is no longer routinely used.

Consider imaging with an MRI-brain to assess the pituitary. If an ectopic source of ACTH is suspected based on serology, consider CT-chest, -abdomen and -pelvis.

Management

Patients are not normally admitted for investigation of Cushing's syndrome; however, it may be detected incidentally in the inpatient population (especially on rotations such as Rheumatology who like to use a lot of prednisolone!).

The definitive management of Cushing's syndrome is very much determined by the underlying aetiology. For example, in exogenous Cushing's the steroids should be slowly weaned to cessation (the longer the patient has been on steroids, the slower the weaning). This is not always possible (e.g. in the case of refractory inflammatory bowel diseases), but should remain the target.

If steroids cannot be ceased completely, the patient's risk factor should be optimised to minimise the risk of complications (see above), and they should be monitored regularly by an endocrinologist. Patients should have ongoing osteoporosis screening with 2-yearly BMD scans and a regular HbA$_{1c}$, and should commence a lipid-lowering agent. Side effects such as hypertension, osteoporosis and lowered libido should be managed if they occur. Non-pharmaceutical management should include optimisation of diet (consider dietitian review), tobacco and alcohol cessation and exercise.

If the patient's Cushing's is due to neoplasia, then definitive management would be resection of the tumour, and surgical referral should be made promptly with simultaneous medical optimisation of the patient to improve surgical outcomes. Medical therapy with metyrapone, mitotane or ketoconazole could be considered in patients who have no known primary, are not fit for surgery or continue to have increased cortisol despite prior surgical management. Radiotherapy applied to the tumour may also be effective, but side effects of hypopituitarism are common. These are all consultant-level decisions.

SYNDROME OF INAPPROPRIATE ANTI-DIURETIC HORMONE SECRETION

Syndrome of inappropriate antidiuretic hormone secretion (SIADH) is a constellation of signs and symptoms characterised by excess release of antidiuretic hormone (a.k.a. ADH or vasopressin). ADH causes retention of water by acting on the collecting ducts and distal convoluted tubules of the kidneys, and the negative feedback loop is closed by the hypothalamus as it measures serum osmolality. The net effect of increased serum ADH is dilutional hyponatraemia. The net effect is impaired water secretion as water is retained, diluting the serum, and increased concentration of urine.

SIADH may be caused by central nervous system pathology (e.g. meningitis, haemorrhage, ischaemia, trauma, surgery), malignancy (small-cell carcinoma of the lung being the 'classic' tumour), medications (including carbamazepine, cyclophosphamide, multiple chemotherapeutic agents, haloperidol, amitriptyline, valproate, methotrexate, interferon, desmopressin, amiodarone, ciprofloxacin and ecstasy), hypopituitarism, adrenal insufficiency, hypothyroidism and HIV infection. It may be idiopathic, particularly in the elderly.

SIADH is often suspected when hyponatraemia is discovered. It is most common in the elderly and patients who are hospitalised. SIADH is also a very common cause of hypo-osmolality. Complications of SIADH include hyponatraemia, seizures, confusion, coma, respiratory arrest and death. If the sodium is corrected too rapidly, the patient is at high-risk of **central pontine demyelination**, an irreversible CNS disorder that has close to 100% mortality. The mortality of severe hyponatraemia is very high.

Diagnosis

Patients may report anorexia, nausea, vomiting, myalgias, myasthenia, tremor, altered breathing, dysarthria, confusion, seizures and lethargy. These symptoms are exaggerated with a more rapid onset of hyponatraemia. At end stages, SIADH can lead to delirium, cerebral oedema and, ultimately, coma. The history should cover common presentations of malignancy and stroke.

Examination may be normal; however, neurological signs (including hyporeflexia, myoclonus, asterixis, dysarthria and confusion) are not uncommon. Carefully note the patient's vitals and **volume state**. If an indwelling catheter (IDC) is in situ, note the concentration and volume of the urine. Inspect for signs of common and serious causes of SIADH including meningitis, subarachnoid haemorrhage, malignancy and hypothyroidism. Classically, SIADH occurs in euvolaemic patients without blood pressure abnormality, ascites, chest crackles or peripheral oedema.

Investigations

Serology should include an FBE, UEC (to quantify the hyponatraemia and assess renal function), CMP, TSH and CRP (as a baseline inflammatory marker). A spot BSL may be performed to exclude the pseudo-hyponatraemia seen with hyperglycaemia. A 'paired osmolality' – i.e. serum and urine osmolality – should be sent as close together as possible. Typical features of SIADH include hyponatraemia, urine osmolality >100 mosm/kg, serum osmolality <275 mOsm/kg and the absence of hyperglycaemia or fluid depletion. Consider testing adrenal function with serum cortisol to exclude adrenal insufficiency. Although plasma ADH can be tested, it is not performed routinely as urinary osmolality >100 mOsm/kg is usually evidence enough to demonstrate excess circulating ADH.

Imaging should include a CXR (to exclude an ACTH-producing lung tumour and infection), with consideration given to an MRI-brain if the clinical suspicion of a pituitary tumour, stroke or trauma is high. If the clinical suspicion of malignancy remains high in the absence of thoracic neoplasia, consider completing the patient's 'pan-scan' with a CT-abdomen/pelvis. An ECG should be requested. A method for excluding alternate diagnoses is outlined in Fig. 39.1.

Management

Treatment is dependent on the patient's symptoms and the underlying aetiology, with correction of volaemic state and sodium levels being the priority. Chronic hyponatraemia rarely carries neurological sequelae and should be corrected gently. Symptomatic hyponatraemia should be assessed promptly. Patients with moderately severe hyponatraemia (i.e. <120 mmol/L) can have serious neurological consequences including altered cognition, seizures and coma. As always, begin your management of the patient by assessing their 'ABC' (airway, breathing and circulation) and escalating their care if necessary. A plan for managing a patient with SIADH may include the following:

1 Admission under an Endocrinology or General Medical unit with regular medications and DVT prophylaxis:

   a discuss with your registrar regarding withholding 'salt-losing' medications (e.g. thiazide diuretics, selective serotonin reuptake inhibitors, carbamazepine and some other anti-epileptic agents, MAO inhibitors, ACE inhibitors and NSAIDs) as the risk of ceasing these may outweigh the benefits, particularly the anticonvulsants.

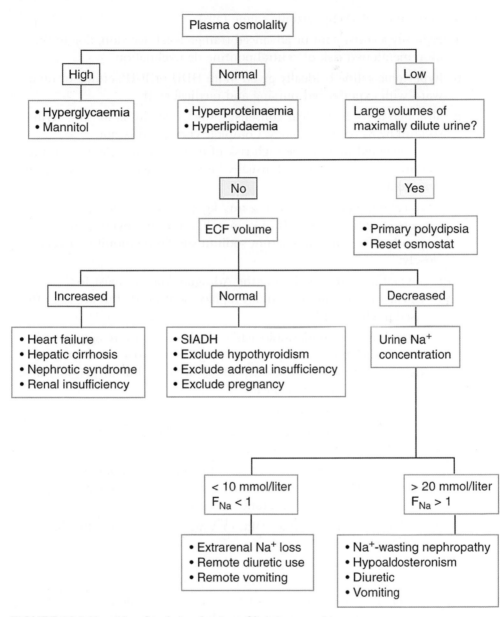

FIGURE 39.1 Algorithm for the evaluation of hyponatraemia.

Adapted from: Singer GG, 1998. Fluid and electrolyte management. In: Carey CF, Lee HH, Woeltje KF, eds. The Washington Manual of Medical Therapeutics, 29th ed. Philadelphia: Lippincott-Raven, p. 44.

2 Commencing an 800–1000 mL oral fluid restriction with a strict fluid balance:

  a note that, in some cases (e.g. haemorrhagic stroke), fluid restriction may not be appropriate.

3 Treatment of the underlying cause, if known (e.g. empirical antibiotics for meningitis or pneumonia).

4   Consideration of IV hypertonic saline (3%):

a   typically a consultant or advanced trainee level decision, due to the aforementioned risk of central pontine demyelination

b   hypertonic saline is ideally given in an HDU or ICU setting, or on a ward with experienced nursing and medical staff

c   although there is no clear consensus, the usual aim is to raise serum sodium by 8–10 mmol/L/day. Complete correction is not recommended (due to the high risk of over-correcting) with a serum sodium of 120–125 mmol/L usually being sufficient to prevent further symptoms

d   a typical regimen would be 1–2 mL/ kg 3% saline over 1 hour, expected to raise sodium by 1–2 mmol/L/hour, but every patient responds differently and serum sodium should be monitored very closely:

i   several formulas, including the Adrogue–Madias, exist for calculating a patient's sodium replacement needs but are not often used in clinical practice

ii   intensivists or endocrinologists may choose to more aggressively correct sodium (e.g. 3–4 mL/kg/day 3% saline over an hour) for patients with severe neurological disturbance, but this should **never** be initiated as a junior doctor.

5   Dietitian review re: high sodium diet.

6   Consideration of a loop diuretic (e.g. 20 mg IV frusemide) to increase water excretion and lower urine osmolality.

7   Consideration of urea (e.g. 10–40 g/day) to enhance osmotic diuresis and water excretion. Note that this concoction tastes pretty foul, and is poorly tolerated – try diluting it with orange juice.

8   Serial pathology slips for either UEC or VBG to closely monitor the changing electrolytes.

IV saline should be ceased immediately if the serum sodium rises >12 mmol/L in less than 24 hours. Vasopressin receptor antagonists (e.g. the V_2 receptor antagonist tolvaptan) do not yet see regular use in clinical practice when treating SIADH. Patients will often need to remain on their fluid restriction on discharge, be it on a more relaxed scale (e.g. 1200–1800 mL/day). They should be encouraged to remain on a high-sodium diet.

CHAPTER 40

NEUROLOGY

Joseph M O'Brien

Neurology is a beast of a rotation. Many people find neurology a challenging specialty, but there are fantastic learning opportunities available and it is often considered one of the 'essential' rotations in the lead-up to physician's exams. In larger hospitals, the Neurology team is often divided into 'General Neurology' and 'Stroke' due to the large volume of work for the latter. Key areas to review prior to your rotation include neuroanatomy, localisation of lesions and the acute stroke protocol for your hospital.

You will have the opportunity to perform many lumbar punctures (LP), hone your clinical examination skills and become proficient at interpreting neuroimaging. You will likely have a larger role to play in the management of outpatients in the Medical Day Unit (MDU) as you chart intravenous immunoglobulins (IV Ig), natalizumab and other infusions and review these patients if required.

Neuroradiology meetings are common, and in many cases it is the resident's responsibility to prepare the list for these weekly or fortnightly sessions. You will work closely with the Ophthalmology, Palliative Care, Allied Health and Rehabilitation teams. For information about outpatient management of patients with neurological illness, please refer to Chapter 61, 'Neurology outpatients'.

STROKE

The World Health Organization's definition of stroke is, 'Rapidly developing clinical signs of focal (at times global) disturbance of cerebral function, lasting more than 24 hours or leading to death with no apparent cause other than that of vascular origin'. Stroke may be broadly divided into ischaemic (80%) or haemorrhagic (20%), which in turn may be subarachnoid or intracerebral depending on the source of bleeding. The term 'cerebrovascular accident' is no longer encouraged, although the abbreviation CVA remains commonplace.

In an ischaemic stroke, blood supply to an area of brain parenchyma is cut off due to an embolic event (i.e. particles from elsewhere obstructing an artery), hypoperfusion or thrombosis (i.e. in situ arterial obstruction from atherosclerosis or dissection). Conversely, in haemorrhagic stroke rupture of a blood vessel results in bleeding within the cranial vault. This may be primary (i.e. spontaneous rupture) or secondary (i.e. due to malignancy, vascular deformity, coagulopathy, vasculitis, substance abuse or sepsis).

Risk factors for stroke include dyslipidaemia, hypertension, obesity (specifically waist to hip ratio), atrial fibrillation, diabetes, prior transient ischaemic attacks (TIA), smoking, sedentary lifestyle, depression, intravenous (IV) drug use, alcohol abuse, family history (especially relatives <55 years old), male gender and advanced age.

Stroke is a common presentation and the second leading cause of death in Australia with over 50,000 people suffering from a stroke per year. Stroke survivors also place significant burden on the healthcare system, requiring extensive periods of rehabilitation, modified equipment and potentially lifelong assistance with completing their activities of daily living (ADLs). In 2012, the estimated yearly cost of 'stroke' was estimated to be $5 billion in Australia alone. Annually, 15 million people endure strokes worldwide.

Diagnosis

Most patients will be able to tell you the classic presentation of a stroke, thanks to the successful public health campaign 'FAST' – facial droop, arm weakness, slurred speech and time sensitivity to treatment. The symptoms of ischaemic stroke may come on suddenly, or have a more insidious, slow progression depending on the size of the vessel occluded and the degree of blockage and collateral flow. Some of the most commonly found stroke syndromes include hemiplegia with or without signs of focal higher cerebral dysfunction (such as aphasia), visual field deficit, hemisensory loss or brainstem deficit. Loss of consciousness is rare. Some tips for localising strokes include the following:

- Embolic strokes and subarachnoid haemorrhages (SAH) due to an aneurysm tend to have a sudden onset, but aneurysmal SAH rarely has focal neurology.

- Fluctuant symptoms suggests thrombotic disease.

- Stepwise progression of symptoms suggests multiple small vascular events.

Examination findings are dependent on the arterial territory affected. As well as completing a thorough peripheral neurological and cranial nerve examination, assess the cardiovascular system (particularly noting body mass index, hypertension, irregular rhythm, carotid bruit, postural changes, altered heart sounds and peripheral oedema) and inspect for signs of hypercholesterolaemia (e.g. xanthelasma). Note the patient's level of consciousness, speech, presence of neglect and pupillary reaction. The clinical examination is vital in localising the stroke, especially where there will be a delay to neuroimaging.

An excellent resource for the documentation of stroke symptoms is the National Institutes of Health Stroke Scale (NIHSS), available freely online (as well as a tutorial for examining stroke patients). This is used in the clinical decision-making process and should be completed by someone at the registrar level. If you are on the Stroke Unit, consider keeping blank copies of this form with you.

Natural history

A transient ischaemic attack (TIA, known colloquially as a 'mini-stroke') is a temporary episode of arterial blockage that lasts <24 hours. The symptoms are the same as a stroke in that vascular area. The presence of neurological signs that are worsening classifies the stroke as a 'stroke in evolution' or 'progressing stroke'. Classically, anterior strokes have completed evolution by 24 hours and posterior strokes by 72 hours. Although not specific, typically ischaemic strokes and subarachnoid haemorrhages have a rapid onset and intracerebral haemorrhages slowly progress (as blood accumulates). Large strokes can result in death.

With ischaemic stroke, there is often an attempt to open anastomotic pathways and institute homeostatic measures to increase oxygenation of the affected territory after an occlusion has occurred. Symptoms of stroke tend to occur when post-lesion flow is <50% and revascularisation is time-sensitive to provide optimal recovery.

The pattern of symptoms seen with various territory infarcts is related to the underlying neuroanatomy, outlined briefly in Table 40.1. Ischaemic strokes may

TABLE 40.1 Stroke syndromes

STROKE SYNDROME	NOTES
Lacunar (NB: *lacune* means 'little lake')	• Refers to deep penetrating arteries surrounding the circle of Willis • Strongly associated with hypertension • Majority are purely motor, with hemiplegia on the contralateral side of the body to the lesion
Pontine (a.k.a. 'brainstem strokes')	• A medial pons lesion produces weakness and internuclear ophthalmoplegia • A lateral pons lesion produces sensory loss and cerebellar signs (e.g. gait disturbance and vertigo) • May exhibit symptoms from a particular cranial nerve, allowing further localisation • Severe pontine strokes may result in 'locked-in syndrome'
Watershed	• Occur in areas with poor vascular supply between cerebral artery territories • Proximal arm weakness with distal sparing and Broca's aphasia • Often due to hypotension • Divided into cortical zone or internal border zone

continued

TABLE 40.1 Stroke syndromes—cont'd

STROKE SYNDROME	NOTES
Cerebellar haemorrhage	• Headache, vomiting and gait disturbance • Strength and sensation usually normal • May have 6th nerve palsy
Anterior cerebral	• Presentations include contralateral hemiplegia (arm spared more than leg), apraxia and cortical sensory loss in the leg only • Frontal lobe findings such as incontinence, slow mentation, perseveration and grasp and suck reflexes may be present
Middle cerebral	• Contralateral hemiplegia, aphasia, facial weakness, lateral gaze weakness, facial sensory loss and sided neglect and ipsilateral gaze preference • Greater dysfunction in the arm and face than leg • Isolated superior MCA will have expressive aphasia (Broca's); isolated inferior MCA stroke will have receptive aphasia (Wernicke's)
Posterior cerebral	• Homonymous hemianopia (without motor paresis), prominent sensory loss, alexia (without agraphia), inability to name colours, visual agnosia, prosopagnosia (inability to recognise known faces) and recent memory loss

Adapted from: Canavan, M., McGrath, E. & O'Donnell, M., 2012. Chapter 147: Stroke. In: Hoffman, R., Benz, E.J., Silberstein, L.E., et al., Hematology: Basic Principles and Practice, 6th ed. Philadelphia: Saunders, pp. 2067-2075. Crocco, T.J. & Goldstein, J.N., 2014. Chapter 101: Stroke. In: Marx, J., Hockberger, R. & Walls, R., Rosen's Emergency Medicine, 8th ed. Philadelphia: Saunders, pp. 1363-1374. Harvey, R.L., Roth, E.J., Yu, D.T., et al., 2010. Chapter 50: Stroke syndromes. In: Braddom, R.L., ed. Physical Medicine and Rehabilitation, 4th ed. Philadelphia: Saunders, pp. 1177-1222.

undergo what is known as rebound haemorrhage or 'haemorrhagic conversion', classically at day 3. This is due to ischaemia of the vascular endothelium. Infarcted tissue swells slowly with mass effect becoming a possibility after 48 hours. Eventually, the infarct is reabsorbed and the patient is left with a well-demarcated, fluid-filled cavity evident on neuroimaging.

If haemorrhagic strokes are allowed to continue, the blood fills the space normally occupied by cerebrospinal fluid (CSF). A subarachnoid haemorrhage will quite quickly raise the intracranial pressure (ICP), resulting in coma or death if unrelenting.

Long-term complications of stroke depend on the area involved, and include dysarthria (inability to produce speech properly due to motor dysfunction), dysphasia (inability to produce speech clearly for another reason), dysphagia (altered swallow), persistent weakness (including hemiparesis in severe cases), incontinence, acalculia (inability to process numbers), agraphia (inability to write), cognitive impairment, visual changes, seizures, sleep disorder, complex pain syndrome, personality changes, pseudobulbar affect (i.e. sudden outbursts of crying or laughter) and depression.

Investigations

Stroke is most often diagnosed on clinical examination, but an urgent CT- or MRI-brain is essential for diagnosis and to measure the extent of infarction or bleeding. Blood work should also be sent urgently, with a full blood examination (FBE); urea, electrolytes and creatinine (UEC); calcium, magnesium and phosphate (CMP); liver function tests (LFT); coagulations studies; C-reactive protein (CRP); and blood sugar level (BSL). If the patient is of childbearing age (remembering any woman aged 10–60 years is pregnant until proven otherwise), request a beta-HCG, as tissue plasminogen activator (tPA) is teratogenic. In young patients (e.g. <35 years) you may consider a thrombophilia screen.

Fasting lipids and glucose (or alternatively HbA_{1c}) should be requested for the following morning. Depending on your history, you should also consider blood alcohol concentration (BAC), thyroid-stimulating hormone (TSH), arterial blood gases (ABG; to assess hypoxia) and a toxicology screen. If fever is present, order a urine microscopy/culture/sensitivities (M/C/S) and blood cultures.

An electrocardiogram (ECG) is essential to review for atrial fibrillation (AF) and concurrent cardiac ischaemia, a contraindication to thrombolysis. A chest X-ray (CXR) should be performed to exclude infection. Consideration should be given to a lumbar puncture (LP) if SAH remains a highly suspected diagnosis in the setting of clear CT-brain, as blood may be evident in the CSF (NB: LP prevents administration of tPA). If a CT-brain is clear at the time of diagnosis, consider escalating to a CT-brain perfusion study or even MRI-brain as in the acute phase (i.e. first 72 hours) an ischaemic stroke may be very difficult to identify.

A transthoracic echocardiogram (TTE) should be ordered to review for a left ventricular thrombus and atrial fibrillation, but does not need to be completed as an inpatient. Electroencephalography (EEG) may be indicated with ongoing seizures. Doppler ultrasound should be performed on both carotid arteries to review for atherosclerosis.

Management

If a person is suspected of having a stroke, quickly assess their 'ABC' (i.e. airway, breathing and circulation) and escalate their care if haemodynamically unstable. A typical plan for a patient with an ischaemic may read as follows:

1 Admission under General Medicine or Stroke team with regular medications and deep vein thrombosis (DVT) prophylaxis, ideally in a Stroke Unit:

a   discuss withholding warfarin in the setting of large strokes with your registrar or consultant.

2 Correction of hypoglycaemia, application of supplemental oxygen if hypoxic and treatment of fever with paracetamol (1 g IV up to QID).

3 Consideration of thrombolysis with administration of recombinant tissue plasminogen activator (tPA, a.k.a. alteplase) once haemorrhage has been excluded on CT-brain:

    a   this is a consultant-level decision; if you are in a rural or remote hospital, you may be able to teleconference to a neurologist for advice

    b   can only be used if it is <4.5 hours since the onset of symptoms

    c   patients must be consented to the risk of haemorrhagic conversion with permanent disability or death

    d   exclusion criteria include age >80 years, oral anticoagulant use (regardless of INR), coma, SBP >180 mmHg, septic emboli, advanced liver disease or right heart failure, platelets <100 × 10^9/L, hypoglycaemia and a past history of stroke in <3 months; relative contraindications include head trauma, AMI in past 3 months, resolving Sz or multi-lobar infarction (i.e. > ⅓ of the hemisphere)

    e   better outcomes are seen with younger patients, given tPA within 90 minutes, with mild to moderate neurological signs

    f   don't give antiplatelet agents *and* thrombolysis – withhold 24 hours.

4 Consideration of antiplatelet agents in those in whom thrombolysis is contraindicated, and in all patients within 48 hours:

    a   typical regimen would be aspirin 300 mg PO oral stat, or in the case of *true* aspirin allergy clopidogrel 75 mg PO stat.

5 Consideration of mechanical intervention (e.g. clot retrieval):

    a   currently available in a limited number of specialist centres across Australia, and should be discussed with the Stroke registrar; if you are in a rural centre, your consultant or the neurologist by teleconference may agree upon transfer for this intervention.

6 Monitoring of blood pressure, with a target of >160 mmHg but <220 mmHg. The BP targets can be a point of controversy and it is best to clarify with your Stroke Unit what is preferred:

    a   moderate hypertension may seem paradoxical, but it allows the brain to achieve the optimal cerebral perfusion pressure (CPP)

    b   if the patient is symptomatic or there are or signs of end-organ damage, consider treatment at a blood pressure <220 mmHg

    c   example agents include labetalol, hydralazine, esmolol, nicardipine and enalapril as these act quickly and have short half-lives.

7 Starting a lipid-lowering agent (e.g. atorvastatin 40 mg PO mane).

8 Regular neurological observations.

9 Request bilateral carotid Doppler ultrasound, TTE and fasting lipids and glucose.

10 Urgent referral to Speech Pathology, nil by mouth (NBM) in the meantime (with fluids as appropriate). In those with severe dysphagia as per the speech pathologist, consider dietitian referral for alternate nutrition.

11 Consideration of in dwelling catheter (IDC).

12 Consideration of an MRI-brain if the CT-brain is normal but infarction remains a highly likely diagnosis.

13 Urgent referral to Neurosurgery if intracranial pressure appears to be rising uncontrollably for consideration of craniotomy.

14 Optimisation of secondary risk factors (e.g. dyslipidaemia, hypertension, obesity and diabetes)

15 Avoid sedative agents as it makes measurement of the GCS difficult.

16 Counselling to quit smoking if necessary.

If the patient is in atrial fibrillation, they will require long-term anticoagulation (in the absence of contraindications) as their CHADS$_2$VASc score will be $\geq$2 if they have had a stroke. Similarly, anticoagulation will be required for 3–6 months if a thrombus is detected in the left ventricle on TTE. Referral to Vascular Surgery may be necessary if a large degree of carotid stenosis is detected on Doppler. Patients who have experienced a stroke should be referred to Neurological Rehabilitation as soon as possible.

The consultant may choose to add clopidogrel 75 mg PO daily to the patient's medication list, or to switch the patient to another form of antiplatelet agent called Asasantin SR. This is a combination pill containing 25 mg aspirin and 200 mg dipyridamole. It is taken PO BD, but may cause headache and gastrointestinal (GI) upset so is usually introduced as one tablet nocte with aspirin 100 mg PO mane for a week, then up-titrated with the mane aspirin ceased. The headache usually responds to paracetamol. The choice of clopidogrel vs Asasantin SR depends mostly on patient tolerance.

Haemorrhagic stroke patients should have ongoing neurological observations in a Stroke Unit with referral to Neurosurgery if necessary, monitoring of hypertension, reversal of anticoagulation and consideration of transfusion of pools of platelets or cryoprecipitate.

Patients should have ongoing monitoring for long-term complications with their GP after discharge. People who have had a stroke are at high risk of depression. Those started on anticoagulation should have this reviewed regularly.

MENINGITIS AND ENCEPHALITIS

Meningitis refers to inflammation or infection of the meninges, or the membranes surrounding the brain and spinal cord. Encephalitis implies acute inflammation of the brain itself. There is significant overlap in the way these two conditions

SECTION IV

present to the GP or Emergency Department, with the classic constellation of nuchal rigidity (neck stiffness), photophobia (light sensitivity), fever and headache seen in only ˜50% of patients.

Meningitis and encephalitis may be bacterial or viral. 'Aseptic meningitis' refers to disease where a causative pyogenic *bacterium* cannot be identified with cultures, despite clinical and biochemical evidence of meningeal irritation. It is often self-limiting. The most common bacterial pathogens are *Streptococcus pneumoniae* and *Neisseria meningitides* (known colloquially as 'Meningococcal'). *Listeria monocytogenes* meningitis is more likely in alcoholics, pregnant females and the immunosuppressed.

Atypically, patients may have meningitis due to *Cryptococcus* or Gram-negative bacilli (e.g. *Escherichia coli*, or *Klebsiella* or *Pseudomonas* species). In immuno-compromised patients, rarer infective agents such as *Tuberculosis* or fungi may be the causative organism. The most common viral pathogens are enteroviruses, herpes simplex virus (predominantly HSV-2), HIV and varicella zoster virus (VZV). In rare cases meningitis may result from *Mycobacterium*, fungi, malignancy or drugs.

Meningitis is uncommon in Australia, with approximately 650 cases reported annually. There are two peak incidences, in the neonatal group and in the 10–25 years age group. Older patients had a higher morbidity and mortality with a fatality rate of 3.4%.

Risk factors for bacterial meningitis include extremes of age, splenectomy (especially from encapsulated organisms), alcohol abuse, pregnancy, diabetes, immunocompromised, human immunodeficiency virus (HIV), neurosurgery and head trauma.

Diagnosis

Symptoms may include headache, lethargy, fever, rigors, nuchal rigidity, photophobia, phonophobia (sensitivity to sound), nausea, vomiting, rashes, confusion, seizures and irritability. In rare cases, patients may exhibit aphasia, hemiparesis or other focal neurology. These are typically of acute onset. Your history should cover preexisting infective illnesses (e.g. pneumonia, otitis, pharyngitis) as this may provide clues as to the causative organism. Travel, social, pharmaceutical and illicit drug histories are also very important.

Cerebral signs and symptoms can be used to differentiate encephalitis from meningitis, which should spare brain functions such as mental state, sensorimotor deficit or personality change. Note seizures may be caused by either meningitis or encephalitis. Elderly patients may present atypically. New psychiatric symptoms are more suggestive of encephalitis (particularly due to HSV) than meningitis.

Examination findings may be normal. Fever and tachycardia are common, with hypotension often signifying serious disease. Inspect the patient's whole body for new rash – a petechial rash has high specificity for *Neisseria* meningitis. Note the patient's Glasgow Coma Scale (GCS).

Two specific signs often noted by Emergency physicians include Kernig's sign and Brudzinski's sign. Kernig's sign is performed by flexing the hip and knee at 90°, with distal extension of the knee. Pain is a 'positive' Kernig's, and is indicative of meningism (i.e. irritation of the meninges), which can be due to meningitis or subarachnoid haemorrhage. Brudzinski's includes multiple eponymous signs of meningism, but the most frequently performed involves involuntary flexion of the hip when bringing a patient's head off the examining table when lying supine.

Natural history

Acute meningitis sets in over hours to days, and rarely recurs. Chronic meningitis lasts >4 weeks, with symptoms that often fluctuate. In a small percentage of patients, an abscess may form. For viral meningitis, the median time taken to resolution of symptoms is ⁻9.5 days regardless of intervention.

Despite prompt antimicrobial therapy, bacterial meningitis carries a high 30-day mortality that varies with causative agent (<5% for *Haemophilus influenzae* b, 10% with meningococcal and up to 20% in pneumococcal). People with bacterial meningitis may require admission to the Intensive Care Unit (ICU) for inotrope support, intubation and mechanical ventilation. Most viral meningitides are benign, with <1% having complications.

Several bacteria that can cause meningitis can be vaccinated against, including some strains of *Neisseria meningitides*, *Haemophilus influenzae* type B (Hib) and some strains of *Streptococcus pneumoniae*.

Long-term complications of bacterial meningitis include persistent neurological sequelae including altered behaviour, an acquired brain injury, visual loss, hearing impairment, difficulty concentrating, gait disturbance and epilepsy, headaches, permanent physical disability from septic emboli and fatigue.

Investigations

Due to its occasionally subtle presentation, clinicians must always keep the diagnosis of meningitis in mind with an undifferentiated patient with fever. Basic blood work should be sent; include an FBE, UEC, CMP, CRP, ESR, LFT, BSL, TSH and blood cultures. If there is not a clear source, also request a urine M/C/S and CXR. Obtaining a lactate on arterial or venous blood gases (ABG or VBG) may also be of benefit, as elevated lactate correlates with mortality.

The gold standard of diagnosis remains analysis of cerebrospinal fluid (CSF) obtained via lumbar puncture (LP). Contraindications for LP include anticoagulation, evidence of lumbar infection or skin lesion over the intended lumbar space, thrombocytopenia $<80 \times 10^9$/L and raised intracerebral pressure (ICP). The patient should be assessed clinically for indicators of potentially raised ICP, including a history of CNS disease, focal neurological signs, new seizures, papilloedema on fundoscopy, immunocompromise or altered conscious state. If not confident in your ability to assess these parameters, a CT-brain could be performed to exclude raised ICP prior to performing the LP.

Interpretation of LPs is covered in Chapter 13, 'Investigations: other'. The CSF request form should have adequate clinical history and ask for M/C/S, cytology, cell count, glucose, protein and, if viral meningitis is suspected, polymerase chain reaction (PCR) for at minimum HSV, VZV and enterovirus.

Management

Meningitis should be handled as a medical emergency due to its high mortality rate. Begin by assessing the patient's 'ABC', and escalate if unstable or if the patient has a significantly decreased GCS. Recall a patient cannot maintain their airway with a GCS <8.

Ideally, cerebrospinal fluid is obtained prior to commencing empirical antibiotics. However, if this is going to cause a delay of >30 minutes (e.g. a clearly very difficult LP), antibiotics will typically be commenced at the expense of 'raw' cultures. A typical plan for a patient with meningitis or encephalitis may include the following:

1   Admission under a General Medical or Neurology unit with their regular medications and DVT prophylaxis.

2   Urgent commencement of intravenous antibiotics:

  a   empirical antibiotics are 4 g IV ceftriaxone daily or 2 g IV BD

  b   if *Listeria* is suspected (due to pregnancy, alcohol abuse, immunocompromise, or age >50 years), consider adding benzypenicillin 2.4 g IV Q4H

  c   if Gram-positive diplococcic or *Staphylococcus*-resembling bacteria are seen on Gram stain, if otitis media is present or if the patient has recently had a course of beta-lactam antibiotics, add vancomycin 1.5 g IV BD (renally-adjusted if necessary)

  d   in the setting of penicillin allergy, replace ceftriaxone with vancomycin or 400 mg IV moxifloxacin daily.

3   Dexamethasone should be given as a 10 mg stat dose, *before or with the first dose of antibiotic*, then Q6H for 4 days.

4   Consider empirical antiviral cover (with acyclovir 10 mg/kg IV Q8H for 14–21 days with confirmed viral meningitis from VZV or HSV). This should be converted to ganciclovir (5 mg/kg IV BD for 14 days) if cytomegalovirus (CMV) is isolated on CSF.

5   If necessary, volume replacement with intravenous fluids and correction of electrolytes.

6   Regular neurological observations and consideration of the need for isolation room or High Dependency Unit (HDU).

7   Chasing the CSF report to narrow the antibiotic spectrum:

  a   *Listeria* – ampicillin 1 g IV QID for 21 days total, with gentamicin 6 mg/kg for the first 7 days

  b   *Neisseria meningitides* – ceftriaxone 2 g IV daily for 7 days c *Hib* – ceftriaxone 2 g IV daily for 10 days

   d *Streptococcus pneumoniae* – ceftriaxone 2 g IV daily for 2 weeks.

8 An early Infectious Diseases (ID) referral.

9 Contact tracing should be completed. Chemoprophylaxis for close contacts (determined by ID) for both *Neisseria* and Hib is often rifampicin 600 mg PO BD for 2 days.

10 If an abscess is detected on neuroimaging, urgent Neurosurgery referral.

The spectrum of antibiotics should be narrowed when possible. Repeating the LP is not routine, but may be indicated if there is no improvement after 48 hours treatment, or if fever persists for >8 days without an alternative cause. Patients should be followed up closely by their GP.

EPILEPSY

Epilepsy refers to a heterogeneous group of illnesses that result in long-term predisposition to unprovoked, recurrent seizures. Not all patients who have a seizure are epileptic. Status epilepticus refers to a seizure disorder where a patient either seizes for >5 minutes *or* has two seizures without complete resolution of symptoms between them. Epilepsy is a consequence of hypersensitive neuronal pathways in the cerebral cortex.

Types of seizures include generalised (involving multiple brain regions) or focal (a.k.a. partial, arising from a particular cerebral region). The most commonly used classification is that of the International League Against Epilepsy, a pictorial summary of which can be found in Fig. 40.1.

Absence seizures refer to those where a patient is 'spaced out', often staring *absently*. In old terminology, these were referred to as 'petit mal'. 'Grand mal' refers

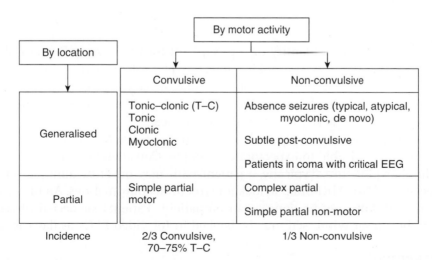

FIGURE 40.1 Classification of seizure type.

Mercadé Cerdá, J.M., Toledo Argani, M., Mauri Llerda, J.A., et al., 2016. The Spanish Neurological Society official clinical practice guidelines in epilepsy. Neurologia 31(2), 121-129.

to tonic–clonic seizures, so named because they have a tonic phase (with muscular rigidity) and a clonic phase (rhythmic jerking of muscles). Simple partial seizures involve no loss of consciousness, whereas patients with complex partial seizures do have altered level of consciousness.

Some patients experience an 'aura' or warning sign, which may manifest as an uncertain feeling, nausea, altered cognition, light-headedness, presyncope or unusual smell, taste, sound or visual changes. Post-ictal (i.e. post-seizure) symptoms include persistent headache, short-term memory loss, disorientation, myalgia (often described as feeling like they've run a marathon), weakness and incontinence. Patients may have injuries from their seizure, either inflicted by their environment or due to tongue-biting.

Risk factors include head trauma, intracranial malignancy, stroke, toxin exposure, meningitis or encephalitis, systemic infections (including HIV, TB and malaria), autoimmune diseases in their activation phase, metabolic dysfunction and family history.

Precipitating factors for seizures in a known epileptic include sleep disturbance, stress, alcohol withdrawal, infection, malignancy, metabolic diseases, hypo- or hyperglycaemia, electrolyte imbalance and autoimmune crises.

Epilepsy is a very common neurological disorder with 3% of people being diagnosed at some stage in their life, and seizures are a frequent referral for the Neurology team.

Diagnosis

The history and examination findings expected in epilepsy are outlined in Chapter 61, 'Neurology outpatients'. If reviewing a patient with epilepsy in the acute setting, look for signs of injury from previous seizures, incontinence, tongue-biting and potential triggers for their seizure.

Investigations

Investigations focus on identifying a precipitant for the seizure. Request bloods, including FBE, UEC + CMP (looking for electrolyte disturbance), LFTs (alcohol abuse), inflammatory markers and blood alcohol level. Consider a toxin screen. If the patient is on an anti-epileptic drug (AED), request serum levels (phenytoin, levetiracetam or valproate) to establish compliance.

If the patient is febrile request blood cultures, a urine M/C/S and a CXR with a sputum M/C/S if able to expectorate a sample. Consideration should be given for a lumbar puncture. Typically, a patient with new onset of multiple seizures will receive a CT- or MRI-brain to look for structural abnormalities. An EEG should be requested, but may be done as an outpatient. Patients suspected of having seizures but never witnessed may be booked in for video EEGs as day cases.

Management

Patients with epilepsy require careful monitoring. Status epilepticus is an emergency, with patients often unable to maintain their airway. When reviewing a patient who has had a seizure, always begin with ABC and escalate if necessary.

If a patient is having a seizure, remove obstacles from around them and ensure their airway is secure. Administer lorazepam (2–4 mg IV) as soon as possible, repeated at 5–10 minutes if still seizing. Consider escalating to a levetiracetam or phenytoin loading dose. If a patient is post-ictal, consider special nursing and neurological observations.

If a patient is experiencing status epilepticus, call for help. Secure the airway, apply oxygen, obtain IV access and simultaneously send bloods (including BSL) and administer further AEDs. The patient should be reviewed by ICU staff. Give dextrose if necessary. Consider phenytoin loading the patient with 1 g IV phenytoin, but note this cannot be given quicker than 50 mg/min due to cardiac side effects.

Not all patients presenting with seizures require ongoing drug therapy. A consultant will decide whether or not a patient requires on going anti-epileptics. Common choices include valproate 10–60 mg/kg PO daily given in divided doses if >250 mg, phenytoin 4–6 mg/kg PO daily given BD, levetiracetam 500 mg PO BD, carbamazepine 100 mg PO BD or topiramate 50 mg PO BD. Absence seizures may be managed with ethosuximide 500 mg PO daily. Carbamazepine is a common choice for partial seizures.

Patients should be linked in with a neurologist, if they do not already have one. If this is their first presentation, many hospitals have dedicated First Seizure Clinics they may be referred to. It is rare that a patient will get their EEG as an inpatient, so ensure this referral has been received and a booking made.

Patients should be informed that they may continue to have minor seizures at home, and typically only need to represent if they are having multiple seizures per day, not recovering between seizures or also having fevers or persistent neurological symptoms.

Patients commenced on anti-epileptics will need a follow-up FBE, UEC and LFT to monitor for side effects in 1–2 weeks. Patient education is vital, explaining the likely course of their illness. Advise them not to have baths, swim alone, walk on roofs or participate in activities that would otherwise place themselves or others at risk (e.g. operating machinery).

Remember to remind patients that they cannot drive for a period of time, as outlined by your state's guidelines. Lastly, it is **vital** to warn patients commencing lamotrigine or carbamazepine to beware a rash (potentially an early sign of the deadly skin condition Stevens–Johnson syndrome) and to contact the Neurology registrar or present to ED urgently.

MIGRAINES

Migraines are covered extensively in Chapter 61, 'Neurology Outpatients'. This section outlines only the management of refractory migraine that cannot be managed as an outpatient or in the short stay section of the Emergency Department.

then 40 mg PO daily for a further 5 days) and antiviral therapy with acyclovir (400 mg PO five times daily for 7 days) or valaciclovir (500 mg PO daily for 7 days). Patients without contraindication should have regular simple analgesia with paracetamol and NSAIDs.

As patients are often unable to close their eye properly, provide them with artificial lubrication for their affected side and tape their eyelid shut with a patch over the top (especially nocte) to prevent corneal irritation and ulceration. Surgical referral for transmastoid decompression of segments of the facial nerve is rarely warranted. Referral for rehabilitation with physical therapy and consideration of injection of botulinum toxin should be considered on a case-by-case basis.

There is no need for specialist follow-up of Bell's palsy in clinic, unless an alternate diagnosis remains considered. Follow-up with the patient's GP at the end of their course of steroids and antivirals is appropriate, with repeat bloods to review liver function, FBE and blood sugars.

MYASTHENIA GRAVIS

Myasthenia gravis (MG) is an autoimmune disorder of the neuromuscular junction characterised by myasthenia (i.e. muscular weakness) and fatigability of skeletal muscles. Antibodies are produced against either the acetylcholine receptor (AChR; present in 80–90% of patients) or muscle-specific kinase (MuSK), although both ultimately reduce postsynaptic activity. 10% of patients are seronegative for both MuSK and AChR.

Risk factors include concurrent autoimmune disease (e.g. rheumatoid or scleroderma), female gender and the genes HLA-88 and DR$_3$. There is an association with thymus hyperplasia (60–80%) and thymoma (15%). Myasthenia gravis is not uncommon, affecting 1.4 in 10,000 Australians.

Diagnosis

The classic history of a patient with MG is a person experiencing fluctuant muscle weakness around the eyes, limbs and chest wall that improves with rest, and is exacerbated by movement. Patients may initially report diplopia (double vision), ptosis (droopy eyelids) or bulbar muscle weakness (manifest as dysphagia, dysarthria and fatigable mastication), but as the disease advances any skeletal muscles may be affected. The distribution of weakness varies and is often described as being worst in the afternoon or evening, and may be aggravated by infection, anxiety or menstruation.

Proximal myopathy is more frequently encountered than distal. It is an emergency if the patient's *respiratory muscles* are involved, particularly if they report dysphagia, and an urgent referral to ICU should be made. Take a complete medical, past, social and family history.

Examination often demonstrates a patient with ptosis and reproducible weakness of skeletal muscles. A visual examination and inspection of the ocular cranial nerves should be completed to review for diplopia, obvious ocular weakness or other abnormality. Interrogate upward gaze for 2 minutes. Auscultate the chest, as patients with respiratory muscle involvement are predisposed to pneumonia. Percuss the chest and examine for a mediastinal mass, potentially indicating a thymoma. Note muscle atrophy or fasciculation, dysarthria, facial tics or altered swallow. Reflexes are typically normal.

Natural history

Subtypes of myasthenia gravis exist, including ocular (i.e. only affecting ocular muscles and unlikely to progress if stable for ≥2 years) and generalised MG with AChR antibodies, MuSK antibodies or neither AChR nor MuSK antibodies. The association with thymoma is strong enough to warrant screening in new diagnoses.

Initially patients may experience days to weeklong periods of time symptom-free, but typically 'flares' intensify in frequency and disability with a peak progression within 5–7 years of onset. MG can be thought of in three phases – an active phase, with the peak severity of symptoms; a stable phase, with possible resolution of symptoms and subsequent tapering of medications; and a third phase marked by either remission without immunosuppressant therapy, or relapse.

A myasthenia crisis is a medical emergency that occurs in 10–20% of patients with MG, where the patient's level of weakness involves the oropharyngeal muscles and necessitates intubation to maintain their airway. This may be the first presentation of MG in some people and is commonly triggered by infection, surgery, pregnancy or tapering of medications.

Investigations

The diagnosis of myasthenia gravis is confirmed by the presence of antibodies against acetylcholine receptors (AChR-Ab) or muscle-specific kinase (MuSK-Ab). Patients should also have a baseline FBE, UEC, CMP, LFT, CRP and ESR. Consider anti-striated muscle antibody (anti-SM) for thymoma screening and a rheumatological screen for concurrent autoimmune disease (e.g. TSH for thyroid, HbA_{1c} for diabetes, anti-CCP for rheumatoid arthritis etc). If the patient is febrile, perform a CXR and get cultures of blood, urine and sputum to look for an infective source and potential trigger.

An electromyogram (EMG) of the facial muscles should also ideally be obtained at the time of diagnosis. If clinical history is provided, the Neurology Lab will provide repetitive nerve stimulation (RNS) and single fibre studies. RNS often shows a decremental response >10%, and single fibre studies may show 'jitter' or variability in time between action potentials.

Request a CT- or MRI-brain if there is an unclear diagnosis and stroke or malignancy remain potential diagnoses. If a mediastinal mass is suspected clinically or seen on CXR, request a CT-chest simultaneously. Respiratory function tests (RFTs) should be requested if the patient is experiencing difficulty breathing.

Lastly, a bedside test called the 'Tensilon' (or edrophonium) test may be performed if a patient has symptoms obvious enough to observe potential improvement. Patients are given 2 mg of a fast-acting, short-duration ACh inhibitor called edrophonium, and the prolonged presence of ACh in the neuromuscular junction *should* rapidly demonstrate improved strength in affected muscles. This test can be repeated to a maximum of 10 mg, with the most frequent response seen between 4 and 6 mg. Risks include exacerbation of asthma, COPD and cardiac disease and as such these are relative contraindications. Atropine should be drawn up (0.4–0.6 mg) ready to administer if severe side effects occur.

Management

If a patient with MG shows signs of respiratory distress, rapidly assess their ABC and escalate as required. The emergency care of a myasthenic crisis involves intubation to maintain their airway, transfer to ICU, treatment of the underlying precipitant and high-dose steroids. Consideration of plasmapheresis or intravenous immunoglobulin (IVIG) should be given. In an otherwise well patient with MG, a plan template may include the following:

1 Admission under General Medicine or Neurology with regular medications and DVT prophylaxis.

2 Trial of pyridostigmine (30–60 mg four to five times daily) after confirmation of AChR antibodies.

3 ICU referral if respiratory function appears compromised:

a consideration of plasmapheresis.

4 Addition of prednisolone if symptoms break through pyridostigmine, with escalation to azathioprine, cyclosporine or mycophenolate as guided by your consultant.

5 If failing oral medical therapy, consideration of IVIG.

6 Speech Pathology review for swallow safety.

7 If respiratory function is a concern, serial peak flows.

8 If a thymoid tumour has been detected, referral to Thoracic Surgery for thymectomy, with consideration of radiotherapy by Radiation Oncology.

9 Outpatient optometrist referral for ocular MG.

10 Opportunistic vaccinations with influenza and pneumococcal vaccines.

Patients should be followed up regularly by both a neurologist and their GP. If an immunomodulator has been started the patient should have monitoring for side effects as required.

GUILLAIN–BARRÉ SYNDROME

Guillain–Barré syndrome (GBS) is a term applied to a group of immune-mediated, predominantly motor polyneuropathies. The classic description of GBS is an acute, progressive, symmetrical myasthenia with significant hyporeflexia that follows an acute infective illness. Risk factors include advanced age, male gender, recent surgery/trauma, bone marrow transplantation and lymphoma.

GBS is relatively uncommon, with an incidence of 2–8 per 100,000 people in Australia.

The pathophysiology remains poorly understood, but is believed to be due to immune-mediated damage to the myelin of peripheral nerves triggered by bacterial or viral infection. Antecedent infections may be reported 1–4 weeks prior to onset of neurological symptoms. *Campylobacter jejuni* is the most common, but other provocative agents include HIV, influenza, CMV, EBV, *Mycoplasma pneumoniae* and, more rarely, *E. coli, Haemophilus influenzae*, hepatitis C, varicella zoster and HSV.

Diagnosis

The presentation of GBS can be variable, but common features include a symmetrical, progressive weakness with hyporeflexia that usually (but not always) starts in the lower limbs and 'ascends' to affect higher myotomes. Dyspnoea, tachypnoea, hypoxia or chest wall weakness are signs the patient may need mechanical ventilation and these people should be reviewed by ICU urgently.

Ask about dysphasia, dysphagia, lumbar pain, paraesthesia, postural dizziness, altered bowel habit, incontinence, diplopia, the speed with which symptoms set in and palpitations. Rarely, some patients present purely with autonomic symptoms.

GBS is often preceded by infection, and your history should cover common antecedent causes (e.g. diarrhoea for *Campylobacter*). Take a complete medical, family, social and travel history. Exposure to toxins such as heavy metals, aerosolised paints and vapours may mimic GBS. Sensory symptoms without motor involvement makes GBS unlikely.

Examination is variable, but commonly demonstrates hyporeflexia (with reflexes often completely absent), ataxia, bilateral muscle weakness ('flaccid paralysis'), altered sensation and facial paralysis. There may be some signs of autonomic dysfunction (dysrhythmia, postural hypotension, urinary retention). Auscultate the chest for signs of infection. Monitor the vitals carefully. Perform bedside measurement of FEV_1.

Natural history

GBS is an acute disease, with maximal symptoms reached by 4 weeks. Subtypes of GBS exist, including acute inflammatory demyelinating polyradiculoneuropathy (AIDP; the most common), Miller Fisher syndrome (MFS), acute motor axonal neuropathy (AMAN) and acute sensorimotor axonal neuropathy (AMSAN).

Patients with GBS are hospitalised for an average of 1 week with ˜25% requiring mechanical ventilation for airway support. The majority of patients recover completely, however one-fifth of patients have persistent neurological symptoms, with 10% of all GBS patients left with serious disability. Despite maximal medical therapy mortality remains at ˜3%, with higher mortality seen amongst the elderly and those with rapid-onset or severe symptoms. AIDP has a chronic equivalent known as chronic inflammatory demyelinating polyneuropathy (CIDP).

Long-term complications of GBS include permanent disability, dyspnoea and predilection to respiratory infection, paraesthesia, autonomic dysfunction (orthostasis, dysrhythmia, altered bowel motility, incontinence) and complex pain syndromes. Patients who are bedbound are at higher risk of venous thromboembolic events (VTE). Unfortunately, up to 10% of patients experience a relapse of the disease.

Investigations

Patients with suspected GBS should be reviewed promptly with urgent blood work requested including FBE, UEC, CMP, LFT, TSH and inflammatory markers (CRP and ESR). Although not routinely requested, consider investigating heavy metals, serum protein electrophoresis (SPEP), serum immunoglobulins (as IgA deficient patients cannot have IVIG), HIV, Quantiferon Gold (QFG) and creatine kinase (CK; to exclude rhabdomyolysis) if there is a history of exposure or risk factors.

Specific antibodies against different glycolipids in the nerve exist and are related to different GBS subtypes, including anti-GQ1b, anti-GT1a, anti-CD1b, anti-GM1, anti-GD1a, anti-GalNac-GD1a and anti-GD1b. These are not ordered routinely due to their expense and unclear interpretation in the clinical setting.

If the patient is febrile, request a urine M/C/S, CXR and serial blood cultures. If the patient has diarrhoea, consider a faecal M/C/S (noting ?*Campylobacter* in the clinical history). All patients with suspected GBS should also have a lumbar puncture reviewed for elevated protein and mononuclear leucocytes. If suspected clinically, consider also requesting HSV, enterovirus and/or VZV PCR on the CSF. Note that CSF may appear normal in the first 7–14 days of disease.

Nerve conduction studies (NCS) should also be requested. These may also be normal in the acute phase of GBS. Typical findings include prolonged H-reflexes (absent in severe disease), increased distal latency, conduction delay or block, prolonged F-waves and temporal dispersion in multiple nerves. Rarely, a nerve biopsy may be required to provide the diagnosis. Nerve biopsy would be expected to demonstrate demyelination in segments with axonal loss and T-lymphocyte infiltration.

Neuroimaging should be considered with either CT- or MRI-brain. MRI is preferred and may show nerve root thickening and enhancement. Contrast should be used with either modality if renal function and allergies are non-prohibitive. An ECG should be requested to review for dysrhythmia.

Management

GBS with respiratory involvement is a medical emergency. Begin by assessing every patient's 'ABC'. If airway or breathing is compromised, immediately escalate care and refer to ICU for consideration of intubation and mechanical ventilation. 25–30% of patients will need respiratory support. If your patient is stable, a typical plan for admission may include the following:

1 Admission under Neurology or General Medicine with regular medications and DVT mechanical and chemical prophylaxis.

2 Chasing nerve conduction studies, if not formally reported (often access to this service is quite delayed).

3 Administration of IVIG at 0.4 mg/kg/day IV for 5 days (if IgA levels are normal).

4 Alternatively, plasmapheresis may be performed with best response if started within 7 days of symptom onset.

5 Close monitoring of respiratory function with serial peak flow measurement:

   a indications for referral for mechanical ventilation include a patient unable to clear sputum, aspiration, a quickly decreasing vital capacity, an FVC <15 mL/kg or hypoxia on VBG/ABG.

6 If paralysis is severe, nursing care should include frequent positional changes and standard pressure sore prevention measures.

7 Maintenance of fluid balance and optimisation of electrolytes.

8 Postural blood pressures BD (if patient can tolerate), consider withholding antihypertensives.

9 Consideration of telemetry, if dysrhythmia is detected on ECG.

10 Consideration of gabapentin or low-dose tricyclic antidepressants for neuropathic pain.

11 Antiemetics and simple analgesia PRN.

12 Full Allied Health assessment from physiotherapy, OT and social work and speech pathology if dysphasia or dysphagia present.

Patients with GBS should receive an early referral to Rehabilitation, especially if they required admission to ICU. Elements of autonomic dysfunction should be managed as appropriate. Repeating NCS after a few days to weeks may help determine the subtype of GBS. If persistent chest wall dysfunction is suspected, consider outpatient respiratory function tests. It is advised that patients avoid immunisation for 1 year after GBS unless essential. People who have had GBS as an inpatient should be reviewed by the GP within 1 week after discharge and should ideally see their admitting specialist within 2–4 weeks.

CHAPTER 41

INFECTIOUS DISEASES

Joseph M O'Brien

Infectious Diseases (ID) is not a rotation many junior doctors will have the fortune to complete. Few jobs exist for interns and residents and, when ID is available, it often comes paired with another specialty. Infectious Diseases is a rotation that complements all future careers, being of particular use to those considering a career in physician's training as no medical registrar can function without a solid understanding of microorganisms and their antimicrobial management.

Infectious Diseases is a broad specialty, and it would be apt to write an entire textbook on ID alone (in fact, many people have!). This chapter aims to give junior doctors a solid foundation for some common scenarios and a guide for more difficult cases.

In most hospitals, Infectious Diseases is a largely consult-based service. In addition to any inpatients, you and your team will likely complete several specific rounds including your standard consults, antimicrobial stewardship rounds (where you get to politely rouse on everyone using antibiotics inappropriately!) and transplant patient consults. Another great learning opportunity on ID rotations is the 'microbiology round', where the microbiologist of the week teaches using interesting recent pathology and discusses difficult cases with their peers.

Clinics will play a large role in your job as an ID resident. These may be subdivided into classes of disease (e.g. Hepatitis Clinic covering all viral causes of liver inflammation), disease-specific (e.g. HIV or Tuberculosis Clinics) or Travel Medicine (both preparing travellers for their trips and investigating fever in the returned traveller). Consultants and registrars also attend these clinics and, due to the specialist nature of their content, it is best to always run your opinion by a senior before making management decisions or discharging the patient.

TRAVEL MEDICINE AND FEVER IN THE RETURNED TRAVELLER

A very common problem for the medical registrar (or admitting resident) is determining the source of fever in the returned traveller. As globalisation continues and people have access to more remote locations, the variety of presentations continues to increase requiring doctors to have an improved understanding of exotic organisms.

Many patients take greater risks while travelling, with trauma being the most common cause of presentation. The majority of people will seek medical attention within 1 month of travel. While not truly exhaustive, consider asking about the following factors when taking a history from this patient cohort:

- Where did you travel to, and on what exact dates? Who travelled with you? Did you have any stopovers and, if so, what did you do while you were there?

- Did you have any symptoms while travelling? How long after returning home did they begin?

- Have you had diarrhoea, respiratory symptoms, fevers, weight loss, rigors or arthralgias? Were you in any accidents? Take a systematic history based on their response.

- Did anyone who travelled with you develop the same issues? Has anyone at your current residence?

- What style of accommodation did you stay in (e.g. tent or 5-star hotel)? What was the purpose of your journey (e.g. business, volunteering, pleasure)?

- What did you do while travelling? What type of environment were you in (e.g. jungle, desert)? Did you travel by plane, boat, car or elephant? Did you scuba dive, visit schools or orphanages, hike, travel to high altitude or swim (specifically in rivers, sea or still water)? Were you bitten by or did you have close contact with any insects or other animals? Where did you source your drinking water? What kind of food did you eat (note in particular meat, seafood, dairy products and foods with high water content [e.g. salads])?

- Did you see a travel doctor prior to going overseas? Did you require any immunisations or prophylactic medications? Less than 50% of patients in a USA study had seen a doctor prior to travelling to developing countries.

- If in a malaria-endemic region, did you use insect nets at night or wear insect repellent?

- What is your complete medical and past history? Are you on regular medications? Are there any conditions that run in the family? Did you require any treatment overseas (e.g. requiring injection or surgery)? If female, were you pregnant at the time of travel?

- Do (or did) you smoke tobacco or other drugs? How much alcohol did you drink? Did you use intravenous (IV) drugs? If working overseas, were there any occupational exposures? Did you get any new tattoos or have acupuncture?

- *If appropriate rapport has been established*: did you have sexual intercourse with other people overseas? Were they male, female or both?

SECTION IV

BOX 41.1 Remembering the risk factors in returned travellers

ID-FOOLS
Immunocompromise
Drugs (both prescribed and recreational)
Food
Overseas and remote travel
Occupational exposures
'**L**overs'
Sick 'contacts', including people, animals, environment, water etc
Source: Acronym supplied by Dr Kerry Jewell, MBBS, BMedSc.

> Did you use a barrier method of contraception? Do you know which country your partner was from? Has there been any dysuria, frequency, haematuria, discharge, pruritus or skin changes?

Note the mnemonic in Box 41.1 that will help you remember the risk factors in returned travellers.

The most common presenting issues are diarrhoea, respiratory symptoms (cough and dyspnoea), fever and skin conditions. If reviewing this type of patient, remember to perform a very thorough physical examination taking note of the patient's general appearance (pallor, jaundice, cachexia), vitals and temperature, lymphadenopathy, hepatosplenomegaly, dermatological conditions and altered heart sounds or changes in the lung fields. Examine the genitalia if indicated by the history (not routine). If PR bleeding is occurring, consider a digital rectal examination (DRE). Remember, people who have just been overseas can coincidentally present with non-infective disease (e.g. inflammatory bowel disease)!

If the patient is well, no investigations may be necessary. However, if the illness is prolonged, affecting the patient's ADLs or causing confusion, lethargy, hypotension, focal neurology, significant discomfort, pain or fever, strongly consider sending pathology and requesting imaging. A good starting point would include FBE, UEC, CMP, LFT, inflammatory markers (CRP ± ESR), beta-HCG in women 10–60 years old and blood cultures if febrile. If the patient has been in a tropical area, consider thick and thin films for malaria or dengue 'NS1'. Dependent on history, also consider human immunodeficiency virus (HIV), hepatitis (A, B, C and, if travelling in endemic regions, E), Epstein-Barr virus (EBV) and cytomegalovirus (CMV) serology.

If there are urinary symptoms or a fever, ask for a urine microscopy/culture/sensitivities (M/C/S). If the patient has respiratory symptoms, request a CXR, nasopharyngeal airway (NPA) swab for respiratory multiplex PCR and a (preferably early morning) sputum M/C/S with consideration of atypical culture, silver stain (for fungi and *Pneumocystis jirovecii*) and Ziel-Nielssen stain (for tuberculosis). Consider a stool M/C/S with *Clostridium difficile* toxin (CDT) if on antibiotics and ova, cysts and parasites (OCP) as guided by history.

If seen in clinic, discuss admitting unwell patients with the consultant. Patients should be re-booked within an appropriate time to follow-up on the results of the investigations requested, and a plan should be in place for any critical results (e.g. a planned admission if malarial thick and thin films are positive). Review Chapter 20, 'Notifiable diseases', to see if a positive result requires reporting to the Health Department in your state.

Resources for Travel Medicine include the Centers for Disease Control (which, although American, provides current information about worldwide disease outbreaks and patterns), GeoSentinel (a global surveillance network established by the International Society of Travel Medicine to monitor patterns of illness) and the Victorian Government's 'Blue Book' guidelines for infectious diseases. Additionally, Massachusetts General Hospital has developed a website where you can input the patient's age and destinations to generate a suggested list of vaccinations and potential exposures (http://gten.travel/trhip/trhip).

The most common cause of fever in a returned traveller is viral upper respiratory tract infections, and the most common cause of traveller's diarrhoea is enterotoxigenic *Escherichia coli*.

IMMUNISATIONS

Questions about immunisations are very common on ID, and some hospitals even run specialised Immunisations Clinics. The childhood and young adult immunisation schedule for Australia is reproduced in Fig. 41.1. It is quite likely you had to memorise this for your Paediatrics term!

More relevant to the junior doctor working in adult medicine, recommendations for adults include the following:

- Patients in high-risk groups (including those with chronic illness, Indigenous Australians, Torres Strait Islanders and immunosuppressed patients) should receive influenza vaccine (Fluvax®) annually and the 23-valent pneumococcal vaccine (Pneumovax 23®) every 5 years.

- Hepatitis A vaccination should be given to Indigenous Australian and Torres Strait Islander children living in high-risk areas (Queensland, Northern Territory, Western Australia and South Australia).

- Human papillomavirus (HPV) vaccination is currently recommended for all adolescents aged 12–13 years.

- Groups such as childcare workers, healthcare workers and those working in public health should consider having the annual influenza vaccine.

Prevention is the best cure, but you will still encounter patients throughout your clinical practice who do not believe in the efficacy, safety or necessity of vaccination. When interacting with these people, remember to maintain your cool demeanour, respect their right to their autonomous opinion and calmly and rationally explain the rationale behind vaccinations. Many people will be convinced of the value in vaccination after a conversation where they are allowed to express their concerns, and are not readily dismissed.

SECTION IV

Child programs	
Age	**Vaccine**
Birth	• Hepatitis B (hepB)
2 months	• Hepatitis B, diphtheria, tetanus, acellular pertussis (whooping cough), *Haemophilus influenzae* type b, inactivated poliomyelitis (polio) (hepB-DTPa-Hib-IPV) • Pneumococcal conjugate (13vPCV) • Rotavirus
4 months	• Hepatitis B, diphtheria, tetanus, acellular pertussis (whooping cough), *Haemophilus influenzae* type b, inactivated poliomyelitis (polio) (hepB-DTPa-Hib-IPV) • Pneumococcal conjugate (13vPCV) • Rotavirus
6 months	• Hepatitis B, diphtheria, tetanus, acellular pertussis (whooping cough), *Haemophilus influenzae* type b, inactivated poliomyelitis (polio) (hepB-DTPa-Hib-IPV) • Pneumococcal conjugate (13vPCV) • Rotavirus
12 months	• *Haemophilus influenzae* type b and Meningococcal C (Hib-MenC) • Measles, mumps and rubella (MMR)
18 months	• Measles, mumps, rubella and varicella (chickenpox) (MMRV)
4 years	• Diphtheria, tetanus, acellular pertussis (whooping cough) and inactivated poliomyelitis (polio) (DTPa-IPV) • Measles, mumps and rubella (MMR) (to be given only if MMRV vaccine was not given at 18 months)
School programs	
10–15 years (contact your State or Territory Health Department for details)	• Hepatitis B (hepB) • Varicella (chickenpox) • Human papillomavirus (HPV) • Diphtheria, tetanus and acellular pertussis (whooping cough) (dTpa)

FIGURE 41.1 Australian childhood and young adult immunisation schedule.

© 2016 Commonwealth of Australia as represented by the Department of Health.

INFECTION CONTROL

Infection control refers to the prevention of nosocomial (i.e. hospital-contracted) infection via application of epidemiological principles. A common issue of contention between medical and nursing staff is the proper conduction of isolation and infection control measures. Doctors are notoriously bad at complying with certain infection control measures (e.g. in one large trial observational study 7.6% of doctors completed hand hygiene as per policy), and junior doctors are often unsure when to isolate patients and when these barriers can be removed.

The following section is intended as a guide, based on recommendations made by the National Health and Medical Research Council (NHMRC). You should also refer to your hospital network's specific policy on isolation and infection control techniques.

- There are various levels of isolation – standard precautions, contact precautions, droplet precautions, airborne precautions and isolation for immunocompromise.

- Standard precautions involve the basics of routine hand hygiene (the 'five moments' being before touching a patient, before a procedure, after a procedure or exposure risk, after touching the patient and after touching the patient's surroundings), with soap and water used for visibly soiled hands or those exposed to *Clostridium difficile* or norovirus, personal protective equipment (gloves, gowns, goggles, mask) when appropriate, sterile gloves for aseptic procedures, safe handling of sharps with appropriate disposal, routine environmental cleaning and specific decontamination after exposure to bodily fluids.

- Contact precautions incorporate the above principles and add wearing gloves and a gown before entering the patient environment, and using patient-specific equipment (e.g. a stethoscope confined to that patient's room until cleaned). Examples of patients requiring contact precautions include those with multi-resistant *Staphylococcus aureus* (MRSA) or suspected infective diarrhoea. Ideally, the patient is placed in a single room or, in the setting of MRSA infection, a room with other patients confirmed to be MRSA colonised.

- Droplet precautions aim to prevent transmission of secretions from the respiratory tract and involve wearing a mask, goggles if 'splash-back' is likely and a single room. The patient should wear a mask when being moved through hallways and the door should be closed when possible. Examples of patients requiring droplet precautions include those with rubella, *Neisseria meningitidis, Bordetella pertussis,* influenza, adenovirus, *Haemophilus influenzae type b* and *Mycoplasma pneumoniae.*

- Airborne precautions involve the use of properly-fitted P2 respirators and negative-pressure rooms. Examples include patients with measles, active respiratory tuberculosis and pulmonary varicella.

- A patient with severe immunocompromise (e.g. absolute neutropenia) should have droplet precautions in a positive pressure room (i.e. to push air *out* of their room).

- Additional precautions exist for special diseases:
  - Patients with infective diarrhoea should ideally be the only person using a toilet.
  - People immune to preventable diseases (e.g. varicella) should preferably nurse those with said illnesses.
  - Patients should not be moved unless necessary.

- Patients with bloodborne illness require only standard precautions, as all patients should be treated as though they have the capacity to cause illness in the treating team if exposed to their bodily fluids.

- The exact length of isolation required for specific infectious agents is in the NHMRC *Guidelines for the Prevention and Control of Infection in Healthcare,* available free of charge online.

SECTION IV

COMMON SEXUALLY TRANSMITTED INFECTIONS

Sexually transmitted infections (STIs) are not a common presentation in an inpatient setting, with the exceptions of Adolescent Medicine and Obstetrics and Gynaecology. As an intern, you may encounter patients with symptoms suggestive of STIs in the Emergency Department (particularly 'fast track' cubicles) or incidentally on the wards. Table 41.1 outlines some of the common features seen in the most frequently encountered and most clinically relevant STIs.

Risk factors for STIs include sexual activity in early adolescence, multiple partners, men who have sex with men (MSM), intercourse with new partners, inconsistent use of the barrier method, and consumption of alcohol or drugs. Note

TABLE 41.1 Sexually transmitted infections

DISEASE	ORGANISM	TREATMENT	NOTES
Chlamydia	*Chlamydia trachomatis*	Azithromycin 1 g PO stat OR doxycycline 100 mg PO BD for 10 days NB: Doxycycline is contraindicated in pregnancy	• May be asymptomatic, especially in men • Males may have clear discharge • Females may have intermenstrual bleeding, mucopurulent discharge, dysuria or pelvic pain • Can cause pelvic inflammatory disease if left untreated and result in female infertility • Increasing in incidence in Australia • Diagnosed with urine PCR
Gonorrhoea	*Neisseria gonorrhoea*	Ceftriaxone 500 mg IM stat + azithromycin 1 g PO stat	• Diagnosed on urine PCR or a positive culture • May present with discoloured discharge, cervicitis, bleeding or dysuria • Incidence in Australia increased from 2008 to 2012

TABLE 41.1 Sexually transmitted infections—cont'd

DISEASE	ORGANISM	TREATMENT	NOTES
Trichomoniasis	*Trichomonas vaginalis*	Tinidazole 2 g PO stat OR metronidazole 400 mg PO TDS for 5 days	• The classic sign is the 'strawberry cervix' with discharge and malodour • Clinical diagnosis, can be confirmed with wet smears from a high vaginal swab • Present but asymptomatic in some people
Syphilis	*Treponema pallidum*	Benzathine penicillin 1.8 g IM stat	• Rarely presents as primary disease (with ulcer or chancre) as it is self-limiting • Secondary syphilis may present with constitutional symptoms, truncal rash and, rarely, neurological signs • Tertiary syphilis is now very rare but may include cardiological or neurological disease • Diagnosed with RPR on serum or a swab/biopsy of lesions
Genital herpes	Herpes simplex virus-2	Symptomatic relief, although in rare circumstances antiviral treatment with acyclovir 400 mg PO TDS or valaciclovir 500 mg PO BD for 5–10 days may be appropriate	• Diagnosed with dry swab of lesions • Spread by skin-to-skin contact • May present with malaise, vesicular lesions, erythema and pruritus • May recur during stress, menstruation or pregnancy • May also be present in mouth or anus • Vertical transmission is possible

continued

TABLE 41.1 Sexually transmitted infections—cont'd

DISEASE	ORGANISM	TREATMENT	NOTES
Hepatitis	Hepatitis A, B, C, D or E viruses	Differs depending on species of virus from symptomatic management to antiviral therapy	• Covered in Chapter 58, 'Gastroenterology outpatients'
Genital warts	Human papilloma virus	Symptomatic relief	• A large family of viruses • Carcinogenic, can lead to dysplasia • May present with warts • Can be spread vertically • Best prevented with the Gardasil® vaccine
HIV	Human immunodeficiency virus	Refer for anti-retroviral therapy at an appropriately skilled HIV Centre	• Covered more extensively later in this chapter

Adapted from: Workowski, K.A. & Bolan, G.A., 2015. Sexually transmitted diseases treatment guidelines, 2015. Morbidity and Mortality Weekly Report, Recommendations and Reports 64(3), 1-137. Atlanta, GA: Centers for Disease Control and Prevention.

that some of the following infections are not purely transmitted by sexual activity, e.g. hepatitis and HIV.

When taking a sexual history from a patient, be direct and non-judgemental. Counsel about risk-taking behaviour (e.g. lack of contraception) as appropriate and inform patients to avoid sexual activity during treatment. If completing an examination of the patient's genitalia, strongly consider an escort of the same gender as the patient.

Investigations are based on the suspected organism but, with non-specific symptoms (e.g. urethritis), may include urine M/C/S with chlamydia and gonorrhoea PCR (best sent early in the morning) and serum FBE + UEC + syphilis RPR (rapid plasmin reagin) ± herpes simplex virus (HSV) ± HIV (if indicated; requires patient consent). If abdominal pain is present, request LFTs and if deranged consider hepatitis A (HAV) + hepatitis B core antibody and surface antigen + hepatitis C (HCV). If there are lesions, dry swabs can be sent for PCR for gonorrhoea, chlamydia and genital herpes. Chancres (i.e. painless ulceration) can be biopsied for inspection for syphilis infection. Note this is usually not necessary for diagnosis and understandably unpopular with patients! It is common to have multiple STIs at once. Discuss opportunistic Pap smear screening with the patient if taking high vaginal swabs. Imaging is rarely necessary, except a transvaginal (TV) ultrasound in suspected pelvic inflammatory disease (PID).

Many patients prefer single-dose treatment, and this is particularly useful in patient groups who may be less compliant (e.g. adolescents). Partner tracking should be completed for most STIs, and notification to the State Health Department is required for chlamydia, gonorrhoea, HIV and syphilis. There are websites (such as www.letthemknow.org.au), which allow people to anonymously notify previous partners. Partners of people known to be affected by chlamydia or gonorrhoea are often treated presumptively. Patients will require sensitive counselling when informed of their diagnosis.

The peak incidence of these diseases remains in the 15–25 years age group. There are special circumstances and potentially adverse outcomes for pregnant women with STIs, and these results should be referred (with consent) to their treating obstetrician.

FEVER OF UNKNOWN ORIGIN

Fever of unknown origin (FUO; alternatively, pyrexia of unknown origin or PUO) is a frequently misused term. The technical definition requires three criteria to be met: 1) a fever $\geq 38.3°C$ on several occasions, 2) the fever should last ≥ 3 weeks and 3) the diagnosis remains unclear despite a week of *appropriate* inpatient investigations.

Febrile illness for investigation is a common inpatient admission, with the majority of cases determined to be due to connective tissue diseases, infection and malignancy. However, up to 50% remain undiagnosed on resolution of symptoms. The infective group are most likely to have a discrete illness such as tuberculosis (TB) or a walled-off abscess. Neutropenic patients with fever are covered separately in Chapter 42, 'Medical Oncology'.

Diagnosis

Identifying the source of an FUO is the aim of admission. History should hence be very thorough, and cover a wide range of topics including a full medical history (noting in particular known inflammatory conditions and malignancy), past medical history (e.g. recent surgery or hospitalisation), travel history, social history, sexual history and family history. Ask about fever, rigors, chills, sweats, weight loss, anorexia, lethargy, cough, chest pain, dyspnoea, abdominal pain, nausea and vomiting, change in bowel habit, joint pains, haematuria, dysuria, urinary frequency and calf pain or swelling. If there are any positive findings, hone in on them and interrogate the topic further. Box 41.2 offers a mnemonic to prompt discussion, with common sources of fever in a hospitalised surgical patient.

BOX 41.2 Mnemonic for postoperative fever: the 6 Ws

Wind	Hospital-acquired pneumonia
Water	Urinary tract infection
Walking (lack of)	Pulmonary embolism/DVT
Wound	Surgical sites and lines inserted
'Wonder drugs'	Drug-induced fever
Wonder why?	Abscesses or walled-off source

Source: Old medical school anecdote.

Examination should similarly be broad. Note the vitals – how recently were they febrile, and what pattern are the fevers? Are they haemodynamically stable? Look for any localising signs of infection, auscultating the heart sounds for new murmurs and the chest for accessory noises. Inspect the teeth for possible abscesses. Palpate the sinuses, temples (for temporal arteritis), abdomen and the calves. Subtle signs such as peripheral stigmata (e.g. splinter haemorrhages), rashes or lymphadenopathy may indicate the underlying pathology. If there are any wounds or lines (e.g. cannulas or catheters), inspect for tenderness, bleeding and discharge. Note the volume state. Consider fundoscopy. Perform a digital rectal examination if indicated (but avoid if neutropenic).

Investigations

Investigation into fever with no known source typically begins with a 'septic screen' including an FBE, UEC, CMP, LFT, CRP, ESR, venous blood gas (VBG) for lactate, blood cultures (ideally from three separate sites and using an aseptic technique), urine M/C/S (± *Legionella* antigen), stool M/C/S with CDT, sputum M/C/S and NPA swab with respiratory multiplex PCR. Any wounds should be swabbed. Consider requesting viral serology (HIV, HAV, HBV, HCV, VZV, EBV, CMV and HSV) and QuantiFeron® Gold (for TB). If autoimmune disease is looking like a possible cause, request thyroid-stimulating hormone (TSH), vitamin B12, anti-nuclear antibody (ANA), anti-neutrophil cytoplasmic antibody (ANCA), rheumatoid factor (RF), anti-CCP and complement (3 and 4) levels.

Imaging should include at bare minimum a CXR with an abdominal ultrasound or CT-abdomen/pelvis if indicated. If significant renal symptoms are present consider a renal tract ultrasound. If fevers persist with respiratory symptoms, a high resolution CT (HRCT)-chest may be indicated. If risk factors are present send three morning sputum samples for acid-fast bacilli (AFB) to exclude TB and a silver stain to inspect for fungi or *Pneumocystis jirovecii* pneumonia (PJP).

If tachypnoeic, dyspnoeic, hypoxic and/or tachycardic, consider investigating the diagnosis of pulmonary embolism with a CT-pulmonary angiogram. Unilateral calf swelling or pain should prompt a Doppler ultrasound. Bony tenderness could be investigated with a bone scan (looking for osteomyelitis). Neurological signs suggest an urgent need for CT-brain and consideration of a lumbar puncture.

Persistent fevers may require investigation with whole body PET scan, bronchoscopy or bone marrow aspirate and trephine.

Management

Management aims to identify the cause and treat the underlying pathology. If a patient is unwell broad-spectrum antimicrobials are usually commenced. However, if the patient is stable a period of non-treatment would be considered to allow the process to present itself. There is some evidence non-specific treatment delays diagnosis and results in worse outcomes. The exception is neutropenic patients with fever, who should be immediately 'pan-cultured' and commenced on high-dose, broad-spectrum antibiotics within 20 minutes.

The prognosis in FUO is dependent on the precipitant of the fevers. Malignant causes and elderly patients have the highest mortality. Even without diagnosis, the majority of patients will experience spontaneous resolution of symptoms and a good outcome. Non-steroidal therapy is trialled in some patients with ongoing fevers and no contraindications for symptom control.

CELLULITIS

Cellulitis is inflammation of the deeper dermis and subcutaneous fat. It typically presents with erythema, swelling, tenderness, warmth and, occasionally, loss of function of the affected area. Erysipelas is a similar disease that is limited to the upper dermis and lymphatics.

The two most common causative organisms are *Staphylococcus* species and *Streptococci* (especially the Group A beta-haemolytic strains), but other causes include *Pseudomonas aeruginosa* (particularly in IV drug users or patients who are regularly admitted), fungi (e.g. *Cryptococcus*) and Gram-negative rods (e.g. *Serratia*). Multi-resistant *S. aureus* (MRSA) presents an additional hurdle for treatment and should always be suspected in current or recent inpatients. In coastal Victoria and far north Queensland, consider *Mycobacterium ulcerans* as a cause for non-healing skin wounds.

An important differential diagnosis is necrotising fasciitis, an infection of the deep fascia that is rapidly progressive, principally painful and carries a very high morbidity and mortality requiring antibiotics and either hyperbaric treatment or amputation of the affected area. Other differentials include lipodermatosclerosis (the inverted champagne bottle sign, often mistaken for 'bilateral cellulitis', which is an incredibly rare phenomenon), thrombophlebitis, lymphoedema, a localised abscess, osteomyelitis (infection of the underlying bone), septic arthritis (severe joint infections), drug reactions, vasculitis and peripheral vascular disease.

Risk factors include obesity, diabetes, immunocompromise, smoking tobacco, intravenous drug use, lymphoedema, skin pathology (e.g. psoriasis, shingles or dermatitis), past history of cellulitis and preexisting wounds and injuries. Animal and insect bites may also cause cellulitis. Cellulitis is a very common cause for admission as an inpatient on General Medical rotations. Once a patient is stable, they tend to be good candidates for transfer to Hospital in the Home to complete their IV antibiotics.

Diagnosis

Diagnosis is made clinically based on the swollen, red and tender area of skin. The lower limbs are affected more regularly than the upper limbs, but cellulitis may develop anywhere in the body. Periorbital cellulitis is particularly serious, as in rare cases it can be complicated by septic cavernous sinus thrombosis (i.e. an infected clot in the cavernous sinus).

When taking a history, ask about the timeline of the erythema and swelling, fevers, rigors, chills, sweats, loss of function, current mobility and effort tolerance, level of pain and prior skin integrity. Ask about previous episodes of cellulitis and how they've responded to treatment. Take a full medical, past, social and family history. Quantify their tobacco exposure and offer 'Quit' counselling as required.

Examination should include general inspection, interrogation of the affected area, vital observations, chest auscultation, assessment of fluid status, palpation of the abdomen and calves and assessment of pulses distal to the erythematous region. Note any discharge or bleeding, affected hair follicles, abscesses, sinuses or animal/insect bites. Erysipelas is often more sharply demarcated than cellulitis due to its more superficial nature.

Investigations

Investigations should include basic blood work (FBE + UEC + CMP) with an inflammatory marker (usually CRP) to monitor response to therapy. If the patient is febrile, order blood cultures. If gout is suspected, request uric acid. If there is exudate or an open wound, send a wound swab for M/C/S. Anti-streptolysin O (ASLO) titre may be of use in separating *Streptococcus* infection from other organisms but is rarely performed. Imaging is not necessary unless necrotising fasciitis (CT or MRI or affected area + urgent surgical review) or DVT (Doppler ultrasound) are suspected.

Management

A typical admission plan for cellulitis severe enough to be managed as an inpatient may include:

1 Admit under General Medicine with regular medications and DVT prophylaxis.

2 Commence IV antibiotics. Typical regimens include 1 g IV flucloxacillin QID or 2 g IV cefazolin TDS (1 g is not an effective dose). In the setting of penicillin allergy, chart vancomycin with a 1.5 mg IV BD loading dose and trough level after three doses for titration. Mild MRSA infection may be managed with oral trimethoprim/sulfamethoxazole (160/800 mg PO daily). Ideally, antibiotics continue for a *minimum* of 14 days.

3   Elevate and immobilise the affected area, ideally higher than the level of the heart. If significant oedema is present apply tight support stockings.

4   Mark out the affected area with a permanent marker and *date the line*. Note there is some fluctuation in the cellulitic area and an early increase in erythema does not indicate treatment failure.

5   Physiotherapy + Occupational Therapy review.

6   Chase cultures sent at admission.

7   Daily bloods, with second-daily CRP.

8   Depending on the duration of antibiotics required, consider converting to a slow-pump infusion or less regular medications (e.g. higher, split doses) to facilitate transfer to Hospital in the Home (HITH).

Patients with cellulitis do not necessarily require outpatient specialist follow-up and could be reviewed by their local GP with bloods prior in 1 week after discharge. If the patient was particularly unwell they could be seen in the General Medicine Outpatients Clinic in 2–4 weeks.

Recurrent cellulitis is a common issue. Patients should be taught good skincare and when to re-present. Consider sending the patient home with a bottle of 4% chlorhexidine to do special washes to remove skin colonisation.

HUMAN IMMUNODEFICIENCY VIRUS

Human immunodeficiency virus (HIV) was once synonymous with acquired immunodeficiency syndrome (AIDS). However, progress in the treatment of HIV infection in the earlier stages has now rendered them two separate ends of a spectrum of disease.

HIV is a retrovirus that infects dendritic cells, monocytes, macrophages and, most famously, $CD4^+$ T-helper lymphocytes. Once the $CD4^+$ T-cell count falls below a certain level, the host loses the cell-mediated wing of their immune response. To understand the concept of HIV/AIDS, several definitions are necessary:

- *Early HIV infection* – refers to the approximately 6-month period after initial infection, prior to symptoms. Also known as 'viral transmission' or recent or primary HIV infection.

- *Acute HIV infection* – symptomatic HIV disease.

- *Clinical latency* – sometimes referred to as 'chronic' HIV, after the acute phase has settled.

- *AIDS* – a $CD4^+$ cell count of <200 cells/μL; or a $CD4^+$ cell percentage of total lymphocytes <15%; or the presence of AIDS defining illnesses. Some of the AIDS-defining illnesses are listed in Table 41.2.

The cardinal symptoms of infection with HIV are weight loss, asthenia (i.e. weakness) and diarrhoea. The retrovirus is transmitted primarily via sexual intercourse, but may also be spread via IV drug use, pregnancy and childbirth (i.e. vertical transmission), lactation and, rarely, by needlestick injury, blood

TABLE 41.2 AIDS-defining illnesses

DISEASE	NOTES
Pneumocystis jirovecii pneumonia (PJP)	• Also known by its previous name, *Pneumocystis carinii* (and hence sometimes still contracted to PCP, especially in the USA) is a fungus • Many patients will be on prophylaxis with trimethoprim/sulfamethoxazole
Candidiasis of oesophagus, bronchus, trachea or lungs	• Pathogenic candidal infection (due to any species of the *Candida* yeast) in any area other than the vagina likely represents immunocompromise
Cryptococcus (extrapulmonary)	• A fungal infection usually contracted by respiratory exposure
Cytomegalovirus infection	• Usually reactivation • Affecting areas other than liver, spleen or lymph nodes • Retinitis in particular is seen in patients with HIV, and requires antivirals
Coccidioidomycosis	• Fungal illness
Chronic intestinal cryptosporidiosis	• Lasting >1 month
Herpes simplex virus causing chronic ulcers	• Lasting >1 month • Alternatively, if HSV is causing bronchitis, pneumonitis or oesophagitis
HIV encephalopathy	• Long-term leads to 'HIV dementia' • Thought to be a direct effect of the HIV retrovirus toxins
Disseminated or extrapulmonary histoplasmosis	• Caused by the fungus *Histoplasma capsulatum*, most commonly manifests as a respiratory illness
Chronic, intestinal isosporiasis	• Lasting >1 month • *Isospora belii* is a parasite, classically seen in tropical areas
Kaposi's sarcoma	• Tumours often seen as violaceous plaques • Due to human herpes virus 8 (HHV8) • May also have internal involvement • Typically seen on upper back, face, trunk and oral mucosa

TABLE 41.2 AIDS-defining illnesses—cont'd

DISEASE	NOTES
Lymphoma	• Especially Burkitt's, but also primary CNS lymphoma or immunoblastic lymphoma • Burkitt's is particularly aggressive
Mycobacterium avium complex (MAC) or other *Mycobacterium* species	• If extrapulmonary or disseminated • *Mycobacterium* are Actinobacteria
Progressive multifocal leukoencephalopathy	• A severe, rare, slow-onset, demyelinating inflammation of the white matter of the brain due to JC virus • Diagnosed clinically with evidence from neuroimaging • Supportive management only
Salmonella septicaemia	• If recurrent or refractory to antibiotics
CNS toxoplasmosis	• Protozoal disease contracted from exposure to infected meat or affected animals' faecal matter (e.g. cats) • Diagnosed with serum antitoxoplasma IgG. Cerebral oedema may be evident on CT
HIV wasting syndrome	• Weight loss of >10% prior body mass, often associated with diarrhoea and lethargy

Adapted from: Buehler, M.D. & Berkelman, M.R.L., 1990. 1993 revised classification system for HIV infection and expanded surveillance case definition for AIDS among adolescents and adults. Morbidity and Mortality Weekly Report, Recommendations and Reports. Atlanta, GA: Centers for Disease Control and Prevention.

product transfusion or transplant. The receptive partner during anal sex is at greatest risk (due to microtears in the mucosa), followed by women in heterosexual intercourse and oral sex. Risk factors include intravenous drug use, risky sexual behaviour, tattoos (especially overseas or 'backyard') and blood transfusions or medical infusions overseas (or in Australia <1985, when screening began).

HIV transmission was decreasing in Australia, but has seen a recent resurgence in incidence leading to increased promotion of prevention. In Australia, 88% of people with new diagnosis HIV are men who have sex with men, 9% contract the virus through heterosexual intercourse and 1% via intravenous drug use. Globally, HIV and AIDS remains a pandemic – particularly in sub-Saharan Africa, South-East Asia, Eastern Europe and increasingly Latin America. In these regions heterosexual sex and vertical transmission have overtaken the rate of homosexual male transmission. Unfortunately, HIV continues to be associated with intense social stigma despite significant advances in treatment.

Diagnosis

Making the diagnosis of HIV can be difficult and, due to the large number of potential presentations and serious consequences of late diagnosis, the possibility of HIV infection should never be dismissed in unusual cases or people presenting with severe flu-like illness, signs of immunocompromise (including the diseases outlined above), generalised lymphadenopathy or renal or liver disease of unknown aetiology. When taking a history from a patient with HIV try to cover:

- When were they diagnosed with HIV? How did they present? Are they aware of how they contracted the disease? Do they attend an HIV Clinic and, if so, how regularly? Who monitors their $CD4^+$ count? Do they know their highest and lowest $CD4^+$ cell count, or their count at diagnosis?

- Have they reached the point where they require treatment? If so, do they know their regimen? Did they experience any complications of this therapy? Important side effects include mood disturbance, fatigue, dermatological changes (including Stevens–Johnson syndrome), GI upset, renal toxicity, myelosuppression and liver disease.

- Have they had any of the opportunistic infections? If so, detail when and the treatment received. Discuss the more common ones with the patient. These are more likely in a patient who is non-compliant with their therapy.

- What is their full medical and past history? Is there a family history of any diseases?
  - If considering treatment, do they have ischaemic heart disease, dyslipidaemia, hepatitis or psychiatric issues? These may interfere with or even preclude anti-retroviral therapy.

- If they are taking treatment, detail their regimen and how many doses they have missed in the past month. Ask about side effects of the therapy, and previous regimens and why they were changed. Ask if they have ever had a resistance test.

- Ask about screening for concomitant STIs, and the frequency of anal or vaginal pap smears. If female, a full obstetric and gynaecological history is suggested.

- Who is at home with the patient? What is their occupation? Is there a risk of exposure to their clients or co-workers and, if so, what measures do they take to prevent this? Do they have a criminal history? Do they have pets (and who cleans up after them)? Quantify their tobacco and alcohol consumption. Clarify if they use intravenous drugs. Ask about exercise and diet. Consider a travel history.

- Do they have regular dental appointments? Do they have an optometrist and have they had an eye-test with dilatation in the past year? Are their vaccinations up to date?

- Ask about how the patient is coping, and screen for symptoms of anxiety or depression. If the patient is not already aware of their services, offer to link them with an HIV support group.

Examination should be very thorough, reviewing for signs of progression of disease and (if started) complications of therapy. A formal weight and set of vitals is necessary. Inspect for cachexia, pallor, fevers, joint swelling or tenderness, myopathy, peripheral fat atrophy, nail changes (including clubbing and cyanosis), oral mucosal sores, oral thrush, state of dentition, pharyngeal lesions, thyroid changes, lymphadenopathy, changes in chest auscultation, breast masses, gynaecomastia, altered heart sounds, abdominal masses or distension, organomegaly (consider measuring liver span), bruising and rashes. In men, consider examination of the penis, testicles and scrotum for lesions or discharge. Women should ideally have a speculum examination annually. If indicated by the history, complete a thorough central and peripheral neurological examination. Consider formal optometry review for visual acuity, fields and fundoscopy (especially with low CD4$^+$ cell count).

Natural history

The natural history of HIV begins with exposure to the retrovirus. The symptoms at seroconversion at 1–4 weeks post-exposure are often described as similar to Epstein–Barr virus, with fever, malaise, pharyngitis, lymphadenopathy, arthralgias and/or a rash. This brief illness is often self-limited, so some people may not present to a healthcare service.

At this point, patients have a high viral load and the HIV spreads with the body developing antibodies against HIV at 2–4 months after initial exposure. Patients experience an asymptomatic period, the length of which is highly variable and depends on the person's genetics, HLA subtypes, age and overall health and wellbeing. This may be as long as 8–10 years. HIV replicates quite rapidly and is prone to errors, resulting in a virus that is very difficult for our immune systems to clear and providing it with a mechanism for drug resistance.

Opportunistic infections begin with increasing frequency as the virus continues to replicate and the patient's level of circulating CD4$^+$ cells decreases. The types of opportunistic infections contracted by the patient give clues as to the degree of immunosuppression (e.g. PJP is common at a CD4$^+$ count <200 cells/mm^3). If treatment is not commenced, patients usually succumb to an opportunistic infection.

Investigations

In the acute phase, HIV is diagnosed based on the presence of HIV RNA in serum as HIV-specific antibodies do not begin circulating immediately. On diagnosis, a patient should have HIV antibodies, CD4$^+$ count (repeated once at baseline and then 6-monthly), CD4$^+$ percentage of total cells, quantitative assessment of HIV RNA (i.e. a 'viral load', done at baseline and regularly when on treatment) and basic blood work to assess the patient's overall health and preclusion to treatment (FBE + UEC + CMP + LFT + coagulation studies + fasting glucose and lipid profile; repeated every 3–6 months). A urinalysis with protein-to-creatinine ratio (PCR) should be done at baseline and repeated annually.

Prior to commencing treatment, patients should also have screening for: pregnancy (beta-HCG); other STIs (syphilis RPR, urinary chlamydia and gonorrhoea

PCR ± trichomoniasis swab); hepatitis A, B and C; Epstein–Barr virus; varicella; herpes simplex; cytomegalovirus; and tuberculosis (with serology ± CXR). A cervical Pap smear is recommended at baseline and repeated at 6 months, with no such current guideline for anal Pap smears. Discuss with the consultant whether toxoplasmosis IgG (past exposure) is necessary.

Management

Management of a patient who has been potentially exposed to HIV in an acute setting (i.e. >72 hours) should include urgent ID review with consideration of post-exposure prophylaxis with anti-retroviral therapy. Patients with a confirmed diagnosis should be referred to your state's HIV Clinic.

Any acute issues should be managed during the patient's first presentation (e.g. acute kidney injury, myelosuppression, encephalopathy) as they would be for any other person. HIV patients often require the input of specialists from many fields of medicine, and you should have a low threshold for referral. Opportunistically screen for general health problems (e.g. diabetes, thyroid dysfunction, dyslipidaemia, common malignancies) and other STIs as outlined above.

During the admission, give lifestyle advice about prevention of spread of HIV in a non-judgemental manner. Consider opportunistic vaccination (if the $CD4^+$ cell count is >500 for live viral vaccines) for influenza, pneumococcal, tetanus, HPV, varicella and hepatitis A and B. Offer assistance with cessation of alcohol, tobacco or other drugs. If the patient has not yet completed their family, make a referral to an appropriate obstetrics and gynaecology centre and discuss the concept of vertical transmission.

Prophylaxis against common opportunistic organisms should be discussed with your consultant as the patient becomes increasingly prone to disease. Generally, prophylaxis is given against PJP and toxoplasmosis with trimethoprim/sulfamethoxazole 160/800 mg PO daily when the $CD4^+$ count is <200, and against MAC with 1.2 g PO weekly azithromycin when the count is <50 cells/mm^3. Histoplasmosis prophylaxis with itraconazole 200 mg PO daily should be considered if *Histoplasma capsulatum* is endemic in the patient's region.

On discharge, in addition to referring the patient to HIV Clinic they should also receive referrals to an optometrist, dentist, dietitian and good GP. If necessary, place the patient in touch with Psychology or Psychiatric services. Patients should be seen in clinic in 2–4 weeks if they have required hospitalisation.

Highly active anti-retroviral therapy (HAART) is the term given to the current therapy for HIV. There are many different classes (including nucleoside reverse transcriptase inhibitors, protease inhibitors, non-nucleoside reverse transcriptase inhibitors and integrase inhibitors) given in various combinations. HAART should be considered for all patients *at diagnosis* to both improve long-term outcomes and prevent further transmission by reducing the host's viral load. Patients usually use a combination of drugs with three different mechanisms in HAART, all of which are chosen and monitored carefully by their ID consultant. If reviewing a patient in clinic or during an admission, it is a good idea to review their

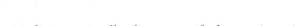

medications in the *Australian Medicines Handbook* to see if the patient is experiencing any of the common adverse effects.

TUBERCULOSIS

Tuberculosis (TB, known historically as 'the consumption') is a bacterial infection caused by the microorganism *Mycobacterium tuberculosis*. Although common in developing countries (particularly South-East Asia and the Western Pacific), it is now relatively rare in the Western world. It is described by the World Health Organization as a 'disease of poverty', with risk factors for tuberculosis include proximity to a known TB patient, travel to areas where TB remains endemic, low socioeconomic status, tobacco use and immunocompromise (e.g. from chemotherapy, malignancy, or HIV).

TB is one of the leading causes of death due to a preventable illness. It is hugely prevalent on a global scale, with some estimates reporting that one-third of the world's *entire population* are latently infected with TB. In Australia, TB is seen not uncommonly in people of Indigenous Australian or Torres Strait Islander heritage.

A serious problem is the emergence of multiple drug-resistant tuberculosis (MDR-TB), as some strains of the bacteria fail to respond to the standard four-agent therapy. MDR-TB involves resistance to at least isoniazid and rifampicin, is worsened by inappropriate management (e.g. not completing prescribed courses of antibiotics) and requires different, second-line agents for a longer duration.

Extensively-drug resistant tuberculosis (XDR-TB) refers to a form of TB that does not respond to first- or second-line therapy and is unfortunately becoming increasingly abundant. The majority of cases have been in Russia, China and India.

Diagnosis

Tuberculosis should be considered in all febrile patients from endemic areas, with or without the presence of cough or dyspnoea. The classic symptoms of cough (± haemoptysis), fever, chills, night sweats, anorexia and weight loss are not always present. When taking a history from a patient with known or suspected TB, cover:

- When did the symptoms begin? Have they formally been diagnosed with TB and, if so, was it based on blood work, sputum or radiological findings?

- Have they commenced treatment? Are they compliant? Have they experienced any side effects of the antibiotic regimen?

- If still suspected – what is their home living situation? Have they travelled to an endemic region? Are they elderly (TB was endemic in Australia until the1950s)? Have they ever had a similar illness in the past? A full travel history is necessary.

- What is their full medical and past history? What is their occupation? Quantify their tobacco consumption. Have they ever used IV drugs? What is their full medication list?

Examination is primarily of the respiratory system, but note also the patient's vitals (particularly looking for fever, tachycardia, hypoxia and tachypnoea), cachexia, pallor, lymphadenopathy, skin changes, the colour and nature of any sputum, joint involvement, bony tenderness, added heart sounds, organomegaly and peripheral oedema. Tuberculoid meningitis is a rare but serious medical condition – if indicated, examine for signs of meningism (nuchal rigidity, photophobia) and consider progressing to lumbar puncture (LP).

Natural history

Tuberculosis is spread via droplet inhalation as people expel particles into the air. People are contagious while they have active, untreated respiratory infection. Not everyone exposed will become infected (dependent on the bacterial load, generation of aerosol, ventilation, duration of exposure and host's immunity) and 90% of those who are infected will never develop active disease. Factors that make active disease more likely include immunosuppression, advanced age or infancy, smoking, malnutrition, diabetes, malignancy and concomitant airways disease.

In those 10% of people infected who do develop active disease over their lifespan, the majority will experience symptoms within the first 1–2 years. Some infected patients only have active disease after a period of low immunity (i.e. 'reactivated disease').

After infection via the respiratory tract, tuberculosis can undergo widespread haematogenous dissemination to cause 'extra-pulmonary' or 'miliary' TB, so named because of its radiological resemblance to millet seeds on CXR. This involves active infection of the urinary tract, bones and joints (when involving the vertebral column it is known as Pott's disease), lymph glands, gastrointestinal tract, central nervous system (CNS) or, rarely, skin or breast. Complications of TB include acute arthralgias and joint destruction, respiratory failure, pleural effusions, meningitis (rare), renal impairment, hepatic damage and cardiac tamponade.

Investigations

Diagnosis of TB requires a combination of serology, culture or imaging. If TB is suspected, in addition to basic blood work (FBE + UEC + CMP + LFT) and inflammatory markers (i.e. CRP and ESR), request an interferon gamma release assay (e.g. QuantiFeron Gold, or QFG). QFG is specific to antigens expressed by *Mycobacterium tuberculosis*, as opposed to other methods of testing that will produce a false positive with other species of *Mycobacterium*. QFG is as sensitive as tuberculin skin testing and more specific for active infection, and appears to be equal in sensitivity for latent infection. Strongly consider requesting HIV antibodies simultaneously.

If QFG is unavailable in your area, an alternative for diagnosis is the tuberculin skin test. The Mantoux method involves intradermal injection of tuberculin and objectively measuring the area of induration (*not* erythema) at 72 hours. There are many issues with the tuberculin test – false negatives and positives occur not infrequently, they are assessor-dependent and past vaccination with the BCG vaccination for TB will produce a false positive.

A CXR is normally requested when a tuberculin skin test is positive or with a suspected active infection. CXR may show consolidation or cavitating lesions, typically in the upper lobes, and occasionally with hilar lymphadenopathy. CXR is suggestive but not diagnostic of TB, but could be used to exclude pulmonary TB in a person with a positive skin test. Progression to CT-chest is not always necessary and should be discussed with your registrar.

Sputum cultures should be sent for 'acid-fast bacilli', ideally in the morning, with at least one sent prior to commencing antibiotic therapy. Cultures remain the gold standard of diagnosis but can take 3–6 weeks to return. Sputum is examined with a Ziehl–Neelsen stain. Blood cultures should be sent if the patient spikes a fever.

Bronchoscopy may be used if no sputum can be expectorated and TB remains highly suspected. If meningitis is suspected, an LP is necessary (and TB PCR can be requested on the cerebrospinal fluid). Similarly, if destructive bony lesions or lymphadenopathy are suspected of being tuberculoid, core biopsy can be performed with CT guidance. Caseating (i.e. 'cheese-like' necrotised tissue) granulomas are classic of tuberculosis on histopathology.

Management

Patients with active tuberculosis can be very unwell, particularly if experiencing complications such as effusions, respiratory failure, tamponade, arthralgias or meningitis. Any patient suspected of having active TB infection should be placed in droplet isolation **as soon as possible**. A typical plan may include:

- Admission under General Medicine, Respiratory or Infectious Diseases in a droplet isolation room with regular medications and deep vein thrombosis (DVT) prophylaxis.
- Complete three early morning sputum cultures, requesting acid-fast bacilli (AFB).
- Chase cultures, sent as soon as possible.
- Daily bloods.
- Blood cultures if febrile.
- Commence antibiotic therapy (after discussion with a consultant)
   o The first-line regimen is 'RIPE' – i.e., rifampicin, isoniazid, pyrazinamide and ethambutol.
   o Treatment is typically commenced in patients empirically if unwell while waiting for cultures to return.
- Social worker + physiotherapist (for chest physio) + dietitian ± occupational therapist review.
- Advice on smoking cessation if necessary.
- Notification to the Department of Health.

TABLE 41.3 RIPE therapy for tuberculosis

DRUG	DOSE
Rifampicin	10 mg/kg PO daily, maximum 600 mg/day Causes bodily secretions to turn orange, and interferes with metabolism of several common drugs including the pill and warfarin
Isoniazid	15 mg/kg PO daily, maximum 300 mg/day Can cause liver damage – avoid alcohol
Pyrazinamide	Weight based; contraindicated in liver disease and gout 40 to 55 kg: 18.2–25 mg/kg PO daily, maximum 1 g 56 to 75 kg: 20–26.8 mg/kg PO daily, maximum 1.5 g 75 to 89 kg: 22.2–26.3 mg/kg PO daily, maximum 2 g
Ethambutol	Weight based; contraindicated in people who can't report visual disturbances and people with optic neuritis 40 to 55 kg: 14.5–20 mg/kg PO daily, maximum 800 mg 56 to 75 kg: 16–21.4 mg/kg PO daily, maximum 1.2 g 75 to 89 kg: 17.8–21.1 mg/kg PO daily, maximum 1.6 g

Adapted from: Ferri, F.F., 2015. Tuberculosis. In: Ferri, F.F., Ferri's Clinical Advisor. Philadelphia: Mosby.

The RIPE medications (outlined in Table 41.3) are used in combination due to the rate of single- and dual-drug resistance. As isoniazid interferes with vitamin B6 (pyridoxine) metabolism, it should be co-administered to prevent neuropathy and neurological dysfunction. It begins with a 2-month induction, with ethambutol ceased on confirmation of sensitivity to the remaining three agents. They then progress to the 4-month continuation phase with rifampicin and isoniazid (given once, twice or thrice weekly). This phase may be extended to 7 months in people with cavitary lesions on CXR, a positive sputum culture after induction or contraindications to pyrazinamide. Drug-resistant strains **must** be discussed with an ID specialist and all patients with TB should be referred to an ID service.

Patients with active pulmonary TB do not necessarily require admission. If compliance is likely, they have a confirmed plan for follow-up, there are no children <4 years old or immunocompromised people in their home and they agree to remain housebound until the sputum smear is negative, the patient may be able to be managed as an outpatient.

CHAPTER 42

MEDICAL ONCOLOGY

Joseph M O'Brien

This chapter will run in a slightly different format to previous inpatient chapters, as the way an intern or resident functions in Medical Oncology is unique. Rather than go into detail about the medical conditions you will encounter on this rotation, this chapter aims to cover some of the trickier complications seen in Oncology patients, as most treatment-based decisions will come from a consultant level.

The majority of Oncology admissions will be to manage complications of treatment, or progression of disease. Medical Oncology is one of the busiest rotations available to junior doctors, with the majority of patients being very sick and prone to sudden deterioration. Fortunately, senior Oncology clinicians are well aware of this and tend to provide a lot of support to their junior staff. Have a low propensity to escalate situations with Oncology patients.

Oncology registrars are required in clinic for a large portion of the day, resulting in an increased level of responsibility for junior doctors. In larger centres, Oncology services may be split into 'streams' (e.g. Sarcoma, Breast and Lung, Gastrointestinal). Depending on your unit, you may be asked to present patients at multidisciplinary meetings (MDM) – see Chapter 33, 'Unit meetings', for a guide on how to prepare for these presentations.

Oncology patients will need daily bloods, with 'tumour lysis bloods' (i.e. FBE + UEC + CMP + LFT + coagulation studies + uric acid + LDH) for those at high risk. Oncology is a fantastic rotation for learning about common and rare malignancies, and how to become comfortable with unwell patients.

FEBRILE NEUTROPENIA

Febrile neutropenia ('feb neut') is defined as a person with a fever $\geq 38.3°C$ in the setting of an absolute decrease in circulating neutrophils $\leq 1.0 \times 10^9/L$; *or* a patient with known neutropenia who is systemically unwell with a high suspicion of sepsis. Severe neutropenia is $\leq 0.5 \times 10^9/L$, and profound neutropenia $\leq 0.1 \times 10^9/L$. Notably, fever is not an essential component of 'febrile' neutropenia, with many people not being able to mount the immune response necessary.

Different organisations have different definitions for these patients (some more conservative, e.g. using a neutrophil cut-off of $<1.5 \times 10^9/L$) but the principle

TABLE 42.1 Low- vs high-risk patients with febrile neutropenia

LOW-RISK	HIGH-RISK
Solid tumours	Haematological malignancy
Haemodynamically stable	Myelosuppression
No comorbidities	Advanced age (>60 years)
Normal cultures	Bone marrow infiltrate
Normal chest X-ray	Steroid dose >25 mg/day
No sign of line sepsis	Significant mucositis (grade 2+)
No mucositis	Currently receiving radio- or chemotherapy
	Surgical wounds
	Comorbidities (e.g. diabetes)
	Malnutrition
	Prior neutropenia
	Neutropenia expected to last >7 days
	Recent inpatient admission with infection
	Haemodynamic instability

Adapted from: Gippsland Oncology Nurses Group, 2010. Management of febrile neutropenia in adults: Gong cancer care guidelines. <https://www.scribd.com/document/45908611/Febrile-Neutropenia -Management-Guidelines-0210.pdf>.

remains the same – these patients are very sick, and require urgent care with international guidelines recommending a 'time to antibiotics' <60 minutes, carrying the same urgency as 'time to needle' for stroke patients.

Febrile neutropenia is a medical emergency, and patients are classified as low or high risk (see Table 42.1). Both have the potential to progress to septic shock if not treated urgently. Fevers in a patient with malignancy undergoing treatment may be due to the disease itself, the direct effect of treatment (some melanoma therapies in particular are associated with fevers) or infection secondary to lowered host immune defences.

The majority of infections are believed to be due to chemotherapy-induced mucositis of the gastrointestinal system. Bacteria remain the most common cause, with viruses a close second and fungi a distant third. Although rare, polymicrobial bacteraemia is possible.

Diagnosis

Diagnosis of febrile neutropenia requires a set of observations revealing a fever, and bloods demonstrating neutropenia. When taking a history from the patient (or a collateral if the patient is too unwell), discuss:

- How long have they felt unwell? Is this their first fever? Have they had rigors, chills or sweats?

- Do they have any localising symptoms – headache, photophobia, nuchal rigidity, dental pain, cough, wheeze, chest pain, abdominal pain, altered bowel habit, melaena, PR bleeding, dysuria, urinary frequency or haematuria?
- Have they had signs of pancytopenia (e.g. other minor infections, spontaneous bruising, exertional dyspnoea and fatigue)?
- What kind of malignancy do they have? Do they know its staging? What treatment have they received so far? Have they had surgery and, if so, where and when? Where are they in their cycles of treatment (usually expressed as 'REGIMEN Cycle *x* Day *y*,' e.g. 'FOLFOX Cycle 2 Day 3')? Is there further treatment planned?
- Do they have any other medical conditions (e.g. COPD or diabetes)? This would place them in the high-risk group.
- Has the patient been compliant with their anti-fungal (e.g. fluconazole), antiviral (e.g. valacyclovir) and *Pneumocystis jirovecii* pneumonia (e.g. Bactrim® DS) prophylaxis?
- Do they have any known allergies?

Examination should similarly focus on identifying complications of the patient's chemoradiotherapy or localising signs of infection. Observations should be taken regularly and, if ≥2 breach clinical review criteria (e.g. hypotension and tachycardia), the patient should be urgently started on antibiotics. Take particular notice of any lines in situ (PICC lines, ports, catheters, even boring old cannulas) as these may harbour infection.

Auscultate the chest carefully, palpate the abdomen, and inspect **any and all** surgical sites. Do not forget to examine the patient's mouth, looking for neutropenic ulcers (i.e. painful ulcers that may provide a route of infection) and mucositis. Similarly, it may be indicated to inspect the perianal region – however, it is still advised that you do **not** perform a digital rectal examination (DRE) due to the risk of bacterial seeding via fragile mucosa.

Natural history

Febrile neutropenia rapidly progresses to septic shock if untreated. Regardless of optimal medical care, overall in-hospital mortality still approaches 10% in adults. Long-term complications are rare, but a patient who has had an episode of febrile neutropenia remains at high-risk for subsequent infections.

Investigations

Since febrile neutropenic patients may not mount a complete inflammatory response, history and clinical examination may not provide many clues as to the underlying cause of sepsis. As such, this patient cohort requires a 'shotgun' approach to investigations to narrow the possible diagnoses.

Blood cultures are the most urgent and important investigation and should be sent to the laboratory immediately (see Chapter 14, 'Investigations: other' for a guide on how to take blood cultures using an aseptic technique). Three sets of blood cultures of ≥20 mL volume from separate sites should be drawn with daily cultures until three consecutive are negative. Ideally, *at least* one set of cultures should be drawn prior to commencing antibiotics. If the patient has a long-term access site (e.g. central line), one set of cultures should be drawn through this avenue (**without** being flushed prior).

An initial serology panel should include FBE, UEC, CMP, LFT, LDH, CRP coagulation studies, uric acid and serum lactate (available quickly on a venous blood gas or 'VBG'). A lactate >2.0 is a poor prognostic marker. An urgent chest X-ray should be requested.

The idea with a febrile neutropenic patient is to 'pan-culture' them, so request a nasopharyngeal airway swab for respiratory multiplex PCR, a sputum M/C/S (microscopy/culture/sensitivities), a urine M/C/S and a stool M/C/S (with *Clostridium difficile* toxin if they have recently been on antibiotic therapy). Swab any wounds or surgical sites and request an M/C/S. Unless clinically indicated, a lumbar puncture (LP) is not required before discussion with a registrar or consultant.

In patients whose fever persists, more specialised investigations may be appropriate. These include a high resolution CT (HRCT) chest to investigate fungal infection or *Pneumocystis jirovecii* pneumonia (PJP), abdominal CT to review for neutropenic enterocolitis (NEC), CT sinuses for sinusitis, serum galactomannan (a polysaccharide found in *Aspergillus* infection) and a whole body positron-emitting tomography (PET) scan. Bronchoscopy with bronchoalveolar lavage may be considered in persistent cases. These are not routine and you will be guided by your registrar or consultant.

Management

The guiding principle of managing febrile neutropenic patients is to get cultures off as soon as possible and start antibiotic therapy within 60 minutes (at some centres, the suggested time to antibiotics is 20 minutes!). The antibiotic chosen should cover the suspected and common pathogens. Common choices for hospital policies are piperacillin/tazobactam (sold as Tazocin®) 4.5 g IV QID, meropenem 1 g IV TDS or cefepime 2 g IV TDS. If the suspected source is skin, consider adding in vancomycin at a loading dose (typically 1.5 g IV BD) with titration based on trough 'vanc' levels on day 3.

If gastrointestinal symptoms are present, consider adding metronidazole (500 mg IV BD). If a patient has an allergy to beta-lactams, consider ciprofloxacin 500 mg IV BD with vancomycin. Patients at risk of septic shock should be aggressively fluid resuscitated. A basic plan for a febrile neutropenic patient might read:

1   Admit under Oncology (or Haematology) with regular medications and DVT prophylaxis when platelets >50.

2   Chase urine, sputum, stool and blood cultures.

3   Continue IV antibiotics for 4–5 days, narrowing the spectrum if a source is identified.

4 Appropriate rehydration with IV fluids.

5 Paracetamol as an antipyretic Q4H.

6 Barrier nursing.

7 Close observations every 4 hours.

8 Consider Infectious Diseases review.

Patients at particularly low risk may be able to be treated with oral broad-spectrum antibiotics alone. Patients should be monitored closely for delirium, hypotension and respiratory failure and disseminated intravascular coagulation (DIC) – if any of these syndromes are present, an ICU review is recommended.

Persistent neutropenic fever syndrome exists when a patient continues to have febrile episodes >4 days after initiating antibiotic therapy, usually indicating a pathogen outside the current spectrum of treatment. Differential diagnoses include fungal infection, drug fevers, malignancy-related fever and thromboembolic fevers. At this stage, adding anti-fungal coverage should be strongly considered (but remains a consultant-based decision).

Granulocyte colony-stimulating factor (G-CSF or filgrastim) is a very expensive recombinant isomer of a polypeptide that stimulates marrow to produce granulocytes. Its use is not routinely recommended in febrile neutropenic patients unless the patient is at immensely high risk of poor outcome (e.g. neutropenia >10 days, profound neutropenia, uncontrolled primary disease or presence of multi-organ dysfunction).

Patients are typically de-escalated to amoxicillin with clavulanic acid (Augmentin® Duo Forte) 875/125 mg PO BD with ciprofloxacin 500 mg PO BD as atypical coverage when they are appropriately stable. If the patient has a penicillin or beta-lactam allergy, consider moxifloxacin 400 mg PO daily.

MALIGNANT EPIDURAL SPINAL CORD COMPRESSION

Malignant epidural spinal cord compression (MESCC; sometimes referred to as 'spinal cord compression') is a medical emergency requiring immediate radiotherapy or surgical intervention to prevent irreversible neurological loss of function. It is a displacement or compression caused by malignant cells growing in or near the spinal cord or cauda equina (i.e. the bundle of spinal nerves where the spinal cord terminates).

The most common presentation is with new or worsening back pain, and MESCC should be considered in all patients with severe back pain and known malignancy. Unfortunately, MESCC is a poor prognostic factor with a 72% 12-month mortality.

MESCC is most commonly seen in patients with known bony metastases to the spinal column, with the thoracic spine being most frequently involved. As such cancers of the breast, prostate, lung and kidney carry a higher incidence than other solid tumours. It is also seen in some haematological malignancies (e.g. multiple myeloma and non-Hodgkin's lymphomas). Rarely, cord compression may be caused by collapse of a vertebral body due to pathological fracture.

Diagnosis

Diagnosis is suspected clinically with new or rapidly worsening back pain in a patient with known malignancy. The patient may not have peripheral neurological signs (e.g. radiculopathy). The gold standard investigation remains a magnetic resonance image (MRI) of the affected spinal region. If there is evidence of compression on an MRI but the patient is asymptomatic, it is known as subclinical or 'impending' cord compression.

History should focus on the type of malignancy the patient has, its treatment thus far, the future plan, their medical comorbidities and their level of function (especially in comparison with their pre-morbid state). Patients often describe their pain as worse on reclining, and severe enough to wake them from sleep. Ask particularly about paraesthesia, weakness, confusion, gait disturbance, ataxia, incontinence and imbalance. Examination should be targeted – a thorough neurological examination is essential. Be mindful of the time-critical nature of cord compression (with a high suspicion, send off the imaging request before starting your examination – they take a while to get processed!). Loss of anal tone is a late sign of cord compression, but remember not to do a DRE on neutropenic patients.

Natural history

If MESCC is not treated rapidly, the patient will be left with permanent neurological damage below the affected spinal level.

Investigations

As mentioned above, MRI of the spine is both essential and urgent. If possible, imaging of the entire spine should be performed. If MRI is contraindicated (e.g. the patient has an older pacemaker or significant orthopaedic metalwork), a CT can be used as a substitute, although its sensitivity and specificity are inferior.

Other investigations required would include an FBE, UEC, CMP and CRP. Differential diagnoses include musculoskeletal pain, radiation myelopathy from previous radiotherapy and a spinal cord abscess (patients usually present with more of a septic appearance and have biochemical evidence of infection).

Management

Gold standard management is decompression of the mass placing pressure on the spinal cord. Depending on the location of the mass, the health of the patient and the availability of services, this can be either medical, surgical or radiotherapy.

Once imaging is obtained, the appropriate referrals to Neurosurgery and Radiation Oncology should be made. The consultant or registrar on duty should be notified, and the patient considered for glucocorticoids (e.g. 10 mg dexamethasone intravenously). Steroids should be avoided in the setting of infection. Patients with paralysis >48 hours are not typically considered for surgical intervention. In rare cases, a tumour known to be highly vulnerable to chemotherapy may be treated with chemotherapy and radiotherapy without the need for surgery.

The patient should be admitted under the home unit with ongoing neurological observations. Steroids should be weaned when tolerated. If there is a consideration of osteoporosis, bisphosphonate therapy (e.g. 5 mg IV zoledronic acid administered on discharge) should be considered.

If a patient presents with severe pain suggestive of spinal cord compression, has a significant burden of disease, contraindications to both surgery and radiotherapy and a severe loss of function, a referral to Palliative Care may be appropriate. The decision to make a patient for palliation should always be discussed with a registrar or consultant.

TUMOUR LYSIS SYNDROME

Tumour lysis syndrome (TLS) is a constellation of metabolic derangements caused by large-scale cell lysis, usually after chemotherapy has begun (but occasionally spontaneously). It is an oncological emergency that can be fatal if not prevented or treated. Patients may be asymptomatic, or may feel generally unwell, seize or experience cardiac dysrhythmias.

Patients with high-risk malignancies commencing treatment should have **twice daily** bloods (morning and afternoon) to monitor for the typical biochemical changes seen with TLS. Patients at highest risk of tumour lysis syndrome are those with a high turnover malignancy (e.g. Burkitt's lymphoma, acute lymphoblastic leukaemia, small cell carcinoma of the lung), highly cytotoxic agents and a large burden of disease (see Table 42.2). All Oncology patients should be on TLS

TABLE 42.2 Relative risk of tumour lysis syndrome

RISK	HISTOLOGICAL TYPE OF TUMOUR
Highest	Burkitt's lymphoma
	Non-Hodgkin's lymphoma with high tumour burden
	Acute lymphoblastic lymphoma
	Acute myeloid leukaemia
Moderate	Multiple myeloma
	Low-grade lymphomas undergoing treatment
	Breast cancer with chemotherapy and hormone treatment
	Small cell carcinoma of the lung
	Germ cell tumours
Lowest	Low-grade lymphomas with interferon therapy
	Merkel's cell carcinoma
	GI adenocarcinoma
	Medulloblastoma

Adapted from: Cairo, M. S., Coiffier, B., Reiter, A., et al., 2010. Recommendations for the evaluation of risk and prophylaxis of tumour lysis syndrome (TLS) in adults and children with malignant diseases: an expert TLS panel consensus. British Journal of Haematology 149(4), 578-586.

SECTION IV

TABLE 42.3 Biochemical changes in tumour lysis syndrome

MARKER	CHANGE
Uric acid	Increased
Phosphate	Increased
Potassium	Increased
Creatinine	Increased
Calcium	Decreased

Adapted from: Ferri, F.F., 2015. Tumor lysis syndrome. In: Ferri, F.F., Ferri's Clinical Adviser. Philadelphia: Mosby.

prophylaxis with allopurinol (300 mg PO daily, or 100 mg with poor renal function) and adequate hydration.

Diagnosis

Diagnosis is based on serology. The typical biochemical findings are outlined in Table 42.3.

Patients may have a completely normal physical examination. They may report fatigue, myalgias, palpitation or chest pain. Be sure to note their volume state.

Natural history

If electrolytes and fluid state are not corrected, tumour lysis syndrome is invariably fatal. Aggressive hydration is necessary and urgent to prevent further deterioration. Patients with TLS most frequently die of large volume haemorrhage, renal failure or cardiac arrhythmia.

Laboratory tumour lysis syndrome is ≥2 of hyperkalaemia, hyperphosphataemia, hypocalcaemia and hyperuricaemia. Clinical tumour lysis is the above, plus an increase in serum creatinine ≥1.5× baseline, new cardiac dysrhythmia, seizures or sudden death.

Investigations

Patients at risk of TLS should have twice-daily bloods for 48–72 hours after commencing treatment, which can be stepped down to daily if no disturbance in electrolytes is detected after this time. 'Tumour lysis bloods' include FBE, UEC, CMP, CRP, LDH, LFT, uric acid and coagulation studies. No imaging is required although, if the patient's renal function is deteriorating without the other expected electrolyte changes, the patient should be investigated for acute kidney injury like any other patient (see Chapter 38, 'Renal medicine').

Management

The key to managing tumour lysis syndrome is prevention (if possible). All Oncology patients will likely be on allopurinol as prophylaxis against TLS. Patients in the highest risk group should have IV hydration running prior to commencing their chemotherapy. Close monitoring is essential – consider placing an indwelling catheter to monitor urine output. Place the patient on a strict fluid balance. Any electrolyte abnormalities should be corrected immediately. Daily ECGs should be performed. Consider requesting QID neurological observations due to the risk of seizures.

If a patient begins to experience TLS, the allopurinol dose should be escalated to 600–900 mg per day. IV hydration should be escalated immediately. If a patient is adequately hydrated, a low-dose loop diuretic (e.g. 40 mg PO frusemide) could be considered. Rasburicase, a very expensive recombinant enzyme (urate oxidase), may be used in extreme circumstances to lower the serum uric acid at a dose of 50–100 units/kg/daily for 1–5 days. This is a consultant-level decision. If giving rasburicase, allopurinol should be ceased.

The patient should go onto a potassium-binding resin (e.g. Resonium®) and, if necessary, have calcium gluconate with short-acting insulin (10 units) and glucose (25 mg in 10 mL). Oral phosphate binders may also be needed. Consider a referral to ICU, as the patient may require filtration and would likely benefit from the one-to-one nursing ratio.

EXTRAVASATION OF CHEMOTHERAPY

Extravasation is the leakage of drugs into the extravascular space and, when this is a chemotherapeutical agent (particularly a 'vesicant' or blister-inducing drug), patients may experience long-lasting and severe injury. To prevent this type of injury, chemotherapy is ideally administered via a securely-placed central venous catheter (CVC).

Patients at highest risk are those with chemotherapy via a peripheral line, those who are obese, who move frequently or have preexisting dermatological disease, lymphoedema or sensory deficits. Different chemotherapeutic drugs are classified as either irritants or vesicants, but there is a moderate overlap between these definitions.

Usually a nurse will alert you to a patient they suspect of having extravasation. Inspect the site for swelling, numbness, burning, paraesthesia, erythema, pruritus or tenderness. Signs may have a delayed presentation.

Most hospitals that deliver chemotherapy will have a policy for this situation. If not, ensure the infusion is ceased and the patient has adequate analgesia charted. Elevate the affected area if possible, and apply a cold pack (unless the agent was vincristine or etoposide, which worsen ulceration when exposed to cold). Leave the line in situ – not only can you attempt to aspirate back some of the drug, but chemotherapy agents have an antidote available that could be delivered by the same line (discuss this with a registrar, as it is rarely practiced).

If an ulcer or blistering begins to form, consider a referral to Plastic Surgery for review. If the extravasation is thought to have occurred via a CVC, consider a CT-chest to confirm the leakage. Again, stop the infusion and attempt to aspirate back as much drug as possible.

MUCOSITIS

Mucositis, or inflammation or ulceration of the mucous membranes lining the gastrointestinal tract, is a common adverse effect from chemotherapy and radiotherapy to the head and neck. Certain chemotherapeutical drugs have a higher association with mucositis (including 5-fluorouracil, bleomycin, cytarabine, doxorubicin, etoposide, methotrexate and melphalan) and patients at highest risk are younger patients and those with malnutrition, poor oral hygiene or previous dental disease. Up to 40% of patients who undergo chemotherapy are affected.

Diagnosis

Diagnosis is based on clinical examination, with no imaging or serology necessary. Inspect for bleeding, discharge and/or ulceration. Examine for signs of oral thrush. A basic set of bloods (FBE + UEC + CRP) could be sent to exclude systemic infection and renal injury. If the patient is febrile, blood cultures should be sent as there is a clear route of entry for potential pathogens. History-taking should focus on the duration of symptoms, ability to maintain oral intake and other GI symptoms (diarrhoea, melaena, PR bleeding, nausea and vomiting). Consider swabbing any ulcers if you suspect infection with herpes simplex virus (HSV).

Natural history

If mucositis is severe enough (i.e. grade 3+), it may prevent a person from being able to maintain a sufficient diet. If this is the case, nasogastric (NG) feeds or even total parenteral nutrition (TPN) should be considered to help optimise their nutrition.

One of the two commonly used grading systems, the National Cancer Institute common terminology criteria for adverse events (CTCAE), is outlined in Table 42.4. Mucositis can progress to the point where oral intake is impossible and can even result in death if no intervention is made. Other side effects include electrolyte disturbance, dehydration and subsequent acute kidney injury. Fortunately, mucositis is usually self-limiting. If a patient is particularly prone to mucositis their subsequent chemotherapy doses may be down-titrated.

TABLE 42.4 NCI CTCAE grading of mucositis

GRADE 1	GRADE 2	GRADE 3	GRADE 4	GRADE 5
Asymptomatic or mild Sx, no intervention needed	Moderate pain not interfering with oral intake; soft diet indicated	Severe pain interfering with oral intake; consider NG feeding	Life-threatening consequences; urgent intervention necessary	Death

Adapted from: National Cancer Institute (NCI), 2010. Common terminology criteria for adverse events. <http://evs.nci.nih.gov/ftp1/CTCAE/CTCAE_4.03_2010-06-14_QuickReference_5x7.pdf>.

Management

Ideally, mucositis is prevented with appropriate hydration and diet and good periodontal and oral hygiene. Patients with dentures should remove and clean these regularly. There is a building amount of evidence for chlorhexidine mouth-washes (ouch!) to prevent oral mucositis. Unfortunately, many cases are inevitable. Patients with pain should have adequate topical and systemic analgesia charted. Topical agents include lignocaine viscous 2%, 10 mL PO cocaine 0.5% mouthwash or benzydamine (i.e. Difflam™) mouthwash. Patients should have regular mouth care charted (e.g. Biotene® 2.5 mL PO QID or, if available, 'Peter MacCallum' mouthwash).

Patients with grade 2+ mucositis should be considered for a modified, less abrasive diet. If the mucositis is severe enough to impact upon their diet, they should have an urgent dietitian review with consideration of commencing either NG feeds or TPN to help supplement their oral intake.

Systemic analgesia is equally important. In addition to regular medications, consider charting the patient for subcutaneous or intravenous morphine. If the patient is allergic to morphine, consider fentanyl. If the patient has ongoing issues with pain relief, make a referral to the Acute Pain Service (APS).

NEUTROPENIC ENTEROCOLITIS

Also known as typhlitis, neutropenic enterocolitis (NEC) is a life-threatening and necrotising inflammation of the intestines seen in patients with an absolute neutrophil count of $<1.0 \times 10^9$/L. Seen most commonly in patients with haema-tological malignancy, it is thought to occur secondary to loss of mucosal integrity from chemotherapeutic agents, allowing passage of pathogens into various layers of the bowel wall. Intramural inflammation, oedema and necrosis play a role in causing the symptoms experienced by patients. People with NEC are often concur-rently bacteraemic.

Diagnosis and natural history

Neutropenic enterocolitis should be suspected in a patient known to be neutro-penic with the symptoms of abdominal pain (particularly in the right upper quadrant), fevers and abdominal distension. Patients may also report nausea and vomiting, diarrhoea, cramping and frank PR bleeding.

Examination should focus on the gastrointestinal system, but also aim to exclude other sources of infection. A peritonitic abdomen should lead to an urgent erect chest X-ray and surgical referral due to the risk of perforation.

The differential diagnosis for NEC includes acute appendicitis, acute graft-versus-host disease, cytomegalovirus colitis, ischaemic bowel, cholecystitis and viral gastroenteritis. If neutropenic colitis goes unrecognised or untreated, it can result in death due to perforation, bowel necrosis or overwhelming sepsis.

Investigations

A CT-abdomen is the preferred imaging modality for NEC, ideally with both oral and IV contrast. Basic blood work should be requested (FBE + UEC + CMP + CRP ± LFT if right upper quadrant pain present) and, due to the high incidence of bacteraemia, blood cultures would also be advisable. Stool cultures (with *Clostridium difficile* toxin) should also be considered. Barium enemas and colonoscopy should be avoided acutely due to the risk of perforation.

Management

Management ranges from the supportive to surgical, depending on the clinical state of the patient. Uncomplicated patients should be placed on 'bowel rest' with appropriate IV rehydration, placement of a nasogastric tube, parenteral nutrition, broad-spectrum antibiotics and blood products as required. Regardless, an early surgical referral should be made so the surgical team is 'aware' of the patient.

Surgery is avoided on a patient with acute NEC due to neutropenia and thrombocytopenia but, if the patient has a perforation, it cannot be delayed. Antibiotic regimens are similar to febrile neutropenic patients, and should cover Gram-negative bacilli and anaerobes. A standard choice is piperacillin/tazobactam 4.5 g IV TDS. Severely neutropenic patients may be considered for G-CSF. Patients should have their subsequent cycles of chemotherapy delayed until they have fully recovered from neutropenic enterocolitis.

SIDE EFFECTS OF CHEMOTHERAPY

It is unlikely you will have had a lot of prior experience with chemotherapy as a student or intern. As such, the ward registrars and pharmacists will be valuable sources of information when dealing with these new classes of drugs. Some of the chemotherapeutic agents have 'classic' side effects in addition to the myelosuppression and gastrointestinal upset the majority of them cause. A select few seen with commonly used drugs are listed in Table 42.5.

TABLE 42.5 Specific side effects of common chemotherapeutic agents

CHEMOTHERAPY	SPECIFIC SIDE EFFECTS
5-Fluorouracil	• Mucositis and diarrhoea (can be dose-limiting) • Cardiotoxicity • Mood change • Maculopapular eruptions
Alemtuzumab	• Neutropenia • GI upset • Flu-like symptoms

TABLE 42.5 Specific side effects of common chemotherapeutic agents—cont'd

CHEMOTHERAPY	SPECIFIC SIDE EFFECTS
Arsenic	• Cardiotoxicity – prolonged QT_C
Bevacizumab	• GI upset • Hypertension • Osteonecrosis (very rare)
Bleomycin	• Interstitial pneumonitis
Cetuximab	• Acne-like rash, usually on trunk and face • Flu-like symptoms • GI upset • LFT derangement • Peripheral neuropathy
Cisplatin	• Nephrotoxicity • Neurotoxicity • Haemolytic anaemia • Extreme nausea
Cyclophosphamide	• Haemorrhagic cystitis • Oliguria • Fatigue • Syndrome of inappropriate ADH secretion
Cytarabine	• Neurotoxicity • Mucositis • Keratitis
Doxorubicin (a.k.a. adriamycin) and idarubicin	• Cardiotoxicity with congestive cardiac failure • Typhlitis • Palmar/plantar erythrodysaesthesia
Etoposide	• Haematuria from haemorrhagic cystitis • Secondary and usually refractory leukaemia
Hydroxyurea	• Thrombocytopenia • Leucopenia
Ifosfomide	• Haematuria
Ipilimumab	• Acne-like rash • Diarrhoea • Lethargy • Vitiligo • Infertility • LFT derangement

continued

TABLE 42.5 Specific side effects of common chemotherapeutic agents—cont'd

CHEMOTHERAPY	SPECIFIC SIDE EFFECTS
Methotrexate	• Acute kidney injury (especially if previously hypovolaemic) • 'Methotrexate lung' • Associated with fluid overload (due to mode of delivery) • Myelosuppression
Nivolumab	• Diarrhoea • Malaise • Rash • Infertility • Thyroid disturbance
Oxaliplatin	• Neurotoxicity (progressive, dose-related peripheral neuropathy) • Ototoxicity
Trastuzumab	• Myalgias • Lethargy
Vincristine	• Peripheral neuropathy • Constipation • Hyponatraemia

Adapted from: Australian Medicines Handbook Pty Ltd, 2014. In: Australian Medicines Handbook [Internet]. Adelaide: Australian Medicines Handbook Pty Ltd. <http://amhonline-amh-net-au>.

CHAPTER 43

HAEMATOLOGY

Joseph M O'Brien

Haematology ('Haem') is an excellent learning rotation, where you will encounter very sick patients who need careful management. The majority of inpatients in most units will be patients with a haematological malignancy; however, Haematology also admits patients with other pathologies of blood (e.g. thrombophilias, aplastic anaemia) when necessary. Refer closely to Chapter 42, 'Medical Oncology', for assistance with managing haematological oncology patients with complications (including febrile neutropenia, tumour lysis, spinal cord compression and mucositis).

Haematology patients often require a large amount of blood products. Consent all patients for blood products on admission, ensuring you tick the '12 month' consent option available to Haem patients. Quite often one of the residents will do a 'blood round' in the morning before ward rounds and order the required blood products from the blood bank. Be sure to keep an active crossmatch for all patients who will need blood.

HAEMOLYSIS

Haemolysis refers to a reduced survival of red blood cells (erythrocytes), often resulting in anaemia (i.e. a decreased number of erythrocytes). The normal lifespan of erythrocytes is ⁻120 days. The many causes of haemolysis are generally classified into intravascular or extravascular depending on where the pathology lies. For more in-depth coverage of anaemia, please refer to Chapter 63, 'Haematology Outpatients'.

Intravascular haemolysis refers to destruction of the erythrocytes occurring within the bloodstream, and may be due to conditions such as transfusion reactions, infection, toxins (e.g. copper, snake bites), cold agglutination disease and microangiopathic anaemias.

Extravascular haemolysis is in turn divided into defects in the red cell itself (*intrinsic*) or its environment (*extrinsic*). Intrinsic red cell defects are structural and classified into an issue with the cell membrane (e.g. hereditary spherocytosis, where the red cell ends up misshapen), haemoglobinopathy (e.g. sickle cell) or enzyme deficiencies such as glucose-6-phosphate dehydrogenase (G6PD) deficiency. Abnormally-shaped erythrocytes are unable to 'bend' to fit through the tight splenic cords, leading to their destruction. Extrinsic causes of haemolytic anaemia include splenomegaly, hepatic disease, autoimmune anaemia, infection (e.g. malaria), toxins and large granular lymphocyte leukaemia.

Generally speaking, the higher turnover of red cells leads to an increased amount of circulating bilirubin (a breakdown product of haem), a 'compensation' effect in the marrow where it attempts to generate more erythrocytes (seen on serology as reticulocytosis) and an attempt to 'correct the balance' between cell destruction and production.

Diagnosis

Haemolytic anaemias may present similar to other anaemias, with pallor, fatigue, dyspnoea and lethargy. In addition, patients may report jaundice (due to increased circulating bilirubin from destroyed erythrocytes), palpitations or, in severe or protracted cases, signs of left ventricular failure. Very rarely, prolonged exposure to free haem units can lead to pulmonary hypertension.

Ask about a patient's ethnic heritage (G6PD deficiency principally affects people of African and Mediterranean descent; hereditary spherocytosis northern Europeans; and thalassaemias people from Southeast Asia, India, China, Africa and the Mediterranean). Take a thorough medical history, particularly an accurate medications list. Ask about the patient's family history. Ask about a recent change in diet or recently changed drugs.

On examination, inspect for general, palmar and conjunctival pallor, jaundice, organomegaly, altered heart sounds (e.g. flow murmur), crackles on chest auscultation and peripheral oedema. Listen carefully for mechanical heart valves. Lymphadenopathy may suggest a more sinister underlying cause, particularly in association with splenomegaly. If pulmonary hypertension is present the patient may be tachypnoeic and hypoxic with a split S_2. A rare sign of intravascular haemolysis is darkened urine.

Natural history

In its early stages, haemolytic anaemia will be asymptomatic. As the burden of anaemia becomes higher, patients may present with the symptoms outlined above. Diagnosis may be made incidentally on serology, with a reticulocytosis being the most common finding. As anaemia progresses, patients may also experience recurrent infections, tachycardia and other dysrhythmias, mood disturbance or even ischaemic heart disease – but often jaundice leads them to present before these symptoms begin!

Investigations

The 'haemolytic screen' is outlined in Box 43.1. You will find this is quite commonly requested as investigation into anaemia (even without evidence of haemolysis) on medical rotations, so it is worth committing to memory.

In haemolytic anaemia, the haemoglobin (Hb) will be decreased, the unconjugated bilirubin (i.e. unprocessed by the liver) will be elevated, LDH (a marker of

BOX 43.1 Haemolytic screen

FBE with peripheral blood film (specifically requesting reticulocyte and spherocyte count), UEC, TSH, LDH, LFTs with fractionated bilirubin, direct antibody test (DAT) and haptoglobin ± blood cultures (if febrile)

Adapted from: Dhaliwal, G., Cornett, P.A. & Tierney Jr, L.M., 2004. Hemolytic anemia. American Family Physician 69(11), 2599–2606.

cell turnover) would be expected to be increased and haptoglobin (a carrier protein) *decreased* as it binds with loose haem and is rapidly excreted by the liver. The DAT will be positive with autoimmune causes. Reticulocytes are a form of immature erythrocyte seen when marrow ramps up production to meet demand. Spherocytes are globular erythrocytes that lack the cytoskeleton that makes normal red cells biconcave in shape. They can result from autoimmune haemolysis or hereditary spherocytosis.

If the shape of cells on the peripheral blood film is abnormal, consider a haemoglobin electrophoresis or screening for G6PD deficiency. If the anaemia is normocytic, registrars often will also request iron studies and, if it is macrocytic, consider vitamin B12 and folate. Some infectious disease (including cytomegalovirus, hepatitis, HIV and Epstein–Barr) and malignancies (e.g. chronic lymphocytic leukaemia and non-Hodgkin's) can also cause an autoimmune haemolytic anaemia, but are not routinely screened for.

Every patient with anaemia should have a cardiovascular assessment with an electrocardiogram (ECG) and chest X-ray (CXR), with high-risk patients also screened for dyslipidaemia and diabetes with fasting lipids and glucose. Clinical examination does not always demonstrate splenomegaly so, if suspicion remains high, consider an abdominal ultrasound.

Management

Once an underlying diagnosis is made, treatment aims to manage the cause of the haemolytic anaemia. If the patient's anaemia is symptomatic, their Hb is <70 g/L or they have an anaemia of <90 g/L with serious comorbidities, a transfusion of packed red blood cells (PRBC) may be considered. Patients are rarely given a single bag of PRBC, so consider charting a minimum of two units.

Lifestyle advice is necessary for people with some forms of haemolytic anaemia (e.g. patients with G6PD deficiency should avoid documented triggers [fava beans, certain medications], and autoimmune haemolysis patients should avoid cold weather). If the cause is determined to be autoimmune, steroids or immunosuppressant therapy may be initiated by a consultant.

Plasmapheresis may be an option for some patients, whereby antibodies are filtered from a patient's serum as an outpatient procedure. In severe cases of splenomegaly a referral to surgeons for a splenectomy may be considered. In end-stage cases, patients may even require allogeneic (i.e. donor) marrow stem cell transplants.

Patients diagnosed with haemolytic anaemia should have their FBE monitored on a regular basis by their local GP. Patients with autoimmune causes of anaemia should be referred to a haematologist or rheumatologist.

HAEMOPHILIA

Haemophilia refers to rare, inherited coagulation factor deficiencies. Haemophilia A reflects a deficit in factor VIII activity, haemophilia B (a.k.a. Christmas disease) results from factor IX inactivity and haemophilia C (a.k.a. Rosenthal syndrome) results from factor XI deficiency. Rarely, if a patient has sufficiently low factor levels they may develop auto-antibodies against them (known as inhibitors).

If the family history is unknown and they are not detected on screening, diathesis (i.e. a susceptibility to bleed) is the most common presentation. This may be as a result of minor trauma or a procedure, or haemoarthrosis (bleeding into joints), mucosal bleeding or, more rarely, intracranial haemorrhage.

Due to the predominantly X-linked pattern of inheritance of both haemophilia A and B, they are more common in males. Spontaneous mutations may occur, and females may exhibit the disease if they have an affected father and carrier mother but are much more likely to simply remain unaffected carriers. There are a number of mutations that result in haemophilias and this is believed to partially account for the variance in severity of disease among individuals.

Diagnosis

Presentation varies based on the severity of disease. In some haemophilia patients (especially A), it may present at birth during minor procedures such as circumcision when bleeding is noted to be abnormally prolonged. Spontaneous haemorrhages may occur in patients with severe disease, with common sites including into joints (haemarthrosis), the urinary or gastrointestinal tracts and the cranial vault.

When taking a history from a patient with diathesis, it is important to ask them about the frequency of episodes, time taken to clot and the need for intervention in the past. Discuss the presence or absence of haemoptysis, haematemesis, melaena, haematuria, haematochezia, haemarthrosis, fatigue, dyspnoea, recurrent infections and spontaneous bruising. Ask about fevers, sweats, weight loss, anorexia, chills and rigors. Past history should include transfusions, surgeries and any complications and any history of trauma. A detailed family history is *vital*; consider drawing a genogram. Due to the chronic nature of haemophilia, consider screening for mental health issues.

If the patient is known to have haemophilia, ask what type, when and how they were diagnosed, how frequently they require transfusions, what treatment they have had (especially factor replacement), if they have had any complications of said treatment, if they know whether there is an autoimmune component to their disease, who their haematologist and dentist are, if they have had genetic counselling, if they exercise regularly and how regularly they have bloods (and who checks them). If the patient with haemophilia is older (i.e. was receiving transfusions prior to 1992), ask about their infectious disease history and if they have been screening for hepatitis A, B and C, cytomegalovirus (CMV), Epstein–Barr virus (EBV) and HIV. If the patient is female and considering starting a family, she should be referred to an appropriate obstetrician.

Examination should concentrate on potential sites of bleeding, in particular the skin, GI and urinary tracts and joints. When examining joints note any swelling, bruising, warmth, tenderness, crepitus on movement, range of motion, instability and atrophy of muscles proximal and distal to the joint. Note tachycardia, tachypnoea, hypotension and orthostasis, which might suggest current anaemia or even current going bleeding. A central nervous system (CNS) examination would be advisable if time permits. If the patient is older, review for signs of infection with hepatitis and HIV. If a GI bleed is suspected, perform a gentle digital rectal examination (if not neutropenic).

Natural history

Haemophilia is a genetic condition, and as such is currently incurable. It does not progress as such, but patients should be increasingly aware of their vulnerability to bleed as they age. As people with haemophilia get older, doctors will be tempted to place them on medications that can exacerbate their disease (e.g. aspirin, NSAIDs, anticoagulants) so patient education is vital.

Long-term complications include joint damage (particularly with recurrent haemarthrosis), ischaemic heart disease, infection from transfusions (although now rare, at one stage 70% of haemophiliacs were HIV positive) and intracranial haemorrhage resulting in potentially permanent disability.

Haemophilia is classified as mild, moderate or severe based on the clinical severity and percentage of factor activity as outlined in Table 43.1. Severe haemophilia can be very limiting and the risk of life-threatening haemorrhage is ever-present.

Investigations

All patients with abnormal bleeding should have an FBE, UEC, CMP, LFT, TSH and coagulation studies. Typically, the partial thromboplastin time is prolonged. Factors VIII and IX should be quantified. Consider C-reactive protein (CRP) and erythrocyte sedimentation rate (ESR) if an autoimmune component is suspected.

TABLE 43.1 Classification of haemophilia

CLASS	FACTOR ACTIVITY (%)	HAEMORRHAGE CAUSE
Mild	>5–40	Major trauma; surgery
Moderate	1–5	Mild trauma
Severe	<1	Spontaneous

Adapted from: White, G.C., Rosendaal, F., Aledort, L.M., et al., 2001. Definitions in hemophilia. Thrombosis and Haemostasis – Stuttgart 85(3), 560–560.

If anaemic, request vitamin B12, folate and iron studies and consider a haemolytic screen if jaundiced. Although not routine, consider vitamin K levels if vitamin K deficiency is suspected. Send blood cultures if febrile. If the patient has been transfused prior to 1992, consider requesting hepatitis B core antibody and surface antigen, and hepatitis C and HIV antigens.

If haemarthrosis is suspected, request a plain X-ray or ultrasonography of the joint and refer to Orthopaedics for consideration of arthroscopy or joint aspiration (hips in particular are susceptible to avascular necrosis of the femoral head and tend to be aspirated).

If haemoptysis is present, begin with a CXR but have a low threshold for requesting CT-chest. If there are abnormal neurological signs, consider a CT- or MRI-brain and spinal column (access to CT is typically faster). If gastrointestinal bleeding is suspected, a nuclear red cell scan or CT-angiography could be requested but the patient will likely need Gastroenterology or Surgery referral for endoscopy.

Management

At baseline, patients with haemophilia require close monitoring with some cohorts requiring regular transfusions (i.e. they are transfusion-dependent). Preventative care is important – patients should be advised to build joint and muscle strength with low-impact exercise (e.g. jogging or swimming), undergo regular dental review and avoid situations with a possibility of trauma.

Children with haemophilia should have an emergency plan (similar to a child with asthma) and daycare centres and schools should be notified. If a patient is a new diagnosis, offer to link them with the Haemophilia Foundation. Opportunistic vaccinations for hepatitis B, influenza and pneumococcus are recommended.

Aspirin, NSAIDs, antiplatelet agents and anticoagulants should be avoided and their GP notified. Offer genetic counselling for new patients with a new diagnosis or those planning on beginning a family. Orthopaedic referral may be made for patients experiencing significant joint pain, particularly in the setting of recurrent intraarticular bleeds. Consider osteoporosis screening with bone mineral density scans 2–5 yearly.

Patients with more severe diseases may be on regular factor replacement to achieve levels of >1% factor activity. Factors are either plasma-derived from donor serum or recombinant (i.e. made in a lab). Recombinant factors are much costlier than plasma-derived alternatives. Mild haemophilia A can be managed with desmopressin subcutaneously (0.3 mcg/kg up to 20 mcg maximum), which stimulates release of factor VIII from storage sites in the endothelium.

Acute haemorrhage should be managed like any other patient bleeding. If the patient is unstable (tachycardic, hypotensive) move them to a resuscitation area and escalate. Patients should be consented and transfused PRBC with the same threshold as patients without haemophilia. If the patient is thrombocytopenic (i.e. $<50 \times 10^9$/L and actively bleeding) transfuse pools of platelets simultaneously. Do not forget to activate the massive transfusion protocol if necessary (see Chapter 24, 'Managing fluids and infusions').

Factor concentrate (either VIII or IX) or tranexamic acid may be given to control bleeding in some situations, but initiating this treatment is usually a consultant-level decision. Patients can be taught to self-administer at home to prevent admissions. Referrals to Gastroenterology, General Surgery, Colorectal, Urology and Orthopaedics should be made as required for surgical management of bleeding.

The future for haemophiliac treatment looks bright, with significant advances being made in genetic therapy. A British trial successfully induced production of factor IX in six type B haemophiliacs with a combination of fibroblast gene therapy and immunosuppressants in 2011, with a 100% 2-year response. It is hoped that this will become a viable treatment for patients with haemophilia in years to come.

PANCYTOPENIA

Pancytopenia (*pan* = all; *cyto* = cells, *penia* = not many) is a haematological state characterised by a reduction in the circulating erythrocytes (anaemia), white cells (leukopenia) and platelets (thrombocytopenia). It is not a diagnosis, but rather a condition requiring prompt investigation. Pancytopenia should be differentiated from aplastic anaemia, which despite the presence of anaemia in the nomenclature actually refers to a distinct lack of pluripotent stem cells of haematopoiesis (i.e. blood-generating), possibly due to a lymphocytic autoimmune reaction.

Pancytopenia is not uncommon, with risk factors including chronic viral illness (e.g. HIV), malignancy, certain medications use and prior chemoradiotherapy. It is life-threatening if not managed swiftly. Morbidity and mortality are dependent on the underlying cause, with wide-ranging triggers for pancytopenia. There is a biphasic peak incidence in the 3rd and 7th decades.

Diagnosis

Patients may present with symptoms of failure of each of the three dominant cell lines – erythroid (fatigue, dyspnoea, chest tightness), myeloid (recurrent infection, malaise, fevers) and megakaryocytes (spontaneous or minimal-trauma bleeding). Symptoms of malignancy may also be present (rigors, sweats, chills, anorexia or weight loss).

History should cover any medical history, family history and past history. A medication list is essential, as many drugs can contribute to myelosuppression (including anti-epileptics, chloramphenicol and sulfonamides). Ask about exposure to chemicals, radiation and any recent viral symptoms. Quantify their alcohol and tobacco use. Enquire about the possibility of pregnancy.

Examination similarly should evaluate the extent to which the lack of cell lines has affected the patient. Note pallor, clubbing, organomegaly, petechiae and bruising, lymphadenopathy and bony tenderness. Remember to inspect the oral cavity for mucocutaneous petechiae and neutropenic ulcers. Look for signs of infection

– auscultate the heart and lungs and palpate the abdomen carefully. Note any signs of left ventricular failure. Consider a testicular examination in men and breast examination in women as part of malignancy screening.

Investigations

A full set of bloods sent marked 'urgent' is vital. Consider FBE with blood film (essential for diagnosis), UEC (note renal function), CMP (hypercalcaemia is associated with malignancy), LFT, TSH, LDH, coagulation studies, uric acid, iron studies and peripheral blood flow cytometry (expensive, and potentially unnecessary if you plan on performing a bone marrow). Depending on the history, also consider a nutritional screen (B12, folate, iron studies) and haemolytic screen. If febrile, request blood cultures, a urine M/C/S, faecal M/C/S with *Clostridium difficile* toxin, nasopharyngeal airway swab for respiratory multiplex PCR and a sputum M/C/S.

Imaging should always include a CXR. An abdominal ultrasound is often performed to review the liver and spleen. Consider a CT-abdomen/pelvis if the patient has a significantly tender abdomen to exclude neutropenic enterocolitis (conveniently you will also get measurements of the liver and spleen).

A bone marrow aspirate and trephine (BMAT; also known as bone marrow biopsy) is required to distinguish aplastic anaemia (a direct marrow failure) from a malignant cause. These are performed by advanced trainees in Haematology. If completing a pathology slip, request, 'Morphology + immunohistochemistry + flow cytometry + cytogenetics ± molecular studies', and complete as much clinical history as possible to guide the laboratory registrar. In aplastic anaemia, there is a hypocellular marrow without malignant cells or fibrosis and, if any haematopoietic cells are present, they are morphologically normal. A haematological malignancy will often (but not always) be evident in the marrow.

If there is a very high suspicion of malignancy and the patient appears to be a good candidate for chemotherapy, they will often get respiratory function tests (RFTs), a transthoracic echocardiogram (TTE) to assess their left ventricular ejection fraction (LVEF) and a 24-hour creatinine clearance (CrCl) to assess the dose they will tolerate.

Management

Pancytopenia is a life-threatening condition, which requires a hasty and accurate diagnosis. As such admission for pancytopenia should be reviewed quickly and investigated as a priority. A typical plan may include:

1   Admit in a barrier-nursed bed under Haematology or a General Medical unit with their regular medications and DVT prophylaxis *only* if platelets are >50.

a   Cease any medications known to cause myelosuppression.

b   Cease antiplatelet agents and NSAIDs if platelets <100.

2   Request required imaging.

3 Request an urgent BMAT – consent the patient, complete the pathology slip for the Haematologist and place the paperwork in an obvious place (these get lost far too often!).

4 Transfusion of PRBC if Hb <70 or symptomatic anaemia. Remember to consent patient for blood products.

5 Transfusion of pools of platelets if platelets <10 × 10^9/L (any setting), <20 if febrile or <50 and planned for a minor procedure.

6 Very low threshold for commencing high-dose, broad-spectrum, IV antibiotics (e.g. 4.5 g IV piperacillin/tazobactam QID and vancomycin as per protocol if high suspicion of MRSA).

7 Consideration of antiviral (valacyclovir 500 mg PO daily), antifungal (fluconazole 200 mg PO daily), tumour lysis syndrome (allopurinol 300 mg PO daily) and *Pneumocystis jirovecii* pneumonia (Bactrim® DS or trimethoprim/sulfamethoxazole 160/800 mg PO daily) prophylaxis.

8 Iron infusion (e.g. 1 g iron polymaltose in 250 mL normal saline) if iron deplete.

9 Consider referral for PET imaging.

Once a diagnosis is reached, management concentrates on treating the cause of the pancytopenia. Myelodysplastic syndromes, haematological malignancy and solid tumour malignancy with a marrow-infiltrative component may require chemotherapy, but this is entirely a consultant-level decision. True aplastic anaemia often needs bone marrow transplantation or immunosuppression. Your role as the resident is to ensure these patients are stable until able to receive treatment and specialist opinion.

DISSEMINATED INTRAVASCULAR COAGULOPATHY

Disseminated intravascular coagulopathy (a.k.a. DIC or consumptive coagulopathy) is a life-threatening, acquired disorder of coagulation characterised by over-activation of the clotting cascade and resulting in formation of fibrin and clotting in small and medium-sized vessels. It may present acutely, or as an insidious and subclinical process.

Triggers or 'pro-coagulants' include infection (especially severe sepsis), malignancy, obstetric complications (e.g. preeclampsia), trauma with widespread endothelial damage, pancreatitis, liver failure, envenomation and transfusion reactions with ABO incompatibility. Some people have an inherited predisposition (e.g. protein C deficiency). DIC is common, affecting 1% of patients hospitalised in tertiary centres.

Diagnosis

The diagnosis of acute DIC should be suspected in any patient with severe bleeding with or without widespread clotting, as the consumption of platelets leads to a tendency to bleed faster than the formation of fibrin develops into clinically relevant clots. This alteration in the balance of bleeding and clotting initially leads to prolonged prothrombin time (PT) and activated partial thromboplastin time (aPTT) with thrombocytopenia. Fibrinogen drops, as it and fibrin are consumed and their degradation products increase the level of anticoagulation.

Signs and symptoms may include bleeding (of any source), acute kidney injury, liver injury, acute respiratory distress, shock, VTE or cerebrovascular disease. Chronic DIC may be asymptomatic, with many of the altered parameters outlined above compensated. Patients with chronic DIC are more likely to have a history of malignancy or VTE in the absence of thrombocytopenia. History from a patient should cover:

- complete medical history, especially regarding malignancy, liver disease and medications
- past history, especially recent surgery
- signs of end-organ damage, including urine output, abdominal pain, confusion, angina, dyspnoea and neurological symptoms
- the development of any new rashes
- if pregnant, a complete obstetric history including past births and pregnancies and any complications
- quantification of alcohol and tobacco consumption.

Examination should aim to elicit the cause for DIC, remembering the causes outlined above (transfusion reaction, sepsis, malignancy, trauma and obstetric complications). Note any infusions the patient is on in particular, as heparin may induce a thrombocytopenia that mimics DIC. Examine all lines (including cannulas) for signs of profuse bleeding.

Natural history

The natural course of DIC begins with exposure to a procoagulant and progresses to coagulation as the platelets aggregate and consumes fibrin. When the thrombi formed begin to break down, they release fibrin degradation products that prevent fibrin clot formation and platelet aggregation elsewhere. The alteration in the balance of the clotting cascade can lead initially to bleeding complications, and ultimately to tissue damage from hypoperfusion and venous thromboembolic events.

Long-term complications in survivors depend on the tissues affected. Those people who experience end-organ damage will likely suffer sequelae of those particular insults (e.g. those who have cerebrovascular disease may need stroke rehabilitation).

Investigations

DIC is a syndrome, the cause of which should be determined hastily. Investigations aim to both assess the severity of coagulation disturbance and elicit a cause. An FBE with blood film and coagulation studies are essential – with acute DIC, expect to see thrombocytopenia, prolonged PT, prolonged aPTT and low fibrinogen.

The blood film will often demonstrate schistocytes, that is severed erythrocytes (a subtype of which is famously referred to as 'helmet cells' due to their shape).

Although not necessary for diagnosis, a D-dimer would be expected to be positive. In DIC, the clumped platelets deplete the coagulation factors. Hence in DIC, the PT and PTT are prolonged but, in HUS/TTP, they are normal.

Also request a UEC and CMP to assess renal function, and LFTs to review for liver injury. The FBE and coagulation studies are often repeated serially to monitor progression and response to therapy. A CXR may be used to exclude an infective source, but imaging is not always helpful in managing a patient with DIC.

Management

Treatment for DIC requires diagnosis of the underlying cause (e.g. management of burns or antibiotics for sepsis). Any instigating factor (e.g. blood transfusion or treatment-dose heparin infusion) should be immediately ceased. A typical plan for DIC may include:

1 Admission (if not already an inpatient) under Haematology or General Medicine with regular medications. Heparin VTE prophylaxis should be continued.

2 Urgent transfusion of fresh frozen plasma (FFP) at a rate of 10–15 mL/kg to normalise the INR.

3 Transfusion of pools of platelets if platelets $<10 \times 10^9$/L.

4 Transfusion of cryoprecipitate (dose of 1 international unit/5 kg) if fibrinogen <1.5 g/dL.

5 Consider serial FBE + coagulation studies.

6 Antithrombin-III may be used in dire cases where the patient is believed to be able to survive the episode of DIC with support. It is usually cost-prohibitive, and should absolutely be discussed with a registrar (or even consultant) before consideration of use.

7 Close monitoring of the patient, preferably in an HDU setting.

8 Monitoring for end-organ damage, including acute kidney injury, skin changes, liver dysfunction and neurological damage.

Patients with acute DIC have a very high mortality, with more than 75% of patients dying during the current admission. Those who survive should be monitored closely for complications and will likely require a lengthy hospital stay. Once the insult to the coagulation system has been rectified, the majority of patients will gradually return to normal lab values with no need for long-term monitoring of FBE and coagulation studies once discharged.

HAEMATOLOGICAL MALIGNANCIES

Patients with haematological malignancies will account for a large portion of the inpatients managed by the Haematology team. Haematological cancers include multiple myeloma, leukaemia and lymphoma. This patient cohort tends to be very

CHAPTER 44

RHEUMATOLOGY

Joseph M O'Brien

Rheumatology is a rare rotation for junior doctors; however, few junior doctors would make it through their intern year without encountering numerous patients with rheumatological issues! Many residents perform a shared role between Rheumatology and another specialty, as few patients tend to be admitted under the 'Rheum' bed card.

Rheumatology is a wide-ranging specialty covering diseases of the joints, bones, muscles and other connective tissues. Common referrals include joint pain for investigation, gout and joint effusions, but you will also be exposed to some fascinating, rarer illnesses such as scleroderma and some of the various vasculitides.

Tasks you will need to be familiar with include performing joint aspirations and injections, running efficient clinics and charting outpatient charts (e.g. infliximab or bisphosphonates). A unique job is care of patients who have had yttrium-90 (^{90}Y) joint injections for rheumatoid arthritis (RA), who are admitted for 48 hours after their injection for monitoring and require physiotherapy review prior to discharge. Please note RA and crystal arthropathies are covered in Chapter 64, 'Rheumatology outpatients'.

SERONEGATIVE SPONDYLOARTHROPATHIES

Spondyloarthropathy refers to disease of the joints of the vertebral column and sacroiliac joints, and as such refers to a range of diseases. Spondyloarthritis is inflammation of said vertebral joints. Seronegative spondyloarthropathies (SpA) are a group of often overlapping diseases including ankylosing spondylitis, reactive arthritis (a.k.a. Reiter's syndrome), psoriatic arthritis, enteropathic (i.e. those associated with inflammatory bowel disease) and undifferentiated spondyloarthropathy (with a moderate overlap).

Despite a similarity in presentation, due to the fact rheumatoid factor is negative on serum these diseases are classed separately from rheumatoid arthritis as 'seronegative' spondyloarthropathies. Globally, SpA are quite common affecting up to 2% of the population.

Pathogenesis is complex and not entirely understood, but strongly associated with the presence of the major histocompatibility complex HLA-B27 (although negative serology does not *exclude* SpA). This antigen plays a role in identifying microorganisms to the T cells of the immune system, and is seen more commonly in Caucasians and people of Chinese descent. Inflammation involves the abnormal activation of T cells and cytokine pathways (including TNF-α).

The most common affected sites are the muscular and ligamentous insertion sites into bone (the 'entheses'), inflammation of which is known as enthesopathy. Other common features among the various SpA include extra-articular features (e.g. uveitis, dermatitis and gastrointestinal features), a typically asymmetrical and oligoarthritic (i.e. only a few joints) presentation and familial inheritance. Matrix metalloproteinase-3 (MMP-3) is an enzyme over-expressed in SpA, and hence sometimes used as a marker of disease activity. Identifying features of the various SpA are shown in Table 44.1.

Diagnosis

Patients will most frequently present with joint pain – typically over the lumbar back, but also with soft tissue oedema or joint effusions of the lower limbs with decreased range of motion. Features that may help you differentiate the

TABLE 44.1 Differentiating features of spondyloarthopathies

FEATURE	ANKYLOSING SPONDYLITIS	ENTEROPATHIC ARTHRITIS	REACTIVE ARTHRITIS	PSORIATIC ARTHRITIS
Age	20s–40s	Any age	20s	30s–40s
Sex (M:F)	3:1	1:1	5–10:1	1:1
Sacroiliitis	Symmetrical	Symmetrical	Either	Asymmetrical
Peripheral disease	Less common; lower extremities	Common; lower extremities	Common; lower extremities	Common; *upper* extremities
Spinal disease	Common	Common	Less common, discontinuous	Less common
Dactylitis	Uncommon	Uncommon	Common	Most common
Enthesitis	Classic	Uncommon	Common	Common
Extraskeletal disease	Occasional uveitis, aortic regurgitation	Inflammatory bowel disease, occasional uveitis, aortic regurgitation	Most common uveitis, conjunctivitis, urethritis, occasional aortic regurgitation	Occasional uveitis, conjunctivitis, urethritis
HLA-B27	90% white 50% African	50%	80%	60%

Adapted from: Asghar, F.A., Graziano, G.P. & Kuntz, C., 2011. Chapter 281: Spondyloarthropathies (including ankylosing spondylitis). In: Winn, H.R., Berger, M.S. & Dacey, R.G., Jr., eds. Youmans Neurological Surgery, 6th ed. Philadelphia: Elsevier Saunders, Table 281.1.

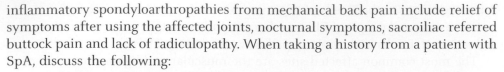

inflammatory spondyloarthropathies from mechanical back pain include relief of symptoms after using the affected joints, nocturnal symptoms, sacroiliac referred buttock pain and lack of radiculopathy. When taking a history from a patient with SpA, discuss the following:

- When and how were they diagnosed with SpA? How old were they? Where was their serology performed? Do they have a rheumatologist or GP managing their condition? Have they ever been hospitalised for their disease? Have they had a joint aspiration?

- Where do they experience pain (i.e. how many and which joints are affected)? Are their joints swollen, tender, warm or deformed? Have they lost function of any joints? What time of day are their symptoms worst? Are they ever woken by their symptoms? Are they relieved or exacerbated by activity?

- Have they ever had any of the extra-skeletal manifestations, such as uveitis (inflammation of the middle layer of the eye), conjunctivitis, costochondritis (inflammation of cartilaginous structures), plantar fasciitis, Achilles tendinitis or urethritis (inflammation of the urethra causing dysuria)? Have they had any dermatological signs (e.g. mucocutaneous lesions)? Do they have a heart murmur (i.e. screening for aortic regurgitation, common in SpA)?

- What treatment have they had for their SpA? Have they experienced any complications or required an escalation of therapy?

- What is their complete medical history, taking particular note of psoriasis, inflammatory bowel disease (IBD) and other rheumatological and autoimmune diseases? Have they ever had surgery?

- What is their occupation? Does their disease affect their activities of daily living (ADLs) at work or home? Are they able to clean, cook, drive, dress themselves and maintain self-hygiene without assistance? Do they use any gait aids? How does their arthritis affect their exercise tolerance?

Examination primarily focuses on the affected joints, but should also cover the common sites of extra-skeletal disease. Note particularly joint effusions, tenderness, erythema, warmth, instability (tested in two planes, e.g. vertical and horizontal), decreased range of motion and loss of function (tested in two manners, e.g. unbuttoning a shirt and putting a key into a lock and unlocking it). Inspect for spinal tenderness, dactylitis (i.e. 'sausage fingers'), chest wall tenderness, enthesitis at the heel (i.e. insertion of Achilles tendon) and signs of long-term steroid use (Cushingoid facies, striae, thin skin, proximal myopathy, cataracts, hypertension), psoriasis (keratinous plaques, alopecia, dactylitis) and inflammatory bowel disease (tender abdomen, cachexia, pallor, fistulae). Listen for a decrescendo diastolic murmur suggestive of aortic regurgitation, which can occur secondary to aortitis. Ask the patient about lesions on their genitalia, and consider examination if appropriate. To identify uveitis properly, a slit lamp examination should be performed.

Natural history

The course of illness for the various SpA is variable, but in general they are chronic conditions interspersed with acute flares. Of note, the patient with an undifferentiated SpA may identify itself as a specific kind of disease as time progresses (e.g. with a first presentation of inflammatory bowel disease). 75% of undifferentiated SpA patients achieved remission at 2 years, in comparison with 10% of ankylosing spondylitis patients and only 2% of patients with psoriatic arthritis.

Investigations

On initial work-up, patients suspected of having a SpA should have basic blood work (FBE + UEC + CMP + LFT) as well as baseline inflammatory markers (erythrocyte sedimentation rate or ESR; and C-reactive protein or CRP). A 'rheumatology panel' should be requested, including rheumatoid factor (RF), antinuclear antibody (ANA), anti-neutrophil cytoplasmic antibody (ANCA), anti-double-stranded DNA (anti-dsDNA) and anti-citrullinated protein antibody (anti-CCP).

If the patient is febrile perform blood cultures, looking for an infective trigger. Consider testing for HIV in patients with risk factors. Discuss with your registrar testing for HLA-B27 – although expensive, it can assist in diagnosis. If a joint effusion is present, consider aspiration and biochemical analysis.

Imaging should include plain films of affected joints. Some classic features include 'bamboo spine' in ankylosing spondylitis (i.e. marginal protrusions called syndesmophytes simulate the appearance of single, long bone in the spine; see Fig. 44.1) and squaring of vertebral bodies. These usually begin in the lumber region and spread superiorly.

A pelvic X-ray should also be requested, specifying sacroiliac views. Typical features include erosive changes at the symphis pubis and 'whiskering' or areas of ossification at the ileum and femoral trochanters. Discitis may also be noted. CT and MRI are *not* always necessary, and tend to show the same changes in greater detail. They may be performed if plain films fail to demonstrate sacroiliitis but the diagnosis remains strongly suspected. Bone mineral density may show a decrease in trabecular bone.

Management

Management should be holistic, involving both non-pharmaceutical and drug treatments to optimise the patient's function. A typical plan may include the following:

1 Confirmation of diagnosis with serology and imaging.
2 Detailed patient education about the nature of SpA.
3 Review by physiotherapy with generation of an exercise plan, avoiding high-impact activities due to the risk of fracture.
4 Continuation of regular medications, and DVT prophylaxis if admitted.

SECTION IV

associated illnesses such as the connective tissue disorders. A neurological exami-nation is strongly advised. Auscultate the heart and lungs carefully. A complete skin check should be performed with particular attention paid to the eyes, face and extensor surfaces, with consideration of clinical photography.

The two 'classic' skin findings associated with dermatomyositis are Gottron's papules (i.e. erythematous papules on extensor surfaces between the metacar-pophalangeal and interphalangeal joints and known as Gottron's sign when on extensor surfaces of other joints) and heliotrope eruption (i.e. red to purple skin changes over the eyelids ± oedema), but may also include facial erythema and poikiloderma (i.e. both hyper- and hypopigmented skin in areas exposed to sun-light). The 'holster sign' is poikiloderma on the lateral thigh; the shawl sign is poikiloderma on the upper back; and the 'v sign' is poikiloderma around the upper chest and neck. Skin changes tend to be violaceous in dermatomyositis. Scalp involvement, nail changes and skin calcification are also seen commonly.

Natural history

Dermatomyositis and polymyositis negatively affect morbidity and mortality. Negative prognostic factors include conduction defects, malignancy, advanced age, delayed treatment >6 months, dysphagia, interstitial lung disease, respiratory muscle weakness and worse myopathy at diagnosis.

Investigations

The gold standard of diagnosis remains a muscle biopsy demonstrating types 1 and 2 fibre necrosis with degeneration and regeneration of fibres and perivascular mononuclear cells in focal collections. Typically, patients will also have an increased CK and the characteristic findings of spontaneous fibrillations, complex repetitive discharges and positive sharp waves on electromyography. Patients diagnosed for the first time should also have basic blood work (FBE + UEC + CMP) with LFT (particularly noting increased AST and ALT), LDH (often increased), TSH, a rheumatology screen (ANA + ESR + CRP ± ENA ± antisynthetase and anti-SRP antibodies) and aldolase (an enzyme found in muscle).

Consider a urine myoglobin (typically increased). Request an ECG to review for conduction defects. MRI may be used to investigate muscle inflammation, but is non-specific. At minimum, a chest X-ray should be done to inspect for interstitial lung disease and, if pulmonary symptoms are present, consider respiratory func-tion tests (RFTs) and a CT-chest. Baseline fasting glucose should be requested if starting steroids. Dysphagia should be investigated with a barium swallow.

Management

Patients presenting with dermatomyositis or polymyositis may need admission due to new-onset weakness. An example admission plan would include the following:

1 Admission under Rheumatology or General Medicine with regular
   medications + DVT prophylaxis.

2 Referral to physiotherapy and occupational therapy (OT) with significant patient education (especially about photosensitivity and falls risk in the elderly).

3 Screening for related conditions.

4 ± Inpatient muscle biopsy.

5 Trial of glucocorticoids at 1 mg/kg/day (maximum 80 mg) for 4–6 weeks, to aim to improve strength and preserve motor function.

6 Consideration of progression to further therapy if required.

7 Pruritus may be subsided with 10 mg PO cetirizine daily.

8 Monitoring for side effects of steroids (including BSL chart).

9 Opportunistic vaccines, particularly prior to starting immunosuppressants.

The patient's prednisolone dose should be very slowly weaned over a year (e.g. by 10 mg/week to 40 mg/day, then tapered by 5 mg/week to 20 mg/day, then after 7 days at 20 mg/day tapered by 2.5 mg/week to 10 mg/day, then after 7 days at 10 mg/day tapered by 1 mg/week to 5 mg/day). Response to therapy at the quadriceps or deltoids should be closely monitored by either their specialist or GP.

If refractory to glucocorticoid therapy, alternative diagnoses should be sought. Continue to monitor in outpatients for malignancy, osteoporosis, infections and side effects of steroid therapy (ironically including glucocorticoid myopathy). Alternative therapies include azathioprine (started at 50 mg/day and up-titrated to 1.5 mg/kg/day and requiring TPMT enzyme testing prior to first dose) and methotrexate (usually started at 15 mg/week with 5 mg PO folate every other day). The optimal duration of immunosuppressant therapy remains unclear.

FIBROMYALGIA

Fibromyalgia (a.k.a. fibrositis) is a chronic pain disorder of unknown aetiology characterised by widespread pain, no identifiable pathology, hyperalgesia and resistance to multiple therapies. Common associated symptoms include extreme fatigue, sleep issues, headaches, irritable bowel syndrome, restless legs syndrome and psychiatric comorbidities such as anxiety and depression. It is thought to be the manifestation of a number of overlapping disorders.

A familial pattern has been noted. Patients with fibromyalgia have physiological responses to painful stimuli, and neuroimaging has demonstrated variance in structure and concentration of neurotransmitters in this cohort. Often clinical examination is normal apart from allodynia (i.e. pain from a normally non-painful stimulus), hyperalgesia (i.e. exaggerated pain from painful stimuli) or diffuse tenderness. Fibromyalgia is quite common, affecting 4% of patients in developed countries with a peak onset between 25 and 55 years. It is six times more frequent in women.

Diagnosis

Patients often present with quite non-specific symptoms, and fibromyalgia remains a diagnosis of exclusion. Common complaints include fatigue, paraesthesia, peripheral numbness, sleep disturbance, headaches and mood disturbances. Some patients describe a 'fogginess' or altered level of concentration and cognition. When taking a history from a patient with fibromyalgia, consider taking a brief psychiatric and detailed social history simultaneously. Be sure to cover their medical, past and family histories in the same detail as any other patient.

Examination may reveal diffuse, *bilateral* tenderness without obvious injury or precipitant, without any inflammation noted in musculature or joints. Perform a thorough physical examination covering joints, abdominal examination and neurological examination of the upper and lower limbs. Previous diagnoses of fibromyalgia required pain at 11 of 18 tender points with pressure firm enough to whiten the nail bed of the examiner's fingertip.

Natural history

The 2010 American College of Rheumatology Fibromyalgia Classification criteria (for research purposes) list the two features of fibromyalgia as: 'chronic, widespread pain in all four quadrants of the body and axial skeleton; and exclusion of other disorders that would otherwise explain the pain'. Symptoms should have been present for >3 months. Fibromyalgia is closely associated with restless leg syndrome, refractory migraines, anxiety, depression and irritable bowel syndrome.

Investigations

Investigations should focus on excluding alternate diagnoses, without being exhaustive and expensive. A standard work-up may include FBE (to exclude anaemia), UEC, CMP, (excluding renal failure and electrolyte disturbance), LFT, TSH (excluding hypothyroidism) and ESR + CRP (as baseline inflammatory markers). ANA and RF are not indicated unless clinical findings are indicative of autoimmune disease.

Management

Management focuses on returning the patient as close to their normal level of function as possible. This is usually achieved with limited success through a multidisciplinary approach to the patient's care, with exclusion of other organic causes for their symptoms, patient education and ample reassurance, development of an exercise program, optimisation of sleep hygiene and referral for cognitive-based therapy (CBT).

If the patient's condition is refractory to these primary steps, then low-dose pregabalin (e.g. 75 mg PO daily to BD), selective serotonin reuptake inhibitor (SSRI) *or* opiate could be considered as symptomatic treatment. Avoid polypharmacy. There is little-to-no evidence for improvement of symptoms with steroids or NSAIDs.

Any coexisting conditions such as anxiety, depression or irritable bowel syndrome should have appropriate referrals made and treatments instigated. Patients with fibromyalgia should have ongoing appointments with their GP and specialist to monitor their condition and continue to encourage and support them. Specialist pain clinics exist for truly refractory cases. If relapse occurs, the cycle begins anew with modest re-investigation and further reassurance and education. Consider a social work referral if a patient's fibromyalgia is impacting upon their activities of daily living.

TABLE 45.1 Examination of the patient with an acute abdomen

General inspection	• Introduce yourself, get an impression of the patient's current medical state • Check the patient's observations • Inspect the abdomen: note previous surgical scars, distension, obvious hernias, bruising, features of chronic disease
Palpation	• Seek to begin palpation away from areas of reported pain • Begin by lightly palpating each quadrant, looking for tenderness, followed by deep palpation. Distraction techniques can be useful, including asking questions or palpating using a stethoscope • Note areas of tenderness; determine if the patient has generalised tenderness (peritonitis) • Examine the flanks for tenderness and always check the groin for hernias • PR examination in patients with bowel disturbances or suggestion of bleeding is mandatory
Percussion	• Useful in certain circumstances including detecting organomegaly and free intra-abdominal fluid
Auscultation	• For patients with distension, checking for bowel sounds can help determine whether the patient is likely to have an obstruction • An abdominal bruit is suggestive of AAA or, less commonly, renal artery stenosis
Special tests	• Focused examination findings based on differential diagnosis (discussed throughout the chapter)

Investigations

- Investigations should be focused dependent on the differential diagnosis in patients who are suitably stable.
- Over time the junior doctor will gain experience assessing patients with an acute abdomen, recognising patterns.
- Even senior surgeons may have difficulties isolating a cause for abdominal pain in some patients, requiring admission for further tests and observation.
- Not all patients referred with abdominal pain will require admission or surgical intervention and can be appropriately followed up in outpatient clinics.
- The art and science of diagnosis relating to the acute abdomen is the subject of entire textbook chapters. We have sought to highlight the

common pathologies and hope that you learn from your experiences, pester your seniors with questions and have an open mind (just like we did!).

APPENDICITIS

Acute (sometimes chronic) inflammation of the appendix, appendicitis typically affects teenagers and young adults, though there are always exceptions.

The classic history is described as central aching abdominal pain that migrates to a sharp right iliac fossa pain, typically associated with nausea, loss of appetite. Patients progressively feel worse.

Examination

There is a wide variety of examination findings dependent on the anatomy of the appendix and severity of the patient's presentation.

- Irritation of the bladder or bowel due to a pelvic appendix can lead to dysuria or diarrhoea, respectively.
- An elongated or retrocaecal appendix may cause discomfort in the LUQ or LLQ. Always correlate the history with examination findings.
- Patients with generalised abdominal pain, fevers and evidence of peritonitis on examination should be suspected as having perforated appendicitis.
- Differential diagnosis includes: mesenteric adenitis (younger patients), ruptured ovarian cysts, pelvic pathology and gastroenteritis.
- Female patients should always have a beta HCG performed in the ED to rule out an ectopic pregnancy.

Investigations

The diagnosis of appendicitis is primarily made on clinical assessment of the patient with investigations playing a supplementary role.

- Serology: increased white cell count and an elevated CRP can confirm the presence of an inflammatory process.
- Imaging: ultrasound and CT may reveal evidence of appendicitis, but do not provide a conclusive diagnosis. CT scans are generally avoided in younger patients but may be indicated in older patients with atypical presentations.

Management

Initial management should include fluid resuscitation, analgesia and IV antibiotics.

Choledocolithiasis

Choledocolithiasis is the presence of gallstones within the biliary duct system. It is a common finding with biliary stones found in up to 10% of patients at the time of cholecystectomy.

Clinical presentation falls largely into three categories:

1 asymptomatic choledocolithiasis, discovered intraoperative for cholelithiasis or due to imaging or deranged LFTs

2 symptomatic choledocolithiasis, in which patients present with biliary type pain in the absence of obvious cholecystitis; some patients may have jaundice due to obstruction

3 complicated choledocolithiasis, manifested as pancreatitis or cholangitis.

Investigations

- LFTs may reveal elevated liver enzymes with a classic 'cholestatic picture' (elevated GGT and ALP) and elevated serum bilirubin.
  - ○ ALT and AST are commonly elevated in early obstruction.
- Ultrasound may detect choledocolithiasis, but visualisation of the entire CBD is often difficult.
- Magnetic resonance cholangiopancreatography (MRCP) provides excellent visualisation of the biliary system (see Fig. 45.5) and is commonly used to work up inpatients for choledocolithiasis.
- Endoscopic retrograde cholangiopancreatography (ERCP; see section below) is both a diagnostic and therapeutic procedure.

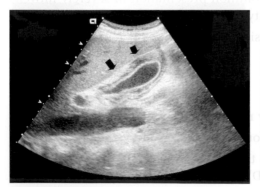

FIGURE 45.4 Abdominal US showing obvious wall thickening in cholecystitis.

Reproduced from: Kelly, K. & Weber, S., 2012. Chapter 31: Cholecystitis. In: Jarnagin, W., Blumgart's Surgery of the Liver, Biliary Tract and Pancreas, 5th ed. Saunders, pp. 487–493, Fig. 31.3.

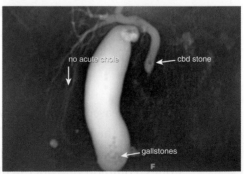

FIGURE 45.5 MRCP demonstrating a stone in the CBD.

Reproduced from: Ahmed, R. & Duncan, M., 2014. The management of common bile duct stones. In: Cameron, J., Current Surgical Therapy, 11th ed. Saunders, pp. 391–395, Fig. 1B.

TABLE 45.2 Assessing the likelihood of choledocolithiasis

PREDICTORS OF CHOLEDOCOLITHIASIS		
Very strong	Strong	Moderate
• CBD stone on abdominal US • Cholangitis • Bilirubin >68 micromol/L	• Dilated CBD on US (>6 mm) • Bilirubin 30–68 micromol/L	• Deranged LFTs (other than bilirubin) • Age >55 years • Gallstone pancreatitis
LIKELIHOOD OF CHOLEDOCOLITHIASIS		
High: any single 'very strong' predictor or both 'strong' predictors. Intermediate: any other combination of 'strong' and 'moderate' predictors. Low: no predictors present.		

Adapted from: Maple, J., Ben-Menachem, T., Anderson, M., et al., 2010. The role of endoscopy in the evaluation of suspected choledocholithiasis. Gastrointestinal Endoscopy 71(1), 1, Table 2.

Management

Management is dependent on the likelihood of choledocolithiasis (see Table 45.2).

- Patients with a high likelihood should have an ERCP
- Patients with an intermediate likelihood can have an MCRP to rule out choledocolithiasis
- Patients with low likelihood of choledocolithiasis can undergo cholecystectomy with an intra-operative cholangiogram

Cholangitis (ascending cholangitis, biliary sepsis)

Infection of the hepatic and common bile ducts is often associated with biliary tract obstruction. It is more common in older patients and those with known cholelithiasis.

Cholangitis carries a high mortality rate in severe infections.

Clinical presentation is classically RUQ pain, fever and jaundice (Charcot's triad):

- Variable, seen in 50–85% of cases.
- Addition of shock and delirium make up Reynolds' pentad.

Choledocolithiasis is the most common cause:

- Patients may have had recent intervention to the biliary system (ERCP) or surgical procedures.
- Infective organism arises from the duodenum with *E. coli* the most common.

There is a range of severity in presentations:

- Septic shock is seen in older patients with other medical comorbidities that may require rapid intensive care input and review.

- Alcohol
  - An alcohol withdrawal scale may be required for patients with dependence.
  - Counselling about the need to reduce alcohol intake is advisable.

Management of complications

- Pancreatic necrosis
  - These patients are at risk of secondary infection of necrotic collections and may require a prolonged course of IV antibiotics. Percutaneous sampling can guide therapy.
- Pancreatic collections
  - Fall into two broad categories:
    - acute pancreatic collections with no definable wall
    - pseudocysts and other walled-off collections.
  - Can be managed without intervention if causing no symptoms.
  - Symptomatic collections may be amenable to drainage via EUS.
  - Larger collections may require drainage via laparoscopy or an open approach.
- Venous thrombosis and pseudoaneurysm
  - May require the draining of adjacent collections before inflammation leads to haemorrhage.

Chronic pancreatitis

Alcohol is the cause in around 80% of patients.

Patients typically report chronic epigastric pain and acute-on-chronic attacks are common.

Patients may present with features of poor nutrition; decreased lipase production leads to steatorrhoea:

- Decreased exocrine production may require supplementation with enzymes such as Creon® (pacrelipase).
- Endocrine dysfunction manifests as diabetes mellitus requiring insulin administration.

Investigations

- Lipase may remain low even in severe acute attacks.
- CT imaging may reveal calcifications consistent with chronic inflammation.
  - Can also aid with the identification of sources of pain such as chronic pseudocysts.

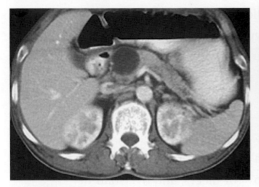

FIGURE 45.6 Pancreatic pseudocyst on CT.

Reproduced from: Rana, S.S., Sharma, V. & Reddy, S., 2015. Combined endovascular and endoscopic management of thoracic aortic pseudoaneurysm, mediastinal pseudocyst, and pancreatic pleural effusion due to chronic pancreatitis. Gastrointestinal Endoscopy 81(6), 1501–1502, Fig. 1B.

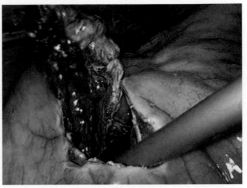

FIGURE 45.7 Laparoscopic debridement showing obviously necrotic pancreatic tissue.

Reproduced from: Ammori, B.J. & Ayiomamitis, G.D., 2013. Chapter 20: Laparoscopic management of pancreatic pseudocysts. In: Frantzides, C., Video Atlas of Advanced Minimally Invasive Surgery. Saunders, pp. 175–182, Fig. 20-9A.

Management

- Alcohol cessation, symptomatic control via analgesia and lipase supplements.
- Management of diabetes.
- Surgical debridement plays a limited role; it is only indicated in patients with severe pain and obvious anatomical abnormality or suspicious lesions (Fig. 45.7).

PEPTIC ULCERS

The role of surgery in peptic ulcer disease has changed in the past few decades, and it is now mostly indicated for treating the emergency complications of ulcer disease.

Emergency presentations of peptic ulcer disease fall into two main categories:

1 upper GI bleeding (see Chapter 37)

2 perforated ulcer.

Peptic ulcer disease refers to both the stomach and the duodenum. Causes include:

- *Helicobacter pylori* is implicated in over 70% of peptic ulcers (90% in some populations).
  - *H. pylori* eradication therapy should be instituted (Chapter 37).
- The overuse of NSAIDs also contributes to the development of ulcers.

Clinical presentations include the following:

- Around a third of patients are asymptomatic.
- Some patients have vague epigastric pain with mild nausea or reflux.
- Hematemesis and malaena.

Perforated ulcer

- Symptoms include sudden onset epigastric or diffuse abdominal pain associated with peritonitis, nausea and vomiting.
- Perforation occurs in around 5–10% of ulcers, and over half of perforations occur in the first part of the duodenum.

Investigations

- Erect CXR: gas under the diaphragm (Fig. 45.8).
- CT can detect a smaller amount (i.e. free gas not visible on plain film).

Management

- Simple peptic ulcers are suited to outpatient management with proton pump inhibitors (PPIs) and gastroscopy.
- Perforated ulcers require urgent management, with intervention desirable within 6 hours for improved outcomes.
  ○ Patients are commenced on high dose PPIs and triple IV antibiotics.
  ○ A nasogastric tube is inserted and the patient is fasted with IV fluids.
- Operative intervention includes direct ulcer repair via omental patch either laparoscopically or by an open approach (Fig. 45.9).
- Conservative management, including the use of antiplatelet medications, with close observation can be utilised in select patients who may have significant medical comorbidities.
  ○ Those who fail to improve may require intervention within 12–24 hours.
- These patients still require *H. pylori* eradication therapy.

DIVERTICULAR DISEASE

Diverticulosis is the presence of protrusions in the wall of the colon, forming sac-like pockets (Fig. 45.10). Particularly common in older populations, it is found in nearly a third of patients aged >50 years.

70% of patients are asymptomatic; the condition is only detected incidentally on imaging or colonoscopy. Around 20% of patients will develop diverticulitis. 95% of affected patients have some form of sigmoid diverticulosis.

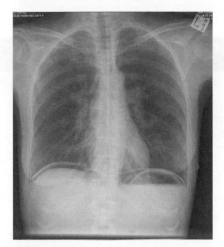

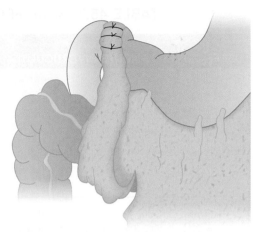

FIGURE 45.8 Erect CXR demonstrating sub-diaphragmatic air consistent with perforated viscus.

Reproduced from: Cadogan, M., Brown, A.F.T. & Celenza, I., 2012. Chapter 37: Abdominal X-ray. In: Cadogan, M., Marshall and Ruedy's On Call: Principles and Protocols, 2nd ed. Elsevier Australia, Fig. 37.4.

FIGURE 45.9 Omental patch repair of a perforated gastric ulcer.

Reproduced from: Teitelbaum, E., Hungness, E. & Mahvi, D., 2017. Chapter 48: Stomach. In: Townsend, C., Sabiston Textbook of Surgery. Saunders, pp. 1188–1236, Fig. 48-11.

Diverticulitis

Diverticulitis is an acute inflammation of diverticular disease. Faecal impaction obstruction leads to erosion of the diverticulum wall resulting in microperforation:

- Most perforations are well contained with the surrounding pericolic fat leading to a localised infection (uncomplicated diverticulitis).
- Severe infections may extend beyond the surrounding fat of the colon leading to larger collections and peritonitis.

Clinical presentation:

- Patients commonly describe LLQ pain associated with a change in bowel habit (diarrhoea or constipation); fever is sometimes present.
- Examination reveals marked tenderness in the left iliac fossa (LIF) in most cases, though diverticulitis can less commonly affect other parts of the colon.
- Patients may present clinically obstructed.

Investigations

- Serology: check inflammatory markers, which are likely to be raised.
- Imaging: CT is particularly useful, allowing for diagnosis and identification of complications in diverticulitis (see Table 45.3 and Fig. 45.11).

TABLE 45.3 The use of CT in acute diverticulitis

CT FEATURES OF ACUTE DIVERTICULITIS	COMPLICATIONS OF DIVERTICULITIS FOUND ON CT
Increased soft tissue density with pericolic fat changes (98%)	Peritonitis (diffuse inflammatory changes, scattered loculated fluid collections)
Colonic diverticula (84%)	Fistula formation
Bowel wall thickening (70%)	Bowel obstruction
Soft tissue fluid collections or abscess (35%)	Diverticular disease is indistinguishable from carcinoma of the colon in up to 10% of patients

Adapted from: O'Keefe, K. & Sanson, T., 2013. Chapter 35: Diverticulitis. In: Adams, J., Emergency Medicine, 2nd ed. Saunders, pp. 299–303, Box 35.2.

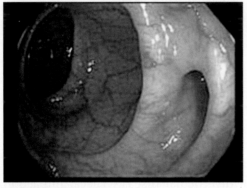

FIGURE 45.10 Diverticulosis on colonoscopy.

Reproduced from: Feuerstein, J.D. & Falchuk, K.R., 2016. Diverticulosis and diverticulitis. Mayo Clinic Proceedings 91(8), 1094–1104, Fig. 2.

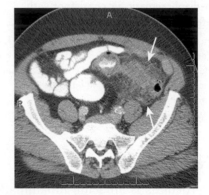

FIGURE 45.11 Sigmoid diverticulitis with fat stranding surrounding the bowel (arrows).

Reproduced from: Balachandran, A., Sagebiel, T. & Silverman, P., 2015. Chapter 111: Mesenteric and omental lesions. In: Gore, R.M. & Levine, M.S., Textbook of Gastrointestinal Radiology, 4th ed. Saunders, pp. 2036–2052, Fig. 111-22.

Management

- Uncomplicated diverticulitis can be treated with IV antibiotics and a period of bowel rest.
- Patients can be prescribed IV fluids for resuscitation and maintenance, though well patients may tolerate clear fluids.
- Larger collections may require surgical drainage.
  - A localised collection may be drained percutaneously under imaging guidance with a drain left in situ.
- Diverticula are a well-known cause of GI bleeding (Chapter 37).

Perforated diverticulum

Severe diverticulitis with gross abdominal contamination requires exploration and washout.

Typically, the perforated segment of the colon (usually sigmoid) is resected and a temporary colostomy created (Hartmann's procedure (see also the section on 'Sigmoid volvulus'). Some select patients may have a primary anastomosis formed ± defunctioning ileostomy (see the section 'Ileostomy').

TRAUMA

General Surgery units provide a trauma service for the hospital.

- Patients who present to ED with high risk injuries (see Chapter 10) activate trauma protocols that page the surgical registrar to attend.
- Primary and secondary surveys are conducted within the ED along with routine bloods and imaging.
- Following the trauma assessment, patients with no apparent injury are admitted for 24 hours of observation and a tertiary survey the following day.
  - Tertiary survey is a complete head-to-toe examination, screening for any missed or delayed injury.
  - Patients with non-life-threatening injuries (limb fractures, deep wounds) who require intervention from another surgical team still remain under General Surgery until a tertiary survey is complete.

See also further discussion of head injury (Chapter 50), thoracic trauma (Chapter 48) and limb trauma (Chapter 46).

Abdominal trauma

History and examination findings help determine the likelihood of an intra-abdominal injury.

The key decision is whether the patient requires urgent exploratory laparotomy (Table 45.4).

Investigations

- FAST (focused assessment with sonography in trauma) scans are a routine component of the trauma assessment, looking for free fluid within the abdomen, though not diagnostic (see Figs 45.12 and 45.13).
- In haemodynamically unstable patients, formal imaging may not be prudent and the patient should be taken to theatre.
- CT scans may assist in diagnosis but may not be able to identify direct injuries, such as those involving the small bowel.

SECTION IV

TABLE 45.4 Abdominal visceral injury

Liver	• Isolated liver injuries do not typically require operative intervention • Over 85% of these cases can be managed expectantly with observation • High resolution CT scans provide excellent visualisation of injury • Interventional radiology plays an important role (embolisation of bleeding vessels, percutaneous drainage of secondary abscesses) • Bile leaks may require ERCP to place a stent for high volume bile leaks
Spleen	• Similarly, over 75% of isolated splenic injuries do not require intervention • Careful monitoring is required as further splenic bleeding will require removal • Splenic preservation can be achieved via angioembolisation of the affected segment or partial splenectomy • Patients with significant splenic haematoma on CT (see Fig. 45.14) or those patients taken for urgent laparotomy typically undergo splenectomy
Bowel	• Most commonly associated with penetrating trauma; as such there is a high index of suspicion during stabbing injuries • Bowel injuries from blunt trauma can be harder to detect, though a high index of suspicion should be held for patients who have suffered high energy trauma
Diaphragm	• Diaphragmatic injuries are closely associated with intra-abdominal injuries • Penetrating diaphragm injuries often involve a thoracic component

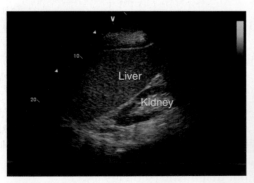

FIGURE 45.12 Negative FAST scan in RUQ, with no free fluid.

Reproduced from: McLean, A. & Huang, S., 2012. Chapter 14: The standard FAST protocol. In: McLean, A. & Huang, S., Critical Care Ultrasound Manual. Sydney: Churchill Livingston, pp. 135–143, Fig. 14.6.

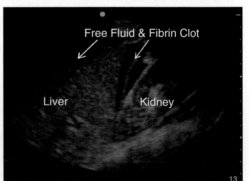

FIGURE 45.13 Free fluid on FAST scan revealed to be a haemoperitoneum.

Reproduced from: Laurich, M. & Tsung, J., 2011. Point-of-care first trimester pelvic ultrasonography for the pediatric emergency physician. Clinical Pediatric Emergency Medicine 12(1), 18-26, Fig. 7.

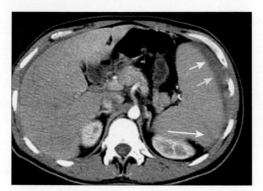

FIGURE 45.14 Subcapsular splenic haematoma on CT.

Reproduced from: Gore, R. & Levine, M., 2010. Splenic rupture. In: Gore, R., High-yield Imaging: Gastrointestinal. Saunders, pp. 764-765, Fig. 1.

Management

- The initial steps of management are instigated during assessment, including analgesia, fluid resuscitation and immobilisation.
- Full set of bloods are sent, include coagulation studies and blood cross match.
- Haemodynamic compromise necessitates rapid access to blood products and close monitoring.
- Patients who meet the criteria for exploratory laparotomy should not have unnecessary delays in transferring to theatre.
- Laparoscopy plays an increasing role in diagnosis, with progression to laparotomy if required.
- Major vascular injuries are common, associated with up to 25% of all major abdominal injuries.
- Exploratory laparotomy (see Box 45.1 for indications)
  - There are management priorities when considering a trauma laparotomy (damage control):
    - control of bleeding
    - control of contamination
    - identification of life-threatening injuries with emergency management.
  - Major trauma is associated with a state of acidosis, coagulopathy and hypothermia.
    - Once life-threatening injuries have been controlled, definitive management of other surgical pathology should be postponed in favour of continuing resuscitation in Intensive Care.
- For intra-abdominal injuries of specific organs, see Table 45.4.

SECTION IV

BOX 45.1 Indications for exploratory laparotomy

- Peritonitis
- Evisceration
- Impaled object
- Haemodynamic instability (documented or suspected intra-abdominal source)
- Associated bleeding from a natural orifice

Adapted from: Britt, L.D., 2014. Abdominal trauma. In: Cameron, J., Current Surgical Therapy, 11th ed. Saunders, pp. 1010–1021, Box 1.

BOWEL OBSTRUCTION

Small bowel obstruction (SBO)

SBO is one of the most common presentations in general surgery.

Intra-abdominal adhesions are responsible for over 75% of small bowel obstructions. Dependent on previous operations some patients have a lifetime risk of 4–30% of developing adhesion-related SBO. Other common causes include hernias and tumour-related obstruction.

Clinical assessment focuses on determining the severity of obstruction and subsequent need for operative management:

- During the initial part of the encounter the patient's current clinical state is important.
- Tachycardia, fever and localised tenderness may indicate severe obstruction.
- Typical symptoms include generalised colicky abdominal pain associated with nausea, vomiting and altered bowel habit. Some patients with recurrent obstructions may recognise their symptoms.
- Examination findings may reveal a distended abdomen with a generalised tenderness. Look for previous surgical scars and always examine for hernias.
- One of the key elements of differential diagnosis to consider is ileus, which is common in recent postoperative patients and those with peritonitis, ischaemia or trauma.
- The severity of the bowel of obstruction is determined by a number of features (see Table 45.5).

Investigations

- Plain film X-rays are often used as a first-line investigation.
- CT abdomen is standard for diagnosis in SBO, allowing for identification of the level and severity of obstruction.

TABLE 45.5 Classification of bowel obstructions

Partial vs complete obstruction	Partial obstruction: lumen still patent with some contents able to pass through Complete obstruction: no passage of contents or air
Open vs closed loop	Open loop: the proximal end of the bowel is open (distal obstruction) allowing for decompression (via NGT) Closed loop: the proximal end of the loop is also obstructed, meaning proximal decompression is not possible
Strangulated	Decreased blood supply leading to bowel ischaemia

Management

- Is dependent on the severity of obstruction.
- Partial obstructions can typically be managed with non-operative treatment, which includes nasogastric tube decompression, bowel rest and IV fluid resuscitation.
  - Careful electrolyte replacement is required.
  - Diet can be slowly introduced once the patient has improved.
  - Some surgeons give oral contrast as a diagnostic and therapeutic technique for partial obstruction.
- Complete, closed loop obstructions and patients with strangulation require operative management.
  - Around 25% of patients with SBO will require operative management.
  - Those patients who fail to improve after a period of non-operative management may require some escalation of care.
  - Laparoscopy can be employed to investigate the viability of the bowel and perform adhesiolysis.
  - Patients with strangulated bowel or several distended large loops may require laparotomy with potential small bowel resection.

Large bowel obstruction (LBO)

Clinical presentations are largely similar to that of small bowel obstruction with abdominal pain and distension. Nausea and vomiting are considered a late symptom of obstruction.

LBOs carry a higher risk of mortality, as high as 18%.

Causes:

- Colorectal cancer is the most common cause of LBO; 15% of all patients with colorectal cancer present as an acute abdomen (LBO).
- Other common causes include diverticulitis, volvulus, faecal impaction, hernias, ileus and adhesions.

Volvulus

Volvulus is the twisting of the colon around the mesenteric vascular supply.

A wide range of presentations is seen dependent on the severity of the obstruction. The symptoms are the same as LBO in the early stages of the condition.

Prolonged volvulus leads to bowel ischaemia, which can result in perforation.

Sigmoid volvulus

- Accounts for less than 10% of LBOs, but has a significantly higher level of mortality.
- It is the more common of the two types of volvulus, typically affecting elderly patients with a history of chronic obstruction secondary to constipation.
- Early recognition allows for decompression via sigmoidoscopy, then definitive surgery.
    - Gangrenous changes to the sigmoid colon will require resection.
    - Hartmann's procedure is a common surgical approach.

Caecal volvulus

- A relatively rare cause of LBO (~1%).
- Management almost always requires surgical intervention with local resection of the affected bowel, which can be performed as a laparoscopic operation in suitable patients.
- The caecum is particularly prone to perforation; rapid intervention is advisable.

Investigations

- Plain abdominal X-rays are a common first-line investigation.
    - Erect chest X-rays can screen for free intra-abdominal air.
- CT abdomen provides a good visualisation of the bowel and allows for categorisation of the obstruction (see Figs 45.15, 45.16 and 45.17).
    - As the most common cause of LBO is colorectal cancer, CT is important for locating the tumour and disease staging.

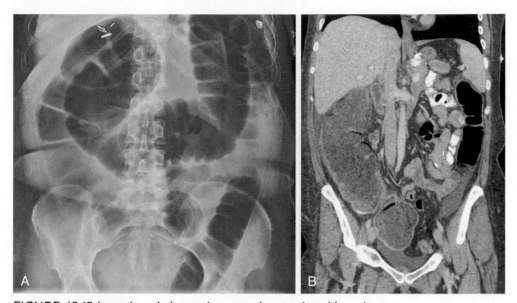

FIGURE 45.15 Large bowel obstruction secondary to sigmoid carcinoma.

Reproduced from: Bornstein, J. & Berger, D., 2014. Large bowel obstruction. In: Cameron, J., Current Surgical Therapy, 11th ed. Saunders, pp. 177–181, Fig. 1.

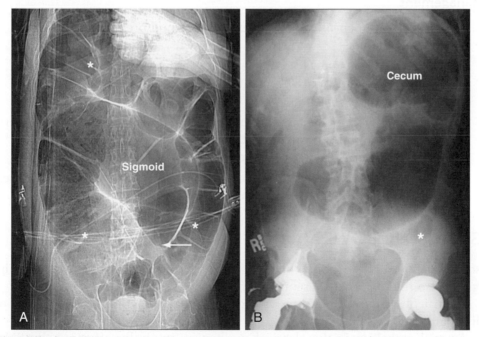

FIGURE 45.16 Plain abdominal X-ray demonstrating sigmoid volvulus (A) and caecal volvulus (B).

Reproduced from: Simmang, C. & McCormick, J., 2013. Chapter 27: Large and small bowel obstruction. In: Bailey, H.R., Billingham, R., Stamos, M., et al., Colorectal Surgery. Saunders, pp. 426–439, Fig. 27.12.

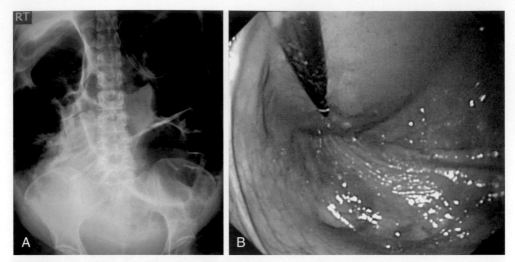

FIGURE 45.17 Sigmoid volvulus on abdominal X-ray; sigmoidoscopy demonstrates a twisted colon.

Reproduced from: Ahmad, A., Shing, K., Tan, K., et al., 2014. Sigmoid volvulus in pregnancy: early diagnosis and intervention are important. American Journal of Emergency Medicine 32(5), 491, Figure A.

Management

- Early management includes IV resuscitation and preoperative IV antibiotics.
- As patients almost always require operative intervention, early medical and anaesthetic team involvement should be sought to optimise the patient for surgery.
- Obstructing tumours should be resected as part of the emergency surgery. Dependent on the clinical presentation, patients should either have a primary anastomosis or a colostomy.
- Patients who are acutely unwell or have significant medical comorbidities may be better suited to colonic stenting via an endoscopic approach.

ISCHAEMIC BOWEL

Ischaemic bowel is the sudden onset of intestinal vascular compromise (see Fig. 45.18), also referred to as mesenteric ischaemia.

A particularly uncommon presentation, it is responsible for less than 0.1% of all inpatient admissions.

Arterial embolism is the classical mechanism, typically affecting the SMA (around 50% of cases). Venous thrombosis can also cause ischaemia. Ischaemia may result from vascular obstruction.

Risk factors include elderly patients, cardiac arrhythmia and valve disease, trauma and hypercoagulable conditions.

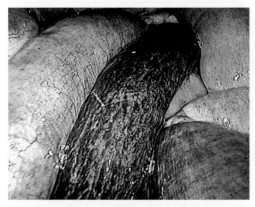

FIGURE 45.18 Ischaemic bowel on laparoscopy.

Reproduced from: Palanivelu, C., Rangarajan, M., Maheshkumaar, G., et al., 2008. Relaparoscopy in the management of acute abdomen due to localized ischemic bowel: a novel technique – case report. International Journal of Surgery 6(6), e89–e91, Fig. 1.

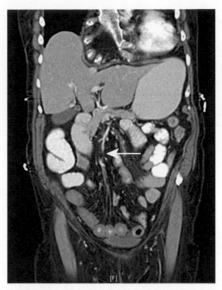

FIGURE 45.19 CTA showing SMA emboli.

Reproduced from: Tryforos, M., 2017. Mesenteric ischemia, acute. In: Ferri, F., Ferri's Clinical Advisor. Mosby, pp. 787–788, Fig. 1M-26.

The classical description of ischaemic bowel is a rapid onset of severe umbilical pain 'out of proportion' to examination findings (i.e. no obvious peritonitis, distension). In late stage presentations patients may present with peritonitis and features of bowel perforation.

Investigations

- CT abdominal angiography is often used to detect emboli associated with ischaemia (Fig. 45.19).
- Venous gas (portal system) is a sign of tissue loss resulting from ischaemia.

Management

- Patients should be fasted and have an NG tube inserted with IV fluids.
- Anti-coagulation therapy should be instituted, with heparin infusions common.
- Early detection in stable patients may allow for endovascular treatment with thrombolysis and stenting.
- Patients with features of bowel gangrene, perforation or haemodynamic compromise should have urgent surgical exploration and mesenteric re-vascularisation where possible and resection of the compromised bowel.

Mortality rates still remain high, around 60–85%.

SECTION IV

ENDOSCOPY

Refers to a wide range of diagnostic and therapeutic techniques using endoscopic cameras allowing for direct visualisation of the mucosal surfaces of the GIT.

Gastroscopy

- Uses a flexible endoscope that can be passed to the duodenum.
- Indications
  - A vast number of indications, including diagnosis of gastrointestinal upset, surveillance of malignancies, treatment of ulcer disease and gastrointestinal bleeding.
- Preoperative
  - Patients are positioned on their side allowing for easy entry of the scope. Sedation is given prior to the procedure.
- Operative
  - The gastroscope is used to inspect the oesophagus, stomach and duodenum (see Fig. 45.20).
  - Biopsies can be taken at each level testing for malignancy, *H. pylori*.
  - Identification of bleeding ulcers allows for intervention: injection of adrenaline and gold probe cautery.
- Postoperative
  - Patients are booked as day cases and discharged home with follow-up in a few weeks to discuss histology results.
- Complications
  - Bleeding and injury to the upper GI tract.

Endoscopic retrograde cholangiopancreatography (ERCP)

- A duodenoscope is positioned allowing cannulation of the duct (see Fig. 45.21).
- Indications
  - Choledocolithiasis, cholangitis, bile leaks, tumours.
- Preoperative
  - Patients should be fasted; the procedure is most commonly performed as an inpatient procedure.
- Operative
  - Once cannulation has been achieved wires, baskets and brushes can be passed into the biliary system allowing for interventions such as stone extraction and biopsies.
  - Cholangiography can also be performed.

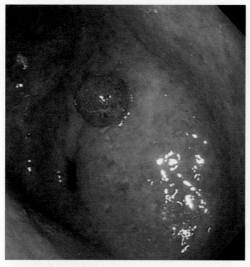

FIGURE 45.20 Benign stomach polyp seen on gastroscopy.

Reproduced from: Liao, Z., Hou, X., Lin-Hu, E.-Q., et al., 2016. Accuracy of magnetically controlled capsule endoscopy, compared with conventional gastroscopy, in detection of gastric diseases. Clinical Gastroenterology and Hepatology 14(9), 1266–1273, Fig. 1.

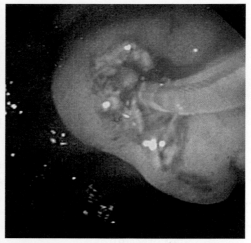

FIGURE 45.21 Cannulation of the CBD during ERCP.

Reproduced from: Canard, J.M., Lennon, A.M., Létard, J.C., et al., 2011. Endoscopic retrograde cholangiopancreatography. In: Canard, J.M., Gastrointestinal Endoscopy in Practice. Churchill Livingstone, pp. 370–465, Fig. 14E.

- ○ Sphincterotomy and stent placement are other therapeutic options to treat bile leaks and cholangitis.
  - – Stenting may be used as a palliative procedure for obstruction secondary to tumours.
- Postoperative
  - ○ Patients may require ongoing treatment and observation of the indication.
  - ○ Bleeding (malaena) following sphincterotomy is sometimes reported.
- Complications
  - ○ Pancreatitis
  - ○ Cholangitis
  - ○ Perforation
  - ○ Stent migration
- Follow-up
  - ○ Patients with stents require future ERCP for removal.

Endoscopic ultrasound (EUS)

- EUS has a large variety of diagnostic and therapeutic applications, as it allows for detection of tissue pathology beyond the visible mucosal layer of the GIT, with US images of adjacent anatomic structures.

- Indications
  - Diagnosis of upper GI and hepatic-pancreatic-biliary (HPB) malignancies, assessment of chronic pancreatitis.
  - Interventions for complications of pancreatitis (i.e. pseudocyst).
- Preoperative
  - Recent imaging is key to help plan the procedure.
- Operative
  - The scope is passed to the area of interest; a variety of instruments allow for tissue biopsies and aspirations.
- Postoperative
  - Patients who are booked for malignancy staging may be outpatient day procedures.
  - Patients with pancreatitis will require ongoing management following the procedure.
- Complications
  - As for gastroscopy, bleeding and perforation.

Colonoscopy

- Endoscopic examination of the large bowel through to the terminal ileum (see Fig. 45.22).
- Alternatives include shorter examination scopes such as flexible sigmoidoscopy or external imaging such as CT colonography.
- Indications
  - Extensive, but include: positive FOBT from bowel screening, PR bleeding, altered bowel habit, diagnosis of inflammatory bowel disease.
  - Flexible sigmoidoscopy is an alternative.

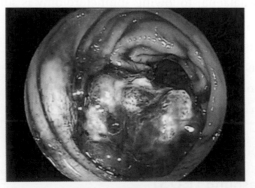

FIGURE 45.22 Obvious sigmoid tumour on colonoscopy.

Reproduced from: Al Beteddini, O.S., Brenez, D., Firket, C., et al., 2012. Colonic angiosarcoma: a case report and review of literature. International Journal of Surgery Case Reports 4(2), 208–211, Fig. 1.

- Preoperative
  - Patients require bowel preparation to ensure adequate visualisation of the colon (see Chapter 37).
- Operative
  - The scope enters the rectum and is manoeuvred around the colon to the caecum, with visualisation of the terminal ileum.
  - Biopsies can be taken of polyps for diagnosis.
  - Polypectomy can be performed on suitably sized polyps using diathermy snare.
  - May be performed in combination with haemorrhoid banding.
- Postoperative
  - Patients are discharged home the same day.
  - Patients should be counselled about the possibility of some rectal bleeding following polypectomy.
- Complications
  - Bowel perforation (1 in 1000).
  - Bleeding following polypectomy or biopsy.

BREAST SURGERY

Breast surgery for the management of tumours is largely separated into two categories: breast conservation therapy (BCT) and mastectomy.

Breast conservation surgery

Involves the excision of the tumour with an acceptable oncological margin, while a significant proportion of breast tissue is left intact.

The approach is known by many names, including lumpectomy, wide local excision (WLE) and quadrantectomy.

- Indications
  - Early stage breast cancer; unilateral disease.
  - Patient agreement to this treatment approach with adjuvant radiotherapy.
  - Benign lesions.
- Preoperative
  - Patient requires complete image staging and tissue diagnosis to determine suitability for BCT.
  - To aid the surgical approach, an image guided wire (hookwire) can be placed into the lesion on the day of surgery in the Radiology Department (Fig. 45.23).

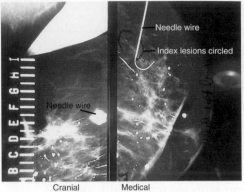

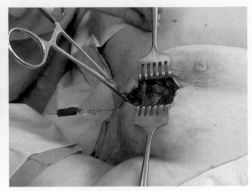

FIGURE 45.23 Hookwire localisation of breast lesion.

Reproduced from: Klimberg, V., Bland, K. & Westbrook, K., 2010. Chapter 7: Needle localization breast biopsy. In: Townsend, C., Atlas of Breast Surgical Techniques. Saunders, pp. 72–87, Fig. 7-3.

FIGURE 45.24 Resection of a tumour as part of a BCT.

Reproduced from: Klimberg, V., Bland, K. & Westbrook, K., 2010. Chapter 7: Needle localization breast biopsy. In: Townsend, C., Atlas of Breast Surgical Techniques. Saunders, pp. 72–87, Fig. 7-9.

- Operative
  - The approach is directly over the tumour; once identified, it is excised with appropriate margins (Fig. 45.24).
  - The tumour is marked with stitches to allow correct orientation of the pathological specimen.
  - This procedure is often combined with a sentinel lymph node biopsy.
- Postoperative
  - Increasingly, these cases are being performed as day cases.
  - Patients should be instructed to wear a sports bra to aid with compression and stability.
  - Discussion at MDM for planning of adjuvant therapy.
- Complications
  - Haematoma, seroma, infection, incomplete excision.

Sentinel lymph node biopsy (SLNB)

This involves the use of a radiotracer substance to identify the earliest draining axillary lymph node for pathological examination. The tracer is combined with a blue dye, which aids visualisation.

- Indications
  - Early stage breast cancer with no clinically palpable nodes.

- Preoperative
  - Prior to the operation the patient is injected with the radiotracer either into the tissue surrounding the tumour or into the tumour itself.
- Operative
  - A handheld gamma probe reads the concentration of dye, usually represented by a corresponding increased pitch in sound from the instrument.
  - The probe will give a 'count' of highest concentration.
  - Once the node has been roughly localised, an incision is made into the axilla to access the node.
  - The probe further aids with direct localisation.
  - A final 'count' is made on the node once it has been excised and the axilla is inspected a final time.
- Postoperative
  - Similar postoperative care as above.
  - A sling can be offered for comfort.
- Complications
  - Seroma, haematoma, infection.

Mastectomy

Mastectomy involves excision of the breast tissue and overlying skin.

- Indications
  - Larger or more centrally placed breast tumours not amenable to BCT.
  - Previous BCT with positive margins.
  - Multifocal breast disease.
  - Patient choice (may include a prophylactic contralateral mastectomy for those with significant risk factors).
- Preoperative
  - Ensure recent imaging and tissue diagnosis are available.
  - The early involvement of breast care nurses for educational and emotional support.
- Operative
  - A number of approaches have been described.
  - The evolution of the principles of oncoplastic surgery has led to the consideration of breast reconstructive options (skin sparing and nipple sparing) when performing mastectomy.

SECTION IV

- For simple mastectomy the overlying skin and breast tissue is excised. The superior portion of the breast is excised followed by the inferior with broad excision of the nipple areola complex.
- Drain tubes are left in situ following the procedure with daily monitoring of outputs.

- Postoperative
  - The patient is admitted for analgesia, observation and drain tube management.
  - The drain tubes typically remain until their daily output drops below an acceptable threshold (such as <30 mL).
  - For patients who have had immediate breast reconstruction (Chapter 52) there should be discussion with the plastic surgery team regarding postoperative care and follow-up.

Axillary lymph node dissection

This involves the excision of all axillary lymph nodes.

- Indications
  - Positive sentinel lymph nodes.
  - Clinically positive nodes on examination.
  - High risk malignancy (inflammatory breast cancer).
- Preoperative
  - Ensure all imaging and tissue diagnosis are available.
  - May be combined with mastectomy.
- Operative
  - Incision over axilla and dissection of axillary structure to identify the lymph node chains.
  - Following dissection, a drain tube is left within the wound cavity.
- Postoperative
  - As with other breast drain tubes, there is careful monitoring and removal once output meets a certain threshold.
  - Keep the arm rested for around 1 week, then introduce exercises.
- Complications
  - Seroma is common, affecting nearly a third of all cases.
  - Nerve injuries are important to recognise. Scapula 'winging' is suggestive of a long thoracic nerve injury. Thoracodorsal nerve injury results in loss of adduction strength.
- Follow-up
  - These patients require close follow-up for monitoring of complications.

HEPATOPANCREATOBILIARY (HPB) SURGERY

Cholecystectomy

Cholecycstectomy is surgical removal of the gallbladder.

- Indications
  - ○ Biliary colic, acute cholecystitis, gallstone pancreatitis, abdominal pain associated with cholelithiasis.
- Preoperative
  - ○ Patients should have US results available showing the presence of gallstones.
  - ○ Preoperative LFTs for baseline and to determine the likelihood of choledocolithiasis.
- Operative
  - ○ Majority completed by laparoscopic approach (Fig. 45.25).
    - Patient is either supine or in lithotomy dependent on surgeon preference of technique.
    - Intraoperative cholangiogram (IOC) is often performed to establish the biliary tree anatomy and to visualise any stones (Fig. 45.26).
    - The presence of duct stones may prompt bile duct exploration.
    - Clips are applied to the cystic duct and artery prior to their division.

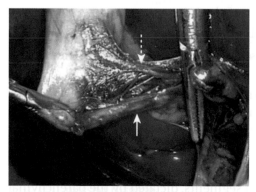

FIGURE 45.25 Dissection of the cystic artery and duct (Calot's triangle).

Reproduced from: Ostlie, D. & Holcomb, G., 2008. Laparoscopic cholecystectomy. In: Holcomb, G., Atlas of Pediatric Laparoscopy and Thoracoscopy. Saunders, pp. 127–133, Fig. 22-4B.

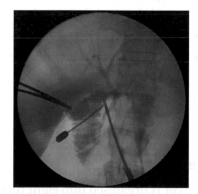

FIGURE 45.26 Normal intraoperative cholangiogram (IOC).

Reproduced from: Rawlings, A., Hodgett, S., Matthews, B., et al., 2010. Single-incision laparoscopic cholecystectomy: initial experience with critical view of safety dissection and routine intraoperative cholangiography. Journal of the American College of Surgeons 211(1), 1–7, Fig. 3.

SECTION IV

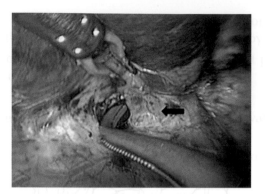

FIGURE 45.28 Dissection of the left hepatic vein during a laparoscopic liver resection.

Reproduced from: Tranchart, H., Gaillard, M., Lainas, P., et al., 2015. Selective control of the left hepatic vein during laparoscopic liver resection: Arantius' ligament approach. Journal of the American College of Surgeons 221(4), e75–e79, Fig. 1.

- Postoperative
  - Patients are admitted for several days for observation and monitoring of potential complications.
  - Patients who have laparoscopic procedures tend to have less pain, and therefore mobilise earlier.
- Complications
  - Haematoma, bile leak (<2%), infection.

Hepatectomy

Dependent on the pathology a patient may undergo a left, right or total hepatectomy, where the latter necessitates liver transplantation.

- Indications
  - Predominantly for malignant tumours of the liver.
- Preoperative
  - As for above, extensive work-up is required due to the stresses of major hepatic surgery.
  - Optimisation of liver functions including clotting.
- Operative
  - Open approach, the liver is mobilised.
  - The vascular supply to the surgical side is identified and ligated, which will result in demarcation of the left from the right liver, giving a guide as to where to commence the division of the specimen from the other side (for simple right or left hepatectomy).
  - Drains are left in the sub-hepatic space for monitoring.

- Postoperative
  - Monitor the patient's LFTs and coagulation studies for evidence of liver failure.
  - Carefully monitor the drain tubes looking for bile or large amounts of blood.
- Complications
  - Haemorrhage, liver failure, bile leak/peritonitis, portal vein thrombosis.

Pancreatectomy

The predominant reason for pancreatic excision is malignancy. Pancreatic cancer most commonly affects the head of the pancreas.

The conventional approach is a pancreaticoduodenectomy involving excision of the pancreatic head, duodenum, CBD and gallbladder (Whipple's procedure). Common variants include pylorus-preserving approaches (Fig. 45.29) to help minimise delays in gastric emptying.

- Preoperative
  - Like most major HPB operations, patient selection is crucial, and those with major medical comorbidities may not be suited to a large operation.

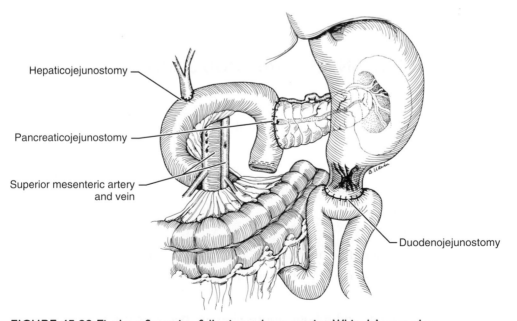

FIGURE 45.29 Final configuration following pylorus-sparing Whipple's procedure.

Reproduced from: Nealon, W., 2010. Chapter 49: Pylorus-saving pancreaticoduodenectomy. In: Townsend, C., Atlas of General Surgical Techniques. Saunders, pp. 545–563, Fig. 49-17.

SECTION IV

- Operation
  - Laparoscopic and robotic approaches are becoming more common; however, the open approach is still widely utilised.
  - The operation can be largely split into two parts:
    - dissection of the pancreas, duodenum and vascular structures to determine resectability
    - reconstruction of the defect once the specimen has been removed.
  - Reconstruction involves mobilising a distal limb of jejunum to form the hepatico- and pancreaticojejunostomies, with a further distal duodenojejunostomy.
  - Multiple drains are placed around the various anastomoses.
- Postoperative
  - Most centres have a specific 'post-Whipple's' protocol that can be followed on the ward.
  - A nasogastric tube should remain in place until output decreases.
  - Drain tube output should be strictly monitored.
  - Regular BSLs.
- Complications
  - Haemorrhage, bile leak, infection.
  - Delayed gastric emptying is a common side effect of the reconstruction.

UPPER GASTROINTESTINAL (UGI) SURGERY

Gastrectomy

Gastrectomy is partial or complete removal of the stomach.

- Indications
  - Gastric cancer.
  - Irretraceable gastric bleeding.
  - Stomach trauma.
- Preoperative
  - Patients should be nutritionally optimised where possible.
  - Pre-admission clinic with anaesthetic input is essential.
- Operative
  - Laparoscopic and robotic approaches are being used more commonly.
  - The open approach is via an upper midline laparotomy.

- The stomach is mobilised by ligating the gastroepiploic vessels and division of the gastrohepatic ligament.
- Total gastrectomy involves excision of the stomach at the distal oesophagus and the distal pylorus.
- Partial gastrectomy typically involves the retention of the upper portion of the stomach, with excision of the pylorus and antrum.
- Following excision, a reconstruction takes place.
  - There are multiple variants including the Bilroth and Roux approaches (Fig. 45.30).
  - Total gastrectomy necessitates the formation of an oesophageal jejunostomy.
- Postoperative
  - Patients require careful monitoring, looking for haemorrhage and anastomotic leak.

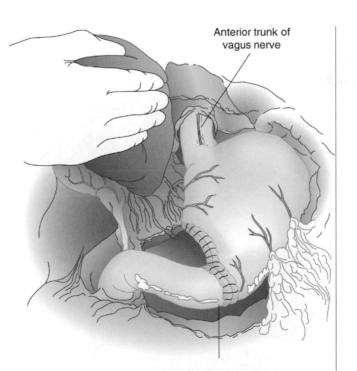

Anterior trunk of
vagus nerve

Billroth I gastroduodenal
anastomosis completed

FIGURE 45.30 Partial gastrectomy with Bilroth I reconstruction.

Reproduced from: Mann, B., 2009. Operation 13: Gastrectomy. In: Mann, B., Surgery: A Competency-based Companion. Saunders, pp. 689–689, Fig. 1.

- Complications
    - Bleeding, anastomotic leak (1–4%), gastric 'dumping' early and late. Smaller meals are more suitable.
    - B12 deficiency.

Fundoplication

Fundoplication involves forming a wrap of the proximal stomach around the lower oesophagus, providing bulk around the lower oesophageal sphincter and helping prevent further reflux symptoms.

- Indications
    - A surgical option for non-obese patients who have persistent symptoms of GORD (Chapter 37) despite optimal medical management.
- Preoperative
    - Patients should have been extensively worked up for GORD including endoscopy.
- Operative
    - Now routinely performed as a laparoscopic procedure (Fig. 45.31).
    - The liver is retracted to reveal the stomach, which is mobilised.

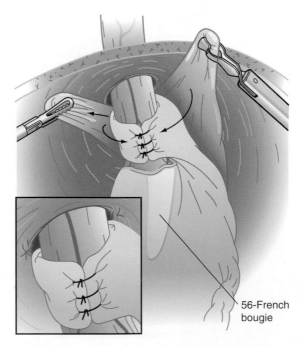

56-French bougie

FIGURE 45.31 Laparoscopic fundoplication.

Reproduced from: Davis, S. & Medbery, R., 2014. Laparoscopic 360-degree fundoplication. In: Cameron, J., Current Surgical Therapy, 11th ed. Saunders, pp.1317–1322, Fig. 7.

- o The stomach is then retracted inferior allowing passage of the distal oesophagus to allow the wrap to be performed.
- Postoperative
  - o Patients are allowed clear fluids postoperatively with commencement of a pureed diet the next day. This diet is maintained for around 3 weeks before solid food can be restarted.
- Complications
  - o Gastric or oesophageal perforation.
  - o Recurrence of symptoms.
  - o Migration of wrap.

Oesophagectomy

Surgical resection of oesophageal cancers is indicated in select patients with invasive tumours. There are multiple laparoscopic and open approaches to oesophagectomy involving access via the thorax and abdomen. Beginning at the hypopharynx in the neck and terminating in the abdomen at the gastro-oesophageal junction (GOJ), the oesophagus has a complicated surgical anatomy.

- Indications
  - o Locally advanced carcinoma without metastatic disease.
  - o Benign stricture disease and dysplastic mucosal changes.
- Preoperative
  - o Tumour or disease is carefully evaluated with endoscopy and CT imaging as required.
  - o Patients require thorough anaesthetic evaluation and ICU involvement postoperatively.
  - o Nutritional supplementation is a key focus of the preoperative stage, typically achieved via NGT feeds in patients unable to tolerate food.
- Operative
  - o Approach is dictated by the location of disease.
  - o Transthoracic oesophagectomy (Ivor Lewis) is commonly used for distal third oesophageal cancers.
    - The traditional open approach includes an upper midline laparotomy and a thoracotomy, permitting access to the oesophagus. Minimal access variants are widely used.
    - Mobilisation of the stomach and oesophagus allows for resection of the tumour with a portion of the proximal stomach (fundus) and oesophagus (see Fig. 45.32).
    - After resection, reconstruction is performed (see Fig. 45.33). One method involves mobilising a portion of the remaining stomach into the chest cavity and performing an end-to-end anastomosis.

- Postoperative
  - NGT is left in situ with IV supplementation.
  - Clear fluids may be commenced from the first postoperative day dependent on surgeon preference with an upgrade in diet once the NGT can be removed.
  - Electrolytes should be monitored daily with IV replacement as required.
- Complications
  - Ileus
  - Infections
  - Anastomotic leak
  - Small bowel obstruction

Ileostomy

Ileostomy is performed as either a temporary or permanent procedure, often in combination with other bowel surgery.

- Indications
  - End ileostomy: following proto-colectomy (most commonly for ulcerative colitis), patients with severe spinal cord injury.
  - Loop ileostomy: temporary to protect a distal large bowel anastomosis.
- Preoperative
  - Where possible patients should be seen by a stomal therapist to help guide placement of stoma.
- Operative
  - Can be performed as a laparoscopic procedure though the approach may be dictated by other parts of the operation.
  - The formation of the stoma site (Fig. 45.34) is the same for end and loop ileostomy.
  - End ileostomy (Fig. 45.35)
    - The proximal end of the small bowel is brought out through the stoma, ensuring that it is correctly orientated.
    - Ileostomy is formed using interrupted sutures.
  - Loop ileostomy (Fig. 45.36)
    - A stoma is formed by passing a loop of the small bowel through the stoma site, with a $\frac{3}{4}$ circumferential incision.
    - The proximal end of the loop forms the ileostomy; an ileostomy rod is used to take pressure off the loop.
    - Can be reversed once the need for diversion has ceased.

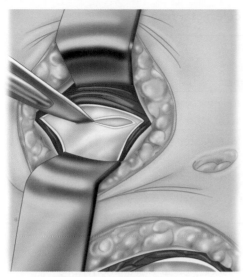

FIGURE 45.34 Forming the stoma site.

Reproduced from: Lin, A., 2013. Chapter 28: End ileostomy and loop ileostomy. In: Fleshman, J., Atlas of Surgical Techniques for Colon, Rectum and Anus. Saunders, pp. 354–362, Fig. 28-1.

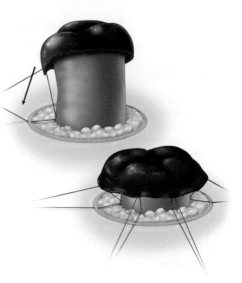

FIGURE 45.35 Forming an end ileostomy.

Reproduced from: Lin, A., 2013. Chapter 28: End ileostomy and loop ileostomy. In: Fleshman, J., Atlas of Surgical Techniques for Colon, Rectum and Anus. Saunders, pp. 354–362, Fig. 28-9.

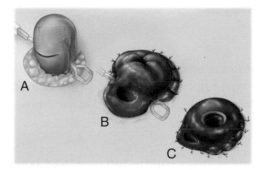

FIGURE 45.36 The process of forming a loop ileostomy.

Reproduced from: Lin, A., 2013. Chapter 28: End ileostomy and loop ileostomy. In: Fleshman, J., Atlas of Surgical Techniques for Colon, Rectum and Anus. Saunders, pp. 354–362, Fig. 28-13.

- Postoperative
  - As for small bowel resection: NGT, clear fluids, diet upgraded once bowel function returns.
  - Ongoing stoma therapy and education.
  - Initially stoma output.
- Complications
  - Stoma complications: retraction, prolapse, high output.
  - General: obstruction, ileus, infection.

TABLE 45.6 Types of colorectal resections

Right hemicolectomy	Excision of the ascending colon, distal ileum, caecum and hepatic flexure. Extended right hemicolectomy is sometimes performed for transverse colon pathology
Left hemicolectomy	Excision of the descending colon, sigmoid colon and splenic flexure. Includes the distal transverse colon
Anterior resection	Performed for pathology related to the sigmoid colon and rectum. In tumours involving the lower part of the rectum, a 'low' or 'ultralow' anterior resection may be required. Indications include tumours, obstruction and diverticular disease
Subtotal/total colectomy	Removal of all of the large bowel. Typically indicated for widespread inflammatory bowel disease (ulcerative colitis), multiple colorectal cancers or familial adenomatous polyposis (FAP) (Chapter 67) Dependent on the health of the surrounding tissue the patient may undergo an ileorectal anastomosis or have an ileostomy

Large bowel surgery

Colectomy

There are many indications and approaches for partial and total excision of the colon. Individual sections can be excised specific to their pathology (Table 45.6). These operations may include a primary bowel anastomosis or be combined with a colostomy.

- Indications
  - Colorectal cancer, diverticulitis, inflammatory bowel disease, polyp disease, trauma.
- Preoperative
  - Recent imaging is essential for planning.
  - Dependent on the disease, contamination of the abdomen and health of the patient, a decision will be made about whether to form an anastomosis or perform a colostomy.
- Operative
  - Laparoscopic assisted approaches are common, though the conventional open laparotomy is still widely used.
  - The affected large bowel is mobilised from its peritoneal attachments and inspected.
  - Control of the mesenteric vascular pedicle is obtained prior to resection of the bowel.

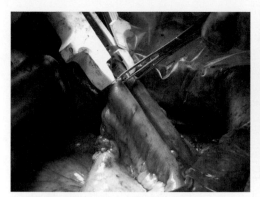

FIGURE 45.37 Side-to-side stapled anastomosis during a right hemicolectomy.

Reproduced from: Hunt, S., 2013. Open right colectomy. In: Fleshman, J., Atlas of Surgical Techniques for Colon, Rectum and Anus. Saunders, pp. 2–11, Fig. 1-10.

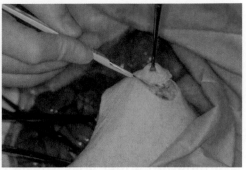

FIGURE 45.38 Formation of a colostomy.

Reproduced from: Albers, B.J. & Lamon, D.J., 2016. Colon repair/colostomy creation. In: Baggish, M.S. & Karram, M.M., Atlas of Pelvic Anatomy and Gynecologic Surgery, 4th ed. Elsevier, pp. 1123–1126.

- An anastomosis can be performed by a stapled (usually side-to-side) or hand sewn (usually end-to-end) technique (Fig. 45.37).
- Postoperative
  - Protocols vary among surgeons, but the common themes are clear fluids postoperatively with an upgrade in diet when the patient feels hungry and demonstrates evidence of bowel activity (bowel sounds, passing flatus).
  - These patients require careful attention to their biochemical results, and should have daily checks with judicious electrolyte replacement.
- Complications
  - Anastomotic leak, intra-abdominal infection.

Colostomy

Colostomy is primarily used to relieve obstruction.

- Indications
  - Faecal diversion (i.e. following surgery).
  - Relief of obstruction.
- Preoperative
  - Where possible patients should be seen by a stoma therapy nurse for making of the optimal colostomy site.
- Operative
  - The colostomy is formed proximal to the site of obstruction (Fig. 45.38).
  - If the obstruction is significant, the distal end of the colon can be fashioned into a mucous fistula to discharge secretions and gas.

SECTION IV

- Postoperative
  - Ongoing stoma nurse care and education.
- Complications
  - Parastomal hernia is common.
  - Watch for retraction and ischaemia of the stoma.

RECTAL SURGERY

Examination under anaesthesia (EUA)

Though perianal disease can be accurately assessed in the outpatient clinic, thorough examination is best completed under a general anaesthetic (GA).

- Indications
  - Large range of indications, including infection, PR bleeding, discharge and/or pain.
- Preoperative
  - If the patient has minimal symptoms at first presentation, a change of diet to facilitate better bowel habits might be worthwhile prior to EUA.
- Operative
  - Under GA the patient is placed in the lithotomy position.
  - A retractor (i.e. Pratt) is used to visualise the rectum.
  - Pathology is localised with reference to the anus as a clock face. Anterior is 12 o'clock; posterior is 6 o'clock.
- Anal fissure
  - See discussion in Chapter 66.
- Anal fistula
  - Probes can be passed through the external opening to locate the internal opening.
  - Fistulas may have a deep and long course; fistulas with more distant external openings may curve around to an internal opening in the posterior midline.
  - Superficial fistulas involving a small amount of sphincter muscle (less than one-third) may be suited to incision and curette (fistulotomy).
  - Larger fistulas involving larger portions of sphincter muscle are not suited to incision initially due to the higher likelihood of developing postoperative incontinence and may have a seton placed.
    - A seton is an elastic band (vessel loops are often used) that is tightened through multiple operations to slowly cut through the sphincter muscle, preventing sudden disruption.
    - Once the fistula is superficial enough, incision may be performed.

- o Some fistulas can be treated with advancement flaps to cover internal openings.
- Perianal abscess
  - o Abscesses localised around the anus that present as erythematous, tender lumps.
  - o The abscess may be well localised to the subcutaneous tissue or spread to the intersphincteric or ischiorectal planes forming fistulas.
  - o Ideal management is early incision and drainage, particularly in patients who display systemic symptoms such as fever.
  - o Patients are kept on IV antibiotics during the perioperative phase.
  - o The wound may be packed with regular dressing changes to prevent re-accumulation of the infection.

Haemorrhoidectomy

An overview of haemorrhoids is given in Chapter 66. Internal haemorrhoids (above the pectinate line) are insensate and suitable to banding. External haemorrhoids are excised.

- Preoperative
  - o Patients may be given an enema prior to the case on the day of surgery.
- Operative
  - o With the patient in the lithotomy position the haemorrhoids are identified, typically found at 4'oclock, 7 o'clock and 11'oclock.
  - o The excision typically begins externally, avoiding damage to the underlying muscle.
  - o Ligation of the base of the haemorrhoid is typically performed, with some surgeons electing to suture the entire wound closed (see also Fig. 45.39, which illustrates ligation of a vascular pedicle).
  - o A dressing is sometimes placed inside the rectum to aid with haemostasis.
  - o A pudendal nerve block is often used for pain management.
- Postoperative
  - o Patients typically experience significant pain and should be prescribed appropriate analgesia.
  - o Most surgeons prefer these patients are discharged with antibiotics (metronidazole) and regular aperients to ease bowel motions.
- Complications
  - o Some patients may experience PR bleeding, which is common and typically self limiting.

SECTION IV

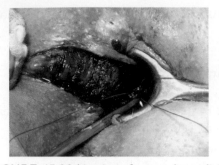

FIGURE 45.39 Ligation of a vascular pedicle following external haemorrhoidectomy.

Reproduced from: Elsevier Inc., 2016. Chapter 35: Hemorrhoidectomy. In: Essential Surgical Procedures. Elsevier, pp. e619–e638, Fig. 35-3-8.

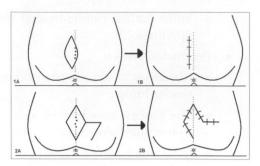

FIGURE 45.40 Karydakis procedure (above) and rhomboid flap (below) for pilonidal excision.

Reproduced from: Ates, M. & Dirican, A., 2011. Short- and long-term results of the Karydakis flap versus the Limberg flap for treating pilonidal sinus disease: a prospective randomized study. American Journal of Surgery 202(5), 568–573, Fig. 1.

Pilonidal sinus

Pilonidal sinus is infection in the natal cleft, typically associated with a tract formed by skin penetration of hair. It is commonly associated with hirsute individuals. Acute infections can present as an abscess in the region of the natal cleft that should be incised and drained, then managed with wound packing dressings. Chronic disease, including the formation of a mature tract (often seen as open pits in the natal cleft), may require excision of the tract and flap coverage of the tissue defect.

- Preoperative
  - As patients are prone under GA for this procedure, they may require review by the anaesthetics team, particularly if they are obese.
- Operative
  - Identification of the full extent of the disease can be aided by the use of methylene blue or hydrogen peroxide to visualise the tracts.
  - The shape of the excision is dictated by the planned reconstruction. Some patients may be left to heal via secondary intention with VAC dressings.
  - The Karydakis or modified Karydakis procedure involves mobilisation of one side of the gluteal tissue to cover the defect, resulting in an 'off-midline' closure (Fig. 45.40).
  - Other approaches include rhomboid (Fig. 45.40) or V–Y advancement flaps to cover the defect, though these may require more tissue recruitment and a large wound.

- o Drains are often placed postoperatively and can be managed by nurses in the community.

- Postoperative

  - o Patients are typically discharged home the next day following excision and may require ongoing dressing support with periodic reviews in clinic.

- Complications

  - o Breakdown of wound, infection and haematoma.

  - o Disease recurrence is a known common complication.

HERNIA SURGERY

Inguinal hernia repair

This is surgical repair of inguinal hernia using mesh.
There are three main approaches:

1 open repair

2 total extraperitoneal patchplasty (TEPP) using a laparoscope (see Fig. 45.41)

3 transabdominal peritoneal patchplasty (TAPP), a laparoscopic operation (within the abdomen).

- Preoperative

  - o The approach should be discussed with the patient: TAPP and TEPP procedures offer faster recovery times as they involve minimal access but carry a higher risk of mortality due to potential major vessel injury.

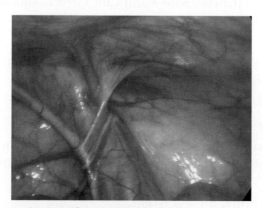

FIGURE 45.41 Laparoscopic view of an inguinal hernia.

Reproduced from: Elsevier, Inc., 2016. Inguinal hernia repair. In: Elsevier, Inc., Essential Surgical Procedures. Elsevier, pp. e1620–e1634, Fig. 85 2-4A.

SECTION IV

- Operative
  - Open repair involves a groin incision down to the external oblique layer, which is then opened to reveal the spermatic cord. The cord is inspected for indirect hernias, with dissection and reduction as required. Direct hernias are often visible deep to the cord on the media side of the epigastric vessels. Mesh is then inset.
  - TEPP involves creating a potential space external to the abdominal cavity using inflating balloons to identify and reduce hernias, allowing for internal placement of mesh.
  - TAPP involves a laparoscopic approach with incision through the peritoneum to allow reduction of the hernia.
  - A common finding is cord lipoma in the absence of a hernia.
- Postoperative
  - Most patients stay at least 1 night for pain control, although these operations are often performed as a day case.
  - Localised pain and inflammation postoperatively can lead to urinary retention and requires careful monitoring.
  - Patients should be advised that they are restricted from any heavy lifting postoperatively (4–6 weeks for open, 3 weeks for laparoscopic approaches).
- Complications
  - Haematoma, infection, recurrence.

Umbilical and paraumbilical hernia repair

- Preoperative
  - These procedures are relatively minor compared to other procedures; nonetheless, patients with significant medical comorbidities still require adequate work-up.
- Operative
  - Often the defects are quite small (<2 cm) and be directly repaired using a large stitch type (i.e. nylon).
  - Larger defects will require mesh repair.
- Postoperative
  - The majority of these patients can be discharged on the same day as their incision is quite small and typically easily managed with oral analgesia.
  - No heavy lifting for 3–4 weeks.
- Complications
  - Infection of the mesh, recurrence.

Epigastric and incisional hernias

Sometimes referred to as ventral hernias, they can be quite large and, in combination with a small defect, are at risk of incarceration (see Fig. 45.42).

These hernias are either approached laparoscopically or via an open approach.

- Preoperative
    - Imaging can sometimes provide valuable information about the number of hernias, and their location.
    - For patients with multiple hernias such that the defect is clinically difficult to isolate, a laparoscopic approach can be helpful.
    - Patients with a single, easily identifiable hernia may still undergo an open approach.
- Operative
    - Open approach involves incision over the hernia with isolation and reduction of the sac before repairing the defect with mesh.

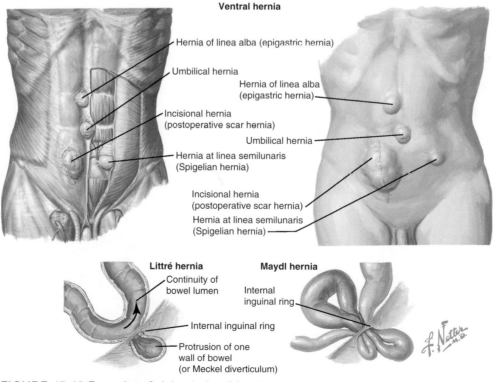

Ventral hernia

Hernia of linea alba (epigastric hernia)

Umbilical hernia

Hernia of linea alba (epigastric hernia)

Incisional hernia (postoperative scar hernia)

Umbilical hernia

Hernia at linea semilunaris (Spigelian hernia)

Incisional hernia (postoperative scar hernia)

Hernia at linea semilunaris (Spigelian hernia)

Littré hernia

Continuity of bowel lumen

Internal inguinal ring

Protrusion of one wall of bowel (or Meckel diverticulum)

Maydl hernia

Internal inguinal ring

FIGURE 45.42 Examples of abdominal wall hernias.

Reproduced from: Soto, F. & Rosenthal, R., 2010. Chapter 89: Ventral hernias. In: Floch, M., Netter's Gastroenterology. Saunders, pp. 228–229, Fig. 89-1.

SECTION IV

- o Laparoscopic involves an off-centre abdominal entry with visualisation of the hernia before placing the other ports.
  - – Dense adhesions may prevent a laparoscopic approach, requiring a conversion to open.
  - – If able to proceed, the hernia is reduced and a mesh is tacked onto the internal abdominal wall.
- Postoperative
  - o Patients should be admitted overnight for analgesia.
- Complications
  - o Bleeding, infection, pain.
  - o Bowel injury from laparoscopic approach.

CHAPTER 46

ORTHOPAEDIC SURGERY

Paul Watson and Lachlan Wight

Orthopaedic Surgery involves the surgical management of bones and joints. With a wide variety of paediatric and adult presentations in both trauma and elective settings, Orthopaedic services have a high volume inpatient workload and multiple weekly clinics. As such the teams will include multiple junior doctors from interns to senior residents to accommodate the workload. Effective and clear delegation of day-to-day responsibilities amongst the junior doctor team is essential to the smooth running of the unit.

Trauma workload from fractures represents the majority of the acute admissions to the Orthopaedic Unit. Patients who are involved in high energy motor vehicle collisions, falls from height or other scenarios with increased risk of multiple injuries will typically have a trauma assessment in ED (Chapter 10) and possible trauma admission to ensure other injury has not been overlooked (Chapter 45).

OPEN FRACTURES

Open fractures are fractures with communication to open air. A patient who presents with a fracture and an overlying wound should be considered as having an open fracture (see Fig. 46.1).

Rapid assessment of the fracture is essential to determine whether there has been a neurovascular injury (see Table 46.1 for classification of open fractures).

Management

- Patients should be given effective pain relief including temporary immobilisation of acceptable positioned fractures. Some fractures will require reduction prior to immobilisation.
- After the necessary examination and investigations, including imaging, the wound should be properly dressed with Betadine® (or other antiseptic substance) and covered with a non-stick petroleum dressing (i.e. Jelonet®).
- Debridement and washout of severe open fractures should occur promptly to avoid the increased risk of deep tissue infection.

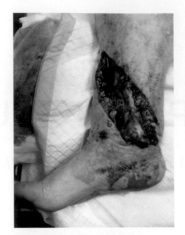

FIGURE 46.1 Right grade IIIB open distal tibial fracture.
Clinical point: patients who have had high-energy limb trauma are at risk of developing compartment syndrome (refer to the section 'Compartment syndrome' later in this chapter).

Reproduced from: Toole, W. & Elliot, M., 2015. Are low-energy open ankle fractures in the elderly the new geriatric hip fracture? Journal of Foot and Ankle Surgery 54(2), 203-206, Fig. 2.

TABLE 46.1 Gustilo-Anderson classification of open fractures

TYPE	DESCRIPTION
I	Open wound <1 cm (not contaminated)
II	Open wound >1 cm and <10 cm without large soft tissue damage
IIIA	Open wound >10 cm with extensive soft tissue damage
IIIB	Open wound that requires flap coverage for exposed bone
IIIC	Open wound with severe vascular injury requiring repair

Adapted from: Gustilo, R.B. & Anderson, J.T., 1976. Prevention of infection in the treatment of one thousand and twenty-five open fractures of long bones: retrospective and prospective analyses. Journal of Bone and Joint Surgery (American) 58(4), 453–458.

- Antibiotic prophylaxis should be commenced, typically IV cephazolin. If washout does not occur within 8 hours of injury, 7 days of antibiotic coverage is recommended.
- Ensure the patient has up-to-date tetanus prophylaxis.

External fixation

- If the fracture site is grossly contaminated, insertion of the permanent metalware is delayed to allow for further washout and preparation of the wound for definitive fracture management.
- The use of an external fixator framework permits temporary reduction of the fracture fragments whereby pins are inserted percutaneously into the bone and held in place by external scaffolding (see Figs 46.2 and 46.3).

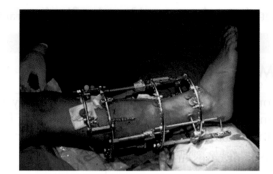

FIGURE 46.2 Example of ring external fixation for a right-sided tibial fracture.

Reproduced from: MacLoed, M., 2010. Proximal tibia fractures: external fixation II. In: Schemitsch, E.H. & McKee, M.D., Operative Techniques: Orthopaedic trauma surgery. Philadelphia: Saunders, pp. 523-542, Fig. 14.

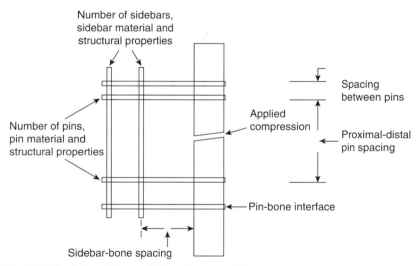

FIGURE 46.3 Principles of the stability of external fixation.

Browner, B.D., 2003. Skeletal Trauma: Basic science, management, and reconstruction, 3rd ed. Philadelphia: Saunders.

- External fixation also plays a role in fracture management where internal constructs will not give adequate reduction or fixation, particularly for comminuted fractures.
- During the postoperative period, the pin sites should be cleaned with normal saline and have a non-occlusive dressing.
- In around 10% of cases the pins show signs of infection, and the bone around the insertion site will show signs of osteolysis.
- If there is persistent infection around any of the pin sites, order investigations to determine if there is an underlying collection and/or evidence of osteomyelitis.

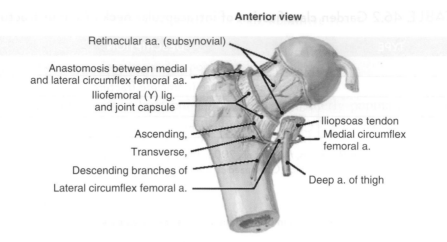

Anterior view

Retinacular aa. (subsynovial)

Anastomosis between medial
and lateral circumflex femoral aa.

Iliofemoral (Y) lig.
and joint capsule

Ascending,

Transverse,

Descending branches of

Lateral circumflex femoral a.

Iliopsoas tendon

Medial circumflex
femoral a.

Deep a. of thigh

FIGURE 46.5 Anatomy of the blood supply of the neck of femur.

Hansen, J.T., 2014. Lower limb. In: Hansen, J.T., Netter's Clinical Anatomy, 3rd ed. Philadelphia: Saunders.

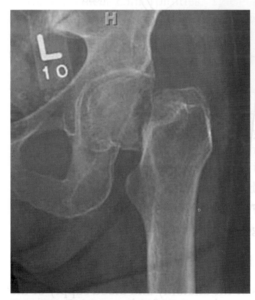

FIGURE 46.6 Subcapital NOF fracture.

Reproduced from: Jackman, J.M. & Watson, J.T., 2010. Hip fractures in older men. Clinics in Geriatric Medicine 26(2), 311-329, Fig. 1.

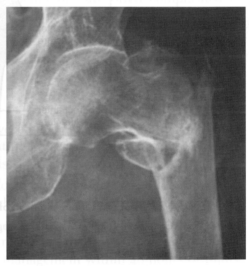

FIGURE 46.7 Extracapsular intertrochanteric NOF fracture.

Reproduced from: Leslie, M.P. & Baumgaertner, M.R., 2009. Intertrochanteric hip fractures. In: Browner, B.D., Skeletal Trauma: Basic science, management, and reconstruction, 5th ed. Philadelphia: Saunders, Fig. 55-3.

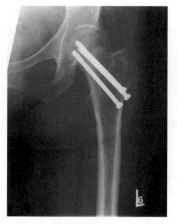

FIGURE 46.8 Cancellous screws placement for an undisplaced subcapital NOF fracture.

Reproduced from: Karanicolas, P.J, Bhandari, M., Walter, S.D., et al., 2009, Radiographs of hip fractures were digitally altered to mask surgeons to the type of implant without compromising the reliability of quality ratings or making the rating process more difficult. Journal of Clinical Epidemiology 62(2), 214-223, Fig. 1.

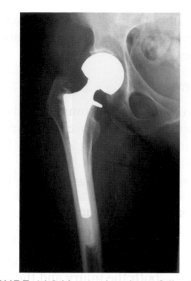

FIGURE 46.9 Hemiarthroplasty following a displaced subcapital NOF fracture.

Reproduced from: Sah, A.P. & Ready, J.E., 2007. Use of oxidized zirconium hemiarthroplasty in hip fractures. Journal of Arthroplasty 22(8), 1174-1180, Fig. 6.

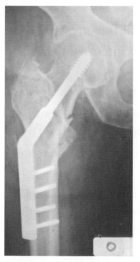

FIGURE 46.10 Dynamic hip screw for intertrochanteric NOF fracture.

Reproduced from: Bartoníček, J., 2011. Trochanteric fractures. In: Waddell, J.P., ed. Fractures of the Proximal Femur: Improving outcomes. Philadelphia: Saunders.

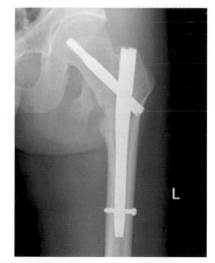

FIGURE 46.11 A short intramedullary nail.

Reproduced from: Bartoníček, J., 2011. Trochanteric fractures. In: Waddell, J.P., ed. Fractures of the Proximal Femur: Improving outcomes. Philadelphia: Saunders.

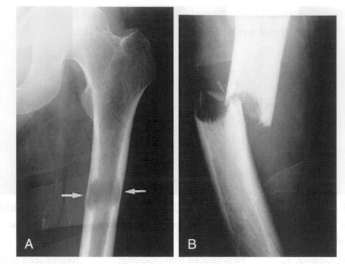

FIGURE 46.16 Pathological midshaft femur fracture (B). Image A was taken 2 weeks prior.

Reproduced from: Mettler, F.A., 2014. Essentials of Radiology. Philadelphia: Saunders, pp. 185-268, Fig. 8-111.

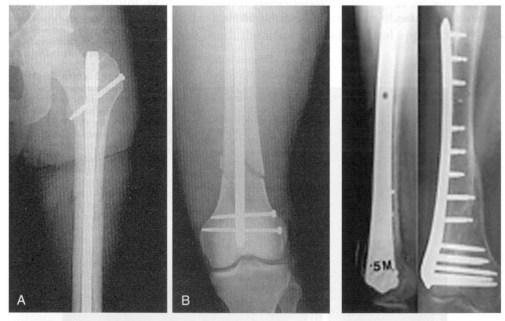

FIGURE 46.17 IM nail for supracondylar distal femur fracture. The cross screws prevent rotation.

Reproduced from: Bucholz, R.W., Heckman, J.D. & Court-Brown, C.M. (eds), 2006. Rockwood and Greene's Fractures in Adults, 6th ed. Philadelphia: Lippincott & Wilkins, p. 1875, Fig. 139-4.

FIGURE 46.18 ORIF of intra-articular distal femoral fracture.

Reproduced from: Krettek, C. & Hawi, N., 2015. Fractures of the distal femur. In: Browner, B.D., Skeletal Trauma: Basic science, management, and reconstruction, 5th Edition. Philadelphia: Saunders, Fig. 59-18.

- Postoperative
  - Pain is an expected complication and may limit mobility in the early stage.
  - Post-op bloods to check haemoglobin and a postoperative X-ray to confirm position of metalware.
  - Patients with fractured NOFs who have had DHS and IM nails can potentially weight bear as tolerated from day 1 postoperatively.
  - Recovery in the elderly patient can be slow, and those presenting from home may need prolonged inpatient subacute care to regain independence.
  - Liaising early with the orthopaedic geriatrics team or the appropriate referring registrar for subacute care can lead to discussion regarding whether or not a patient is appropriate for inpatient rehab.

TIBIAL FRACTURES

- Tibial plateau fractures
  - Include proximal tibia fractures involving the articular surface.
  - Occur during a medial or lateral force and/or axial loading injury.
  - Lead to depression and splitting fractures of the tibial plateau.
  - X-ray can identify the fracture; CT offers superior visualisation of the fracture pattern.
  - Classification systems vary but Schatzker types are commonly used for diagnosis.
  - Management can include external fixation (temporary or definitive), particularly in the instance of open fractures.
  - Fractures can disrupt ligamentous attachments leading to instability.
  - There are many different approaches for ORIF including screw placement for simple split fractures and plates for plating for more extensive condylar fractures. Restoring anatomical contour is the key concern
  - Postoperatively, the non-weight-bearing period is 6 weeks minimum, with an increase in tolerated weight bearing over a further 6 week period.
- Tibial shaft fractures
  - Include fractures in the proximal third of the tibia:
    - due to torsional or high energy impact
    - significant displacement caused by muscle forces from quadriceps and hamstring tendons
    - IM nail performed depending on the amount of proximal tibia and state of communition

- meticulous planning and approach required due to the increased rates of malunion with these fractures.
○ High forces through the tibial shaft can cause fibula fractures (Ring principle), so whole leg X-rays should be requested.
○ Examination should include vascular and neurological status. Be mindful of the possibility of compartment syndrome.
○ Patients can present with large spiral fractures with rotational deformities that can be reduced preoperatively before temporary splinting.
○ Unless there is intra-articular extension the injury can be treated with IM nailing.

Figs 46.19 to 46.23 illustrate various types of tibial fractures and methods of surgical repair.

PELVIC FRACTURES

There are two classic presentations of pelvic fractures:

1 high energy trauma from motor vehicle/motorbike accidents (MVA/MBA)
2 falls in elderly patients.

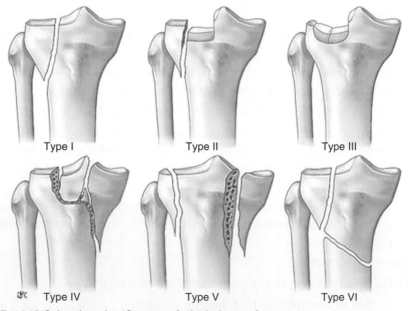

FIGURE 46.19 Schatzker classification of tibial plateau fractures.

Gicquel, T. & Najihi, N., 2013. Tibial plateau fractures: reproducibility of three classifications (Schatzker, AO, Duparc) and a revised Duparc classification. Orthopaedics & Traumatology: Surgery & Research 99(7), 805-816, Fig. 2.

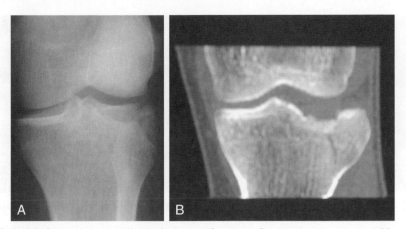

FIGURE 46.20 Schatzker type II tibial plateau fracture. Depression is more readily appreciated on CT scan.

Reproduced from: Langford, J. & Jacofsky, D., 2012. Tibial plateau fractures. In: Scott, W.N., ed., Insall & Scott Surgery of the Knee, 5th ed. Philadelphia: Churchill Livingstone, pp. 773-785, Figs 81-7 A and B.

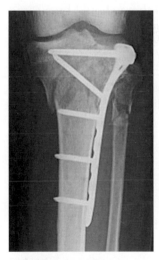

FIGURE 46.21 Tibial locking plate with diaphyseal screw.

Reproduced from: Cronier, P. & Pietu, G., 2010. The concept of locking plates. Orthopaedics and Traumatology: Surgery and Research 96(4 Suppl), S17-S36, Fig. 33A.

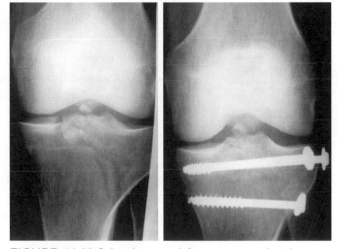

FIGURE 46.22 Schatzker type I fracture treated with diaphyseal screw with anatomical reduction.

Reproduced from: Langford, J. & Jacofsky, D., 2012. Tibial plateau fractures. In: Scott, W.N., ed., Insall and Scott Surgery of the Knee, 5th ed. Philadelphia: Churchill Livingstone, pp. 773-785, Figs 81-4 A and C.

SECTION IV

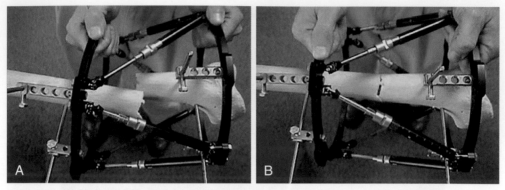

FIGURE 46.23 Ilizarov external fixation device allows for high-tension circumferential fixation.

Reproduced from: Rudloff, M., 2013. Fractures of the Lower Extremity. In: Canale S.T. & Beaty, J.H., Campbell's Operative Orthopaedics, 12th ed. Philadelphia: Mosby, Fig. 54-38.

Due to the potential of life-threatening complications there should be a rapid assessment of pelvic injuries in the trauma setting. There are two key concerns during assessment of a pelvic fracture:

1 Are there any major complications of injury present?
   a Haemorrhage – can be concealed in the large volume of the pelvis and be associated with haemodynamic instability (mortality up to 50%).
   b Neurological injury – L5/S1 in particular.
   c Urological trauma – look for urethral bleeding. Consider urethrogram.
2 Is this an unstable fracture requiring urgent orthopaedic input and management?
   a Unstable fracture patterns are associated with increased risk of haemorrhage.
   b This might include transfer to a centre that offers operative pelvic management.

Examination

- Examination of the pelvis includes palpation of the iliac crests to determine if there is a mechanical instability. This is best performed by an experienced member of the team, and preferably only once.
  - Examination of the perineum and rectum is **essential** in any patient with a suspected traumatic pelvic injury.
  - Trauma patients should have a complete secondary survey performed due to the high association with head and chest injury.

Investigations

- Pelvic X-ray is part of the initial trauma plain films.
- CT scan can help further visualise injury; look for acetabular involvement.

Management

- Initial management in the trauma patient includes appropriate resuscitation as required. If the patient is shocked with pelvic fracture, a pelvic binder should be used.
- Definitive management is dictated by the extent of injury, which determines if the fracture is considered stable or unstable (Fig. 46.24).

Examples of pelvic fractures are shown in Figs 46.25 and 46.26.

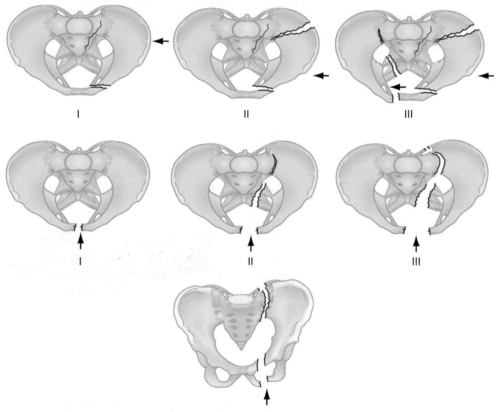

FIGURE 46.24 Young-Burgess classification of pelvic fractures.

- Arrows indicate direction of force.
- Pelvic ligaments help provide stability.
- Stable fractures (APC I and LC I) can be managed non-operatively with protected weight bearing.
- The other fracture patterns are considered unstable requiring operative intervention.

Hak, D. & Mauffrey, C., 2016. Chapter 11: Trauma. In: Miller, M.D. & Thompson, S.R., Miller's Review of Orthopaedics, 7th ed. Philadelphia: Elsevier, pp. 767-855, Fig. 11-21.

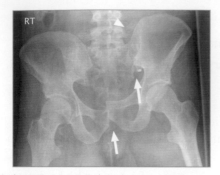

FIGURE 46.25 Pelvic fracture with vertical sheer.

Reproduced from: Morrison, W., Parvizi, W. & Weiss, J., 2012. Pelvic and acetabular fractures. In: Miller, M.D. & Sanders, T.G., Presentation, Imaging and Treatment of Common Musculoskeletal Conditions. Philadelphia: Saunders, pp. 354-365, Fig. 71-10.

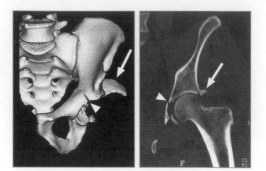

FIGURE 46.26 Acetabular fracture.

Reproduced from: Morrison, W., Parvizi, W. & Weiss, J., 2012. Pelvic and acetabular fractures. In: Miller, M.D. & Sanders, T.G., Presentation, Imaging and Treatment of Common Musculoskeletal Conditions. Philadelphia: Saunders, pp. 354-365, Fig. 71-15.

COMPARTMENT SYNDROME

This is a surgical emergency arising from increased pressure in a fixed body compartment. It most commonly occurs in the limbs but can also affect the abdominal cavity.

Compartment syndrome is commonly associated with limb trauma, particularly of the long bones. Other causes include burns, vascular injuries and crushing mechanisms. A notable indirect cause includes the large volume fluid shift with increased capillary permeability associated with systemic inflammation response syndrome (SIRS) secondary to trauma. Also seen with ischaemia–reperfusion injuries.

Examination

- Examination findings are difficult to demonstrate with early compartment syndrome.
  - The typical early finding is pain out of proportion with clinical findings. Some patients also report paraesthesia. For patients with fractures, immobilisation and reduction should improve pain.
  - Examination may reveal a tense muscle compartment, with pain elicited on **passive** movement of the muscles.
  - Late findings are described as the classic '5 Ps': pain, pallor, pulselessness, paraesthesia, paralysis. This is suggestive of an ischaemic limb (Chapter 47).

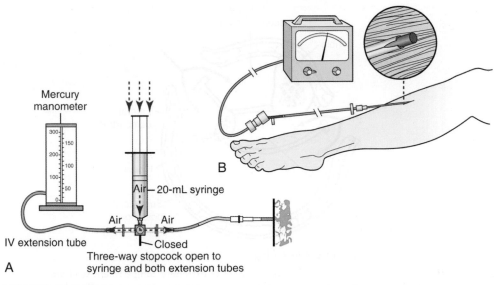

FIGURE 46.27 Using a manometer to measure intra-compartment pressure.

Adapted from: Chung, J. & Mordrall, J., 2014. Chapter 163: Compartment syndrome. In: Cronenwett, J.L. & Johnston, K.W., Rutherford's Vascular Surgery, Philadelphia: Saunders, pp. 2544-2554, Fig. 163-1.

Investigations

- Investigations play a limited role as diagnosis is a clinical one.
- Compartment pressures are sometimes measured using a manometer (Fig. 46.27).

Management

- If the diagnosis is not confirmed or considered unlikely, remove dressings and splints from the affected area and elevate to reduce pressure and oedema.
- **Urgent** surgical release of compartments if the diagnosis is confirmed → fasciotomies (Fig. 46.28). **All** compartments must be released.
- Complications
  - Prolonged ischaemia secondary to compartment syndrome can lead to nerve injury and muscle damage.
  - Muscle damage can have systemic effects due to the release of myoglobulins (nephrotoxic) and hyperkalaemia (cardiac).
  - Permanent muscle and nerve injury may lead to permanent loss of function.
  - The fasciotomy wounds may be too large to close, requiring graft coverage.

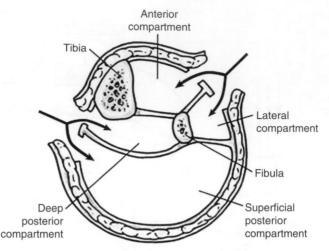

FIGURE 46.28 Fasciotomies of the lower leg.

Ledgerwood, A.M. & Lucas, C.E., 2014. The management of extremity compartment syndrome. In: Cameron, J.L. & Cameron, A.M., Current Surgical Therapy, 11th ed. Philadelphia: Saunders, pp. 1124-1128, Fig. 6.

DISLOCATIONS

Dislocation is the loss of anatomical joint alignment. It can be associated with open injuries and fractures, particularly with high energy trauma. Some patients experience dislocations due to anatomical factors (patella dislocations) or disease of the connective tissue such as Ehlers-Danlos.

The most commonly affected joint is the shoulder, which is the most mobile of all joints. It accounts for around 50% of all joint dislocations.

Presentations are listed in Table 46.3.

Examination

- Examination findings will sometimes reveal an obvious joint deformity with decreased range of motion (ROM). The patient will try and support the limb. Pain is alleviated when the limb is not weight bearing.

Investigations

- Should include plain X-ray to determine the nature of the dislocation.
- CT scan is useful for detecting small fracture fragments (particularly of the elbow).
- MRI scan will help identify ligamentous injuries.

Management

Refer to Table 46.4 for management of specific types of dislocation.

- Reduction should be attempted as soon as feasibly possible. For more difficult cases (knee, hip, elbow), orthopaedic input should be sought.

- **Post-reduction films are mandatory.**
  - Although the joint may appear clinically reduced, fracture fragments or ligamentous injury may have prevented a true reduction.
  - There should be immobilisation of the joint post reduction, with appropriate follow-up organised.

TABLE 46.3 Presentations of joint dislocations

LOCATION	PRESENTATION	MECHANISM
Shoulder	Anterior dislocation >90% Posterior and inferior less common Can be associated with fractures	Direct blow to arm Fall on outstretched hand (FOOSH)
Elbow	Posterior dislocation 90% Usually associated with fracture (particularly radial head) Common paediatric injury	FOOSH
Hip	Dislocation of native hip is rare More commonly seen after arthroplasty though incidence is <2%	High energy impact
Knee	Rare, accounting for <0.2% of all orthopaedic presentations High likelihood of neurovascular injury Ligamentous injury will have occurred (cruciates in particular)	High energy injury
Patella	Lateral dislocation most common	Twisting motion to flexed knee Direct blow to knee

Adapted from: Salata, M. & Wojtys, E., 2010. Chapter 146: Knee dislocation. In: Miller, M.D., Hart, J.A. & MacKnight, J.M. Essential Orthopaedics. Philadelphia: Saunders, pp. 628-632. White, R.E., Forness, T.J., Allman, J.K., et al., 2001. Effect of posterior capsular repair on early dislocation in primary total hip replacement. Clinical Orthopaedics and Related Research 393, 163-167.

TABLE 46.4 Management of common dislocations

Shoulder dislocation	• Reduction can be achieved under sedation
	• Older patients with traumatic mechanisms should give the junior doctor a low threshold for ordering a CT
	   • Look for Bankart fractures involving the glenoid (instability)
	   • Cortical breaches of the humerus are common
	• Multiple methods of reduction; ensure enough staff are present to assist
	   • The approach below involves applying inline traction with counter-traction provided by a sling under the axilla (See Figs 46.29 & 46.30)

continued

TABLE 46.4 Management of common dislocations—cont'd

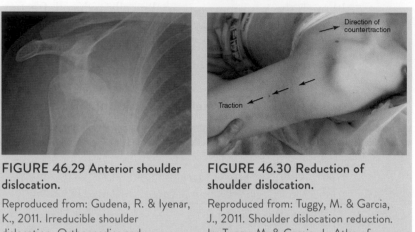

FIGURE 46.29 Anterior shoulder dislocation.

Reproduced from: Gudena, R. & Iyenar, K., 2011. Irreducible shoulder dislocation. Orthopaedics and Traumatology: Surgery and Research. 97(4), 451-453, Fig. 1.

FIGURE 46.30 Reduction of shoulder dislocation.

Reproduced from: Tuggy, M. & Garcia, J., 2011. Shoulder dislocation reduction. In: Tuggy, M. & Garcia, J., Atlas of Essential Procedures. Philadelphia: Saunders, Fig. 52-4.

Elbow dislocation	• Around half of elbow dislocations are associated with a fracture • Difficulties in reduction can be due to fracture fragments • This may necessitate open reduction with fracture fixation (ORIF) • These patients can be evaluated with CT following plain films (see Fig. 46.31) • Reduction is achieved with an assistant as per Fig. 46.32

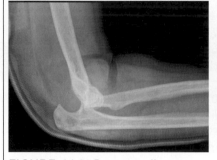

FIGURE 46.31 Posterior elbow dislocation.

Reproduced from: Graham, J.A., 2008. Dislocation reduction of the elbow joint. In: Thomsen, T.W. & Setnik, G.S., eds., Procedures Consult [Internet]. Elsevier, Fig. 2. <www.proceduresconsult.com/medical-procedures/>.

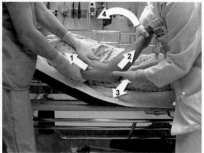

FIGURE 46.32 Reduction of elbow dislocation. Counter traction is provided (1) while traction is applied (2); the elbow joint is palpated to ensure it is appropriately aligned (3) before the elbow is flexed (4).

Reproduced from: Graham, J.A., 2008. Dislocation reduction of the elbow joint. In: Thomsen, T.W. & Setnik, G.S., eds., Procedures Consult [Internet]. Elsevier, Fig. 9. <www.proceduresconsult.com/medical-procedures/>.

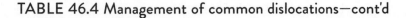

TABLE 46.4 Management of common dislocations—cont'd

Patella dislocation	• Lateral dislocation is most common. Occurs when the patella is forced beyond the lateral femoral condyle, unable to be spontaneously reduced • Can be associated with fractures and cartilage damage (osteochondral defects) – may require CT or MRI assessment • Reduction is achieved as demonstrated in Figs 46.33 and 46.34

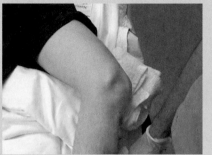

FIGURE 46.33 Dislocated patella.

Reproduced from: Thomsen, T.W. & Setnik, G.S., eds., 2008. Dislocation reduction of the patella. In: Thomsen, T.W. & Setnik, G.S., eds., Procedures Consult [Internet]. Elsevier, Fig. 1. <www.proceduresconsult.com/medical-procedures/>.

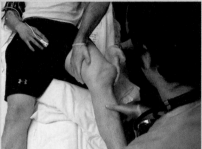

FIGURE 46.34 Reduction of the patella with lateral pressure applied as the knee is extended.

Reproduced from: Thomsen, T.W. & Setnik, G.S., eds., 2008. Dislocation reduction of the patella. In: Thomsen, T.W. & Setnik, G.S., eds., Procedures Consult [Internet]. Elsevier, Fig. 4. <www.proceduresconsult.com/medical-procedures/>.

THE ACUTE JOINT

Acute presentations of swollen and painful joints can be secondary to multiple focal and systemic causes.

Some arthropathies present with multiple affected joints, presenting in either a symmetrical or asymmetrical pattern. These presentations are suggestive of an underlying systemic cause. Acute monoarthritis is often an indication for orthopaedic review.

- History and examination help discriminate between the different processes of single joint pathology.
  - Inflammatory (septic arthritis)
    - Acute onset with erythema and swelling around the joint. Irritable on passive ROM. Septic arthritis (and gout) tend to be monoarthropathies, but can involve multiple joints in some patients.

- Can be associated with fever.
- Examination can reveal joint effusion, particularly with the knee.
  > Painful joints can also arise from an overlying cellulitis or bursitis. This can be differentiated on examination, as these conditions tend to cause a more focal tenderness without the generalised joint irritability.
  > Arthrocentesis can help with diagnosis and isolation of any bacteria.
- Metabolic (gout, pseudogout)
  - Common presentation in great toe, but can affect others including the knee, elbow and wrist.
  - Arthrocentesis will help distinguish between gout, pseudogout and septic arthritis.
  - Treat with anti-inflammatory medication.
- Trauma
  - Fractures of the articular surface can cause profound joint swelling (i.e. tibial plateau) with severe restriction in movement.
  - Disruption to ligament, cartilage and tendon around bone (enthesis) can cause joint effusion.

Investigations

- Always begin with a plain X-ray film to check for foreign body or fracture. These investigations can be supplemented by CT for smaller fractures.
- Bloods to check inflammatory markers are helpful in determining the likelihood of infection; however, in the obviously swollen and erythematous knee, clinical examination findings are more useful.
- Arthrocentesis should be performed.
  - Provides useful information on the cellular make-up of any collection.
  - Collect a sample for cultures prior to giving antibiotics.
  - Identification and collection of a joint fluid sample can sometimes be difficult without imaging; ultrasound guided collections can be organised through the Radiology Department.
  - Early results include the white cell count and glucose level (Table 46.5).

Management

- With a convincing clinical presentation, empirical antibiotic therapy can be started until culture results return, though further samples will be affected.

TABLE 46.5 Joint fluid analysis of multiple acute joint presentations

DIAGNOSIS	APPEARANCE	WBCs/m³	GLUCOSE (% BLOOD LEVEL)	CRYSTALS UNDER POLARISED LIGHT	CULTURE
Normal	Clear	<200	95–100	None	Negative
Osteoarthritis	Clear	<4000	95–100	None	Negative
Traumatic	Straw-coloured, bloody, xanthochromic, occasionally with fat droplets	<4000	95–100	None	Negative
Acute gout	Turbid	2000–50,000	80–100	Negative birefringence; needle-like	Negative
Pseudogout	Turbid	2000–50,000	80–100	Positive birefringence; rhomboid	Negative
Septic arthritis	Turbid, purulent	5000 to >50,000	<50	None	Usually positive
Rheumatoid arthritis	Turbid	2000–50,000	≈75	None	Negative

Adapted from: Schrank, K.S., 2014, Joint disorders. In: Adams, J.G., Barton, E.D., Collings, J., et al., eds. Emergency Medicine, 2nd ed. Philadelphia: Saunders, Table 107.1.

Osteomyelitis (OM)

OM is an infection of bone with either an acute or chronic course. Organisms include:

- *Staphylococcus aureus* (including MRSA)
- *Pseudomonas aeruginosa*
- *Enterobacter* spp.

Source can be from haematogenous spread or direct surgical contamination.

Investigations

- Patient should have FBE and CRP to determine inflammatory marker status.
- Key goal is to establish the causative organism to facilitate targeted therapy.
- Plain X-ray films are sometimes used to detect suggestive signs of osteomyelitis, but MRI is more sensitive and specific regarding location and extent.

Management

- Surgical debridement of affected tissues should take place where possible.
- Current guidelines recommend 6 weeks total treatment with at least 4 weeks of IV therapy.

ARTHROSCOPY

In this technique, a camera (arthroscope) is passed through a small port site into the joint to allow for diagnosis and management of joint pathology.

- Indications
  - o A large number of acute and chronic joint (Chapter 67) pathologies involving the hip, knee, shoulder, ankle and wrist (Table 46.6).
  - o Some procedures are performed with arthroscopic assistance (i.e. ACL reconstruction and rotator cuff repairs).

Management

- Preoperative
  - o Some patients may require pre-admission clinic.
  - o Ensure patients have recent imaging performed prior to the procedure.
  - o Patients can have a range of general, regional and local anaesthetic options.

TABLE 46.6 Common diagnostic and therapeutic uses of arthroscopy

JOINT[a]	DIAGNOSTIC	THERAPEUTIC
Shoulder	Osteoarthritis Synovial biopsy	Rotator cuff repair Labral repair Sub-acromial decompression Washout of infected joint Biceps tenodesis
Hip	Osteoarthritis Labral tears	Washout of infected joint Labral repairs
Knee	Osteoarthritis Synovial biopsy	Meniscal tear repairs Cruciate ligament repairs Washout of infected joint Lateral patellar release Osteochondral defect repair Fracture reduction

[a]Ankle, wrist, elbow arthroscopy are less commonly performed.

- Intraoperative
  - The arthroscope is passed into the joint space.
  - A continuous wash is used, often with a pump mechanism to keep the visual field clear (often a task for the junior doctor!).
  - Other instruments can be introduced to grasp or probe the tissue and cutting tools to trim or shave away loose pieces of cartilage.
  - The surgeon can assess the level of arthritis present by observing wear in the cartilage. Photos can be taken and attached to the report.
- Postoperative
  - Patients who undergo diagnostic arthroscopy are typically booked as day cases.
  - Patients who have undergone a procedure will normally stay overnight.
- Complications
  - Haemarthrosis
  - Infection
  - Failure of procedure

See Figs 46.35 and 46.36 for visualisation and repair afforded by arthroscopy.

JOINT ARTHROPLASTY

The indications for joint arthroplasty are covered in the outpatient assessment (Chapter 67).

There are many prosthetic systems for arthroplasty, each coming with a different surgical approach and set of equipment.

The Australian Orthopaedic Association National Joint Replacement Registry (AOANJRR) produces an annual report that aims to analyse the outcomes for joint arthroplasty, including the rates of revision for patients with a particular type of prosthesis.

Management

- Preoperative
  - Patients are almost always booked electively for these cases.
  - Patients should be reviewed at pre-admission clinic.
- Intraoperative
  - Total hip replacements (THR)
    - The femoral head and acetabular articular surface are replaced by prostheses. These implants are composed of different materials, including mixtures of plastic polymers, metal and ceramic.

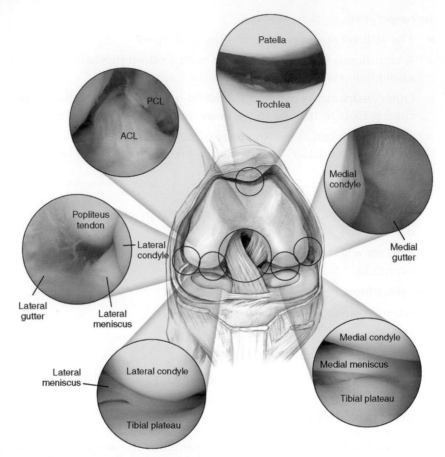

FIGURE 46.35 Visualisation of the knee during arthroscopy.

Miller, M.D. & Hart, J.A., 2010. Knee Arthroscopy. In: Miller, M.D., Chhabra, A.B. & Safran, M.R., Primer of Arthroscopy. Philadelphia: Elsevier, pp. 13-35, Fig. 2-4.

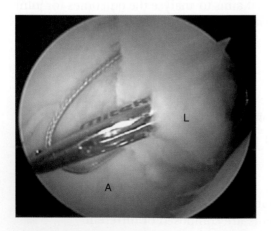

FIGURE 46.36 Arthroscopic repair of labrum (L) tear that has detached from the acetabulum (A).

Reproduced from: Sanchez, V. & Mesa, A., 2015. Chapter 82: Hip arthroscopy. In: Miller, M.D. & Thompson, S.R., DeLee & Drez's Orthopaedic Sports Medicine, 4th ed. Saunders, pp. 953-965, Fig. 82-1c.

- ○ Total knee replacements (TKR)
    - – The knee has three compartments, lateral, medial and patella–femoral. Replacement can be performed on all three, or just one. Arthroplasty on only the medial or lateral knee is termed unicompartmental arthroplasty.
    - – The distal femur and tibial plateau is replaced. Patella resurfacing can include a plastic polymer implant on the posterior patella.
    - – Cutting guide blocks are used to shape the bones for the prosthesis, which are then fitted with testing implants before the permanent prosthetics are inserted.
- ○ Arthroplasty can be offered for shoulder, elbow and ankle joint reconstruction,
- Postoperative
    - ○ Guidelines are surgeon specific, though there is an emphasis on achieving maximum knee extension with physiotherapist input.
    - ○ Early support from Allied Health with their rehabilitation is essential, particularly in patients undergoing bilateral TKRs.
    - ○ Patient should undergo a course of postoperative DVT prophylaxis. The exact course can vary among hospital networks, though commonly patients will receive:
        - – 4 weeks of prophylactic enoxaparin for TKR
        - – 2 weeks of prophylactic enoxaparin for THR
        - – low dose aspirin (150 mg) or rivaroxoban for some.
- Complications
    - ○ Haematoma
    - ○ Infection (see 'Infection of joint prosthesis' below)
    - ○ Dislocation
    - ○ Pain
    - ○ Nerve injury
    - ○ DVT
- Follow-up
    - ○ Usually 2 weeks for wound check, then at 6 weeks review with imaging.
    - ○ Ongoing pain at this stage may be suggestive of poor rehabilitation or problems with the prosthesis.

Examples of TKR and THR procedures are shown in Figs 46.37 and 46.38, respectively.

INFECTION OF JOINT PROSTHESIS

Peri-prosthetic infections are serious postoperative complications from arthroplasty procedures. Infected metalware can act as a reservoir for ongoing further

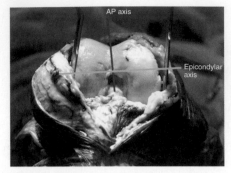

FIGURE 46.37 The patella is retracted to expose the articular surface of the femur. Correctly aligning the axis is a crucial aspect of TKRs.

Reproduced from: Mihalko, W.M., 2013. Arthroplasty of the knee. In: Canale, S.T. & Beaty, J.H., Campbell's Operative Orthopaedics, 12th ed. Philadelphia: Mosby, pp. 376-444.e7. Fig. 7-17.

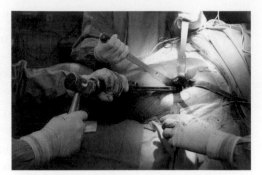

FIGURE 46.38 Cup placement during a THR. Note the junior doctors dutifully holding the retractors!

Reproduced from: Nogler, M., 2009. The direct anterior approach. In: Hozack, W., Parvizi, J. & Bender, B., Surgical Treatment of Hip Arthritis: Reconstruction, replacement, and revision. Saunders, pp. 99-107, Fig. 11-14.

infection necessitating formal washout and potential removal of the prosthesis. There are three broad categories of peri-prosthetic infection:

1 exogenous infections – local sign of infection from wound dehiscence or abscess with tract extending to joint

2 haematogenous spread – can present as new onset pain, irritable joint with fever; collection can be seen on imaging

3 chronic – early loosening of prosthesis perpetuates an inflammatory process that forms a chronic effusion.

Management

The surgical management of these patients (see Fig. 46.39) is dependent on the condition of the tissue surrounding the joint and the antibiotic susceptibilities of the causative organism.

- The recommended empirical regimen for these patients is IV vancomycin, which will also cover for potential MRSA involvement.

- Swabs and tissue samples should be taken at every operation to help identify the causative organism and allow a targeted therapy.

- These patients should be discussed with the Infectious Diseases team for guidance and approval for antibiotics.

- One organism in particular, *Priopionibacterium acnes*, is closely associated with septic arthritis in the shoulder (with or without a prosthetic) and will need coverage in the empirical setting from either vancomycin or benzylpenicillin.

SECTION IV

Condition   **Surgical procedure**

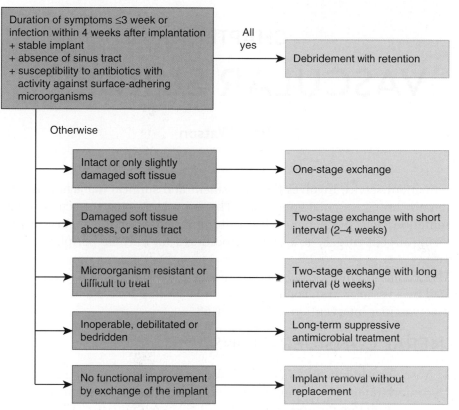

FIGURE 46.39 Surgical treatment pathway for peri-prosthetic joint infection.

Zimmerli, W. & Parham, S., 2015. Orthopedic implant-associated infections. In: Bennett, J.E., Dolin, R. & Blaser, M.J., Mandell, Douglas, and Bennett's Principles and Practice of Infectious Diseases, 8th ed. Philadelphia: Saunders, pp. 1328-1340, Fig. 107.1.

SECTION IV

CHAPTER 47

VASCULAR SURGERY

Paul Watson

The inpatient service involves the assessment and surgical management of both acute and chronic vascular conditions. There is a large range of acuity in patient presentation from the patient with acute limb ischaemia or aneurysm rupture requiring urgent surgery to elective procedures for chronic peripheral vascular disease.

This chapter outlines common emergency presentations and procedures performed by a vascular unit. For a discussion of vascular disease and indications for elective vascular intervention see Chapter 68.

GENERAL CONSIDERATIONS

- Vascular patients are often medically unwell with multiple medical comorbidities that require careful observation and management in the context of a major operation.
- Adequate preoperative assessment in the pre-admission setting including liaising with medical and anaesthetic teams can help with the perioperative management of these patients.
  - Clamping of major vessels, particularly the aorta, create notable cardiac stress; therefore, preoperative assessment of cardiac and respiratory function is essential.
- Most patients will continue on their antiplatelet medications throughout the perioperative period; however, other anticoagulants may need to be stopped. Check with the registrar.
- Vascular Surgery has a close relationship with the Radiology Department including shared responsibility for endovascular procedures.

ACUTE ABDOMINAL AORTIC ANEURYSM (AAA)

AAA is a life-threatening condition involving full thickness (all wall structures) dilation of the abdominal aorta by more than 50%. Though around 75% of AAAs are asymptomatic, any patient >50 years presenting with abdominal pain should have an AAA excluded.

An approach to the asymptomatic AAA is discussed in Chapter 68.

Ruptured AAA

- As this is a surgical emergency, many hospitals have an emergency AAA protocol involving rapid involvement of the inpatient vascular team and access to theatre.
- Patients may present with abdominal/back/flank pain and a clinically palpable, pulsatile mass.
  - A brief history should include whether the patient has a known AAA.
  - The presence of haemodynamic instability (hypotension/tachycardia) is an indication for rapid operative intervention.
- In the emergency setting a rapid bedside ultrasound can help identify the presence of an AAA.
- Initial management is determined by the patient's clinical status.
  - Bilateral wide-bore IV access should be obtained.
  - Bloods include FBE, UEC, coagulation studies and blood group and hold.
  - Though the patient can be haemodynamically unstable, fluid restriction should be limited creating a 'permissive hypotension' that decreases internal haemorrhaging and loss of clotting factors and platelets.
- Patients who are haemodynamically stable can undergo further imaging with CT (with angiography is helpful) to visualise the appearance and dimensions of the aneurysm, aiding in preoperative planning.
- Definitive surgical management is either via open repair or endovascular aortic repair (EVAR; see below).
  - EVAR is increasingly used for patients presenting with a ruptured AAA who have favourable anatomy for endovascular approach. EVAR is only feasible in those patients stable enough to have preoperative CT.

Symptomatic AAA

- Onset of symptoms can be slow; patients may present to ED or GP with abdominal or back pain.
  - Always rule out AAA in patients >50 years with abdominal pain or back pain. Examination may reveal a pulsatile mass.
  - U/S is a useful screening tool for AAA, with some studies suggesting routine screening for patients aged >65 years.
  - CT remains the gold standard for examining AAAs (see Fig. 47.1).
- Symptomatic AAA can be suggestive of rapid dilatation of the aneurysm.

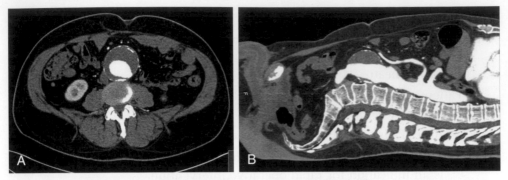

FIGURE 47.1 Transverse and sagittal CT images demonstrating AAA.

Reproduced from: Goldstone, J., 2013. Aneurysms of the aorta and iliac arteries. In: Moore, W.S., Vascular and Endovascular Surgery, 8th ed. Philadelphia: Saunders, Fig. 39-3.

- Inflammatory AAA: CT (± angiogram) is then indicated to determine the size and extent of the aneurysm.

Patients presenting with either a ruptured or symptomatic AAA will require urgent assessment by the vascular team for transfer to theatre.

ACUTELY ISCHAEMIC LIMB

This is a vascular emergency requiring urgent specialist input and management. It more commonly affects the lower limbs.

Acutely ischaemic limb is predominantly caused by three processes:

1. Embolism
   a. Tends to be cardiac in origin, associated with atrial and ventricular thrombus from dysrhythmias (AF), decreased cardiac function following cardiac ischaemia (recent AMI) or infective vegetations.
   b. Particularly common cause of upper limb ischaemia.
   c. Emboli may also come from more peripheral thrombus in the limb.
2. Thrombus
   a. More common for acute ischaemia of the lower limb.
   b. Patients with diffuse atherosclerotic disease (known peripheral vascular disease) are more likely to develop an acute thrombosis, which is thought to be secondary to the decreased and disrupted flow throughout the diseased sections of the vessel.
   c. Prothrombotic conditions can also contribute to the development of acute thrombus.
3. Trauma
   a. Common causes include recent procedures such as access for endovascular cardiac procedures and blunt or penetrating trauma from high energy trauma.

The presentation of an acutely ischaemic limb is classically described by the '6 Ps':

1 **p**ain (out of proportion)

2 **p**ulselessness

3 **p**araesthesia

4 **p**aralysis

5 **p**allor

6 **p**oikilothermia (or perishingly cold).

- History is essential to establish the time of onset and previous vascular history, including previous vascular interventions in the affected limb.
  - Rapid onset with no proceeding symptoms is the common presentation of an embolic event. These cases are more readily associated with the so-called '6 Ps'.
  - Gradual onset with a history of prior ischaemic sounding limb pain is more suggestive of a thrombus.
  - The patient's past medical history is helpful in establishing the potential progression of peripheral vascular disease.

Examination

- Examination should focus on assessing the neurovascular status of the limb (see Table 47.1).
  - Appearance of the limb: colour, coolness.
  - Vascularity of the limb: peripheral pulses, capillary refill.
  - Function of the limb: neurological examination including power and sensation.
  - Examination of the contralateral limb may reveal signs of chronic vascular disease.

Management

- Initial management steps can be instituted while the diagnosis is being confirmed.
  - Patients should have blood tests including CK, blood group and hold with cross-match and coagulation profile.
  - Heparinisation should be promptly commenced to prevent further development of thrombus.
  - Wide bore IV access and fluid resuscitation as needed.
  - Analgesia.

TABLE 47.1 Clinical category of an acutely ischaemic limb

	CATEGORY	DESCRIPTION/ PROGNOSIS	SENSORY LOSS	MUSCLE WEAKNESS	DOPPLER SIGNALS	
					Arterial	Venous
I	Viable	Not immediately threatened	None	None	Audible	Audible
II a	Threatened Marginal	Salvageable if promptly treated	Minimal (digits) or none	None	(Often) inaudible	Audible
II b	Threatened Immediate	Salvageable with prompt revascularisation	More than digits, associated with rest pain	Mild, moderate	(Usually) inaudible	Audible
III	Irreversible	Major tissue loss and/or permanent nerve damage	Profound, anaesthetic	Profound, paralysis	Inaudible	Inaudible

Norgren, L., Hiatt, W.R., Dormandy, J.A., et al., 2007. Inter-Society consensus for the management of peripheral arterial disease (TASC II). European Journal of Vascular and Endovascular Surgery 33(Suppl 1), S1-S75, Table E1.

- The clinical urgency of the ischaemia dictates the extent of investigation before intervention.
  - Bloods including coagulation profile, CK and cross-match can be done during the initial resuscitation stage.
  - If the limb is clinically assessed as IIb, there may not be sufficient time for formal imaging as revascularisation needs to occur rapidly.
    - As the aim is to re-vascularise the limbs within 6 hours, some patients may proceed directly to theatre with an on-table angiogram.
  - Patients with I and IIa category ischaemia have a sufficient intervention window that allows dedicated imaging.
    - CT angiography (CTA) is the most commonly used modality to assess the vessel patency.
- The non-threatened limb may be suited to initial management with thrombolysis.
- Surgical management for reversible ischaemia includes percutaneous transluminal angioplasty (PTA), bypass grafts and open endarterectomy.
- Irreversible ischaemia may necessitate amputation dependent on the level of the occlusion (Figs 47.2 and 47.3).

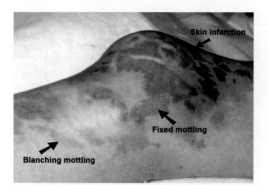

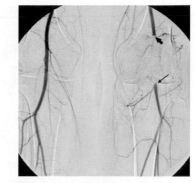

FIGURE 47.2 Skin changes resulting from severe acute limb ischaemia. Fixed mottling of the skin is indicative of non-viability.

Reproduced from: O'Connell, J. & Quiñones-Baldrich, W., 2009. Proper evaluation and management of acute embolic versus thrombotic limb ischemia. Seminars in Vascular Surgery 22(1), 10-16, Fig. 1.

FIGURE 47.3 Arteriogram of the left popliteal artery showing defect. The 'meniscal' cut-off is suggestive of an embolic event.

Reproduced from: Gregory, W., 2009. Acute limb ischemia. Techniques in Vascular and Interventional Radiology 12(2), 117-129, Fig. 18.

ANGIOGRAPHY IN VASCULAR SURGERY

Various of imaging techniques are used to assess and treat vascular disease, though catheter mediated angiography remains the gold standard due to the quality of resolution and fine detail of the images.

- Digital subtraction angiography (DSA) is a process of using contrast to visualise the structure of vessels, with enhancement of the contrast in the images achieved by subtracting bone and soft tissue using the digitised plain film from the contrast injection images (see Figs 47.4 and 47.5).
  - These procedures were traditionally performed in theatre; however, partnerships with the Radiology Department have led to more cases being performed in interventional radiology suites and vascular catheter laboratories.
  - Contrast is administered directly into the artery or vein with rapid acquisition of images.
- Angiography has allowed rapid treatment of vascular disease with many methods of relieving obstruction and restoring flow.
- Patients with poor renal function will need preoperative fluid optimisation to avoid further decline in renal function. It can be useful to liaise with the renal team to obtain a perioperative plan.
- Advances in computed tomography angiography (CTA) and magnetic resonance angiography (MRA) have led to an increased use of these techniques as an alternative to visual arterial occlusion.
  - Doppler U/S can be useful in determining vessel flow.

SECTION IV

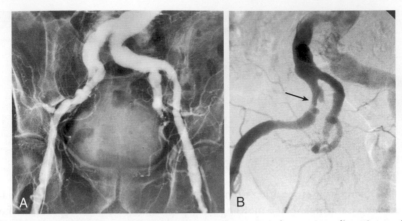

FIGURE 47.4 Though the vessels are apparent, subtracting the surrounding tissue allows for greater visualisation of the flow and blockage of contrast.

Reproduced from: Kaufman, J., 2014. Chapter 2: Fundamentals of angiography. In: Kaufman, J.A. & Lee, M.J., Vascular and Interventional Radiology: The requisites, 2nd ed. Philadelphia: Saunders, pp. 25-55.

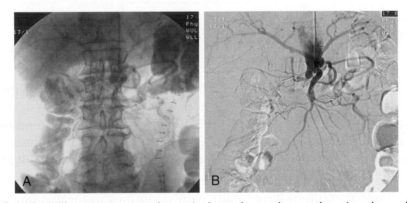

FIGURE 47.5 Midline structures such as spinal vertebrae subtracted to view the coeliac trunk.

Reproduced from: Kaufman, J., 2014. Chapter 2: Fundamentals of angiography. In: Kaufman, J.A. & Lee, M.J., Vascular and Interventional Radiology: The requisites, 2nd ed. Philadelphia: Saunders, pp. 25-55.

- Concepts of vessel patency
  - Inflow
    - An assessment of the blood flow from the proximal system to the affected area (i.e., is a femoral occlusion compounded by an iliac aneurysm?).
  - Run-off
    - Are the distal vessels patent?
    - Important when considering revascularisation surgery of a limb.

– The high resolution images from DSA allow for good visualisation of small vessels in the limb.

AAA REPAIR

- **Preoperative considerations**
  - ○ Anaesthetics review: in pre-admission clinic if elective. In emergency situations call the anaesthetist in charge.
  - ○ Post-op destination: arrange for an HDU/ICU bed by liaising directly with the ICU registrar.
  - ○ Patient should have between 4 and 6 units of cross-matched blood; the use of a 'cell saver' (recycling of erythrocytes) can decrease transfusion requirements.
- The patient should always be prepared for an open AAA repair.
- **Open AAA repair** (Fig. 47.6)
  - ○ Indications
    - – Ruptured or symptomatic AAA, asymptomatic AAA with a diameter >5.5 cm.
    - – Aneurysm not technically suitable for EVAR.
  - ○ Intraoperative
    - – Access to the AAA via a laparotomy or retroperitoneal approach.
      - > For the ruptured AAA, a midline laparotomy approach to the aorta is utilised, allowing for rapid access to the aorta for potential clamping.

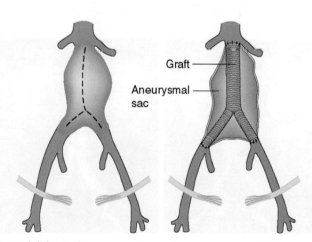

Graft

Aneurysmal sac

FIGURE 47.6 Open AAA repair.

Adapted from: Bradbury, A.W. & Cleveland, T.J., 2012. Vascular and endovascular surgery. In: Garden, O.J., Bradbury, A.W., Forsythe, J.L.R., et al., Principles and Practice of Surgery, 6th ed. Edinburgh: Churchill Livingstone, pp. 345-378, Fig. 21.25.

SECTION IV

> Patients with structural renal abnormalities may require a retroperitoneal approach.

– Clamping of the aorta allows for opening of the aneurysm, removal of any thrombus then placement of the graft. Patients typically receive intraoperative heparin infusion.

- **Endovascular aortic repair (EVAR)**

  o Indications

    – Infra-renal aneurysm with suitable renal and common iliac artery anatomy. Reported rates of suitability are 55–74%.

  o Intraoperative

    – Through femoral access an endovascular stent is passed beyond the proximal limit of the aneurysm and secured distally using the common iliac arteries.

    – Preoperative CTA imaging is required to ensure the patient has suitable anatomy for an endovascular graft (see Fig. 47.7).

    – After placement of the prosthesis imaging is performed to confirm stent position and check for endoleak.

- **Postoperative care** is typically dictated by hospital protocol, though will include:

  o daily bloods to check haemoglobin

  o close monitoring of the patient's neurovascular status; check peripheral pulses in particular

  o drain tube monitoring and removal as per postoperative instructions.

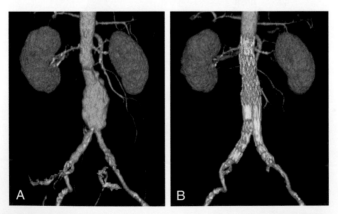

FIGURE 47.7 EVAR of AAA preoperative (A) and postoperative (B) CTAs.

Reproduced from: Isselbacher, E.M., 2013. Aortic disease. In: Antman, E.M., Cardiovascular Therapeutics: A companion to Braunwald's Heart Disease. Philadelphia: Saunders, pp. 606-619, Fig. 40-1.

- Complications
  - Endoleak
    - Blood flow outside the lumen of the graft within the aneurysmal sac.
    - Concern regarding the risk for long-term rupture.
    - May lead to conversion to open repair as secondary procedure.
  - Conversion to open repair from EVAR
    - May occur in the early postoperative period due to device migration.
    - May occur in the later postoperative period due to endoleak.
  - Infected graft
- Follow-up
  - Regular imaging to ensure correct position of graft and monitoring of leakage

MANAGEMENT OF ACUTE ISCHAEMIA

Though each anatomical region presents unique technical challenges, the principles of revascularisation remain the same. In particular, the ultimate goal is to relieve symptomatic arterial occlusions that may progress to total occlusion with significant morbidity.

Patients presenting with acute ischaemia require urgent institution of a management plan dependent on the nature of the occlusion.

- **Pharmacological thrombolysis**
  - Indications
    - Patients who present with a viable acute limb ischaemia of less than 14 days may be suited to initial thrombolytic therapy.
  - Preoperatively
    - Ensure the patient has normal coagulation studies.
    - Treatment is contraindicated in patients with recent surgery or active bleeding due to risk of haemorrhage.
  - Intraoperative
    - Agents such as streptokinase, urokinase and tissue plasminogen activator (TPA) actively break down thrombi.
    - These agents are directly infused into the affected vessel via endovascular catheter.
    - Imaging of the obstruction can help determine the effectiveness of thrombolysis.

- o Postoperative
  - – Patients may require further surgical management if the thrombus is inadequately cleared.
  - – Further imaging can help assess.
  - – Lysis of the clot may lead to more distal emboli, although they are typically asymptomatic.
- o Complications
  - – Postoperative bleeding.
  - – Incomplete thrombus clearance.
- **Thrombo/embolectomy**
  - o Indications
    - – Well circumscribed, acute embolus.
    - – Threatened extremity requiring prompt revascularisation.
  - o Preoperatively
    - – Ensure the patient's coagulation status is checked. Some hospital protocols include the use of preoperative antiplatelet medications.
  - o Intraoperative
    - – The affected artery is incised and directly cannulated with a Fogarty balloon catheter using angiography (see Fig. 47.8).

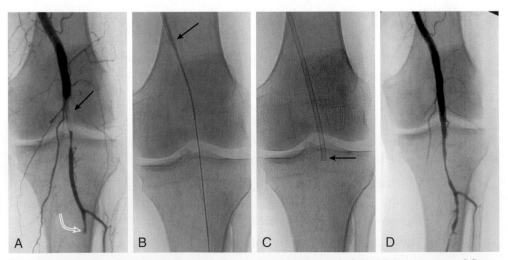

FIGURE 47.8 Aspiration embolectomy for popliteal artery embolus with restoration of flow.
Reproduced from: Kaufman, J.A., 2014. Chapter 4: Vascular interventions. In: Kaufman, J.A. & Lee, M.J., Vascular and Interventional Radiology: The requisites, 2nd ed. Philadelphia: Saunders, Fig. 4-33.

- The balloon is passed beyond the extent of the thrombus, inflated, and the clot is retrieved through the arteriotomy. Repair is by either direct closure or vein graft patch.
  - ○ Postoperative
    - Further postoperative imaging can be useful to determine if underlying chronic thrombosis contributed to acute embolus/thrombus formation.
    - Patients should have the cause of embolus investigated with medical team input and management of vascular risk factors.
    - There is typically a period of postoperative neurovascular observation including toe pressures to determine if there has been an improvement in blood flow.
  - ○ Complications
    - Vessel trauma from the procedure.
    - Pain related to vessel dilatation.

MANAGEMENT OF CHRONIC ISCHAEMIA (ENDOVASCULAR)

There are a number of endovascular and open surgical options in managing chronic arterial disease.

Chapter 68 outlines the diagnosis and investigations of this disease process, with optimisation of medical therapy playing a key role in perioperative and long-term management. Though a chronic ischaemic process can affect the upper limb, these conditions are particularly common in the lower limb and neck (carotid). The TASC II classification gives recommendations on treatment options for lower limb intervention based on anatomical and disease factors.

Percutaneous transluminal angioplasty (TPA) in the lower limb (and/or endovascular stents)

TPA is a common, less invasive approach for approaching mild and moderate peripheral vascular disease.

- Indications
  - ○ Chronic symptomatic ischaemic symptoms.
  - ○ Type A and B TASC II patients and those with Type C lesions with multiple medical comorbidities.
- Preoperative
  - ○ As an elective procedure these patients should all undergo review in the pre-admission clinic with anaesthetics input.

- Intraoperative
  - An endovascular balloon is passed along a guide wire to the site of stenosis via arterial puncture using intraoperative imaging.
  - The balloon is inflated to dilate the vessel and break up the plaque via mechanical stress.
  - Some patients will simply receive PTA with no stent placement; however, stenting can be considered as a primary intervention. The decision of when to place stents primarily and when to perform PTA is dependent on the location and nature of the stenosis/occlusive disease.
  - Patients should receive intraoperative heparin.
- Postoperative
  - Postoperative imaging is typically used to assess the position of the stent and patency of the vessel.
  - The patient should have post-op ABIs performed for comparison with preoperative baseline readings.
- Complications
  - Postoperative pain.
  - Pseudoaneurysm from wall instrumentation.

Carotid artery stenting (CAS)

CAS is an endovascular alternative to carotid endarterectomy. Though carotid angioplasty can be performed alone, stenting carries a more favourable long-term outcome with a reduced risk of embolisation. However, CAS is associated with a higher risk of complications in older patients.

- Indications
  - Patients with severe symptomatic stenosis (70–99%) with no suitable surgical access.
  - Patients unsuitable for invasive surgery due to medical comorbidities.
  - Stenosis following carotid endarterectomy.
- Preoperative
  - Preadmission clinic with anaesthetics input.
  - Dual antiplatelet medications should be continued; check unit protocol or with the registrar.
  - Some surgeons prefer imaging of the entire extra- and intracranial 'overview' imaging for preoperative evaluation.
- Intraoperative
  - Femoral access is still most commonly used.
  - Patients are typically given intraoperative heparin.

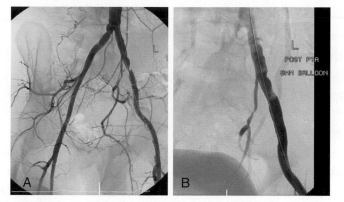

FIGURE 47.9 A focal left external iliac artery stenosis treated with a stent.

Reproduced from: Nicholson, A. & Scott, J., 2014. Intervention for chronic lower limb ischaemia. In: Beard, J.D., Gaines, P.A. & Loftus, I., eds. Vascular and Endovascular Surgery: A companion to specialist surgical practice, 5th ed. London: Saunders, pp. 45-72, Fig. 4.3.

- o Using angiography, stenosis is identified and stent deployed (Fig. 47.9).
- o Some procedures will involve the use of an embolic prevention device (EPD) to prevent stroke.
- Postoperative
  - o Instrumentation of the carotids may stimulate the baroreceptors, which may result in intraoperative bradycardia, requiring atropine. Symptoms may persist in the postoperative period.
  - o Hypertension needs to be carefully observed.
  - o Neurological status should be monitored to detect any evidence of stroke.
- Complications
  - o Stroke, bleeding, haemodynamic instability.

ENDARTERECTOMY

Endarterectomy is most commonly performed for the treatment of carotid and femoral artery disease. However, it can be considered in lower limb chronic ischaemia for patients with unilateral disease.

Carotid endarterectomy (CEA)

CEA is the gold standard for treating atherosclerotic carotid vascular disease with a primary aim of reducing risk of ischaemic stroke.

SECTION IV

- Indications
  - Recently symptomatic and/or severe carotid stenosis.
  - Native carotid with no previous intervention.
  - Selected patients may undergo a prophylactic CEA as they require other procedures associated with a risk of ischaemic stroke (coronary artery bypass).
- Preoperative
  - Patients are typically worked up in the context of recent ischaemic stroke, which should include a dedicated duplex ultrasound.
  - Most patients are commenced on some form of antiplatelet therapy.
- Intraoperative
  - Direct open access to the vessel via a neck incision.
  - Clamps are applied and an incision is made into the vessel (see Fig. 47.10).
  - Atherosclerotic plaque is dissected from the wall of the artery.
  - The vessel can be directly closed although a patch graft is preferred to reduce the risk of postoperative stroke and carotid restenosis.
  - Some techniques involve division of the proximal vessel, facilitating easier removal of plaque via eversion of the vessel, which is then replanted.
- Postoperative
  - Patients will typically be transferred to ICU postoperatively for monitoring.

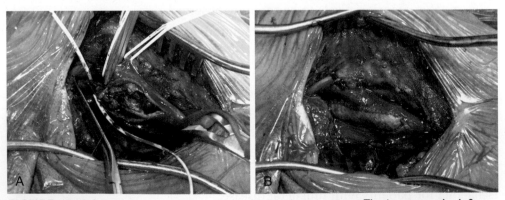

FIGURE 47.10 Surgical exposure for right carotid endarterectomy. The image on the left demonstrates the plaque within the vessel. On the right the vessel has been closed with a bovine graft.

Reproduced from: Beaulieu, R. & Abularrage, C., 2014. Carotid endarterectomy. In: Cameron, J.L. & Cameron, A.M., Current Surgical Therapy, 11th ed. Philadelphia: Saunders, pp. 811-818, Figs 4 and 6.

- Key postoperative observations include BP monitoring (cerebral hyperperfusion), neurological status and local wound.
    - Drain tube management as per post-op orders.
    - Patients should have duplex U/S during Outpatient follow-up as per unit protocol (typically around 3–6 weeks).
- Complications
    - Mortality can be as high as 3%, which should be discussed with the patient during consent.
    - Risk of injury to the glossopharyngeal and vagus nerves, with the latter responsible for postoperative swallowing difficulties.
    - Carotid restenosis.

ARTERIAL BYPASS SURGERY

An open procedure, vascular bypass surgery is reserved for patients with severe peripheral arterial disease (see Chapter 68).

- Bypass surgery is typically performed for disease affecting the distal aorta and lower limbs.
- Synthetic or autologous vein (see Fig. 47.13 later) grafts are used to re-vascularise the limb distal to the level of occlusion.
- The indications and intraoperative approach are dependent on which technique is being used (see Table 47.2).
- Postoperative
    - Patients may have an HDU bed booked dependent on preoperative planning.
    - The patient may be on a heparin infusion for 24–48 hours postoperatively, then be put onto regular aspirin.
    - Measurement of ABI or toes pressures can help confirm re-perfusion.
- Complications
    - Early complications can include bleeding, infection and graft failure. The majority of graft failure in the early setting is due to technical error.
    - Late failure of grafts is typically due to progression of peripheral vascular disease.
- Follow-up
    - Patients should have regular follow-up with U/S scans over graft sites.
    - Any chronic wounds present before intervention should start to be regularly reviewed for signs of healing.

SECTION IV

TABLE 47.2 Indications and approach of common arterial bypass surgeries

TECHNIQUE	INDICATIONS	APPROACH
Supra-inguinal disease		
Aorta-femoral	Distal aortic or iliac disease resulting in severe claudication	Abdominal exposure of the aorta. Any significant thrombus from the vessels is removed. Tunnelling of the graft through to the distal anastomosis site (Figs 47.11 and 47.12)
Femoro-femoral	Unilateral severe iliac disease with patent aorta	A tunnel is created from one femoral artery to another through the abdominal wall (Fig. 47.11)
Axillo-femoral	A measure of last resort for revascularisation for patients who have had previously failed bypass or severe disease	A graft is passed from healthy axillary artery to the femoral anastomotic site. The graft is tunnelled down the chest wall (Fig. 47.11)
Infra-inguinal disease		
Femoro-popliteal	Superficial femoral artery (SFA) or proximal popliteal disease	Exposure may be over the length of the proposed graft or 'stepped' incisions to allow tunnelling of the graft. Local vein grafts can be utilised (Fig. 47.13)

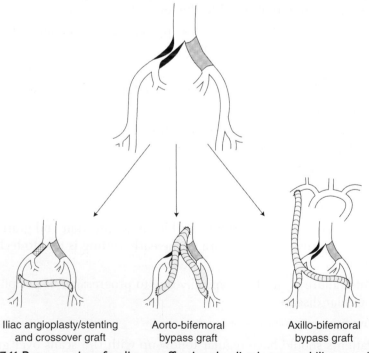

Iliac angioplasty/stenting and crossover graft — Aorto-bifemoral bypass graft — Axillo-bifemoral bypass graft

FIGURE 47.11 Bypass options for disease affecting the distal aorta and iliac vessels (supra-inguinal).

Adapted from: Nicholson, A. & Scott, J., 2014. Intervention for chronic lower limb ischaemia. In: Beard, J.D., Gaines, P.A. & Loftus, I., eds. Vascular and Endovascular Surgery: A companion to specialist surgical practice, 5th ed. London: Saunders, pp. 45-72, Fig. 4.6.

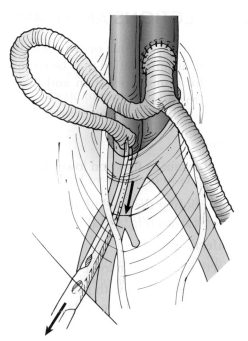

FIGURE 47.12 Tunnelling of the aorto-bifemoral graft.

Adapted from: Menard, M. & Belkin, M., 2014. Chapter 110: Aorto-iliac disease. In: Cronenwett, J.L. & Johnston, K.W., Rutherford's Vascular Surgery, 8th ed. Philadelphia: Saunders, pp. 1701-1721, Fig. 110-12.

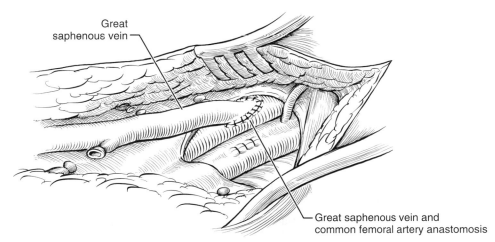

Great saphenous vein

Great saphenous vein and common femoral artery anastomosis

FIGURE 47.13 Femoro-popliteal bypass with end to sided anastomosis with vein graft.

Adapted from: Pounds, L., 2010. Chapter 85: Femoropopliteal bypass. In: Townsend, C.M., Jr. & Evers, B.M., Atlas of General Surgical Techniques. Philadelphia: Saunders, pp. 919-928, Fig. 85-4.

- – Great toe and 5th toe amputations are performed using 'tennis racquet' incisions.
  - – Extensive forefoot necrosis and poor foot perfusion may necessitate a trans-metatarsal amputation.
  - – The wounds are often left open to heal by secondary intention with regular dressings to help prevent further infection.
- Postoperative
  - Patients will need DVT prophylaxis charted, particularly for patients who have had a major amputation.
  - Postoperative pain is especially common; patients are typically given a PCA or epidural.
  - Some surgeons may use drains for their major amputations as stump haematoma is a common complication.
  - Patients who have had toe amputations will require regular dressings. Once the wound contamination has improved, VAC dressings (Chapter 51) are often used.
- Complications
  - Following debridement of diabetic foot wounds, patients remain at high risk of infection due to their micro- and macrovascular disease. Ongoing review is required to determine if the patient requires formal amputation.
  - Stump haematoma, pain and DVT are common complications of major amputation.
  - Phantom limb pain is a well-documented phenomenon in which the patient describes pain sensations of their absent limb.
- Follow-up
  - Patients will require close monitoring of their wounds either with their local GP or outpatient clinic.
  - Patients with major limb amputations will need follow-up with Orthotics to monitor their progression with a prosthetic.
  - The successful use of a prosthetic is influenced by the patient's premorbid mobility and the level of amputation. Typically, patients with BKAs have better functional outcomes that those with AKAs, partly due to the easier use of the prosthetic limb.

VARICOSE VEIN SURGERY

Surgery for the removal of varicose veins is one of the most common elective vascular procedures. Patients can be initially treated with a range of non-operative and conservative methods (Chapter 68).

- Indications
  - Leg pain or swelling associated with obvious superficial venous dilatation.
  - The aesthetic appearance also plays a role in a patient's wish to have surgery.
- Preoperative
  - Mapping of the affected veins via duplex U/S in combination with clinical examination.
  - Prior to the procedure the veins are marked, including incision sites.
- Intraoperative
  - Multiple technical methods are used.
  - **Venous stripping**
    - Used predominantly for the great saphenous vein (GSV) (Fig. 47.16).
    - Involves ligating the vein close to the common femoral vein and a vein stripping device passed distally through the vein down to either the knee or ankle level.
    - The vein is then ligated distally and the stripper is retracted, pulling the vein away, through the initial incision site.
    - Similar procedure can be used for the small saphenous vein.
    - There are widespread variations of this approach.
  - **Stab avulsions**
    - Multiple incisions are made over the vein, and the pieces of the vein are removed through the skin (Fig. 47.17).

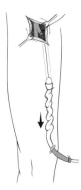

FIGURE 47.16 Stripping of the GSV via a distal to proximal approach.

Adapted from: Ma, H. & Iafrati, M.D., 2014. Varicose vein stripping and ambulatory phlebectomy. In: Chaikof, E.L. & Cambria, R.P., Atlas of Vascular Surgery and Endovascular Therapy. Elsevier, pp. 684-693, Fig. 59-2.

SECTION IV

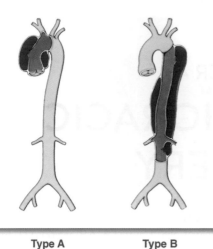

FIGURE 48.1 Type A and B aortic dissection patterns.

Reproduced from: Baliga, R., Nienaber, C., Bossone, E., et al., 2014. The role of imaging in aortic dissection and related syndromes. JACC: Cardiovascular Imaging 7(4), 406–424, Fig. 3.

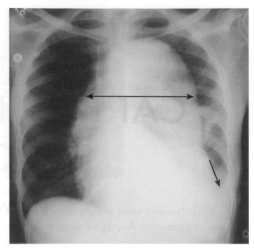

FIGURE 48.2 Widened mediastinum consistent with aortic dissection.

Reproduced from: Herring, W., 2016. Chapter 13: Recognizing adult heart disease. In: Herring, W., Learning Radiology, 3rd ed. Saunders, pp. 114–128, Fig. 13-23.

- These dissections sometimes present as a chronic issue with a slow onset of symptoms.

Investigations

- Initially, a plain CXR may be ordered in the undifferentiated patient with chest pain that may reveal the classical finding of a widened mediastinum (Fig. 48.2).
- Haemodynamically stable patients can undergo a CT aortogram.
- Haemodynamically unstable patients may have diagnosis confirmed by bedside TTE.

Management

- All patients are treated with medications to help maintain haemodynamic control and prevent further propagation of the dissection, with beta-blockers commonly used.
- Type A dissection: open surgical repair is required unless patients have severe medical comorbidities.
  - Repair includes excision of affected aortic tissue (Fig. 48.3).
  - Disruption of the aortic valve may necessitate repair or replacement.

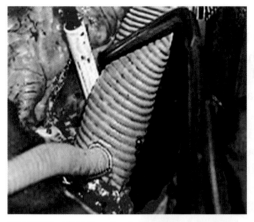

FIGURE 48.3 Proximal aortic replacement with a synthetic graft.

Reproduced from: Alexious, C. & Sosnowski, A., 2007. Tube-graft inversion for the construction of an "open" distal anastomosis during ascending aortic replacement. a new technique. Annals of Thoracic Surgery 83(1), 326-328, Fig. 3C.

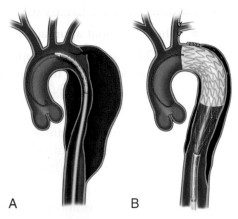

A   B

FIGURE 48.4 Endovascular treatment of a type B aortic dissection.

Reproduced from: Conrad, M. & Cambria, R., 2014. Chapter 138: Aortic dissection. In: Cronenwett, J., Rutherford's Vascular Surgery, 8th ed. Saunders, pp. 2169–2188, Fig. 138-6.

- Type B dissection: non-operative management is the classical approach although there has been an increasing role for endovascular approaches in patients with symptoms (Fig. 48.4).

CORONARY ARTERY BYPASS GRAFTS (CABGs)

CABG involves myocardial revascularisation using graft vessels to bypass diseased sections of the coronary arteries.

- Indications
    - PCI vs CABG (see Chapter 69).
- Preoperative
    - The overall management approach is usually discussed at a combined Cardiology/Cardiac Surgery case conference with review of images and recent angiography results. Ensure that patients are listed on the meeting and that their investigations are available for review.
    - Patients require extensive work-up to ensure they are fit enough to undergo major surgery.
    - Antiplatelet agents should be ceased at least 1 week prior, but all other cardiac medications should be continued.
    - Patients will require elective admission to the ICU postoperatively; the junior doctor is usually required to ensure the bookings are made.

- Postoperative
  - Patients spend around 24–48 hours in ICU post-op.
  - Constant observation of heart rate and rhythm is essential to monitor for arrhythmias.
    - Atrial fibrillation is common.
  - If the patient remains haemodynamically stable, extubation is performed early.
  - Daily bloods should be checked with electrolyte replacement where necessary.
  - Blood pressure and cardiac function are typically more stable in patients who have off-pump CABG.
- Complications
  - Cardiac arrhythmias, ventricular dysfunction, cardiogenic shock.
  - Complications from CPB: electrolyte disturbances, clot formation.
- Follow-up
  - Patients require close observation to determine ongoing graft patency.
  - Arterial grafts have a higher long-term patency rate than venous grafts.

CARDIAC VALVE SURGERY

The treatment of valvular pathology represents up to 20% of all cardiac surgical interventions.

Surgical management can be offered for management of disease affecting any of the cardiac valves; however, the aortic and mitral valves are more commonly affected. The options for management include valve repair (valvuloplasty) and replacement. Aortic valvuloplasty has limited uses, and is generally not advisable in patients with severe, calcified valves.

Aortic valve replacement (AVR)

- Indications
  - Symptomatic aortic stenosis and regurgitation (Chapter 69).
  - Asymptomatic patients in select cases, though the inclusion criteria are a source of debate.
- Preoperative
  - Patients require extensive work-up to determine suitability for valve replacement surgery (Chapters 56 and 69).
  - Discussion at Cardiac Surgery case conference regarding optimal perioperative management.

- Operative
  - There are multiple approaches and techniques for replacing the aortic valve.
    - The age and cardiac function of the patient play a role in the decision making.
    - Autografts such as the Ross procedure are considered in young patients.
    - There is increasing use of transcatheter approaches, avoiding an open operation: transcatheter aortic valve implantation (TAVI).
  - Approach is via median sternotomy.
  - The patient is put on CPB with cross-clamping of the aorta.
  - Access to the aortic valve is made by aortomy (Fig. 48.7).
  - The leaflets are resected, but the fibrous ring (annulus) is left intact to allow for inset of the new prosthetic valve (Fig. 48.8).
  - There are different categories of prosthetic valves (see Table 48.1).
  - Once the prosthesis is secure, the patient is weaned from CPB and a TOE is used to assess the function of the valve and ventricle, assessing for any leak around the new valve.
- Postoperative
  - Patients are monitored in ICU.
  - Patients with longstanding severe aortic stenosis may experience fluctuations in blood pressure as the degree of volume loading is altered.
  - Patients are commenced on oral anticoagulation around 48–72 hours postoperatively.
- Complications
  - Bleeding, infection of the valve (uncommon in mechanical), aortic dissection, atrial fibrillation, perivalvular leak.
  - Long-term risk of embolic events (stroke), thus the need for anticoagulation.

Mitral valve repair and replacement

- Indications
  - Severe/symptomatic mitral stenosis (Chapter 69).
- Preoperative
  - Patients attend pre-admission clinic and are extensively worked up with an anaesthetics review.
  - The patient is discussed at a Cardiology/Cardiac Surgery case conference.

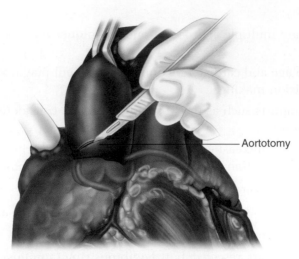

FIGURE 48.7 Exposure of the aortic valve via an aortomy.

Reproduced from: Rodriguez, R. & Sellke, F., 2010. Chapter 9: Aortic valve replacement. In: Selke, F., Atlas of Cardiac Surgical Techniques. Saunders, pp. 121–131, Fig. 9-2.

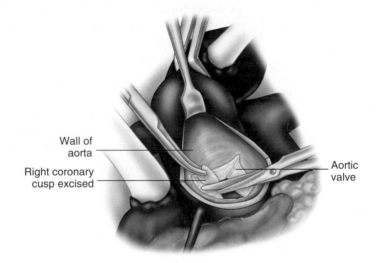

FIGURE 48.8 Excision of the aortic valve.

Reproduced from: Rodriguez, R. & Sellke, F., 2010. Chapter 9: Aortic valve replacement. In: Selke, F., Atlas of Cardiac Surgical Techniques. Saunders, pp. 121–131, Fig. 9-3.

- Operative
  - Following median or partial sternotomy and initiation of CPB the mitral valve is exposed via an arteriotomy.
  - Inspection of the valve can then take place, determining whether a repair or replacement is required.
    - Isolated flail segments may be amendable to resection and repair (Fig. 48.9).

TABLE 48.1 The use of bioprosthetic vs mechanical heart valves

TYPE	DESCRIPTION	RECOMMENDATION FOR USAGE
Bioprosthetic valve	• Includes xenograft (porcine, bovine), homograft and allograft (pulmonary valve – Ross procedure) • Decreased durability • Anticoagulation not required	• Select patients between 60 and 70 years of age • Patients >70 years of age • Patients not suitable for anticoagulation
Mechanical valve	• Variety of products exist • Superior durability • Requires lifelong anticoagulation	• Select patients between 60 and 70 years of age • Patients <60 years of age

General considerations:

Anticoagulation is achieved via the use of warfarin.

Target INR is 2.5–3.5 for patients with mechanical cardiac valves.

Patients may require close follow-up with home nursing services (i.e. hospital in the home [HITH]) to ensure they are coping.

Adapted from: Nishimura, R.A., Otto, C.M., Bonow, R.O., et al., 2014. AHA/ACC guideline for the management of patients with valvular heart disease: a report of the American College of Cardiology/American Heart Association Task Force on Practice Guidelines. Journal of the American College of Cardiology 63, e57.

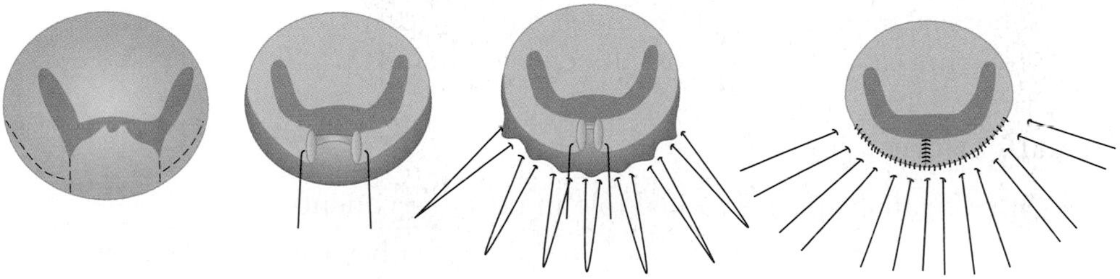

FIGURE 48.9 Process of repairing a flail segment of the mitral valve.

Reproduced from: Rosengart, T. & Anand, J., 2017. Chapter 60: Acquired heart disease. In: Townsend, C., Sabiston Textbook of Surgery. Saunders, pp. 1691–1719, Fig. 60-13A.

- More diffuse disease necessitates replacement with a prosthetic valve; this is usually supplemented with an annuloplasty ring to maintain normal valvular dimensions.
  ○ Once the valve is secured, the atrium is closed and the patient is weaned from CPB with TOE monitoring of valve function.
- Postoperative
  ○ ICU monitoring postoperatively, though patients can be quickly downgraded if they progress well.
  ○ Patients are commenced on oral anticoagulation 48–72 hours post-op.

- Complications
  - Similar to that of AVR, close observation for perivalvular leak is required.

CHEST TRAUMA

Traumatic injuries to the thoracic area account for around 25% of all trauma-related deaths. The most common mechanism is blunt trauma (90%), though only 1 in 10 require surgery.

Screening for thoracic injuries during trauma assessment begins during the primary survey as thoracic injuries have the potential to affect airway, breathing and circulation.

Rapid identification and management of life-threatening injuries is key to reducing the mortality and morbidities of these injuries.

Examination

- Clinical diagnosis is key; careful examination of the chest can reveal obvious flail segments, penetrating trauma, chest wall wounds and bruising. Look for tenderness on palpation.
- Auscultation can reveal decreased air entry on either or both sides suggestive of fluid or air collection.
- Haemodynamic compromise, decreased heart sounds and distended neck veins are classical features of pericardial tamponade.
- Thoracic trauma needs to be ruled out in patients with persistent tachypnoea and hypoxia despite oxygen therapy.

Investigations

- Investigations play a limited role in unstable patients.
  - Plain X-ray films performed in the trauma bay can help identify pneumothorax (Fig. 48.10) or haemothorax (Fig. 48.11), though may not reveal all injuries.
  - FAST scans may reveal pericardial effusions.
  - Formal investigations can wait until the patient is stable.

Management

- Life-threatening injuries must be prioritised (Table 48.2).
- Patients with high-risk mechanisms and evidence of chest trauma should be considered for an emergency thoracotomy.
  - Cardiac tamponade.
  - Penetrating injury with involvement of mediastinal structures (oesophagus, great vessels).

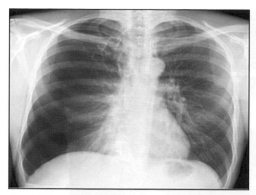

FIGURE 48.10 Right-sided simple pneumothorax.

Reproduced from: Seif, F., Samaha, A., Tannous, G., et al., 2010. Acute onset of dyspnea in an HIV patient. American Journal of Medicine 123(11), 999–1000, Fig. 1.

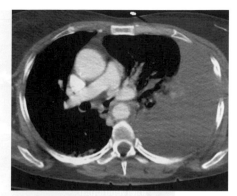

FIGURE 48.11 Large left-sided haemothorax with mediastinal displacement. Requires urgent drainage.

Reproduced from: Miller, L. & Mirvis, S., 2015. Chapter 8: Blunt chest trauma. In: Mirvis, S., Problem Solving in Emergency Radiology. Saunders, pp. 172–216, Fig. 8-21.

TABLE 48.2 Severe chest injuries and initial management

PATHOLOGY	SIGNS AND SYMPTOMS	INITIAL MANAGEMENT
Tension pneumothorax	Hypoxia and tachypnoea Decreased air entry on affected side Tracheal deviation	Needle decompression of 2nd intercostal followed by ICC insertion
Massive haemothorax	Decreased air entry Bruising CXR evidence	Insertion of an ICC Pay attention to output; if >1500 mL consider thoracotomy
Tracheal rupture	Rare Associated with pneumothorax with persistent air leak despite ICC Patient may have bruising or pain in upper chest/neck	Bedside flexible bronchoscopy to confirm
Aortic dissection/ transection	High mortality with 85% of patients dying before reaching hospital	Permissive hypotension If sufficient time move to angiography for stent placement
Pericardial tamponade	Hypotension, distended neck veins FAST positive (Fig. 48.12)	Thoracotomy and drainage

- Operative
  - An endoscopic camera is placed in a laterally positioned patient. The lung is deflated by the anaesthetist allowing manipulation of the tissue.
  - Additional port sites allow for passage of other instruments.
  - Biopsies and wedge sections can be taken using a variety of stapling and electrocautery devices (Fig. 48.13).
  - Pleurodesis is commonly performed with VATS.
    - Performed for recurrent pneumothorax or pleural effusion.
    - Most common methods are mechanical abrasion and chemical pleurodesis.
    - The idea is to obliterate the pleural space, preventing any future collection.
    - Requires that the lung is capable of fully inflating against the chest wall.
  - Once the procedure is completed, an ICC is inserted under vision, with some surgeons choosing to place a pleural catheter for analgesia.
- Postoperative
  - Patients can normally return to a high dependency bed on the ward postoperatively.
  - There is regular observation of the ICC and daily CXRs are performed.
  - These drains are usually connected to suction initially, which can be ceased early postoperatively if there is no evidence of a large air leak.
    - Air leaks manifest as bubbling in the underwater seal drain compartment.
    - Some patients may display subcutaneous (or surgical) emphysema, a normally harmless phenomenon.
  - Once the ICC drain output is less than 100–150 mL in a 24-hour period, it can be removed with a final CXR 4 hours post removal.
- Complications
  - Haemothorax, collections.
  - Pneumothorax, ongoing air leak from lung tissue.

Lobectomy and pneumonectomy

Involves resection of lung tissue for the treatment of lung tumours. Lobectomy is the removal of a single anatomical lobe, whereas pneumonectomy is excision of the entire lung. Both fall under the category of major pulmonary resection.

- Indications
  - Lung cancer (see Chapter 69).

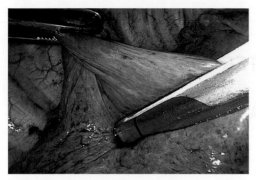

FIGURE 48.13 VATS lung wedge resection using a stapling device.

Reproduced from: Sciortino, C., Mungo, B. & Molena, D., 2014. Video-assisted thoracic surgery. In: Cameron, J.L. & Cameron, A.M., Current Surgical Therapy, 11th ed. Saunders, pp. 1418– 1422, Fig. 4.

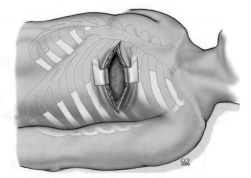

FIGURE 48.14 Anterior thoracotomy.

Reproduced from: Murthy, S., 2008. Chapter 10: Thoracic incisions. In: Patterson, G., Pearson's Thoracic and Esophageal Surgery, 3rd ed. Churchill Livingstone, Fig. 10-9.

- Preoperative
  - As for patients undergoing VATS, RFTs are essential for any patient undergoing lung resection.
  - Resection cases are usually discussed at thoracic MDM meetings to determine the best management strategy.
- Operative
  - These procedures are increasingly performed via VATS, though some patients may not be suited and require thoracotomy.
  - Thoracotomy involves rib retraction to allow access to the operating field (Fig. 48.14).
  - The region of lung to be resected is mobilised and important vascular structures are dissected out and divided as required around the hilum.
  - Testing of the closure is performed by re-inflating the lung and testing for leaks.
  - An ICC is left in situ along with an extra pleural catheter for analgesia.
- Postoperative
  - These patients may require a period of observation in the ICU.
  - The chest drain is not left on suction, and daily CXRs look for a rise in the fluid level in the post-pneumonectomy space.
- Complications
  - Infections, haemothorax, collections.
  - Bronchial stump breakdown.
  - Slow respiratory recovery.

SECTION IV

CHAPTER 49

EAR, NOSE AND THROAT (ENT) AND HEAD AND NECK SURGERY

Paul Watson

ENT TRAUMA

Nasal fracture

- Fracture results from nasal trauma from either the front or side.
- Identification of the deformity (Fig. 49.1) and reduction should be performed before the swelling increases, obscuring the normal anatomy.
- If swelling is prominent, reduction can be performed after 5–7 days.
- A splint is used to hold the nose in place (thermoplastic splints are commonly used).
- Septal haematoma (Fig. 49.2)
  - Should be drained either by needle aspiration or incision.
  - Packing the nose after drainage will help prevent re-accumulation of haematoma.
  - Progressive septal haematoma will progress to necrosis of the cartilage.
  - Oral antibiotics are recommended to prevent infection; severe infection can lead to cavernous sinus thrombosis, a potentially fatal complication.

Ear trauma

- Lacerations to the ear
  - Can involve the underlying cartilage.
  - Contaminated wounds require extensive washout to prevent chronic inflammation.

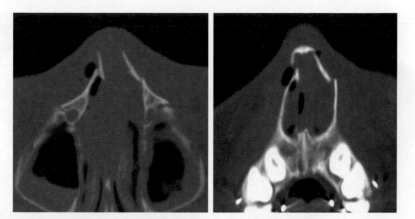

FIGURE 49.1 Axial facial bone CT demonstrating nasal fractures.

Reproduced from: Lo Casto, A., 2012. Imaging evaluation of facial complex strut fractures. Seminars in Ultrasound, CT, and MRI 33(5), 396–409, Fig. 3.

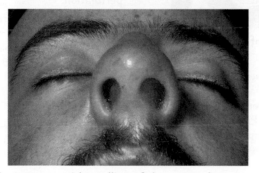

FIGURE 49.2 Septal haematoma with swelling of the external nose.

Reproduced from: Dhillon, R.S. & East, C.A., 2013. Chapter 2: Nose and paranasal sinus. In: Dhillon, R.S. & East, C.A., Ear, Nose and Throat and Head and Neck Surgery, 4th ed. Elsevier, Fig. 2-30.

- ○ Exploration of the wound is required to ensure no haematoma is present.
- ○ Potential complications include chondrodermatitis nodularis helicis (CDNH), a painful, benign nodularity of the cartilage, as well as necrosis secondary to haematoma.
- ○ Repair of the laceration can take place in the ED with a local anaesthetic block (Fig. 49.3) if the laceration is simple with minimal tissue loss.
- • Tympanic perforation
  - ○ Direct injury resulting from sharp object/cotton bud or from significant barotrauma (high energy blunt force/diving; see Fig. 49.4).
  - ○ Infections with middle ear collections can affect the membrane.
  - ○ Patient has initial onset of pain that is associated with some hearing loss and tinnitus.

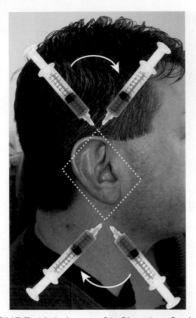

FIGURE 49.3 Areas of infiltration for local anaesthetic ear blocks.

Reproduced from: Khodaee, M. & Kelly, B.F., 2011. Chapter 8: Peripheral nerve blocks and field blocks. In: Pfenninger, J.L. & Fowler, G.C., Pfenninger and Fowler's Procedures for Primary Care, 3rd ed. Saunders, pp. 45-51, Fig. 8-8.

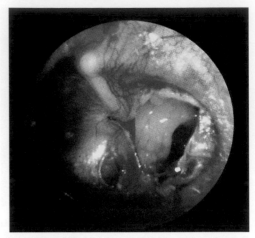

FIGURE 49.4 Obvious defect and external canal bleeding consistent with tympanic perforation.

Reproduced from: Buttaravoli, P. & Leffler, S., 2012. Chapter 37: Perforated tympanic membrane. In: Buttaravoli, P., Minor Emergencies, 3rd ed. Saunders, pp. 145-146, Fig. 37-1.

- ○ Otoscopy can reveal a tympanic defect allowing for assessment of the size of injury.
- ○ Small defects will heal spontaneously (typically within 2 months)
  - – Patient should keep the ear clean and dry during this time.
- ○ Larger defects may require surgical correction with tympanic flap or myringoplasty.

Laryngeal trauma

Laryngeal trauma is uncommon owing to the relative mobility of the laryngeal structures and protection offered by the surrounding neck tissue.

- • Suspected laryngeal trauma is a management priority due to impending airway loss and should be immediately addressed.
- • The most common mechanisms are:
  - ○ blunt force trauma from a direct bow to the throat
  - ○ penetrating trauma
  - ○ burns (inhalation and caustic).

- Patients with minor trauma who are conscious and able to breathe normally without stridor may be suitable for observation and steroid therapy to reduce oedema.
- Patients with obvious respiratory distress require a secured airway either by intubation or tracheostomy.
- Patients with burns involving the larynx may have a delayed inflammatory response; early intervention may be required.
- Patients with high energy trauma leading to laryngeal injuries are at high risk of cervical spine injuries.
- Once the airway is secure CT imaging can be performed to assess the extent of the damage and allow for definitive management.

EPISTAXIS

Nose bleeds (epistaxis) are a common ED presentation that usually arises from irritation of the mucosal membrane.

- Ask the patient about recent trauma, history of epistaxis or any polyps/lesions that have been present.
- Get an estimation of blood loss as epistaxis can result in significant bleeding. Check if the patient has a history of haemophilia or is on any anticoagulant therapy.
- If the patient takes warfarin, it would be advisable to check the INR.
- The first step to approaching epistaxis is first aid:
  ○ Compress the nose over the base of the nose; clasping the bridge of the nose has no real benefit. The patient should sit upright and lean forward.
  ○ This should help alleviate bleeding from Kisselbach's plexus, the most common site of bleeding in the anterior part of the nasopharynx.
- Co-phenylcaine nasal spray offers the dual benefits of local anaesthesia and vasoconstriction.
- Warm saline washout may allow visualisation of the bleeding vessel under speculum examination, allowing cauterisation with silver nitrate.
- Packing of the nose with a nasal tampon (Fig. 49.5) or inflatable balloon (such as RapidRhino®; see Fig. 49.6) can tamponade bleeding.
- Packs can be left in for 48 hours, and then removed for checking for persistent bleeding. Broad spectrum antibiotic cover is recommended.
- If the vessel cannot be identified and packing is not sufficient to control the bleeding, suspect the vessel could be in the posterior nasopharynx. In this case, a posteriorly placed balloon may have a greater effect.
- If substantial bleeding persists an exploration in theatre may be required to find and control the source.

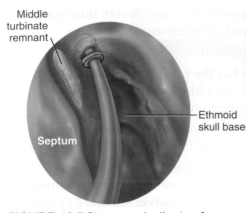

FIGURE 49.7 Sinus punch allowing for culture collection and drainage.

Reproduced from: Ramikrishnan, V.R., 2013. Chapter 15: Extended frontal recess dissections. In: Palmer, J.N., Atlas of Endoscopic Sinus and Skull Base Surgery. Saunders, pp. 135-150, Fig. 15-14.

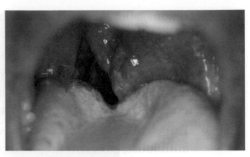

FIGURE 49.8 Large left-sided peritonsillar abscess displacing the uvula.

Reproduced from: Waage, R., 2011. Chapter 80: Peritonsillar abscess drainage. In: Pfenninger, J.L. & Fowler, G.C., Pfenninger and Fowler's Procedures for Primary Care, 3rd ed. Mosby, pp. 506-510, Fig. 80.3A.

- ○ Infections are typically bacterial.
- ○ Topical drops are first-line treatment, but IV or oral antibiotics can be indicated for severe infections.

Pharyngeal infections

- Though *tonsillitis* is most commonly associated with children, bacterial tonsillitis can still affect young adults.
  - ○ The presence of a large amount of pus is largely suggestive of a bacterial infection, though those with viral tonsillitis can still present with marked swelling and tenderness.
  - ○ Some patients will not tolerate oral intake during this period and present to ED for review.
  - ○ Analgesia and oral steroids can aid with symptoms relief but thorough examination is indicated to rule out serious pharyngeal pathology.
- *Peritonsillar abscesses* (Fig. 49.8) have a much broader age presentation.
  - ○ Also known as quinsy, these patients can present with fever, pain (specifically trismus) and dysphagia.
  - ○ In cooperative patients with accessible collections, needle aspiration under local anaesthetic (spray and needle) can be used for collection; if symptoms improve without re-accumulation the patient may be treated with antibiotics.
  - ○ However, persistent symptoms, respiratory compromise and patients at risk of bleeding should have formal incision and drainage in theatre.

- Patients who are immunocompromised should have cultures taken for possible fungal involvement.
- Epiglottitis
    - Though primarily affecting children, epiglottitis can occur at any age, due to bacterial infection (*Haemophilus influenzae*).
    - Supraglottic inflammation leading to airway obstruction.
    - Stridor is a striking feature of this condition; patients can quickly become hypoxic as the condition has rapid onset.
    - Management priorities include securing the airway with an urgent Anaesthesiology and ENT review:
        - intubation ± tracheostomy
        - low threshold for code blue due to impending total airway obstruction.
- Ludwig's angina
    - Rapidly progressive cellulitis of the neck affecting the floor of the mouth.
    - Increased intraoral swelling leads to tongue displacement and obstruction.
    - The classic examination findings are bilateral submandibular swelling with an elevated tongue.
    - Broad spectrum IV antibiotics should be commenced with a low threshold for intubation.

TONSILLECTOMY AND ADENOIDECTOMY ('Ts AND As')

This involves surgical removal of the tonsillar and/or adenoid tissue via an intraoral approach.

- Indications
    - Recurrent tonsillar infection or peritonsillar abscess.
    - Airway obstruction, sleep disruption from hypertrophic tonsils and adenoids.
    - Malignancy.
- Preoperative
    - Patients may require Anaesthesiology review prior to the procedure, with particularly close attention paid to the patient's dental health.
- Intraoperative
    - The patient is positioned supine and is approached from overhead with the tongue retracted to reveal the tonsils and adenoids.
    - Tonsils are typically removed with some form of diathermy (Fig. 49.9).

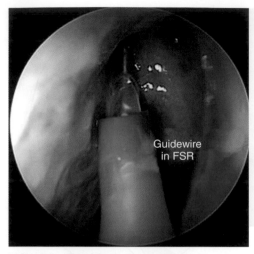

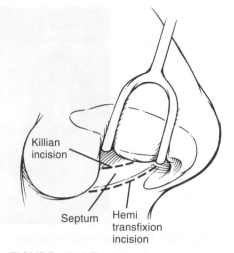

FIGURE 49.12 Access to the frontal sinus recess using a guidewire during FESS.

Reproduced from: Lal, D., Stankiewicz, J., et al., 2015. Chapter 49: Primary sinus surgery. In: Flint, P.W., Haughey, B.H., Lund, V.J., et al., Cummings Otolaryngology, 6th ed. Saunders, pp. 752-782, Fig. 49-26B.

FIGURE 49.13 Traditional approaches to open septoplasty.

Reproduced from: Ramakrishnan, J.B., 2016. Chapter 27: Septoplasty and turbinate surgery. In: Scholes, M.A. & Ramakrishnan, V.R., ENT Secrets, 4th ed. Elsevier, pp. 184-191, Fig. 27-1.

- Postoperative
  - Patients are admitted overnight for observation, often with nasal packing that is removed the following morning.
- Complications
  - A small amount of bleeding is common; however, it seldom requires intervention (<1%).
  - Damage to the orbit and skull base are uncommon but serious complications.

Septoplasty

Septoplasty is surgical correction of the nasal septum, related to congenital acquired deformities. It is commonly performed in combination with inferior turbinectomy.

- Indications
  - Septal deviation leading to obstructive symptoms.
- Preoperative
  - Thorough history and examination are essential to determine if a patient is suited to septoplasty for obstructive symptoms.
- Operative
  - A nasal approach is used, via an inferior mucosal incision (Fig. 49.13) allowing access to the septum.

- The septum is repositioned with resection of the bony septum and cartilage as required.
- Some surgeons utilise an endoscopic approach.
- Postoperative
  - Patients are admitted overnight with nasal packing to aid with haemostasis.
  - Patients are typically positioned head up at 30°.
  - Discharge is day 1 post-op after removal of nasal packing; regular washings of the nose are prescribed.
- Complications
  - Infection and bleeding are common complications. Septal haematoma is of particular concern, requiring urgent drainage.

Turbinectomy

Inferior turbinate hypertrophy (Fig. 49.14) is a common cause of a nasal obstruction, often secondary to septal deviation.

- Indications
  - Obstructive symptoms related to mucosal inflammation of the inferior turbinate.
  - Middle turbinates are less commonly implicated due to the smaller amount of mucosal tissue.
- Preoperative
  - Preoperative CT imaging can help determine the nasal anatomy for surgical planning.
- Operative
  - Turbinectomy procedures are usually performed on the inferior turbinates.
  - The key objective is to reduce the size of the turbinate while preserving function (mucosal tissue); therefore, a submucosal resection of the turbinate is performed either by surgical resection or ablative techniques.
- Postoperative
  - As for septoplasty, removal of nasal packing after an overnight admission.
- Complications
  - As with all nasal surgery, bleeding is a common but not typically serious complication.

Uvulopalatopharyngoplasty (UPPP)

UPPP is performed to treat an obstruction that involves the soft palate, tonsillar pillars and uvula.

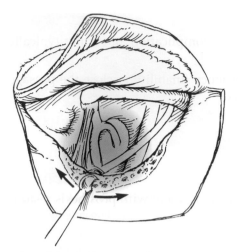

FIGURE 49.16 Access to the stapes via a tympanomeatal flap.

Reproduced from: House, J. & Cunningham, C., 2015. Chapter 144: Otosclerosis. In: Flint, P.W., Haughey, B.H., Lund, V.J., et al., Cummings Otolaryngology: Head and neck surgery, 6th ed. Saunders, pp. 2211-2219, Fig. 144-8.

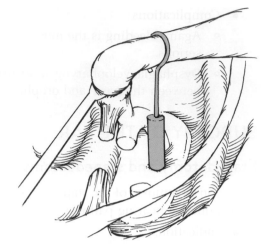

FIGURE 49.17 'Piston' prosthesis following drilling into the stapes footplate.

Reproduced from: House, J. & Cunningham, C., 2015. Chapter 144: Otosclerosis. In: Flint, P.W., Haughey, B.H., Lund, V.J., et al., Cummings Otolaryngology: Head and neck surgery, 6th ed. Saunders, pp. 2211-2219, Fig. 144-13.

Myringoplasty and tympanoplasty

Myringoplasty refers specifically to repair only of the tympanic membrane (TM); tympanoplasty includes surgical intervention to the membrane and the ossicles. The goal of the procedure is to restore normal anatomy and improve hearing.

- Indications
  - Myringoplasty is typically performed in acute tympanic membrane perforation, usually resulting from trauma as the surrounding tissue is likely to be healthy.
  - Tympanic perforation from chronic disease may include disease of the surrounding middle ear and mucosa requiring intervention.
  - Chronic tympanic membrane perforation secondary to cholesteatoma is a specialised case, requiring consideration of a mastoidectomy.
- Preoperative
  - Audiometry can characterise and assess the severity of hearing loss.
  - Imaging is not typically utilised.
  - The approach is dictated by the size and location of the perforation as seen on otoscopy.

- Operative
  - Repair of the TM involves placing a graft on the 'inside' surface (medial grafting) or the outside surface (lateral grafting) with the latter approach often preferred.
  - A key step of the procedure is to remove all squamous epithelium (Fig. 49.18) from the middle ear to prevent development of a cholesteatoma.
  - Myringoplasty includes direct access to the membrane via the external canal. The flaps of the tympanic membrane are approximated and a covering graft is placed over the TM (Fig. 49.19).
  - Tympanoplasty may necessitate an approach involving exposure of the ossicles, such as a postauricular incision.
  - The temporalis fascia often serves as useful donor tissue for grafting. Conchal flaps are another commonly described approach.
- Postoperative
  - Patients will typically have an external ear packing for at least 7 days to protect the graft.

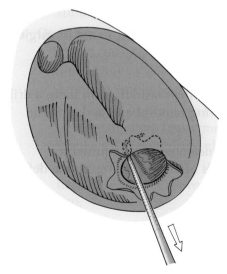

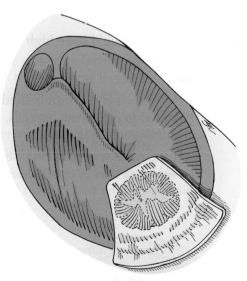

FIGURE 49.18 The flaps of the perforation are pulled outwards from the middle ear, removing squamous epithelium.

Reproduced from: Hirsch, B., 2008. Chapter 113: Myringoplasty and tympanoplasty. In: Myers, E., Operative Otolaryngology: Head and neck surgery, 2nd ed. Saunders, pp. 1133-1145, Fig. 113-2.

FIGURE 49.19 A graft placed over the tympanic membrane.

Reproduced from: Hirsch, B., 2008. Chapter 113: Myringoplasty and tympanoplasty. In: Myers, E., Operative Otolaryngology: Head and neck surgery, 2nd ed. Saunders, pp. 1133-1145, Fig. 113-3.

SECTION IV

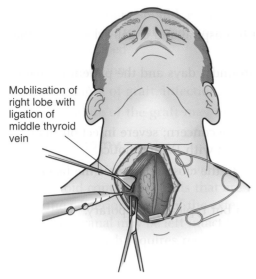

Mobilisation of right lobe with ligation of middle thyroid vein

FIGURE 49.21 Initial approach to thyroidectomy.

Reproduced from: Townsend, C.M. & Beauchamp, R.D., 2015. Chapter 36: Thyroid. In: Townsend, C.M., Bauchamp, R.D., Evers, B.M., et al., Sabiston Textbook of Surgery, 20th ed. Saunders, Fig. 36-24.

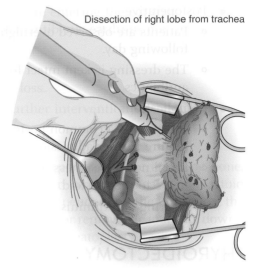

Dissection of right lobe from trachea

FIGURE 49.22 Principles of dissection in thyroid surgery include reflecting the lobe to dissect from the trachea under direct vision.

Reproduced from: Townsend, C.M. & Beauchamp, R.D., 2015. Chapter 36: Thyroid. In: Townsend, C.M., Bauchamp, R.D., Evers, B.M., et al., Sabiston Textbook of Surgery, 20th ed. Saunders, Fig. 36-30.

- Review by the Endocrinology inpatient team is useful for guidance of thyroid replacement therapy.
- The junior doctor should be clear on the postoperative management plan, including whether radio-iodide ablation therapy is planned, which may alter the timeline for thyroid replacement.
- Complications
  - Hoarseness and voice changes are associated with injury to either the recurrent laryngeal nerve or the superior laryngeal nerve.
  - Though great care is taken with the dissection around the nerve, the patient should be appropriately counselled preoperatively regarding the potential risk of voice changes.

TRACHEOSTOMY

- Indications
  - Elective tracheostomies are performed prior to major oral and pharyngeal operations, particularly those involving excision of tumours and reconstructions.

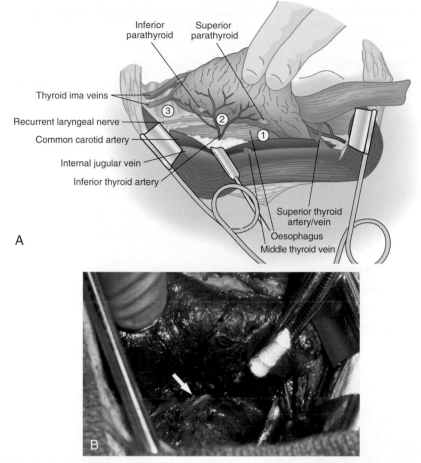

FIGURE 49.23 Illustration (A) and intraoperative image (B) of RLN (3) in close relation to the inferior thyroid artery.

Reproduced from: Townsend, C.M. & Beauchamp, R.D., 2015. Chapter 36: Thyroid. In: Townsend, C.M., Beauchamp, R.D., Evers, B.M., et al., Sabiston Textbook of Surgery, 20th ed. Saunders, Fig. 36-29.

- ○ Patients who have had a prolonged period of intubation will also be considered for tracheostomy.
- ○ Emergency airway access: airway swelling, obstruction or severe trauma.
- Operatively
  - ○ Laryngeal operations may begin with intubation, followed by direct tracheal access.
  - ○ Direct approach to the trachea is exposed after retraction of the strap muscles and ligation and division of the thyroid isthmus.
  - ○ Exposure of the trachea by opening the overlying fascia allows access into the airway under direct vision.

- ○ The trachea is incised (see Figs 49.24, 49.25 and 49.26) and a series of dilators are used to expand the aperture to permit passage of the tube (Fig. 49.27).
- Postoperatively
  - ○ The constant danger is accidental decannulation of the tracheostomy. If suspected the securing dressing should be checked.
  - ○ Management of the tracheostomy includes daily cleaning of the dressing site, checking that the tube is secured and suctioning of any excessive mucus build-up. The patient will have daily reviews by the hospital tracheostomy management service.
  - ○ When the patient is alert, comfortable and postoperative swelling has reduced, the patient can be safely de-cannulated on the ward. Two trained members of the nursing staff will deflate the cuff and remove the tube under exhalation.
- Complications
  - ○ Haematoma from vascular injury, trachea-oesophageal fistula and tube obstruction secondary to mucus or blood clots, subcutaneous emphysema.

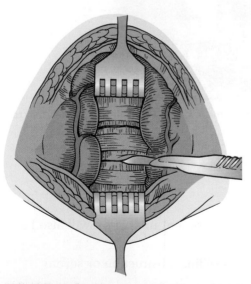

FIGURE 49.24 After exposing the trachea, an incision is made between the second and third rings.

Reproduced from: Kost, K., 2008. Chapter 68: Tracheostomy. In: Myers, E., Operative Otolaryngology: Head and neck surgery, 2nd ed. Saunders, Fig. 68-3.

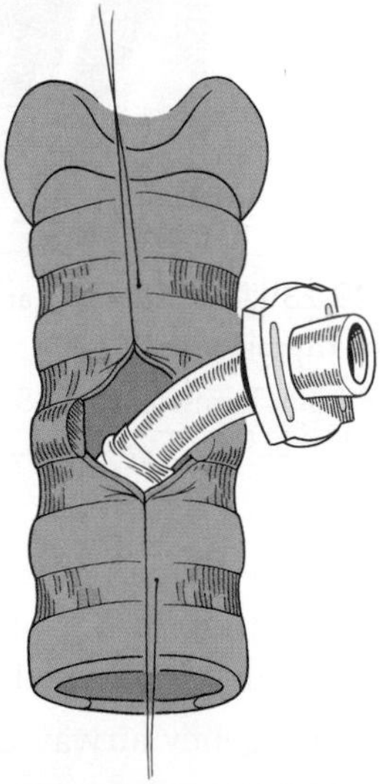

FIGURE 49.25 Traction sutures aid passage of the tube into the aperture, and allow easy identification of the tracheostomy in the event of accidental removal.

Reproduced from: Kost, K., 2008. Chapter 68: Tracheostomy. In: Myers, E., Operative Otolaryngology: Head and neck surgery, 2nd ed. Saunders, Fig. 68-7.

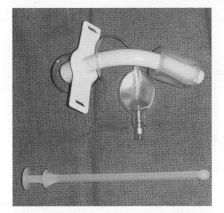

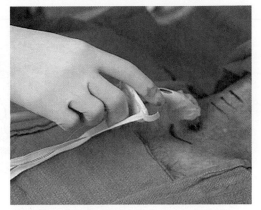

FIGURE 49.26 A plastic tracheostomy tube.

Reproduced from: Chan, T. & Devaiah, A.K., 2009. Tracheostomy in palliative care. Otolaryngologic Clinics of North America 42(1), 133-141, Fig. 2.

FIGURE 49.27 The tracheostomy tube is introduced into the stoma via the dilator.

Reproduced from: Mallick, A., Bodenham, A.R., 2014. Percutaneous tracheostomy and cricothyrotomy techniques. Anaesthesia and Intensive Care Medicine 15(5), 215-220, Fig. 9.

- Although risks of pneumothorax and pneumomediastinum are reported, they are most commonly associated with paediatric patients.

LARYNGECTOMY

Laryngectomy is primarily undertaken for confirmed laryngeal malignancy.

- Indications
  - Locally advanced or panglottic disease typically requires total laryngectomy.
  - Early stage laryngeal carcinoma may permit localised excision of the affected cord or section of glottic tissue via partial laryngectomy, with flap reconstruction for larynx preservation and coverage for any associated defect.
- Operative
  - The approach to laryngectomy is via the anterior neck with complete exposure of the hypopharynx via division of the strap muscles (Figs 49.28 and 49.29).
  - The thyroid is carefully divided and reflected off the trachea, making sure to keep the vascular pedicle intact.
  - Extension of the tumour into the thyroid is an indication for thyroid lobectomy.
  - Refer to Fig. 49.30 for an example of a total laryngectomy specimen.

SECTION IV

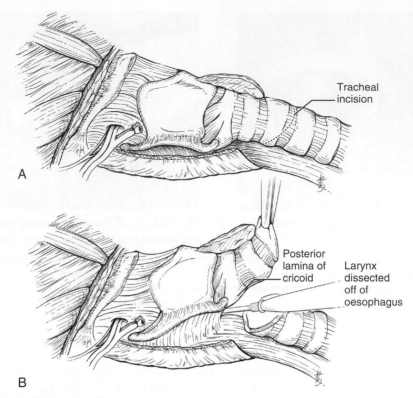

FIGURE 49.28 Division of the constrictor and infrahyoid muscles exposes the larynx; the tracheal incision is made and specimen is excised.

Reproduced from: Holsinger, C. & Bhayani, M., 2011. Chapter 37: Total laryngectomy. In: Cohen, J.I. & Clayman, G.L., Atlas of Head and Neck Surgery. Saunders, Fig. 37-9.

- When closing, a nasogastric tube is placed and enteral feeding commenced postoperatively.
- Postoperative
  - These patients will require ICU support and monitoring, having already been booked for a high dependency bed in the preoperative setting.
  - Patients with tracheostomies (Fig. 49.31) can commonly become agitated, especially since it impairs their ability to communicate; ensure that a pen and paper are nearby to allow the patient to write.
  - Oral feeding of the patient is often patient and surgeon dependent, but can occur as soon as day 7 postoperatively. The use of pre-feeding gastrografin studies is reserved for those who have had complex reconstructions.
  - Postoperative optimisation of the patient's nutrition should be a key priority for the junior doctor.

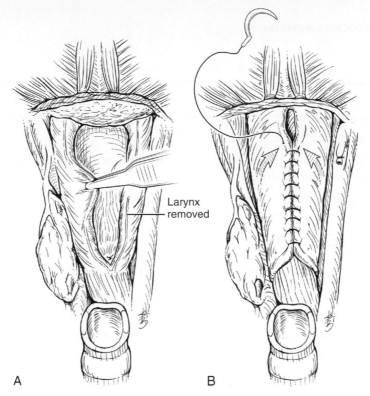

A   B

FIGURE 49.29 After the larynx is excised, the mucosal layer of the remaining hypopharynx is closed.

Reproduced from: Holsinger, C. & Bhayani, M., 2011. Chapter 37: Total laryngectomy. In: Cohen, J.I. & Clayman, G.L., Atlas of Head and Neck Surgery. Saunders, Fig. 37-11.

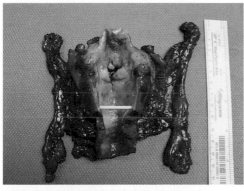

FIGURE 49.30 Total laryngectomy specimen.

Reproduced from: Rassekh, C. & Haughey, B., 2015. Chapter 110: Total laryngectomy and laryngopharyngectomy. In: Flint, P.W., Haughey, B.H., Lund, V.J., et al., Cummings Otolaryngology, 6th ed. Saunders, pp. 1699-1713, Fig. 110-5A.

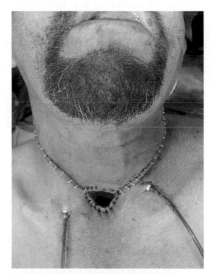

FIGURE 49.31 Closure after total laryngectomy with tracheostomy and drains left in situ.

Reproduced from: Rassekh, C. & Haughey, B., 2015. Chapter 110: Total laryngectomy and laryngopharyngectomy. In: Flint, P.W., Haughey, B.H., Lund, V.J., et al., Cummings Otolaryngology, 6th ed. Saunders, pp. 1699-1713, Fig. 110-5B.

- Complications
  - Late complications can include pharyngeal-cutaneous fistula that may require drainage and regular dressing reviews in outpatients.
- Follow-up
  - Patients will have ongoing review to track postoperative progression with wound healing and nutrition.
  - Appointment in clinic for review of speech aids can be made.

PAROTIDECTOMY

Parotidectomy is partial or complete excision of the parotid gland.

- Indications
  - Benign and malignant tumours.
  - Resection of malignant tumour may also include a lymph node neck dissection for staging and treatment purposes.
  - Recurrent sialadenitis.
- Preoperative
  - The indication for intervention will dictate whether the patient requires a superficial or total parotidectomy.
  - Invasive tumours and surgery for recurrent sialadenitis require resection of the deep lobe and therefore total parotidectomy.
  - High grade malignancy or facial nerve involvement may necessitate a radical parotidectomy with resection of the facial nerve.
  - CT imaging aids in operative planning.
- Operative
  - The parotid is approached posteriorly (Fig. 49.32), allowing for dissection of the facial nerve, which passes through the gland.
  - The use of intraoperative electromyography (EMG) to detect facial nerve fibres is debated.
  - Deep extension of the tumour sometimes necessitates mandibulotomy for access to the tumour.
  - Invasive skin cancers involving the parotid may leave a defect requiring flap reconstruction.
  - A drain is placed during closure to prevent haematoma, supplemented with a compressive dressing.
- Postoperative
  - Patients are admitted to the ward, with observation of drain tube output and facial nerve function.
  - Once the drain has been removed the patient is discharged home.

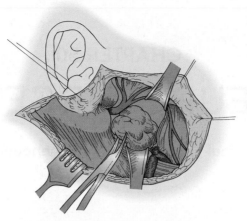

FIGURE 49.32 Parotidectomy begins posteriorly, which allows for early visualisation of the facial nerve.

Reproduced from: Johnson, J., 2008. Chapter 62: Parotidectomy. In: Myers, E., Operative Otolaryngology: Head and neck surgery, 2nd ed. Saunders, Fig. 62-12.

- Complications
  - Bleeding leading to haematoma.
  - Facial nerve weakness and damage (3–5%).
    - The nature of facial nerve damage will determine the outcome. Neuropraxia from compression has a reasonable chance of at least partial recovery.
    - Transection of the nerve typically has a poorer outcome.

CHAPTER 50

NEUROSURGERY

Paul Watson and Rami Shenouda

INCREASED INTRACRANIAL PRESSURE (ICP)

Increased ICP is a common neurosurgical issue that can manifest as a sudden acute issue or secondary to a chronic process. ICP is normally around 10–15 mmHg.

There is a direct relationship between volume and pressure within the skull, which defines a fixed volume of intracranial space; increased volume leads to a proportional increase in pressure. Increased intracranial volume arises from three areas:

1 blood – intracranial bleeding, venous obstruction
2 CSF – hydrocephalus
3 brain – intracranial tumour, cerebral oedema; abscesses from CNS infections can also lead to increased ICP.

Clinical manifestations can be split into global symptoms and focal signs:

- Global signs – headache, decreased GCS, papilloedema.
- Local signs – largely dictated by the cause of increased pressure (i.e. herniation, haematoma). However, signs can be falsely localising (CN VI palsy).
- Cushing's reflex is a classical response to increased ICP – bradycardia, hypertension and respiratory depression.

There are two potential major effects of increased ICP:

1 Reduction in cerebral blood flow (CBF)
   a Cerebral perfusion pressure (CPP) is substituted as a measurement of CBF.
   b CPP = MAP − ICP, where MAP is mean arterial pressure.
   c In chronic elevated ICP there is some auto-regulation, via increased blood pressure (increase in MAP).
   d Leads to tissue hypoxia, decreased conscious state.
   e Chronically elevated CPP can lead to hypertensive encephalopathy.

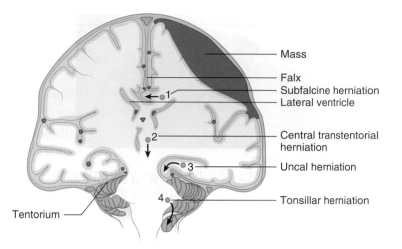

FIGURE 50.1 Herniations of the brain.

Reproduced from: Mirvis, S., Kubal, W., Shanmuganathan, K., et al., 2015. Chapter 3: Craniocerebral trauma. In: Mirvis, S., Problem Solving in Emergency Radiology. Saunders, pp. 20–52, Fig. 3.14.

2 Herniation

   a Brain tissue herniation (see Fig. 50.1) is one of the most devastating complications of increased ICP.

   b Meningeal barriers (falx cerebri, tentorium) form compartments within the brain. Increased pressure from a mass forces tissue from one compartment into another leading to herniation.

   c Transtentorial and uncal herniation lead to brainstem compression, resulting in haemodynamic and respiratory compromise, followed swiftly by death if left untreated.

Investigations

- CT brain is usually the first investigation in patients stable enough to be taken to Radiology and can identify haem.

Management

- Initial management includes rapid identification of the cause (head trauma, intracranial bleeding, hydrocephalus, see sections below) and prevention of further increases in ICP.
- Patients should be sat up to 30°, with an infusion of mannitol 0.5–1 g/kg.
- Patients with low GCS should be prepared for intubation, and an initial hyperventilation to lower PCO_2. IV glucocorticoids are not recommended.
- Patients with suspected TBI or post surgery benefit from constant ICP monitoring, most commonly via an external ventricular drain (EVD), shown in Fig. 50.2. An alternative is a pressure transducer.

SECTION IV

TABLE 50.1 Management of intracranial tumours

TUMOUR SUBTYPE	SURGERY	CHEMOTHERAPY AND RADIOTHERAPY (RTx)	PROGNOSIS
Tumours of the meninges			
WHO Grade I (benign meningioma)	• Small lesions <2 cm suited to observation • Excision of larger or symptomatic tumours in suitable patients where possible	Partially resected or non-resectable tumours should be considered for therapy	>90% 5-year survival
WHO Grade II (atypical meningioma)	Resection where possible	Adjuvant RTx Significantly higher percentage of local recurrence compared to Grade I	73% 5-year survival
WHO Grade III (malignant meningioma)			42% 5-year survival
Glial tumours			
Glioblastoma (IV)	Maximal resection with preservation of neurological function in suitable patients	Temozolomide is often used in combination with surgery, or alone RTx with a schedule suited to the patient	<5% 5-year survival 35% 1-year survival
Astrocytoma (I–III)	Maximal resection with preservation of neurological function in suitable patients Re-resection is considered in Grade I disease	Adjuvant RTx for patients with Grade II–III Unclear benefit from chemotherapy	Excellent prognosis for Grade I with complete resection, often considered curative Grade II median survival around 7.5 years Grade III median survival about 5 years

TABLE 50.1 Management of intracranial tumours—cont'd

TUMOUR SUBTYPE	SURGERY	CHEMOTHERAPY AND RADIOTHERAPY (RTx)	PROGNOSIS
Sellar tumours			
Pituitary tumours	Transphenoidal resection in patients with neurological symptoms and where medical hormone treatment has failed	Ongoing hormone therapy if required	Microadenomas have the best cure rate, but recurrence is known Recurrence more common for macroadenomas
Other tumours			
Acoustic neuroma	• Can involve a retromastoid or middle fossa approach to preserve hearing • Surveillance is an option for smaller lesions though associated with progressive hearing loss	• Stereotactic radiosurgery can be used • No clear evidence for best radiotherapy modality	Prognosis is good in tumours that are completely excised
Metastatic tumours	Single metastases with local effects can be offered excision, provided patient is suitable	• Stereotactic radiosurgery for patients with a small number of lesions • Whole brain radiotherapy for patients with multiple lesions	• Palliation may be considered for patients with poor function or diffuse, non-controlled primary disease • Even with optimal disease factors median survival is ~7 months

- The decision to intervene is often difficult and requires close and frank discussion with the patient and their family about the likely outcomes.
  - Multidisciplinary meetings allow for the formulation of management plans and junior doctors will be expected to make sure all imaging is available for discussion.

SECTION IV

- The decision is whether these patients require an operation to evacuate the haematoma or should have a period of observation.
  - Patients with features of increased intracranial pressure should have evacuation of the haematoma.
  - On CT a midline shift of >5 mm or clot thickness <10 mm is often thought to be an indicator for surgery.
    - Patients on anticoagulants will need reversal.
  - The patient's medical comorbidities should be considered when making this decision; those with poor quality of life and large haematomas are unlikely to have a good outcome from operative intervention.

Subarachnoid haemorrhage (SAH)

- The textbook presentation is a sudden onset severe headache secondary to a ruptured cerebral aneurysm.
  - Some patients experience a loss of consciousness and seizures; the latter are associated with poor outcomes.
- Mortality from this condition approaches 50%.
- Brain CT may not reveal any obvious haematoma and be reported as normal.
- LP can detect blood within the CSF aiding diagnosis (though be mindful of false positives!).
- Between 10% and 23% of patients will experience a rebleeding event.
- Management includes close monitoring in ICU for signs of increased ICP.
- Operative management options are limited.
  - If further aneurysm is identified the patient may be suitable to undergo aneurysm clipping.

ACUTE HYDROCEPHALUS

For an overview of hydrocephalus refer to Chapter 71.

Acute hydrocephalus is usually the hallmark of an obstructing tumour. Unlike the insidious onset of chronic hydrocephalus, these patients tend to feel acutely unwell with headaches, nausea and vomiting with fluctuations in their conscious state.

Investigations

- Full neurological is warranted to look for other signs of increased intracranial pressure.

- Initial investigations should include a CT brain, which will reveal the presence of hydrocephalus.
  - However, MRI provides superior resolution and is more sensitive in identifying potentially obstructive tumours.

Management

There are two main approaches to treating acute hydrocephalus:

1. Third ventriculostomy
   a. Endoscopic third ventriculostomy (ETV) is a procedure that involves perforating the 3rd ventricles into the subarachnoid space to facilitate easing of pressure.
   b. The role of ETV is still not clearly defined; some surgeons use it as an alternative to shunting.
2. Shunts
   a. Multiple variants exist but the principles remain the same.
   b. A one-way flow catheter is inserted into a lateral ventricle with the distal end opening into another bodily cavity at lower pressure.
      i. Peritoneum (ventriculoperitoneal shunt) and right atrium (ventriculoatrial shunt) are two common examples.
   c. Shunts only allow passage of CSF once ventricular pressures reach a certain level.
   d. Mechanical failures of the shunt are a known complication; this may lead to inadequate drainage and recurrence of symptoms requiring another drain to be placed.

SPINAL TRAUMA

The provision of acute spinal services is often split between Orthopaedics and Neurosurgery. Acute spine services are only available at major trauma and tertiary hospitals. Patients presenting to more peripheral hospitals will require discussion and possible transfer to a hospital offering a spinal service. Junior doctors are often tasked with liaising with the spinal registrar including transferring the necessary images to the recipient hospital for review.

Around 80% of spinal cord injuries are due to trauma, with 15–24-year-olds most commonly affected (30%). 74% of these injuries result from either motor vehicles accidents (MVAs) or falls. Motorcycle riding and diving into shallow water are considered particularly high-risk mechanisms. 85% of spinal injuries will involve a fracture, 10% will be related to ligamentous injuries and 5% will affect only the cord.

Cervical spine trauma

- Any patient presenting to ED under a 'trauma' call will have a cervical collar fitted until spinal injury has been excluded.
- Trauma assessment including primary and secondary survey is covered in Chapter 10.
- Conscious patients may report neck pain, neurological disturbances (i.e. paraesthesia, weakness). Inspect and examine the neck for midline tenderness.
  - The ability to take an accurate and complete history may be limited if the patient is not alert and cooperative.
  - Similarly, examination of the patient is only feasible in the awake and non-intoxicated patient.
  - The threshold for imaging in these patients to exclude spinal fracture is low.
- All trauma patients must have cervical spine imaging unless they meet all of the Nexus criteria (Box 50.1).
  - Initial imaging will typically include AP and lateral plain X-rays, some with open mouth views of the upper cervical vertebrae.
  - CT C-spine provides good views of the bony anatomy of the vertebrae, allowing for identification of fractures and abnormalities in the contour of the spine (dislocation/subluxation).
  - MRI is not used during initial trauma assessment, but may provide useful information regarding ligamentous injury at a later stage.
- Cervical spine fractures are largely classified into two groups:
  - Atlanto-axial fractures (Table 50.2)
    - Involve C1 (atlas) and C2 (axis).
    - The joint contributes a significant portion of the rotation of the cervical spine.

BOX 50.1 Nexus guidelines for non-utilisation of C-spine imaging in trauma patients

- No posterior midline cervical spine tenderness
- No evidence of intoxication
- A normal level of alertness
- No focal neurological deficit
- No painful distracting injuries

Adapted from: Liew, S., Jain, A., Rosenfeld, J., et al., 2012. Injury to the spine and spinal cord. In: Rosenfeld, J., Practical Management of Head and Neck Injury. Elsevier Australia, pp. 98-135, Box 6.1.

SECTION IV

TABLE 50.2 Atlanto-axial cervical spine fractures

Occipitocervical dislocation	• Separation of the skull from C1 • Found in around 1 in 5 fatal C-spine injuries • Often missed on plain X-ray • Evidence of instability/dislocation can be found on CT • May be associated with occipital fracture • Almost always requires operative management (posterior occipital-cervical fusion)

C1 (atlas) fractures	• Two main mechanisms of injury:
	   • axial loading – leading to lateral mass and burst fractures
	   • hyperextension – anterior and posterior fractures
	 • The transverse ligament is an important stabilising structure (Fig. 50.5); if ruptured it causes atlanto-axial instability (Fig. 50.6) and will likely require C1–C2 posterior fusion
	 • Atlas fractures with intact transverse ligaments can be managed with immobilisation such as halo traction devices (Fig. 50.7)

C2 (axis) fractures	• The most clinically important fractures involve the odontoid process (dens) • Fractures through the waist of the dens carry risk of non-union via avascular necrosis • May require posterior fusion due to risk of non-union

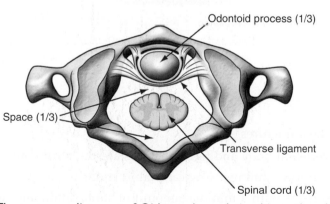

FIGURE 50.5 The transverse ligament of C1 has a close relationship to the odontoid process.

Reproduced from: Reiter, M. & Basra, S., 2008. Chapter 17: Atlas fractures. In: Kim, D., Atlas of Spine Trauma. Saunders, pp. 173–182, Fig. 17.1.

SECTION IV

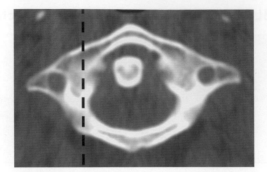

FIGURE 50.6 Transverse ligament rupture leading to displacement of the odontoid process.

Reproduced from: Gire, J., Roberto, R., Bobinski, M., et al., 2013. The utility and accuracy of computed tomography in the diagnosis of occipitocervical dissociation. Spine Journal 13(5), 510–519, Fig. 12.

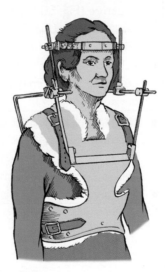

FIGURE 50.7 Halo vest traction device.

Reproduced from: Dandy, D. & Edwards, D., 2009. Chapter 10: Injuries to the face, head and spine. In: Dandy, D. & Edwards, D., Essential Orthopaedics and Trauma, 5th ed. Churchill Livingstone, pp. 145–165, Fig. 10.16.

- ○ Subaxial fractures
  - – Vertebral body and facet fractures are the most common.
  - – Perform a full neurological examination.
  - – Patients with a minimal amount of subluxation and no symptoms can be managed conservatively with immobilisation for 6–12 weeks.
- • Watch for spinal shock: hypotension, bradycardia with absent bulbocavernosus reflex.

Thoracic and lumbar spinal trauma

- Thoracic and lumbar spinal injuries (Table 50.3) are commonly associated with high energy trauma, particularly with other thoracic and lumbar injuries.
- It is important to consider the possibility of multiple sites of injury. Thoracolumbar spinal fractures have a 5–20% risk of a secondary fracture. A full spinal CT series is required in these patients.

TABLE 50.3 Thoracolumbar spinal injuries

Compression fracture	• Generally stable fractures of the anterior column that can be managed conservatively
Burst fracture	• Caused by axial loading with flexion • Higher risk of associated spinal cord injury and secondary fracture. Make sure to get a CT • Stable fractures may only involve the anterior and middle column and can be potentially managed with an orthosis (TLSO) • Unstable fractures involve all 3 columns (see Figs 50.8 and 50.9) and may require fixation if there is significant disruption to the posterior ligament complex or neurological symptoms
Fracture-dislocation injury	• Most commonly occur at the thoracolumbar junction • Disruption of all 3 columns with facet joints • Highly unstable, significant association with spinal cord injury • Likely to require operative management
Chance fracture	• Classical mechanism is from a lap seatbelt during trauma • Extreme flexion forces place excessive tension through the middle and posterior columns • Up to 50% of patients have an associated intra-abdominal injury • If the posterior ligament complex is compromised patients generally require operative intervention ('non-bony' chance fracture)
Cauda equina syndrome	• Though more commonly associated with disk herniation, fracture fragments may impinge on the lumbrosacral canal • Bilateral leg pain, bladder dysfunction and 'saddle paraesthesia' are classical symptoms • Patients require urgent spinal decompression with restoration of the canal space

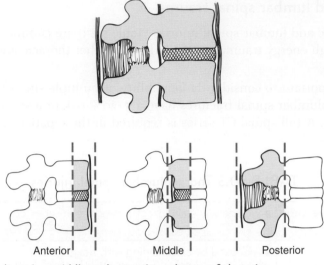

Anterior | Middle | Posterior

FIGURE 50.8 Anterior, middle and posterior columns of the spine.

Reproduced from: Smirnov, E., Anderson, G., Albert, T., et al., 2012. Chapter 57: Thoracic and lumbar spine fractures. In: Devlin, V.J., Spine Secrets Plus, 2nd ed. Mosby, pp. 386–398, Fig. 57-2.

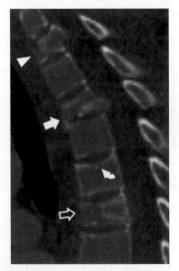

FIGURE 50.9 Unstable burst fracture associated with multiple fracture sites.

Reproduced from: Bensch, F., Kolvlkko, M., Koskinen, S., et al., 2012. Multidetector computed tomography of spinal fractures. Seminars in Roentgenology 47(4), 330–341, Fig. 1.

- Patients should be immobilised on a spinal board until assessment and investigation has ruled out spinal injury.
  - Assessment can include log roll with midline palpation in conscious and cooperative patients.
- The key step is first determining if neurological injury is present, then definitive imaging to see if the patient has an unstable fracture pattern.

MANAGEMENT OF THE CHRONIC SPINE

Laminectomy

Laminectomy involves removal of one or both lamina of a vertebral body.

- Indications
  - Spinal stenosis (most commonly lumbar) that has not improved with conservative therapies or demonstrates progressive neurological symptoms with clear anatomical correlation.
- Preoperative
  - Patients should attend pre-admission clinic and have an anaesthetic review.
- Operative
  - The classic approach is a midline incision over a prone patient in a specialised frame with hip flexion, reducing the curve of the lumbar spine.
  - The vertebra is then accessed with visualisation of the laminae.
  - This exposure allows for pedicle-to-pedicle resection.
  - This procedure can be combined with a posterior fusion if required.
- Postoperative
  - Patients are encouraged to mobilise early.
  - There are typically restrictions on bending, lifting and twisting movements for 8–12 weeks.
- Complications
  - Dural tears, neurological injury, epidural haematomas.
  - Wound infections.

Discectomy

Discectomy is surgical intervention for the management of herniated intervertebral discs.

- Indications
  - Herniated or prolapsed intervertebral discs (commonly lumbar) associated with pain or neurological deficit.
- Preoperative
  - As for laminectomy.
- Operative
  - Multiple techniques have been described including minimally invasive approaches such as microdiscectomy (using a microscope).
  - Open discectomy involves gaining access to the herniated disc via a posterior approach.

- o The spinal canal is entered and the nerve root retracted to allow dissection of the disc.
- Postoperative
  - o Patients may be discharged the next day if they recover well from surgery.
  - o Typically, there are restrictions on lifting for 4 weeks.
- Complications
  - o Wound infection, pain.
  - o Epidural haematoma, neurological injury.

CHAPTER 51

PLASTIC AND RECONSTRUCTIVE SURGERY

Paul Watson

TRAUMA

General considerations

Patients who present with large or deep wounds, particularly on the face or limbs, form the bulk of Emergency and inpatient referrals for the plastic surgery team. A simple wound sustained in a clean environment and free from foreign body or haematoma should heal without the need for specialist involvement.

There are specific situations in which the plastic surgical team will consider further intervention, as follows:

- There are important anatomical structures deep to the wound that have been/may have been damaged requiring exploration or repair (especially in the hands – see below).
  - The depth of a knife injury is not always appreciable on clinical examination due to the 'shelving' nature of the blade (Fig. 51.1). A careful examination is required.
  - Glass has a tendency to shatter on impact with tissue: the deeper the injury, the more likely a foreign body will be present (Fig. 51.2). **X-ray is essential.**
  - Extensive soft tissue damage may require extensive debridement of non-viable tissue, which may leave a tissue defect requiring coverage (Fig. 51.3).
  - Wounds contaminated with foreign material may require exploration and washout in theatre (especially animal and human bites; see Fig. 51.4).
  - Human and animal bites present an increased infection risk due to the presence of bacteria in the oral cavity. Bites on the hands are of

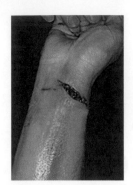

FIGURE 51.1 Laceration over volar wrist from a knife. Carries risk of tendon and vascular injury.

Reproduced from: Klatt, E.C., 2015. Chapter 16: The skin. Robbins and Cotran Atlas of Pathology, 3rd ed. Philadelphia: Saunders, pp. 409-446, Fig. 16-106.

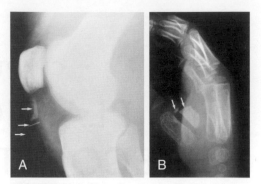

FIGURE 51.2 Glass foreign bodies initially missed on ED presentation due to lack of imaging investigations.

Reproduced from: Quick, C.R.G., Reed, J.B., Harper, S.J.F., et al., 2014. Chapter 17: Soft tissue injuries and burns. In: Quick, C.R.G., Reed, J.B., Harper, S.J.F., et al., Essential Surgery: Problems, Diagnosis and Management, 5th ed. London: Churchill Livingstone, pp. 232-244, Fig. 17.1.

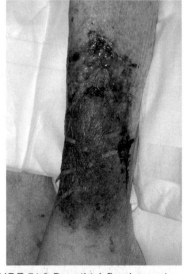

FIGURE 51.3 Pre-tibial flap laceration, requiring debridement.

Reproduced from: Lo, S., Hallam, M.J., Smith, S., et al., 2012. The tertiary management of pretibial lacerations. Journal of Plastic, Reconstructive and Aesthetic Surgery 65(9), 1143-1150, Fig. 3.

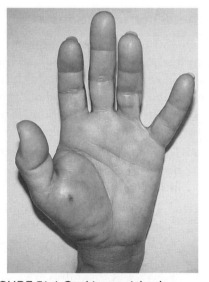

FIGURE 51.4 Cat bite on right thenar eminence leading to gross oedema and infection of the right thumb.

Reproduced from: Madsen, D.L. & Forthman, C.L., 2014. Hand infections. In: Cameron, J.L. & Cameron, A.M., Current Surgical Therapy, 11th ed. Philadelphia: Saunders, pp. 724-732, Fig. 10.

particular concern due to the ability of sharp teeth to pierce into deeper soft tissue seeding infection.

- ○ Elderly patients can sustain wounds that lead to lifting of the skin off the underlying tissue, forming a 'flap' of tissue. The flap may appear easy to suture; however, there is often extensive soft tissue damage and the overlying skin is not viable. Debridement and grafting is often required.

Hand trauma

- Injuries to hands require thorough history and examination to fully evaluate the potential impact on function.
- All dressings should be taken down and the wound fully exposed.
- Pain relief in the form of oral analgesia and/or local anaesthetic (after neurological status has been assessed) are helpful.

Finger trauma

Fingers are common sites of injury in both the domestic and workplace settings. Lacerations with knives and blunt force 'crush injuries' are typical presentations.

Crush injuries

Trauma to the tips of the fingers can result in disruption of the nail bed.
- Nail bed injuries can be associated with fractures of the distal phalanx. X-rays should be obtained.
- Treatment includes removal of the nail under local anaesthetic with wound washout and direct repair of the nailbed.
- Crush injuries involving extensive loss of tissue (partial amputations/ de-tipping injuries) may require soft tissue reconstruction.

Fractures

Hand fractures commonly result from crush or direct blow injuries.
- Acute closed hand fractures can have streamlined referrals to acute plastic outpatient clinic (Chapter 72) provided the patient has no other injury.
- Open hand fractures will need admission for IV antibiotics and wound washout.

Tendon injuries

All deep lacerations involving the hand and forearm have the potential to injure muscle and tendons. Injuries from sharp thin blades such as knives have the capacity to injure tissue deeper than the appearance of the skin wound.

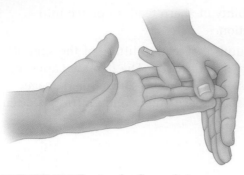

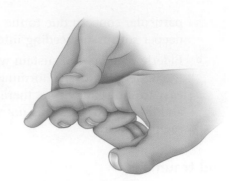

FIGURE 51.5 Testing for flexor digitorum superficialis (FDS). FDS and FDP are isolated in the other digits.

Cannon, D., 2013. Chapter 66: Flexor and extensor tendon injuries. In: Canale, S.T. & Beaty, J.H., Campbell's Operative Orthopaedics, 12th ed. Philadelphia: Mosby, pp. 3247-3304, Fig. 66-4.

FIGURE 51.6 Testing for flexor digitorum profundus (FDP).

Cannon, D., 2013. Chapter 66: Flexor and extensor tendon injuries. In: Canale, S.T. & Beaty, J.H., Campbell's Operative Orthopaedics, 12th ed. Philadelphia: Mosby, pp. 3247-3304, Fig. 66-3.

- Careful examination using correct technique can help identify which tendon may have been affected.
  - Active range of motion of the fingers should be performed under controlled conditions, with the examiner stabilising the hand to examine specific joints (see Figs 51.5 and 51.6).
- The 'zone of injury' of the injured tendon can help.
- Flexor tendon repairs are performed in theatre. The depth of injury to the tendon is often expressed as a percentage and influences postoperative care.
  - Simply put, the technique involves joining the ends of the tendons using multiple passes of the suture, with each pass known as a 'strand'.
- Potential risks include infection and tendon re-rupture requiring close follow-up with hand therapy.

Neurovascular injury

Penetrating injuries to the palm of the hand and lacerations to the sides of the digits are commonly associated with damage to neurovascular structures.

- Examination of the sensation of the fingers can help determine injury to the common and digital nerves.
- Lacerations should raise suspicion of injury to the digital artery, necessitating exploration of the wound.
- Repair of the vessels may require a microsurgical approach (outlined below).

Amputations

The term amputation is widely used (and at times imprecisely used) to describe finger and hand injuries resulting in loss of tissue.

Fingertip injuries resulting in loss of the tip are termed 'de-tipping' injuries and are common with workplace and domestic blade-based injuries. These injuries may result in exposed bone with insufficient soft tissue for primary closure. They sometimes necessitate local flap coverage with or without grafting.

Partial amputation refers to a deep wound that has compromised several important structural components, though the tissue distal to the injury is still attached.

- Traumatic amputations of the digits, particularly the thumb, can undergo *re-implantation* with bony fixation and microvascular repair of the neurovascular bundles provided the digit and the hand have otherwise minimal soft tissue damage.
- The re-implanted digit is treated as for a free flap in the postoperative period.

WOUND MANAGEMENT AND DRESSINGS

The variety of tissue defects created by trauma- or excision-related nonviable tissue can present a reconstructive problem-solving challenge.

Understanding the basic tools of reconstructive surgery can help the junior doctor appreciate the approach a plastic surgeon takes when considering how to repair a defect. This approach is referred to as the 'reconstructive ladder' (Fig. 51.7). The intention is to aid the surgeon to decide on a reconstructive option by considering the least invasive option suitable for correction of a defect. Each step is progressively more invasive, requiring the use of more complex surgical techniques.

Principles of reconstruction

Free flap
Distant flap
Local flap
Grafting
Primary intention (closure of wound)
Secondary intention (dressings)

FIGURE 51.7 The reconstructive ladder.

Slimman, R., 2009. Wound closure and the reconstructive ladder in plastic surgery. Journal of the American College of Certified Wound Specialists 1(1), 6-11.

Dressing selection

Dressing selection is made after assessing the patient's wound and considering the phase of wound healing.

- Ultimately the goal is to promote optimal wound moisture to permit the easy removal of nonviable tissue and promote healing.
    - Wounds that are too dry impair the breakdown and removal of necrotic tissue. This delays granulation and epithelisation of healthy tissue.
    - Wounds that are too moist similarly interfere with the normal epithelisation process.
    - The dressing should keep the wound sterile from outside microorganisms.
- Wounds can become chronic requiring long-term dressing with ongoing outpatient support and review.
- Though some patients may be capable of changing dressings by themselves or have family members to assist, outpatient nursing services may be required to provide dressing changes.
    - Local GPs with nursing staff support can also provide this service.
    - Hospital networks may provide home visiting services through HITH or district nursing.
- The expense of the dressing may affect patient compliance with the dressing regimen and needs consideration when developing a discharge plan.
- When managing a contaminated deep wound, there are a number of dressing techniques to aid with reducing microbial presence and debriding non-viable tissue:
    - Initial wound swabs should be taken to identify the pathogen.
    - Empirical IV antibiotics are given in the interim, typically IV cephazolin for trauma unless there is a risk of dirty wound contamination, then broad-spectrum cover such as piperacillin–tazobactam (Tazocin®) is recommended. (See Appendix IV for dosages.)
    - Deeply contaminated wounds can undergo packing with betadine or normal saline soaked gauze that can be changed up to 4 times a day.
    - Each time the dressing is removed, the gauze will remove the necrotic tissues and slough, promoting healthy wound healing.
    - Ensure patients have sufficient analgesia for each scheduled dressing change.

Vacuum assisted closure (VAC) devices

- VAC dressings are temporary foam-based dressings that use negative pressure to clear exudate, interstitial fluid and bacterial load from a wound (see Fig. 51.8). They promote wound granulation.

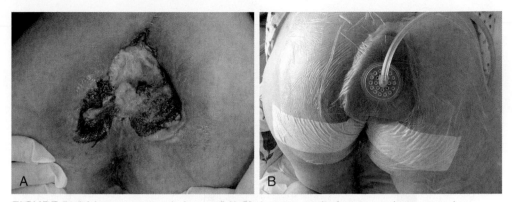

FIGURE 51.8 Vacuum assisted closure (VAC) dressing applied to a sacral pressure ulcer.

Reproduced from: Aydin, U. & Ozgenel, Y., 2008. A simple solution for preventing air leakage in VAC therapy for sacral pressure sores. Journal of Plastic, Reconstructive and Aesthetic Surgery 61(10), 1267-1269, Figs 1 and 4.

- ○ The foam component of the dressing can remain intact for up to 72 hours, then requiring change. Changing a VAC dressing is often performed in theatre allowing examination of the wound, washout and debridement under anaesthetic.
- ○ VAC dressings can be used as a longer term temporary measure prior to definitive reconstruction, particularly with abdominal defects.
- The junior doctor is often tasked with organising the VAC pump 'machine'.
- ○ Typically, surgical wards will keep a supply. If not, the operating theatre suites or Hospital in the Home (HITH) services may store them.

A summary of all types of surgical dressings is given in Table 51.1, which includes Figs 51.9 to 51.14.

GRAFTS

Grafts can be made from all tissue types including bone, although skin grafting is more readily associated with Plastic Surgery. Grafts involve the transfer of tissue without a vascular supply. Neovascularization occurs at the graft site after 48 hours. During this avascular period the graft survives by diffusion of oxygen and nourishing substances from the graft bed. The thickness of the graft (see Fig. 51.15) will influence how much nutrient supply the graft requires to survive. This process is known as 'take'.

As grafts require a vascularised tissue bed capable of providing a blood supply, bare bone, tendon and cartilage are not suitable for grafting and soft tissue coverage is achieved via flap reconstructive options. Before reconstruction can be commenced, patients need to have a clean wound bed, free of infection, sometimes

TABLE 51.1 Types of surgical dressings

TYPE OF DRESSING	DESCRIPTION	EXAMPLE
Non-adherent tulle/mesh gauze Non-stick dressing that can be applied directly to the wound, covered with other dressings such as gauze and crepe	• Used as a protective dressing for traumatic, healing wounds and grafts (see below) • Examples include: Jelonet®, Bactigras®, Inadine®, Mepitel®, Xeroform®	 **FIGURE 51.9 Non-adherent gauze dressing.** Reproduced from: Khunger, N. & Lihiri, K., 2010. Vitiligo surgery. In: Robinson, J.K. Hanke, C.W., Siegel, D.M., et al, Surgery of the skin, 2nd ed. London: Mosby, Fig. 42.8.
Hydrogel Moisture-donating dressing that enables granulation and autolytic breakdown of non-viable tissue	• Used for wounds with dry slough, necrosis and eschar requiring moisture for removal • This requires a secondary dressing over the top for support • Examples include Comfeel®, Intrasite®	 **FIGURE 51.10 Hydrogel dressing.** Reproduced from: Menaker, G. & Mehlis, S., 2012. Dressings. In: Bolognia, J.L., Jorizzo, J.L. & Schaffer, J.V., eds., Dermatology, 3rd ed. London: Saunders, pp. 2365-2379, Fig. 145.8.

Hydrocolloid

Occlusive dressing that combines with exudate to form a gel and maintain wound moisture

Hydrates and promotes breakdown of slough

- Used for wounds that are producing some exudate to encourage granulation and epithelisation
- Available as sheet dressings and gels
- Examples include Tegasorb®, Duoderm®

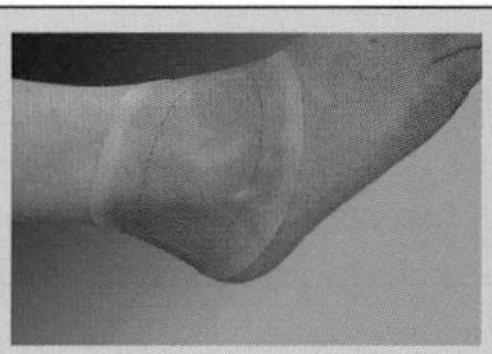

FIGURE 51.11 Hydrocolloid dressing.

Reproduced from: Menaker, G. & Mehlis, S., 2012. Dressings. In: Bolognia, J.L., Jorizzo, J.L. & Schaffer, J.V., eds., Dermatology, 3rd ed. London: Saunders, pp. 2365-2379, Fig. 145.10.

Foam-based dressing

Mostly comprised of polyurethane

Absorbent dressings that can be cut and shaped to provide wound protection in pressure care

- Either used as support for other dressings such as hydrogels, mesh and packing dressings or to protect fragile wounds and pressure ulcers
- Combination based products are available (such as Mepilex®) that use a silicone layer as wound interface in high exudate wounds

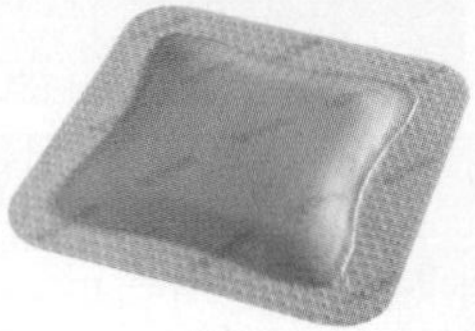

FIGURE 51.12 Combination silicone foam dressing.

Reproduced from: Chilcott, M., 2011. Wound dressing. In: Pfenninger, J.L. & Fowler, G.C., Pfenninger and Fowler's Procedures for Primary Care, 3rd ed. Philadelphia: Mosby, pp. 278-284, Fig. 44.6.

continued

SECTION IV

TABLE 51.1 Types of surgical dressings—cont'd

TYPE OF DRESSING	DESCRIPTION	EXAMPLE
Absorbent fibre dressing • Common types include alginate and hydrofibre • Can be used to pack wounds • Some alginate-based dressings have haemostatic properties • Capable of absorbing high amounts of exudate • Dressings can be changed multiple times a day to aid in debridement of tissue and removal of excess moisture absorbed in dressing	• Commonly used in cavitating wounds as a packing dressing • Supported by a foam or gauze dressing • Haemostatic properties of calcium alginate dressings make them useful for dressing split skin graft (SSG) donor sites • Examples include: Kaltostat® Algisite® (alginate), Aquacel® (hydrofibre) • Alginate dressings tend to form a gel with wound exudate that can be mistaken for slough when the wound is cleaned between dressing changes	**FIGURE 51.13 Alginate dressing.** Reproduced from: Levin, Y., Brown, K.L. & Phillips, T.J., 2015. Wound healing and its impact on dressings and postoperative care. In: Robinson, J.K., Hanke, C.W., Siegel, D.M., et al., Surgery of the Skin, 3rd ed. London: Mosby, pp. 114-133, Fig. 8.5.
Silver-based dressings • Dressings impregnated with silver. • Demonstrate broad-spectrum antibacterial properties • Some formulations of the dressing allow for weekly dressing changes, beneficial in patients with chronic wounds	• Used in treatment of ulcers, colonised, burns and chronic wounds • Supported by other tape-based dressings	**FIGURE 51.14 Silver-based dressing.** Reproduced from: Levin, L. & Kovach, S., 2014. Soft Tissue Reconstruction for the Foot and Ankle. In: Coughlin, M.J., Saltzman, C.L. & Anderson, R.B., Mann's Surgery of the Foot and Ankle, 9th ed. Philadelphia: Saunders, pp. 794-827, Fig. 17-8B.

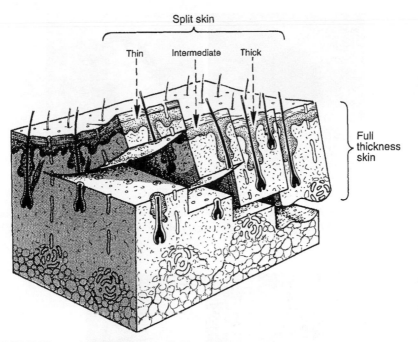

FIGURE 51.15 The varied thicknesses of skin grafts.

McGregor, A. & McGregor, I.A., 2000. Chapter 3: Free skin grafts. In: McGregor, A. & McGregor, I.A., Fundamental Techniques in Plastic Surgery, 10th ed. London: Churchill Livingstone, Fig. 3.1.

necessitating that a patient undergo formal theatre washout prior to definitive grafting.

A skin graft will always include the epidermis and a variable amount of dermis.

Full thickness skin grafts (FTSG)

An FTSG includes the entire epidermis and dermis. Harvesting of the entire dermis allows retention of the collagen support structure of the skin, giving a superior cosmetic appearance due to the prevention of contracture. The use of FTSG from local areas also allows for close skin colour matching (see Fig. 51.16).

This technique leaves a secondary defect on the donor site. The donor site of the FTSG will require primary closure or an SSG dependent on location. The amount of full thickness skin that can be harvested for grafting is thereby limited. There are higher metabolic requirements for a successful take.

Split skin grafts (SSGs)

SSGs are a partial thickness graft containing the entirety of the epidermis and a partial thickness of dermis (see Fig. 51.17). The loss of dermal support structures leads to contraction of the graft. Poor skin colour matching makes an SSG a poor choice for the face.

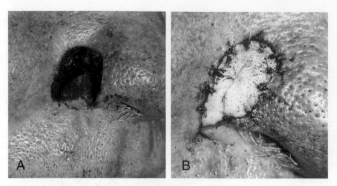

FIGURE 51.16 Nasal alar skin defect covered with an FTSG.

Reproduced from: Acosta, A.E., Aasi, S.Z., MacNeal, R.J., et al., 2015. Chapter 19: Skin grafting. In: Robinson, J.K., Hanke, C.W., Siegel, D.M., et al., Surgery of the Skin, 3rd ed. London: Mosby, Fig. 19.3.

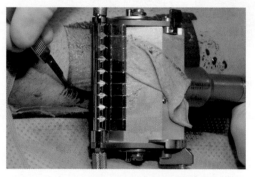

FIGURE 51.17 Use of a powered dermatome to take an SSG from the thigh.

Reproduced from: Smith, M.H. & MacIver, C., 2016. Skin grafting. In: Kademani, D. & Tiwana, P., Atlas of Oral and Maxillofacial Surgery. St Louis: Saunders, pp. 1247-1260, Fig. 120-6 B3.

As the layer of dermis is left intact on the donor site, it will heal spontaneously. The site can be reused in the future for a further SSG if required. SSGs require a lower metabolic load during take.

Meshing of the skin graft allows for a larger graft size (see Fig. 51.18) and allows exudate to pass through the graft, though the healed site has poor cosmesis.

Graft complications

Graft failure

- Caused by haematoma under the graft site.
  - Haematoma will lift the graft from the wound bed, preventing take.
  - Haemostasis on the graft site before the graft inset can help reduce the chances of this occurring.
- Shearing forces over the graft site disrupt the formation of fibrin.

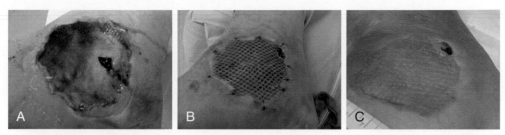

FIGURE 51.18 Meshed SSG for management of a chronic foot wound. **B** demonstrates intraoperative inset of the graft with well taken graft 4 weeks postoperatively in **C**. Note there is a small area that will heal via secondary intention.

Reproduced from: Simman, R. & Phavixay, L., 2011. Split-thickness skin grafts remain the gold standard for the closure of large acute and chronic wounds. Journal of the American College of Certified Wound Specialists 3(3), 55-59, Fig. 4.

- Pressure dressings help keep the graft in place.
- VAC dressings are sometimes used for cavitating wounds with grafts, particularly on the lower limb.

Graft infection

Skin grafts are considered low risk of infection. Patients typically receive prophylactic antibiotic coverage.

Graft dressings

At the end of the procedure a compression dressing will be applied to hold the graft on the wound bed. A properly moulded and secured dressing is essential to prevent complications as described above.

Dressings differ dependent on the location of the graft:

- Face (FTSG)
    - A 'bolster' dressing involving non-stick gauze can be moulded to fill the 3-D nature of the graft inset (see Fig. 51.19).
    - The donor site (usually preauricular, postauricular or supraclavicular) is typically small enough to be closed directly.
- Trunk/abdomen (SSG)
    - Non-adherent gauze over graft, then dressing gauze and sheet adhesive (polyester-based products such as Mefix® and Hypafix® are common)
- Limbs (typically SSG though FTSG are used on the hands)
    - Non-adherent gauze, dressing gauze and crepe bandage.

FLAPS

Flaps involve the transfer of tissue with an intact blood supply. Flaps don't necessarily involve skin; they can include any type of tissue, including muscle and bone,

SECTION IV

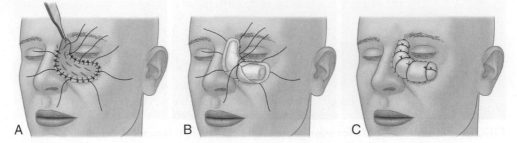

FIGURE 51.19 An FTSG secured with a tie-over bolster dressing. The fenestrations as depicted in A permit wound ooze through the graft, preventing haematoma build-up under the graft.

Scherer-Pietramaggiori, S.S., Pietramaggiori, G. & Orgill, D.P., 2013. Chapter 17: Skin graft. In: Neligan, P.C., Plastic Surgery, 3rd ed. Saunders, Fig. 17.10.

for complex reconstructions. Fascial, muscle and bone flaps can be utilised in a standalone approach.

Flaps also have a number of uses aside from providing soft tissue converge, including providing sensation, muscle function and tissue expansion.

Local flaps

- Small local flaps can be raised without a known or named blood supply due to the small area of tissue that has been mobilised.
- These flaps are also used in various other parts of the body with a length-to-width ratio of around 1:1; this does limit the size and application of the flap if not based on a known vascular supply.
- Local flaps provide superior function and appearance to FTSG, particularly when the donor site can be closed primarily.
- These flaps require a simple dressing; an antibacterial ointment on the face (such as chloramphenicol) is popular.
- These procedures are performed as day cases and the patient can be reviewed in 1 week with pathology (if for malignancy) and flap review. The patient should avoid placing any unnecessary pressure on the flap.
- Complications include haematoma under the flap, necrosis of the tip (especially if poorly designed) and wound dehiscence.

Regional flaps

- Regional flaps exploit the known blood supply of the tissue to raise large flaps.
- These flaps can include fascia and muscle, with impressive pedicle (blood supply) lengths allowing for coverage of distant defects.

- There are a number of commonly used regional flaps:
  - delto-pectoral: used for facial defect coverage
  - trapezius: for posterior neck and scalp coverage
  - latissimus dorsi: for breast reconstruction.
- These flaps leave a significant secondary defect at the donor site, which, if not amenable to primary closure, can be covered with a skin graft.
- Complications are largely the same as those of local flaps. although regional flaps with a long vascular pedicle may develop features of congestion if the patient has poor vascular status or pressure is applied around the flap.

Free flaps

- Free tissue transfer involves the transfer of a flap from a donor site with division of the vascular supply and then anastomosis with recipient vessels at the graft site.
- Extensive preoperative planning is involved in identifying the donor vascular vessels, sometimes requiring CT angiography to ensure patent supply to the potential flap.
- During the operation (see Fig. 51.20) the vascular supply of the flap is anastomosed (see Fig. 51.21) to selected grafts vessels at the recipient site using microsurgical tools and a microscope.

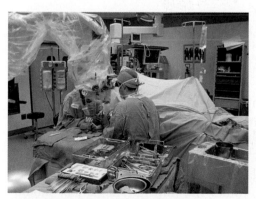

FIGURE 51.20 Typical set-up for microvascular surgery.

Reproduced from: Dzwierzynski, W., 2013. Chapter 11: Replantation and revascularization. In: Neligan, P.C., Plastic Surgery, 3rd ed. Saunders, Fig. 11.2.

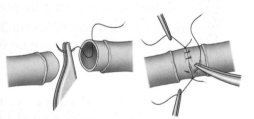

FIGURE 51.21 Illustration of microsurgical arterial anastomosis.

Kwei, S.L., Weiss, D.D. & Pribaz, J.J., 2009. Chapter 9: Microsurgery and free flaps. In: Buyuron, B., Eriksson, E., Persing, J.A., et al., Plastic Surgery: Indications and practice. London: Saunders, pp. 79-94, Fig. 9.2A and F.

SECTION IV

- Free flaps offer versatile tissue coverage involving skin, fascia, muscle and bone. Common examples include:
  - Radial forearm free flap (RFFF) – a fascio-cutaneous flap based on the radial artery
    - Preoperative Allen's test will assist in determining if the radial or ulna artery is dominant in the hand.
    - The donor site is covered with an SSG, protected with a splint until the graft is reviewed.
  - Anterolateral thigh (ALT) flap – a myocutaneous flap based on the lateral femoral circumflex artery with a wide range of uses for traumatic and elective defects
    - The donor site can be closed primarily, typically with drains due to the large size of the wound.
    - Patients can weight bear as tolerated postoperatively.
  - Deep inferior epigastric (artery) perforator (DIEP) flap – a large fascio-cutaneous flap based on the aforementioned artery
    - Used in breast reduction following mastectomy.
    - Donor site closed primarily with drains.
    - Patients should wear an abdominal binder to protect the donor site.

The postoperative free flap

- In the initial postoperative period the flap requires close monitoring. The first 48 hours of monitoring are considered critical. The junior doctor will frequently receive pages from the ward regarding the free-flap patients that should be answered promptly.
  - Hand-held Doppler ultrasound is used at the end of the case to locate and mark the position of the vascular supply. Checking of 'the Doppler' is regularly performed by the nursing staff on the ward.
  - The nursing staff will also complete regular 'flap observations' which include maintaining a specialised observation chart with particular emphasis on the patient's vital signs and the appearance, temperature and capillary refill of the flap.
  - Maintaining perfusion to the flap is critical, with a suggestion that systolic blood pressure is kept around 100 mmHg. The patient should have regular haemoglobin checks.
  - If possible, the flap should be visible, with care taken to avoid pressure placed on the pedicle and flap inset.
  - Patients should receive subcutaneous heparin while an inpatient to reduce the risk of anastomotic thrombosis.

- Complications
  - Patient factors
    - Factors such as cardiovascular disease, smoking, hepatic disease, diabetes and poor nutrition can all lead to flap compromise.
    - Adequate pre-admission optimisation of medical comorbidities can help reduce their impact on outcome, particularly in relation to nutritional status and glycaemic control.
  - Haematoma
    - Large haematomas can place pressure on the vascular pedicle.
  - Anastomotic leak
  - Arterial insufficiency
    - Flap will appear cool, pale and demonstrate reduced capillary refill.
    - Doppler is typically absent, though may be faintly present.
  - Venous congestion
    - Flap will appear oedematous, often described as a 'bruised' appearance.
    - Doppler is typically present.
    - Congested flaps can be treated with medicinal leeches, which will draw congested blood from the flap. Leeches need to be placed directly on the flap. Ciprofloxacin prophylaxis is recommended.

Figs 51.22 to 51.24 show various flap procedures.

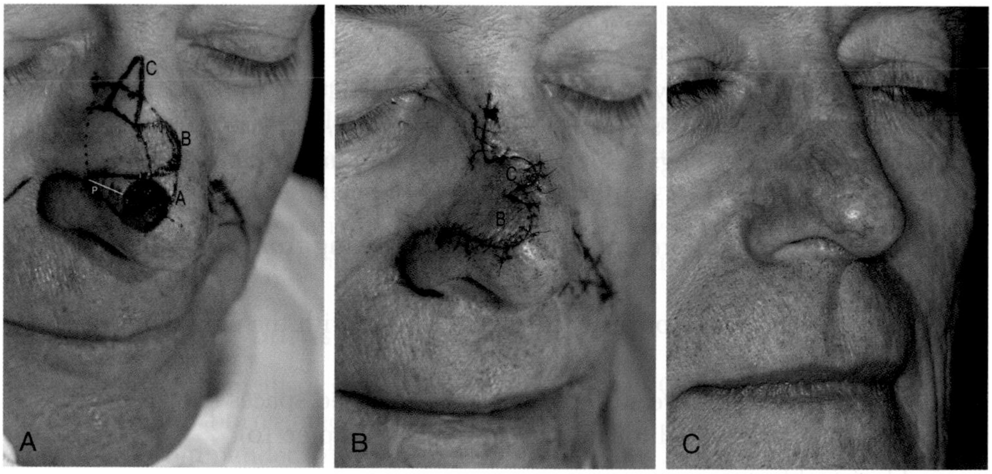

FIGURE 51.22 Local bilobe flap to cover a nasal defect following excision of a skin lesion. **C** shows long-term follow-up with good cosmetic outcome.

Reproduced from: Minsue Chen, T., Wanitphakdeedecha, R. & Nguyen, T.H., 2009. Flaps. In: Vidimos, A.T., Ammirati, C.T. & Poblete-Lopez, C., Dermatologic Surgery. Elsevier Health Sciences, pp. 163-180, Fig. 13-17.

TABLE 51.2 Depth of burn injury classification

DEPTH	APPEARANCE AND CHARACTERISTICS OF SKIN	
Epidermal burn	• Also called 'superficial', this type of burn only affects the epidermal layer of skin • Appears erythematous and dry • Painful • Blanches with pressure • Commonly associated with sunburn and hot water scalding • Will typically heal within 1–2 weeks • Capillary refill: normal • Sensation: intact	 **FIGURE 51.25 Epidermal burn.** Reproduced from: Rawlins, J., 2011. Management of burns. Surgery 29(10), 523-528, Fig. 4 a, b, c and d.
Superficial dermal	• Affects the epidermis and upper part of the dermis • Appears red with blister formation • Painful • Occasionally lead to scarring • Heal within 2–3 weeks • Capillary refill: present • Sensation: intact	 **FIGURE 51.26 Superficial dermal burn.** Reproduced from: Rawlins, J., 2011. Management of burns. Surgery 29(10), 523-528, Fig. 4 a, b, c and d.
Deep dermal	• Extends to the deep dermis • Has a variable waxy and blotchy red appearance • Not painful, but can be tender on examination • Capillary refill can be difficult to assess • Usually scars, will cause functional issues if around joints • Heals in around 2–4 months • Capillary refill: absent • Sensation: absent	 **FIGURE 51.27 Deep dermal burn.** Reproduced from: Rawlins, J., 2011. Management of burns. Surgery 29(10), 523-528, Fig. 4 a, b, c and d.

TABLE 51.2 Depth of burn injury classification—cont'd

DEPTH	APPEARANCE AND CHARACTERISTICS OF SKIN	
Full thickness	• Total loss of epidermis and dermis • Typically appears as grey/white leathery burns • Burns do not blanch and sensation is absent • Scarring is severe, and causes significant contracture • A layer of eschar forms over the top of the tissue • Capillary refill: absent • Sensation: absent	**FIGURE 51.28 Full thickness burn.** Reproduced from: Rawlins, J., 2011. Management of burns. Surgery 29(10), 523-528, Fig. 4 a, b, c and d.

Adapted from: Australian and New Zealand Burns Association (ANZBA), 2013. Chapter 5: Burn wound assessment. In: Emergency Management of Severe Burns. Melbourne: ANZBA. Rice, P. & Orgill, D., 2014. Classification of burns. In: UpToDate [Internet]. <http://www.uptodate.com/>.

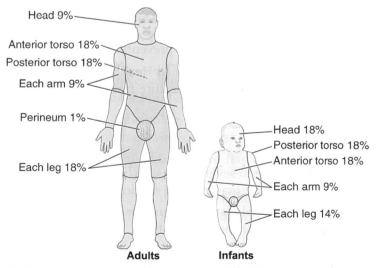

Head 9%
Anterior torso 18%
Posterior torso 18%
Each arm 9%
Perineum 1%
Each leg 18%

Adults

Head 18%
Posterior torso 18%
Anterior torso 18%
Each arm 9%
Each leg 14%

Infants

FIGURE 51.29 Estimation of total body surface area (TBSA) for assessing extent of burn injury.

Ferri, F.F., 2017. Burns. In: Ferri, F.F., Ferri's Clinical Advisor. Philadelphia: Mosby, Fig. 1B-60.

- – Following the procedure, the expander is periodically filled in outpatients percutaneously with saline (or air) until the desired size has been reached (patient has most input).
- Dependent on breast cancer staging patients can either undergo an immediate or delayed reconstruction.
  - ○ Immediate breast reconstruction direct to implants can be considered for select patients.
  - ○ It's important to ask patients if they will require chemo- or radiotherapy as this can alter the approach of the reconstruction.
- Postoperative
  - ○ Post-op free flap – each surgeon may have their own post-op protocol.
  - ○ Patients who have undergone tissue expansion require observation for 1–2 days to watch for haematoma.
  - ○ Drain tubes can be left in with outpatient nursing monitoring.
- Complications
  - ○ Bleeding (potentially leading to haematoma).
  - ○ Infection – deep infection involving an expander or implant may lead to removal.
  - ○ Rupture of implants or expanders.
  - ○ Flap complications.

Breast reduction

Breast reduction surgery involves reducing the volume of the breast.

- Indications
  - ○ Physical pain from large breasts, asymmetry, oncological resection, cosmetic.
  - ○ Patients may undergo reduction during a contralateral mastectomy and reconstruction to maintain symmetry.
- Preoperative
  - ○ The patient and the surgeon should discuss the procedure and develop an understanding of the likely outcome.
  - ○ Patients with obesity who smoke are at higher risk of complications. Patients with high BMIs may require a delay of surgery until they have lost weight.
- Intraoperative
  - ○ Multiple approaches used with different 'patterns' of reduction.
  - ○ Reduction greatly affects the shape of the breast, which may require repositioning of the nipple and breast contouring (mastopexy).
  - ○ Care must be taken to retain adequate vascular supply to the nipple.

- Postoperative
  - Drains are sometimes left in postoperatively, removed as per surgeon instructions.
  - Patients may wear a soft bra initially, allowing time for healing.
- Complications
  - Infection, haematoma, pain are common complications. Nipple necrosis is a potential complication necessitating close follow-up of the patient.

Figs 51.30 to 51.33 illustrate various aspects of breast reconstruction.

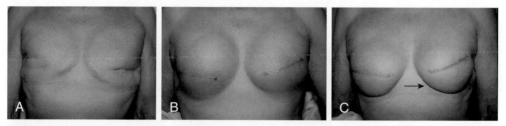

FIGURE 51.30 Tissue expanders (B) used for reconstruction post bilateral mastectomies (A). After exchange of tissue expanders for implants, the final shape is apparent with restoration of the inframammary fold (C).

Reproduced from: Nahabedian, M.Y. & Mesbiah, A.N., 2009. Breast reconstruction with tissue expanders and implants. In: Nahabedian, M.Y., ed., Cosmetic and Reconstructive Breast Surgery. Saunders, pp. 1-19.

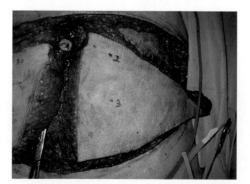

FIGURE 51.31 Raising the abdominal deep inferior epigastric perforators (DIEP) flap.

Reproduced from: Mathes, D.W. & Neligan, P.C., 2010. Preoperative imaging techniques for perforator selection in abdomen-based microsurgical breast reconstruction. Clinics in Plastic Surgery 37(4), 581-591, Fig. 6B.

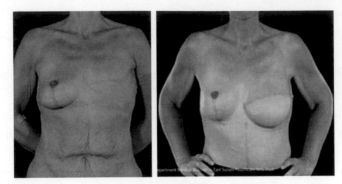

FIGURE 51.32 Preoperative and postoperative DIEP reconstruction.

Reproduced from: Salim, F., Adlard, R. & Pickford, M.A., 2013. The fleur-de-lis DIEP - introducing a 5th zone for DIEP reconstruction. Journal of Plastic, Reconstructive and Aesthetic Surgery 66(10), 1424-1427, Figs 2 and 4.

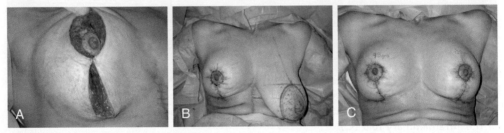

FIGURE 51.33 Approach to breast reduction: the pattern of reduction with tissue excised from the inferior breast. The next two images show final appearance of the breast compared to the left and after bilateral completion.

Reproduced from: Hammond, D.C., 2009. Chapter 7: Breast reduction. In: Hammond, D.C., Atlas of Aesthetic Breast Surgery. London: Saunders, pp. 147-182, Fig. 7.15 M, U and X.

CHAPTER 52

UROLOGY

Paul Watson and Todd Galvin Manning

THE ACUTE SCROTUM

Testicular torsion

The most common urological emergency, testicular torsion predominantly affects younger males (<25 years), with over 60% of cases occurring between the ages 12 and 18, but it can occur at any age. The most common mechanism relates to a twisting of the spermatic cord, although trauma (including minor knocks and bumps) can be the causative agent for a small proportion of cases, and further clinical suspicion should arise if this is mentioned when taking a history.

History is critical and classically reveals a sudden onset severe unilateral testicular pain that is unrelenting with sudden onset swelling. Paediatric history is also of significant importance with predisposing factors including cryptorchidism and 'bell clapper' deformity. It is also worth noting that a good history should include an accurate timeline of onset until presentation. Although it can be dangerous to rely on this, it may indicate further urgency for operative intervention.

Examination

- Examination should focus on determining the position of the testicle, with the classical description of a high riding testicle with a transverse lie. Additionally, the testicle may feel firmer in comparison to the contralateral side and the cremasteric reflex may be absent.

Investigations

- Clinical judgement should determine diagnosis, with investigations playing a minor role.
- If there is **any** suspicion that torsion is present, **DO NOT** delay surgical exploration in an attempt to confirm with imaging. The gold standard diagnostic test is surgical exploration given the time critical nature of the condition.

- Ultrasound with Doppler is seldom used and may cause unnecessary delays in treatment.
- The majority of testis remain viable if detorsed within a 6-hour time window (with very few remaining viable past 24 hours), but keep in mind the delay until presentation and additionally the delay until surgical review.

Management

- Management of suspected testicular torsion includes surgical exploration via scrotal approach (Fig. 52.1).
  - Exploration allows for the inspection of both testis, correction of the malrotation (if present) and fixation of the affected *and non-affected* testicle in the correct position via a three-point fixation technique (orchidopexy).
  - Bilateral orchidopexy is always performed as the contralateral testis may be at risk of subsequent torsion.
- Complications are predominantly due to delayed presentation or management of testicular torsion (>6 hours) can lead to irreversible ischaemia and necrosis (Fig. 52.2).
  - A non-viable testicle may require orchidectomy.
  - As such any patient who is to undergo a scrotal exploration for testicular torsion should be counselled about the possibility of the orchidectomy and loss of fertility.

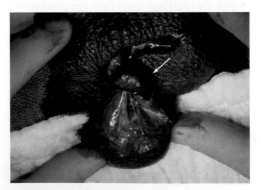

FIGURE 52.1 Exploration of the scrotum reveals a twisted cord with surrounding oedema.

Reproduced from: Smith, T.G. & Coburn, M., 2017. Chapter 72: Urologic surgery. In: Townsend, C., Sabiston Textbook of Surgery, 20th ed. Elsevier, pp. 2068-2106, Fig. 72.26.

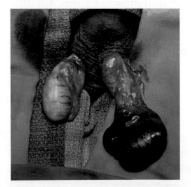

FIGURE 52.2 Ischaemic necrosis of the left testicle.

Reproduced from: Ferri, F.F., 2009. Chapter 225: Testicular torsion. In: Ferri, F.F., ed. Ferri's Color Atlas and Text of Clinical Medicine. Philadelphia: Saunders, pp. 752-753, Fig. 225.2.

Epididymitis and orchitis (epididymo-orchitis)

Orchitis seldom occurs without epididymitis. Sexually transmitted infections (STIs) such as *Neisseria gonorrhoeae* and *Chlamydia trachomatis* are the most common organisms in younger patients, with *Escherichia coli* prevalent in older patients. Non-infectious epididymitis is thought to be predominantly a chronic condition related to autoimmune or vascular disorders.

History includes scrotal swelling and tenderness, and patients can report fever, chills and dizziness in severe cases.

Examination

- Examination usually reveals a unilateral swollen and erythematous scrotum with tenderness over the epididymis.
- Some patients may develop a hydrocele secondary to inflammation.

Investigations

- Investigations should include genital swabs to determine if the patient has an STI and urine M/C/S.
  - Ultrasound may be used to confirm hyperaemic changes consistent with infection and its extent/severity, although this rarely changes management, and if torsion is suspected surgical exploration should be strongly considered.
  - U/S may be advantageous, however, in identifying occult malignancy if there are other clinical features present.

Management

- Treatment should include IV antibiotics (usually broad spectrum until cultures are returned and including coverage for STI) in acutely unwell patients, **elevation and ice**.
- Patients typically require good analgesia and anti-emetics.

UROLOGICAL INFECTIONS

The presence of infection in the genitourinary tract does not necessitate input from the Urology inpatient team. Low grade, uncomplicated infections of the urinary tract are routinely managed in the primary care setting where basic outpatient pathology services are capable of confirming the presence of a micro-organism, which allows targeted treatment.

Patients who develop systemic features of urinary tract infections such as fever, rigors and nausea may require short periods of observation and treatment until their symptoms have improved, and the patient can be discharged on oral therapy. Identification of these patients in the ED and appropriate management can reduce the number of patients who need to be admitted.

Acute bladder infections (acute cystitis)

Patients often present with dysuria (particularly describing a burning sensation on urination), increased urinary frequency, lower abdominal pain, fever and/or retention.

Most UTIs can be treated in an outpatient setting with oral antibiotics – antibiotic guidelines for the treatment of urinary tract infection are widely available. As they are less common in males, an STI screen should be considered.

Recurrent UTIs suggest an underlying anatomical abnormality.

Pyelonephritis

This is an infection involving the upper urinary tract (ureters and kidneys). Presentations are more common among women.

Patients often present with flank pain and lower abdominal pain. There is sometimes a history of a trial of oral antibiotics from their GP.

Investigations

- Investigations should include FBE, UEC urine, FWT and blood and urine M/C/S.
- The decision to order further imaging (CT) is determined by concern for non-improving infection vs harm from radiation exposure.

Management

- Routine cases of pyelonephritis can be managed with a short course of IV antibiotics.
- Ongoing fevers and pain, with worsening inflammatory markers, may require further imaging to investigate if the patient has developed a renal abscess.
- Pyelonephritis in a renal transplant patient or solitary kidney patient is of critical importance and requires formal urological review.

Renal abscess

Arising from within the renal parenchyma, renal abscess is often a result of advanced pyelonephritis. Classical symptoms include vague abdominal pain with ongoing fevers and sweats.

Investigations

- They can be visualised via ultrasound or CT imaging.

Management

- Smaller abscesses (<5 cm) are treated with prolonged IV antibiotics.
- Larger abscesses can be managed with imaging guided percutaneous drainage with a drain tube left in situ.

- Only if the abscess is causing obstruction of the urinary tract is surgical intervention considered.

Perinephric collections

It is important to distinguish renal abscess from perinephric collections as the latter are separate from the urinary tract, potentially developing from haematogenous spread.

Obtaining a sample is key to developing a treatment regimen. Patients may require a long course of IV antibiotics. Consult Infectious Diseases.

Prostatitis

Prostatitis is associated with UTIs and anatomical abnormalities.

History will initially include symptoms of UTIs (sometimes recurrent despite treatment), in particular dysuria and increased frequency, with patients frequently becoming systemically unwell with fevers, nausea and vomiting.

- The classic examination finding is a striking and unforgettable level of tenderness on rectal examination as well as a 'bogginess' to palpation of the prostate.
- Treatment is similar to other urinary tract infections, with *E. coli* the most prevalent organism, followed by *Staphylococcus aureus.*
- Some centres have utilised PSA testing as an adjunct to monitor the progress of infection in patients with infective prostatitis; however, this remains controversial.
- Prostatic abscesses are an uncommon complication of prostatitis, associated with anatomical abnormalities or those patients who are immunocompromised.

See Appendix III for a more complete list of common organisms implicated in urological infections.

URINARY RETENTION AND URINARY CATHETERISATION

Urinary retention refers to an inability to voluntarily pass urine. It is particularly common in elderly patients, affecting over a third of patients >80 years, predominantly males.

Common causes of urinary retention are outline in Table 52.1.

The clinical presentation is largely influenced by the acuity of the retention.

Acute urinary retention

The patient will typically describe suprapubic discomfort with a strong urinary urgency.

History should seek to exclude life-threatening causes of acute retention including spinal cord pathology (trauma/epidural abscess).

TABLE 52.1 Common causes of urinary retention

INFLAMMATORY	OBSTRUCTION	NEUROLOGICAL	DRUGS
• UTI • Genital/pelvic surgery	• BPH • Tumour • Constipation • Stenosis/stricture • Trauma • **Clot**	• Multiple sclerosis • Spinal cord injury • Stroke • Neuropathy	• Anticholinergic • Opioids • Calcium channel blockers • Antihistamines

Adapted from: Ban, K. & Easter, J., 2014. Chapter 99: Selected urologic problems. In: Marx, J., Hockberger, R. & Walls, R. Rosen's Emergency Medicine, 8th ed. Philadelphia: Saunders, pp. 1326-1354.

Post-surgical patients are especially at risk of urinary retention on the ward. Inflammation may be secondary to surgical intervention in combination with IV fluid hydration leading to increased bladder filling and decreased smooth muscle relaxation from opiate medication.

Bladder over-distension inhibits normal bladder wall contraction and patients may be unable to fully void. Patients can be directed to mobilise, sit-up or take showers to encourage voiding. Patients voiding small amounts should be asked to attempt further voiding to reduce over-distension. Once a patient's bladder contains over 500 mL of urine catheterisation should be considered.

Examination

- Examination can reveal a firm, tender bladder.

Management

- Drain the urine by relieving the obstruction and subsequently achieve pain relief for the patient.
  - Indwelling catheter (IDC): for managing retention, the catheter should be placed to completely empty the bladder.
  - Suprapubic catheterisation (SPC): reserved for patients with contraindications to IDC (prostatitis, urethral traumas and strictures or repeated failed attempts at placing an IDC) (Fig. 52.3).
  - Some patients who are not suited to IDC (cognitive impairment) may have an intermittent catheterisation ('in and out').
  - Patients with chronic urinary retention can be educated to perform catheterisation themselves (self-intermittent catheterisation [SIC]), which eliminates the need for permanent catheterisation.
- Treat the underlying cause (Table 52.1).
- Prescribe a 'fluid chase' and monitor electrolytes.

- Post-obstructive diuresis is a relatively common phenomenon and denotes the significant polyuria that follows relief from obstruction.
- Although often self-limiting it can cause significant complications for the patient if unmanaged, including altered mental state and sometimes substantial haemodynamic instability.
- A 'fluid chase' ensures that the patient's fluid intake is maintained in balance to their urine output.
  - It is essentially IV normal saline given at a rate of 50% for each mL of urine output.
  - It may be easily charted by asking the nursing staff to record hourly urine outputs and to match the IV rate for the next hour at 50% of what was recorded.
  - Ensuring that this simple process is completed (and correctly) can be the difference between a discharge at 48 hours or an ICU stay (or worse) for your patient.

- Trial of void (TOV)
  - After a period of catheterisation (typically around 24 hours) the IDC is removed and the patient attempts to void normally.
  - Measurement of the urine output needs to be closely monitored in combination with the post void bladder volume residual (PVR).
  - Patients who fail to pass significant volumes of urine while maintaining a high residual (>˜500 mL) may not 'pass' their TOV and require further catheterisation.
    - There are no concrete limits on passing or failing a TOV.
    - Take into account the trend throughout the day. Bladder over-distension prevents complete emptying.
  - If the TOV fails and the patient requires IDC re-insertion, they can be discharged home with the catheter for a repeat TOV with a continence nurse in a day surgery setting. Catheter leg bags (Fig. 52.4) can help with patient mobility and urology nurse specialists should be consulted to help with patient education prior to discharge.
  - The patient should have a Urology review to ensure any obstructive cause such as prostatic enlargement can be managed in a timely manner.

Chronic urinary retention

These patients will usually have a history of urinary retention, commonly associated with prostatic disease. Due to recurrent distension they do not experience the same level of discomfort associated with retention, and can be unaware of their retention until bedside bladder scans are performed. In the outpatient setting patients may report a sensation of incomplete voiding or intermittent

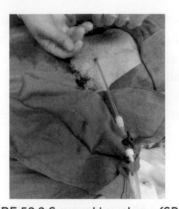

FIGURE 52.3 Suprapubic catheter (SPC).

Reproduced from: Okafor, H.T. & Nsouli, I.S., 2015. Percutaneous bladder catheterization (suprapubic bladder catheterization). Atlas of the Oral and Maxillofacial Surgery Clinics of North America 23(2), 177-181, Fig. 9A.

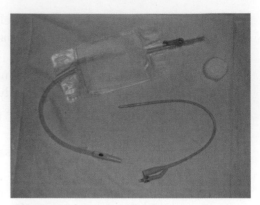

FIGURE 52.4 Urinary catheter leg bag for patients discharged with IDCs.

Reproduced from: Chileshe, C., 2011. Aids to promote urinary continence. European Geriatric Medicine 2(6), 386-390, Fig. 4.

urine stream (lower urinary tract symptoms [LUTS]). Some patients may present with overflow incontinence.

Examination

- Male patients should always undergo a rectal examination to determine prostate size.

Investigations

- Investigation is initiated bedside with a full ward test (FWT) to test for infection and 'bladder scanner' to estimate the volume of urine.
- Note: Although helpful, bladder scanners should not be relied upon for clinical decision making. Suprapubic discomfort and a history of poor or absent voiding should be given more clinical weight than an isolated scanner result.

UROLOGICAL TRAUMA

Urological trauma occurs in up to 5% of all trauma patients.

Renal trauma

Blunt trauma associated with motor vehicle accidents (MVAs) or high energy sporting collisions is the most common presentation. Penetrating trauma is less common, with gunshot wounds accounting for most of these cases.

History should focus on identifying the exact mechanism of injury, particularly the point of impact. Patients may report flank pain, with gross haematuria a feature of high grade injuries, though not entirely reliable. Classification of renal injuries is given in Table 52.2 and Fig. 52.5.

Examination

- Examination of the flanks may reveal tenderness.
- Look for any obvious haematoma.
- FWT is useful to detect microscopic haematuria.

Investigations

- CT scans should be performed in those patients with haematuria or haemodynamic instability with flank pain
- Retrograde pyelogram may demonstrate urinary extravasation and should be completed prior to placement of an IDC if there is any suspicion of lower urinary tract damage.

Management

- Management of renal trauma is described in Table 52.2.
- There has been a push for renal preservation where possible, particularly for paediatric patients.

Bladder trauma

As in renal injuries, blunt external trauma is the most common mechanism. Associated with pelvic fractures (10–30% of cases).

TABLE 52.2 Classification of renal trauma and management

GRADE	DESCRIPTION OF INJURY	MANAGEMENT
Grade I	Subcapsular haematoma, small and non-expanding	Conservative management
Grade II	Renal cortex laceration, without extravasation of urine	
Grade III	Renal medulla laceration, without extravasation of urine	May require surgical exploration and repair
Grade IV	Renal collecting system laceration with extravasation of urine. Can involve vascular injury	Surgical exploration. Vascular injury may need repair
Grade V	'Shattered kidney', which can involve total avulsion of renal hilum	Surgical exploration that may require partial/complete nephrectomy

Barsness, K.A., Bensard, D.D., Partrick, D., et al., 2004. Renovascular injury: an argument for renal preservation. Journal of Trauma 57(2), 310-315.

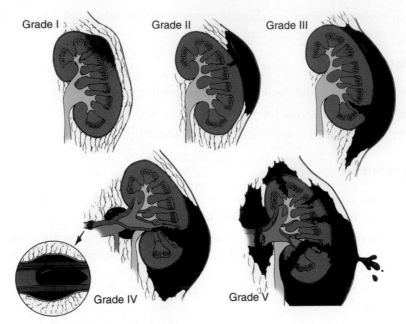

FIGURE 52.5 Classification of renal injuries.

Reproduced from: Santucci, R. & Chen, M., 2016. Chapter 50: Upper urinary tract trauma. In: Wein, A.J., Campbell-Walsh Urology, 11th ed. Elsevier, pp. 1148-1169, Fig. 50.1.

Iatrogenic injuries from abdominal surgery and bladder instrumentation are potential causes and should be excluded during the history. Gross haematuria is particularly common.

Investigations

- FAST scan during the trauma assessment (Chapter 10) may reveal free fluid around the bladder.
- Formal investigations should include CT to determine the classification of bladder injury.
- Contrast can be used through an IDC (cystogram) once lower tract trauma has been ruled out (see above).

Management

- Management of bladder trauma is summarised in Table 52.3.

Testicular trauma

Trauma to the testicle can lead to testicular rupture.

- Patients may present with a bruised hemi-scrotum, swelling, with a palpable collection.
- U/S can help confirm the presence of testicular injury.
- Surgical exploration is indicated where rupture is suspected.

TABLE 52.3 Classifications of bladder injury

GRADE	DESCRIPTION OF INJURY	MANAGEMENT
Contusion	Partial thickness wall injury, associated with blunt trauma	Conservative management with an IDC
Extraperitoneal	Full thickness injuries that do not involve the abdominal cavity	Conservative or surgical repair dependent on the exact nature of injury. Patient can undergo an initial conservative period
Intraperitoneal	Full thickness injury with extravasation of urine into the abdominal cavity (see Fig. 52.6)	Surgical exploration and repair

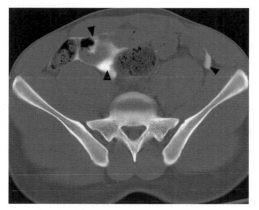

FIGURE 52.6 CT cystogram showing intraperitoneal extravasation of urine.

Reproduced from: Bent, C., Iyngkaran, T., Power, N., et al., 2008. Urological injuries following trauma. Clinical Radiology 63(12), 1361-1371, Fig. 4a.

CYSTOSCOPY AND URETEROSCOPY

Cystoscopy involves passing an endoscopic camera through the urethra to examine the bladder.

Flexible cystoscopy

A short endoscope with flexible tip allows visualisation of the bladder.

- Indications
  - Haematuria, removal of a JJ stent, screening for bladder cancer (Chapter 73).
  - Flexible cystoscopy can be performed for the insertion of indwelling catheters for difficult patients.
  - Can also allow urethral dilatation for patients with stricture.
- Procedure
  - The flexible cystoscope is not much larger than a Foley catheter; therefore only lignocaine gel anaesthetic is required to pass the scope.

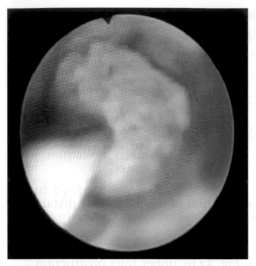

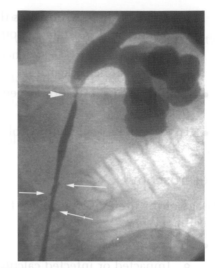

FIGURE 52.9 Ureteroscopy demonstrating a ureteric stone that was removed with a stone extractor.

Reproduced from: Rinaldi, P., Inchingolo, R., Giuliani, M., et al., 2015. Proximal ureteric obstruction caused by glue migration following selective renal artery embolization. Journal of Vascular and Interventional Radiology 26(3), 448-450, Fig. 4.

FIGURE 52.10 Retrograde pyelogram demonstrating ureteric stenosis.

Reproduced from: Zagoria, R.J., Dyer, R., et al., 2016. Chapter 5: The renal sinus, pelvocalyceal system, and ureter. In: Zagoria, R.J., Genitourinary Imaging: The requisites. Elsevier, pp. 146-189, Fig. 5.55.

Investigations

- Plain film can reveal radio-opaque stones (>80%).
- Ultrasound may reveal renal stone disease but is less sensitive than CT; however, US is capable of detecting the complications of calculi, such as hydroureter/hydronephrosis.
- CT kidneys, ureter, bladder (KUB) is the gold standard for measuring and localising stones.
  - Non-contrast scan allows for easy visualisation of calculi.
  - CT can reveal other features such as hydronephrosis (obstruction) and ureteric stranding (infection).
  - As young patients are commonly affected, CT should be used judiciously.
  - The size of the stone dictates the likelihood of spontaneous passing:
    - <5 mm – 70%
    - 5–10 mm – <50%
    - >10 mm – <25%.

Management

- Initial treatment includes analgesia, anti-emetics and IV fluids. Appropriate analgesia should utilise opiates, paracetamol and NSAIDs. PR indomethacin often provides superior relief to other NSAID agents.
- Obstructed stones or patients who display *features of sepsis* may require urgent removal of the stone.
- Stones <5 mm have a good chance of passing, aided by the use of smooth muscle relaxants, i.e. tamsulosin.
- Stones >5 mm should be discussed with the Urology registrar; however, conservative management with medications may still be appropriate if the patient is well and their pain is well controlled without any evidence of renal impairment or obstruction.
- Stones >10 mm have a poor chance of passing and intervention may be required before the stone becomes obstructed.
- Nursing staff and patients should be instructed to filter urine (if possible)
- If a decision for trial of passage is made, patients should be followed up with repeat imaging to ensure clearance.

Surgical management

- Ureteroscopy ± stone extraction or laser ablation if anatomically viable.
  - Stones can be broken up by laser to be extracted in fragments.
- Percutaneous nephrolithotomy (PCNL)
  - Offered to patients with larger calculi (>2 cm, *staghorn*, stones not responsive to lithotripsy).
  - Stone from the kidney is extracted percutaneously over the flank with image guidance (Fig. 52.12).
  - Cases often involve placement of a nephrostomy tube.
- (Extracorporeal) shock wave lithotripsy ([E]SWL)
  - Electrical impulses generate energy waves that fracture calculi.
  - Not particularly useful for large, persistent stones.
- Open stone extraction may be required (rarely) in large, complex calculi that are not amenable to the above approaches.
- Follow-up and recurrence, see Chapter 73.

PROSTATE SURGERY

Transrectal ultrasound (TRUS) biopsy

TRUS biopsies are core biopsies of prostate tissue taken through the rectum.

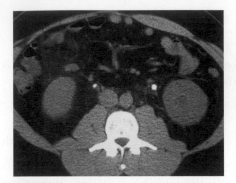

FIGURE 52.11 Bilateral ureteric stones.

Reproduced from: Soto, J., 2011. Ureteral and kidney stones. In: Sahani, D.V. & Samir, A.E., Abdominal Imaging. Maryland Heights, MO: Saunders, pp. 185-189, Fig. 26.5.

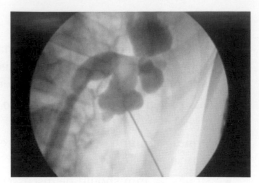

FIGURE 52.12 Intraoperative image of lower calyceal percutaneous access.

Reproduced from: Gamal, W., Moursy, E., Hussein, M., et al., 2015. Supine pediatric percutaneous nephrolithotomy (PCNL). Journal of Pediatric Urology 11(2), 78.e1-5, Fig. 4.

- Indications
  - Enlarged or suspicious lump on PR examination with or without elevated PSA.
  - Follow-up surveillance (Chapter 73).
- Procedure
  - Prior to the procedure the patient should have appropriate antibiotic prophylaxis.
  - The US probe is used to evaluate the size of the prostate.
  - A biopsy needle can be passed through an attachment on the specialised probe.
  - Ideally, 12 cores are taken for pathology in addition to any suspicious lesions.
- Postoperatively patients are discharged home the same day with review in clinic.
- Complications: rectal bleeding, pain, infection (including profound septic shock), prostatitis, urinary infection and retention.
- Follow-up is dictated by biopsy results.
- Transperineal (TP) biopsy is becoming an alternative to obtain core biopsies of the prostate with ongoing research into the infection rates in TRUS vs TP biopsy.

Transurethral resection of prostate (TURP)

- Indications: prostate cancer, benign prostate hyperplasia (Chapter 73).
- Procedure

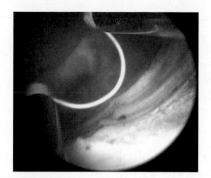

FIGURE 52.13 TURP using the resectoscope.

Reproduced from: Milam, D., 2012. Chapter 71: Transurethral resection of the prostate. In: Smith, J.A., Hinman's Atlas of Urologic Surgery. Saunders, pp. 449-458, Fig. 71.7.

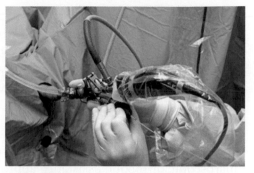

FIGURE 52.14 'Greenlight' photoselective vaporisation of the prostate (PVP).

Reproduced from: Angulo, J.C., Andrés, G., Gimbernat, H., et al., 2015. Laser transurethral resection of the prostate: safety study of a novel system of photoselective vaporization with high power diode laser in prostates larger than 80 ml. Spanish Urology (Actas Urológicas Españolas, English Edition) 39(6), 375-382, Fig. 2.

- Rigid cystoscopy is used to guide the resection scope into the prostate (Fig. 52.13).
- Resection scope is either electrocautery-based (mono/bipolar) or photoselective laser (greenlight) (see Fig. 52.14).
- Ablated prostate is sent for histology.
- Postoperative
  - Patients have IDC inserted post procedure.
  - A continuous bladder washout (CBWO) is used to clear postoperative bleeding; once the output has become clear the patient can undergo a trial of void.
  - When able to pass urine the patient can be discharged.
- Complications
  - Postoperative bleeding.
  - Some ooze is to be expected, though persistent bleeding and failure of CBWO to clear urine may be suggestive of an active bleed with the prostate bed.
  - TUR syndrome, although rare, is significant. It is a result of absorption of hypotonic irrigation fluid from the prostatic venous sinus during resection (especially in longer operations) and can lead to significant electrolyte and fluid derangements, altered mental state and hypertension.

SECTION IV

- Follow-up
  - Patients are typically seen within a few weeks of the procedure to check if symptoms have resolved.
  - Histology is important to determine if the patient requires further discussion at a genitourinary MDM.

Prostatectomy

Prostatectomy is the removal of the prostate and seminal vessels via an open, laparoscopic or robotic assistance approach (see Fig. 52.15).

- Indications: localised prostate cancer.
- Procedure
  - Most commonly a retropubic open approach is used to expose the prostate capsule allowing removal, although perineal approaches are also described.
  - The surgeon may perform the operation as an open, laparoscopic or robot-assisted procedure.
  - The vascular supply and vas are identified and divided.
  - Preservation of the nerves is ideal to conserve sexual function, though not always possible.
  - Reconstruction of the bladder neck and vesiculo-urethral anastomosis with the aid of a Foley catheter is performed (see Fig. 52.16).

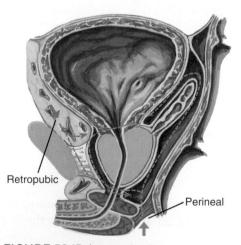

FIGURE 52.15 Approach of prostatectomy with resection margins outlined.

Reproduced from: Tabayoyong, W. & Abouassaly, R., 2014. Chapter 54: Radical prostatectomy. In: Delaney, C., Netter's Surgical Anatomy and Approaches. Saunders, pp. 607-620, Fig. 54.1.

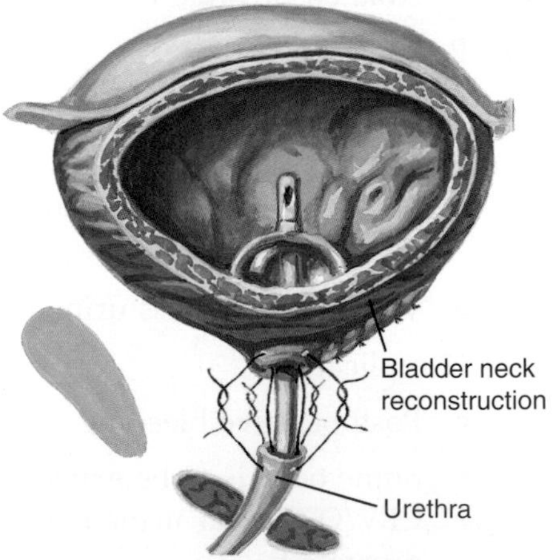

FIGURE 52.16 Vesico-urethral reconstruction with IDC left in situ.

Reproduced from: Tabayoyong, W. & Abouassaly, R., 2014. Chapter 54: Radical prostatectomy. In: Delaney, C., Netter's Surgical Anatomy and Approaches. Saunders, pp. 607-620, Fig. 54.1.

- ○ Often lymph node dissection is also performed.
- ○ Robotic assisted laparoscopic prostatectomy (RALP)
  - – Becoming increasingly popular due to intraoperative vision and precision.
- Postoperative
  - ○ IDC remains for 2 weeks (may vary between hospital protocols) postoperatively, then outpatient TOV.
  - ○ Urological consult should be sought prior to replacement of IDC if the catheter becomes blocked or is inadvertently removed within this period.
- Complications: bleeding from the operative site (check Hb postoperatively), urinary retention (*clots*), loss of sexual function.
- Follow-up: chase pathology for discussion at MDM. Patients should be closely followed up in clinic.

BLADDER SURGERY

Transurethreal resection of bladder tumour (TURBT)

The technique is similar to that for TURP.

- Indications: isolated superficial bladder tumour.
- Procedure
  - ○ Resectoscope used to ablate the urothelial layer of the bladder wall.
  - ○ Continuous bladder wash removes debris, which is collected for histology analysis.
- Postoperative
  - ○ Patients return to the ward with IDC and CBWO.
  - ○ Once washout drainage begins to become clear, washout can be ceased with a TOV soon after when the team is happy the bleeding has subsided.
- Complications: pain, bleeding (clots), infection and retention.
- Follow-up
  - ○ Chase pathology. High grade tumours might require repeat resection or BCG treatment.
  - ○ Cystectomy is considered in refractory cases.

Cystectomy

Cystectomy is surgical removal of the entire bladder. It can be performed as an open or laparoscopic procedure (Fig. 52.17). If the disease involves the prostate, then a cysto-prostatectomy is performed.

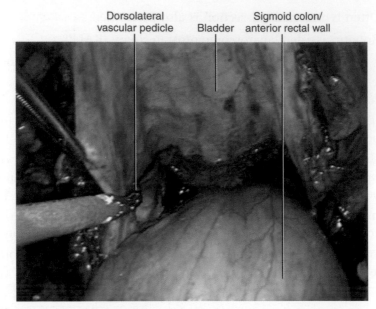

FIGURE 52.17 Laparoscopic cystectomy.

Reproduced from: Chang, S., 2012. Chapter 78: Radical cystectomy. In: Smith, J.A., Hinman's Atlas of Urologic Surgery. Saunders, pp. 501-512, Fig. 78.8A.

The patient requires a form of **urinary diversion** post this radical procedure or complex reconstruction with an orthotopic neobladder to restore excretive passage.

- Indications: invasive bladder cancer, recurrent or incompletely resected superficial bladder tumour.
- Preoperative
  ○ Patient requires extensive cardiorespiratory work-up and anaesthetic review. The patient requires optimal management of medical comorbidities due to the physiological stress of this large operation.
- Procedure
  ○ *Radical cystectomy* involves removal of the seminal vesicles and prostate in males and the uterus, cervix and urethra in females.
  ○ The traditional approach has been via an open laparotomy, though laparoscopic and robotic assisted approaches are used.
  ○ *Partial cystectomy* can be offered to patients with specifically localised disease such as the dome of the bladder.
  ○ Pelvic lymph node dissection is undertaken for complete staging/treatment.
- Urinary diversion/reconstruction
  ○ Once the bladder has been excised, urinary diversion is required, with two common approaches:

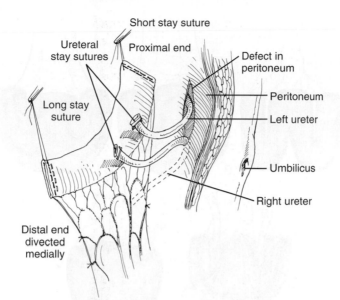

Short stay suture

Ureteral stay sutures

Proximal end

Defect in peritoneum

Peritoneum

Left ureter

Long stay suture

Umbilicus

Right ureter

Distal end divected medially

FIGURE 52.18 Diagram outlining the approach of forming an ileal conduit.
Reproduced from: Scherr, D. & Barocas, D., 2012. Chapter 96: Ileal conduit. In: Smith, J.A., Hinman's Atlas of Urologic Surgery. Saunders, pp. 615-628, Fig. 96.12A.

- Ileal conduit (Fig. 52.18): ureters are anastomosed to a length of separated small bowel that is fashioned into a urostomy (a urine stoma). The patient will require stoma bag coverage as the urostomy is not continent.
- Neo-bladder (Fig. 52.19): an orthotopic (placed anatomically) bladder formed by the reconstruction of bowel (usually ileum but caecum may also be utilised) into a new bladder.
- Ureteric stents and an abdominal drain are left in place.

- Postoperative
  - Patients typically (though not always) have an elective admission to HDU/ICU.
  - Track renal function.
  - Abdominal drain is checked for creatinine to determine if a urine leak is present.
  - Patients should receive education about stoma management.
  - Washout of neo-bladder is performed on ward to remove debris.
    - IDC and SPC are typically used.
    - Though the bladder provides continence, a period of self intermittent catheterisation may be required.
  - Ureteric stents can be removed around 7 days postoperatively.
  - Patients should undergo a cystogram to demonstrate intact anastomosis prior to removal of catheters.

SECTION IV

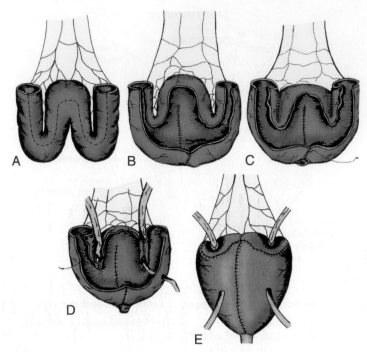

FIGURE 52.19 Diagram outlining the approach of forming an orthotopic neobladder.

Reproduced from: Skinner, E. & Daneshmand, S., 2016. Chapter 99: Orthotopic urinary diversion. In: Wein, A.J., Campbell-Walsh Urology, 11th ed. Elsevier, pp. 2344-2368, Fig. 99.6.

- Complications
    - Death: 30-day mortality rate is 1–2% and 90-day mortality rate is 6–10%. Age compounds this significantly.
    - Anastomotic leak, ileus, collection, bowel obstruction.
    - Stoma complications: necrosis, prolapse.

KIDNEY SURGERY

Nephrectomy

Nephrectomy is removal of the kidney via an open or laparoscopic approach.

- Indications: grade IV/V renal trauma, non-functioning kidney (renal stone disease, recurrent infection, cysts or end-stage renal disease with haematuria/proteinuria), kidney donation, neoplasm.
- *Partial nephrectomy*: sectional excision of renal parenchyma.
    - Small renal cancers (localised) and cysts.
    - Saves more renal tissue for those with decreased function.
    - Often performed laparoscopically; the open approach is decreasingly utilised.

- *Radical nephrectomy*: removal of the kidney with one of: removal of fascia (intact), para-aortic lymph node dissection (RPLND) and/or adrenalectomy.
  - Large tumours or cysts replacing the bulk of the kidney.
  - Tumours with anatomical factors that make partial nephrectomy impractical.
- Preoperative
  - Work-up on renal function including bloods and imaging.
  - MAG-3 nuclear medicine scans use urinary excreted tracers to determine renal function, can give the percentage each kidney provides to renal output.
- Procedure
  - Multiple approaches, including flank (patient in lateral position, most common), anterior (access to larger vessels) and laparoscopic.
  - Lateral approach (Fig. 52.20) may involve 'breaking' the bed to make the flank more prominent.
  - Frozen sections are sometimes used to determine the pathology of the lesion.
  - Tumour may extend into the aorta or vena cava requiring removal and, occasionally, vascular team involvement.
  - *Partial nephrectomy*
    - Mass can be excised as a wedge, or as a 'heminephrectomy' for upper or lower pole tumours.
    - Meticulous haemostasis is required; often a dissolvable sponge-like material (Fig. 52.21) is sutured into the tissue closure. Omental patch flaps are also used.
  - *Radical nephrectomy*
    - The vascular pedicle is ligated to prevent further haematogenous spread.
    - The kidney is removed with an intact Gerota's fascia.
    - Lymph node dissection.
  - *Live donor nephrectomy (LDN)*
    - Commonly performed as a laparoscopic procedure (though some surgeons may use a 'hand-assisted' technique (Fig. 52.22).
    - Donor kidney is retrieved via a lower abdominal incision.
  - Ligation and clipping of the renal vein is illustrated in Fig. 52.23.
- Postoperative
  - Monitor drain tube output as bleeding can be common, especially with partial nephrectomy.

SECTION IV

CHAPTER 53

PRE-ADMISSION CLINIC

Paul Watson

THE PRE-ADMISSION CLINIC

Pre-admission Clinics (PACs) allow review of elective patients who are booked to undergo a complex surgical procedure or those patients with substantial medical comorbidities who require close perioperative management. PAC is coordinated by the theatre liaison nurse for that particular unit, or by dedicated pre-admission nursing staff.

The unit will allocate one of their junior doctors to attend the clinic and review the patient by completing a pre-admission assessment form. The form contains a checklist for clinical information, ordering of investigations and a summary of recommendations including the need for an anaesthetic review. The anaesthetics department run their own PAC, reviewing patients with substantial medical comorbidities or those who will require a specialised anaesthetic or airway approach. In some hospitals the liaison nurse will have already organised an anaesthetics appointment, and the junior doctor will just need to complete the referral section on the PAC form. Timely anaesthetic review allows early identification of medical issues that may otherwise delay procedures and result in cancellations.

The review should encompass a full history and examination of the patient; the classic system review questions (Chapter 11) can provide a good starting point for the new junior doctor. The key is to obtain as much useful clinical information from the patient as possible in combination with correspondence letters from any of the patient's specialists. Luck may be on the junior doctor's side if the patient has had a recent full admission with detailing of the past medical history and a full cardiac and respiratory work-up; however, this may be the first time the patient has been reviewed by any medical staff since they were booked for their procedure.

The junior doctor can also complete other pre-admitting tasks during this appointment such as filling in the patient's regular medications on the drug chart and completing pathology or radiology requests dated for the first post-operative day.

A patient's fitness for a procedure is typically assessed using the American Society of Anaesthesia (ASA) score (Table 53.1).

TABLE 53.1 ASA scoring system for operative risk

CLASS	DESCRIPTION
1	Healthy for age
2	Mild systemic disease
3	Compensated moderate-severe systemic disease that affects level of activity, but not incapacitating
4	Uncompensated disease that is a constant threat to life
5	Critical – unlikely to survive without rapid surgical intervention

Adapted from: Michael, A., Eagland, K., 2012. ASA score in hip fracture patients. European Geriatric Medicine 3 (Suppl 1), S50.

COMPLETING THE PREOPERATIVE ASSESSMENT

Cardiac

- The patient needs to be screened for a past history of:
    - ischaemic heart disease (Chapter 56)
    - cardiac arrhythmias (Chapter 56)
    - angina (Chapter 56)
    - cardiac failure (Chapter 56)
    - valvulopathy (Chapter 56)
    - hypertension (Chapter 56)
    - although these conditions have been previously identified in most patients, a careful history and examination can unearth symptoms suggestive of the above conditions.
- Those patients with a past history of cardiac disease requiring assessment for risk of perioperative cardiac events can undergo stress echocardiography to evaluate potential risk of postoperative ischaemia, which has been shown to demonstrate better risk stratification than ECG alone.
- Patients with mechanical valve replacements will need a carefully considered plan for their anticoagulation medication.
- Patients who have had an acute cardiac ischaemic event in the past 3 months should not have non-emergency surgery.
- Patients who have had recent PCI with bare metal stents should have surgery delayed by at least 6 weeks and ideally 3 months due to increased risk of ischaemic events postoperatively.
- For patients with cardiorespiratory disease, assessing their exercise tolerance in terms of distance or flights of stairs is a useful indicator of functional capacity.

Respiratory

- The patient needs to be screened for a past history of:
  - asthma (Chapter 36)
  - COPD (Chapter 36)
  - PE (Chapter 35)
  - obstructive sleep apnoea.
- All patients who smoke should be counselled on cessation prior to the operation, particularly those patients with established lung disease. Smoking will increase the risk of postoperative respiratory complications and adversely affects wound healing in the longer term. Cessation is recommended at least 4 weeks prior to surgery.
- Patients who are close to their surgery date but are currently unwell with a respiratory tract that presents with persistent cough or sputum production (i.e. infection) should have all nonessential surgery postponed due to the risk of postoperative respiratory complications.
- All patients with chronic lung disease should have a preoperative chest X-ray.

Vascular disease

- Patients at high risk of cerebrovascular events are typically on anticoagulant therapy that will need to be managed (*see below*).
- Patients who are at increased risk of thromboembolic stroke, such as those assessed as a higher CHADS-VASC score (Chapter 35) or who have a carotid bruit on examination, that have not been previously worked up for carotid disease should have a duplex ultrasound and referral for consideration of anticoagulation therapy.

Renal

- Establishing the pattern of a patient's renal function is the key.
- A patient with chronic renal impairment that is stable allows the treating team to understand that the patient is at risk of dehydration and electrolyte disturbances that will need to be carefully managed.
- The patient's blood pressure should be checked to ensure proper control is being achieved with the patient's current medication regimen.
- For younger patients with no history of renal disease, but who present with hypertension, baseline creatinine should be performed to reveal any unsuspected renal impairment.

Endocrine

- Optimal management of diabetes is a key focus of the pre-admission.
- All patients with diabetes should have a recent HbA1c and a full review of any micro- or macrovascular complications.

- ○ History-taking should include how many hypoglycaemic episodes and the frequency.
- ○ Enquire about the patient's daily blood sugar monitoring.

Hepatic disease
- ○ Chronic liver disease has a wide range of effects on the body; three important surgical implications include:
  - – portal hypertension is associated with increased bleeding with major abdominal surgery, and varices make gastric and oesophageal procedures challenging
  - – low albumin production will adversely affect wound healing; in patients who will have decreased oral intake in the perioperative period this can be exacerbated
  - – coagulopathy is common in severe hepatic impairment and has significant implications for surgical mortality if not closely managed; coagulation studies are therefore mandatory in these patients.
- ○ Patients with severe hepatic impairment should have a dedicated outpatient gastroenterology review for perioperative management planning.

Assessment findings need to be clearly documented, with any plans for investigation or other reviews of patients listed in the plan.

PREOPERATIVE INVESTIGATIONS

Routine investigations in the preoperative setting are dependent on the patient's age, medical comorbidities and the type of planned procedure (see Table 53.2). Very few investigations should be considered truly 'routine' and every hospital uses slightly different preoperative investigation guidelines.

Some operations require specific investigations to assist with the technical aspects of the operation. Some of these tests will be organised when the patient is booked from the outpatient clinic; however, it's wise for the junior doctor to check that they have been ordered and that the patient has attended the appointment. Check the notes from the date that the patient was booked for an operation to ensure that there are no outstanding preoperative planning points. Common investigations are discussed in the surgical outpatient chapters and typically include preoperative imaging (such as orthopaedic true size X-rays) or pathology testing.

Anaemia

The preoperative patient who demonstrates anaemia on their blood work should undergo screening for the potential cause (likely iron deficiency) with appropriate treatment in the preoperative setting (Chapter 63). Though the anaemia may not

TABLE 53.2 Suggestions for preoperative investigations

TYPE OF INVESTIGATION[a]	PATIENT <60 YEARS, FIT AND WELL (ROUTINE)	PATIENT >60 YEARS, FIT AND WELL	SPECIFIC INDICATIONS
FBE	Yes	Yes	Routine
UEC	No	Yes	Renal impairment Cardiovascular disease
LFTs	No	Yes	Hepatic disease Upper GI surgery
Coagulation studies	No	Yes	On anticoagulation Hepatic disease
HbA$_{1c}$	No	No (could have fasting glucose as screening)	Established diabetes
Blood group and hold	No	No	For those undergoing large reconstructive, abdominal or cardiovascular surgery
ECG	No	Yes	Cardiovascular disease Abnormal examination findings
CXR	No	No	Patients with respiratory disease Those undergoing thoracic, abdominal or major surgery
Lung function tests	No	No	Patients with respiratory disease Those undergoing thoracic surgery
Echocardiography	No	No	Ischaemic heart disease with no TTE in past 12 months Cardiothoracic surgery

[a]Refer to Chapters 12 and 13.

Thomas, C. & Butler, C., 2011. Chapter 4: The medical vivas, In: Thomas, C. & Butler, C., Examination Anaesthesia, 2nd ed. Sydney: Elsevier Australia.

be symptomatic, the potential blood loss may lower haemoglobin levels further, which could have an adverse effect on a patient with past history of ischaemic heart disease.

Blood transfusion

Patients who are booked for major surgery with a potential for blood loss should be counselled on the indications for perioperative blood transfusions. Most hospitals utilise a specific consent form for blood products that includes an information tear-off sheet for the patient. The discussion regarding blood transfusion should include an explanation of the potential side effects and the need for blood group and hold prior to surgery (Chapter 24).

ANTICOAGULANT THERAPY IN SURGERY

The junior doctor is often required to review a patient's anticoagulant therapy in the pre-admission clinic. It will not always be clear which patients need to cease or change their anticoagulant or antiplatelet therapy in the perioperative period, so speak to your registrar regarding which operations necessitate ceasing antiplatelet medications.

Patients who take warfarin can be put on a therapeutic Clexane® crossover period that involves initiating Clexane therapy while simultaneously discontinuing warfarin. Patients can have their therapy restarted postoperatively with follow-up in the community by HITH to ensure INR is therapeutic before ceasing Clexane crossover. Clopidogrel, the common antiplatelet medication, should be ceased 5 days prior to the operation date.

The more troublesome management issue for the junior doctor involves dual antiplatelets (aspirin and clopidogrel) in patients who have had coronary stenting. Certain elective procedures such as hip and knee arthroplasty have poorer outcomes in the event of postoperative bleeding into the joint and should be delayed until dual antiplatelet therapy can be ceased after:

- a 3-month 'course' for bare metal stents
- a 12-month course following drug-eluting stents.

As there is an increased incidence of in-stent thrombosis for this population group, patients who have ceased antiplatelet therapy (see Box 53.1) should have consideration regarding the location of their procedure, with a recommendation for access to 24-hour PCI services for those patients considered at high risk (see Table 53.3).

These patients should be discussed with their primary cardiologist who can give further insight into the patient's risk of thrombosis and management of their antiplatelet medication (see Table 53.4 for management of NOACs). If not available, discussion with the cardiology registrar on call might be helpful in developing a perioperative management plan for these patients.

BOX 53.1 List of procedures where cessation of antiplatelet medication is recommended

- Spinal
- Intracranial
- Extraocular
- Transurethral resection of the prostate (TURP)
- Major reconstructive surgery
- Orthopaedic arthroplasty

Adapted from: Cardiac Society of Australia and New Zealand, 2009. Guidelines for the management of antiplatelet therapy in patients with coronary stents undergoing non-cardiac surgery. Heart, Lung and Circulation 19(1) 2-10.

TABLE 53.3 Risk factors for coronary stent thrombosis

CLINICAL FACTORS	ANATOMIC FACTORS
• Previous stent thrombosis • Advanced age (>80 years) • ACS indication for stent • Diabetes • Renal impairment • Low ejection fraction	• Left main stenting • Bifurcation stenting • Ostial stenting • Small (<3 mm) stent • Long (>18 mm) stent • Multiple stents

Cardiac Society of Australia and New Zealand, 2009. Guidelines for the management of antiplatelet therapy in patients with coronary stents undergoing non-cardiac surgery. Heart, Lung and Circulation 19(1) 2-10.

TABLE 53.4 Management of novel oral anticoagulants (NOACs) preoperatively

AGENT	PREOPERATIVE INSTRUCTIONS
Rivaroxaban	• Cease 24 hours prior to surgery (if renal function normal) • 48 hours prior if eGFR <50
Apixaban	• Cease 3 days prior to surgery (if renal function normal) • 4 days prior if eGFR <50
Dabigatran	• Cease 3 days prior to surgery (if renal function normal) • 4 days prior if eGFR <50

Cardiac Society of Australia and New Zealand, 2009. Guidelines for the management of antiplatelet therapy in patients with coronary stents undergoing non-cardiac surgery. Heart, Lung and Circulation 19(1) 2-10.

PREOPERATIVE REVIEW REFERRALS

If the patient is to be reviewed by a specialist medical team, a referral will have to be made through the internal hospital process with the request marked as a priority. For patients with surgery in the near future, speaking directly to the liaison nurse who coordinates that clinic may assist in getting the patient a more rapid appointment.

Anaesthetic appointments are normally organised through the PAC staff and will simply require a small written referral outlining the anaesthetic issues with the case (chronic cardiovascular disease, special airway considerations).

The junior doctor should also coordinate with the ICU staff responsible for booking postoperative elective beds for high dependency patients. Those patients having intracranial, major reconstructive or prolonged operations will require careful monitoring and fluid balance postoperatively. Although the bed is 'booked' the availability may change on the day due to increased trauma or emergency demands on the unit, so the team will need to check that the bed is still available on the day of surgery.

CHAPTER 54

INFORMED CONSENT

Paul Watson

WHAT IS INFORMED CONSENT?

Prior to any operation or procedure, patients or their appointed advocates must give their written consent. Patients may only give informed consent if they are deemed 'competent', free from impairment that may affect their judgement or ability to understand information. Otherwise, the next of kin or appointed guardian may give consent for a procedure. Children aged >16 years are able to give consent in Australia.

As part of any informed consent, information regarding the nature of the procedure and possible outcomes will need to be discussed. The Royal College of Australasian Surgeons (RACS) outline discussion points in their position statement on informed consent (see Box 54.1).

CONSENT FORMS

Interns are generally not permitted to complete consent forms with patients; however, residents at PGY2+ experience and higher are commonly expected to 'consent' patients for routine and simple procedures. This can be a daunting task if the patient has significant concerns or questions regarding the proposed intervention. Junior doctors should not complete consent forms with patients when they are unfamiliar with the procedure and expected outcomes.

Hospitals use standardised forms for written consent that must be correctly filled out before the patient may proceed to theatre. The forms differ among hospitals and as such need to be carefully reviewed to ensure the patient and the doctor fill out the correct sections. Some other key points regarding consent forms include the following:

- Clearly specify the site and side for the operation, including writing either LEFT or RIGHT in full as opposed to an abbreviation.
- For elective patients proceeding to theatre, check the consent form to ensure the consent has not expired.
- List the specific complications discussed on the space provided on the form.

CHAPTER 55

MEDICAL OUTPATIENT CLINICS

Joseph M O'Brien

PRINCIPLES OF MEDICAL CLINICS

Medical outpatient clinics are a vital part of the medical system. As you spend more time on the wards you will often begin to notice a common question from the consultant on ward rounds: 'Why is this patient still here?' Many lingering issues are not pressing enough to keep a person in hospital, and can be solved as an outpatient through specialist clinic appointments (common examples include up- and down-titration of medications and reviewing the effectiveness of new therapy at a later point in time). Some patients encountered in outpatient clinics have been referred by GPs or other specialists with a specific issue requiring specialist consideration. Patients who have never been seen in clinic before make excellent practice long cases (but be mindful of the time pressures in clinic).

You will see the management of many chronic illnesses in outpatients – for example, on a Haematology rotation you may not encounter chronic lymphocytic leukaemia on the wards, but will see a lot of these patients being managed in the community. Outpatients helps round out your education as a doctor, involving you in specialist cases you could otherwise miss out on entirely as they are never acute enough to need admission. As a senior student you will be able to watch the specialists monitor the progression of these illnesses, titrate their medications and make further referrals to other specialists for complicated cases.

Another vital role of outpatients is the follow-up of patients who have recently had an inpatient admission. These patients will almost certainly have had changes to their management (or they wouldn't have ended up in hospital), so you need to take a focused history to see how these modifications have made a difference to their condition. Early review clinics bring back recent inpatients in a short period of time – although more common for surgical patients, medical patients who have been discharged from hospital but may still require close attention will be asked to attend these clinics to evaluate their progress. Common examples of specialist early review clinics include 'first seizure clinic' in Neurology and 'endoscopy clinic' for review of pathology from recent scopes on Gastroenterology.

In some clinics, you will have the opportunity to see patients of your own. Typically when helping in clinic you will take the first file off the pile (or go to the next empty room with an appointment slip on the door) to see that patient – take note, no one likes the intern who flicks through to find the easiest cases!

The way you document your interaction will depend on the hospital you are working with – sometimes it is on paper, sometimes digital. Read through the key parts of the previous notes to determine why this patient has come to clinic today. Good sources of information are the most recent (and hopefully completed) discharge summary, operation or endoscopy reports and prior outpatient review notes/letters to their GP from the specialist. Check the pathology and radiology on your hospital's computer to see if they had any bloods or imaging taken prior to this appointment – sometimes discussing these results with a doctor is the only reason the patient is present (e.g. monitoring renal function and symptoms in patients with chronic kidney disease to inform discussions about timing for commencement of dialysis).

You will regularly encounter patients who have not had vital monitoring (bloods or imaging) completed – these can be wasted appointments and, if they can't be completed on the day of their clinic visit, you will need to reschedule them and stress the importance of getting their investigations completed prior to their next appointment. Another common issue is the angry patient. Clinics are typically very busy, and patients are not given an exact appointment time but a 'window' within which they should arrive. These times often slide, and patients and their relatives can get upset, especially when they are without updates in waiting rooms for 2 or more hours. This can be difficult to deal with, but being apologetic and explaining the cause for your delay can sometimes help improve the situation.

Once you feel you understand the patient's case, greet them and lead them into your room (avoid using the overhead speakers for privacy purposes). Explain your role in the team and the purpose of the visit. Many patients will be expecting to see their specialist, and this is not always the case – explain that you are a member of the specialist team, and will discuss their case with the consultant if required (which it often is – if these were simpler issues, there'd be no need for a specialist clinic!).

Even with complex patients, you can reduce the workload on the senior doctors by taking a thorough history, performing a complete physical examination (in particular looking for progression of their illness and complications of their therapy), and being able to report back their salient investigation findings. As a junior doctor or senior student, you should have a plan outlined before you try and contact the consultant or registrar. It is understandable that in some circumstances the issues will be far beyond your level, and no consultant should resent you for that.

Once you've quickly conveyed the history to the consultant (remember, they're in a rush too and will press you for more information if necessary), they will often come in and review the patient with you. If they are happy with your management, they may just ask you to return to the patient, explain the plan to them, and re-book them for another clinic, book them for elective procedures (e.g. scopes) or discharge them from clinic. Don't forget to give your patient any scripts, radiology requests or pathology slips they will need before their next appointment.

Occasionally, you will see a patient in the clinic who is sick enough to require an inpatient admission. In these circumstances, discuss the case immediately with a senior (preferably the consultant who is admitting for that specialty), the bed manager to check the availability of beds and the registrar on ward duty. Many clinics will have admission packs for this situation but, if not, try and cobble together a drug chart, admission note and the pathology and imaging requests you will require.

After clinic, the team has two more jobs. Usually the registrar and the consultant will go through the list of patients who did not attend ('Did not attend' [DNA] or 'Failed to attend' [FTA] as clinic nurses often refer to them) and decide whether they need to be re-booked, or if they should be re-referred by their GP (this has two roles, as it gives the GP an opportunity to discuss the importance of the case with the patient again). It is rare that you would be asked to do this as an intern and, if you are, consider escalating it to your registrar.

Lastly, it is good practice to send a letter to the GP (or other referring doctor) after you have seen a patient in your clinic. This is usually done by dictating a recorded message to the hospital typographers, and using this system can take a bit of adjustment. Like so much of your new job, practice makes perfect and hopefully the typographers will be merciful and adjust your letters to make sense. A good template is:

- three patient identifiers (e.g. name, date of birth and hospital number)
- your own title and name (e.g. Dr Joseph O'Brien, HMO to Dr Gregory House)
- which clinic you are dictating from
- the date of clinic visit and dictation
- the addressee
- any carbon copy recipients and attachments (e.g. for complex patients, to the referring specialist, their GP and any other relevant specialist teams)
- the body of the letter, with the major issues and plan outlined
- a sign off (e.g. 'Thank you for your ongoing management and care')
- your provider number.

This is your only line of communication with the referrer and the GP, so try and be clear and succinct. When dictating, remember that typographers are highly skilled and often have a comprehensive knowledge of medical terms and abbreviations. That said, it is good form to spell out complex medical terms and speak slowly and clearly so your dictation is not the equivalent of a poorly scrawled doctor's note.

CHAPTER 56

CARDIOLOGY OUTPATIENTS

Joseph M O'Brien

Cardiology Outpatients is high turnover, and often streamlined into sub-specialties such as General, Chest Pain (often referred to directly by ED), Electrophysiology/ Pacemaker, Valvulopathy, Risk Reduction (e.g. to assist in management of hypertension and hyperlipidaemia) and Heart Failure Clinics. In some centres they run simultaneously with the Cardiothoracics Clinic to assist in the outpatient work-up of patients with severe problems (e.g. triple vessel coronary artery disease) being planned for surgical intervention.

HYPERTENSION

Hypertension is a silent contributor to cardiovascular disease, described in the literature as the most important modifiable risk factor to cardiovascular disease. It is currently defined as a systolic BP >140 mmHg or diastolic >90 mmHg. However, optimal systolic is <120 mmHg and diastolic <80 mmHg. Stage 2 hypertension is considered systolic >160 mmHg or diastolic >100 mmHg. These figures are not able to be applied generally across all populations however, and for some individuals it may be safe to have pressures higher or lower than the given values.

There is no particular cut-off pressure identified where cardiovascular renal complications begin to occur. Essential hypertension, which accounts for 95% of all hypertensive patients, is hypertension in the absence of renovascular disease, intrinsic renal disease, obstructive sleep apnoea, coarctation of the aorta or endocrine dysfunction (thyroid, aldosteronism, Cushing's, phaechromocytoma).

Patients often query why they need to take medications 'when [they] feel fine'; thus patient education is vital. Hypertension awareness is increasing, but patient compliance is still lagging. Hypertension remains very common, with up to 30% of adults over 20 years being hypertensive. Referrals for refractory hypertension are seemingly randomly divided into Cardiology, Renal and General Medical Clinics.

If asked in clinic to review a patient with hypertension, familiarise yourself with their medical history and see what investigations have already been completed before calling them into the room. Assess their risk factors for hypertension including obesity, insulin resistance/diabetes, high sodium or alcohol intake, a sedentary lifestyle, stress or a low potassium or calcium intake. Ask about previous therapies trialled for their blood pressure and their effects.

Be sure to take the blood pressure yourself (if it has not already been done by the clinic nurse). Compare this with their old records to see what their blood pressure has been like in the past. Remember, you cannot diagnose hypertension from a single reading! Examine them for signs of end-organ hypertensive damage – signs of renal disease, heart failure (particularly left heart failure) and, if feeling particularly keen, ophthalmological changes. If their diastolic is >120 mmHg or you've detected end-organ damage, the patient should be admitted as a 'hypertensive crisis' to exclude life-threatening causes and to treat with parenteral agents.

Basic investigations you can begin with include an FBE and UEC (review for hypernatraemia, hypokalaemia and diminished renal function), fasting lipids and glucose and a 24-hour ambulatory blood pressure monitor (ABPM). Depending on your unit, a renal artery Doppler to review for renal artery stenosis may also be suggested.

ABPM involves a patient wearing a blood pressure cuff and a monitor (about the size of a discman) for 24 or 48 hours, with either 15- or 30-minute interval recordings of blood pressure. They are particularly useful for excluding 'white coat hypertension' (whereby doctor- or measurement-related anxiety briefly increases a person's BP) and detecting intermittent BP changes (e.g. in autonomic dysfunction) and are increasingly becoming the gold standard for diagnosis of hypertension. The following results on ABPM confirm a diagnosis:

1 a 24-hour average of ≥130/80 mmHg

2 diurnal (or waking) average of ≥135/85 mmHg

3 nocturnal (or sleeping) average of ≥120/70 mmHg.

Once the diagnosis has been confirmed, devise a plan for treatment and discuss it with the registrar. Always discuss lifestyle modification in detail – concentrate on weight reduction, increasing exercise, ceasing alcohol and tobacco and reducing sodium intake.

First-line therapy is often a low-dose ACE inhibitor (e.g. perindopril) or an angiotensin-II receptor antagonist (e.g. candesartan), with a calcium channel blocker or hydrochlorothiazide diuretic introduced if necessary. Warn patients (*especially* the elderly) that they may have some orthostatic and post-prandial hypotension in the early course of their treatment and should take care. The right antihypertensive for your patient is the one they actually take – 30–50% of cases respond well. Note beta-blockers (another popular agent) do not appear to provide the same protection against stroke.

The patient should be reviewed either in the clinic or by their GP in 3 months to assess the response to antihypertensive therapy. If hypertension persists, there should be a clear plan for escalation of treatment for the local doctor (e.g. a centrally-acting agent). If the hypertension is truly refractory to medical treatment, other secondary causes of hypertension should be considered.

HYPERLIPIDAEMIA

An elevated serum lipid concentration, or hyperlipidaemia, is known to increase the incidence of cardiovascular disease. The clearest benefit is derived by lowering the low-density lipoprotein cholesterol (LDL, known colloquially as 'bad cholesterol'), with some improvement in rates of cardiovascular disease seen with higher high-density lipoproteins (HDL). If triglycerides are highly elevated, they should also be reduced as a priority to prevent pancreatitis. Similar to hypertension, dyslipidaemia is not diagnosed on a single result and should be confirmed at least 6 weeks later.

When examining your patient, look for external signs of hypercholesterolaemia as well as more widespread signs of cardiovascular illness (xanthomata, xanthelasma, peripheral vascular disease, sternotomy scars, murmurs etc). Ask about their usual diet. Consider secondary causes of hyperlipidaemia, including thyroid dysfunction, cholestatic liver disease, pregnancy, renal disease and certain drugs (e.g. oestrogen, alcohol, aromatase inhibitors, thiazides, steroids, olanzapine and interferon). Particularly important is a family history, both for cholesterol (if known) and cardiovascular events.

First-line management remains lifestyle modification, with a focus on weight reduction and decreased dietary fats. In Australia, PBS restrictions apply to commencing medical therapy for hyperlipidaemia. Patients in the following situations may begin statin therapy:

1 symptomatic coronary artery, cerebrovascular or peripheral artery disease

2 diabetes with microalbuminuria

3 diabetes in Indigenous Australians, or people aged >60 years

4 family history of two first-degree relatives with symptomatic coronary artery disease ≤55 years or one relative symptomatic ≤45 years

5 genetically identified familial hyperlipidaemias

6 males between 35 and 75 years or post-menopausal women with a fasting total cholesterol ≥7.5 mmol/L

7 any patient with a total fasting cholesterol ≥9 mmol/L.

The usual starting dose of atorvastatin is 40 mg PO daily, or 80 mg PO daily post-infarct or stroke. Request LFTs in a fortnight to monitor for liver dysfunction. If statin use is not sufficient (or precluded), consider adding ezetimibe (10 mg PO daily) or a fibrate such as fenofibrate (145 mg PO daily). Ezetimibe has been shown to reduce LDL with or without a statin, but has not been proven to improve mortality.

When starting a statin, consent people to the fact that they may experience muscle pains and should seek GP review. There are no evidence-supported targets for LDL and HDL levels, and instead the intensity of treatment depends on whether the patient is receiving a lipid-lowering agent for primary or secondary prevention.

SECTION V

Investigations should be targeted. All patients at Chest Pain Clinic require an ECG and, depending on the suspicion of coronary artery disease, you may proceed to request blood work (FBE, UEC, troponin, CK, fasting lipids and glucose), CXR, TTE and 'stress testing' ECG or TTE. Some centres may offer CT-coronary angiograms. If the presentation is more typical of a pulmonary embolism, aortic dissection or gastro-oesophageal reflux disease (GORD), request a CT-pulmonary angiogram, CT-aortogram or upper GI endoscopy, respectively.

With multiple cardiovascular risk factors and a history highly suspicious of cardiac chest pain, your registrar may suggest to proceed straight to coronary angiogram. You can help by completing the consent with the patient prior to presenting to the consultant. Risks associated with angiogram include AMI, stroke, arrhythmia, kidney injury, access site haematoma, arterial dissection, excessive bleeding and infection.

CARDIAC TRANSPLANT MONITORING

Very few medical students and junior doctors will have the opportunity to meet patients who have undergone a heart transplant, and they should be thankful for a wonderful and rare learning opportunity. Five centres across Australia and New Zealand perform heart transplants – The Alfred Hospital (Victoria), St Vincent's Hospital (NSW), Prince Charles Hospital (Queensland), Royal Perth Hospital (Western Australia) and Auckland Public Hospital (New Zealand). The half-life of a heart transplant in Australia is 10 years.

If you are considering referring a patient for a transplant, include in your letter:

- the indication – i.e. end-stage heart disease, be it due to cardiogenic shock, refractory heart failure, recurrent and refractory arrhythmias (e.g. as indicated by multiple discharges from an implanted defibrillator) or intractable angina despite maximal medical and interventional therapies
- their age – patients ≥70 years are excluded
- any conditions that could limit the patient's life expectancy to < 5years, including but not limited to malignancy, end-stage disease of another organ system
- any conditions that could prevent the patient's active participation in cardiac rehab postoperatively
- presence of sepsis
- body mass index
- any barriers to compliance with medical therapy
- presence of substance abuse, including alcohol and tobacco.

If you see a transplant patient in clinic, it will likely be a regular review appointment. Ask them about the following:

- What were their preoperative symptoms. Have they resolved? Have they experienced fatigue, chest pain, palpitations, syncope or dyspnoea?

- What is their current effort tolerance, and how does it compare to preoperatively?
- When was their transplant? How regularly do they see their surgeon? How long did they spend in cardiac rehabilitation?
- What is their immunosuppressive regimen?
- Have they experienced any side effects from their medications (e.g. recurrent infections)?
- When was their last echo? What does their current ECG show?

Always discuss these patients with a consultant or registrar before changing any part of their healthcare plan.

- Have they had any presentations for pneumonia? How often do they present to Emergency? Have they ever needed admission to an Intensive Care Unit (ICU), or transfer to a tertiary centre?

- Do they have a personal or family history of asthma, eczema or other atopy (i.e. allergic conditions)?

Your examination should concentrate on the respiratory system, and signs of chronic airways disease. Patients with asthma should have a FEV_1 and FVC recorded each visit. Well-controlled asthma is typified by the following characteristics. Optimal control is associated with decreased rates of hospitalisation and death:

- ability to complete ADLs without interference from symptoms

- diurnal symptoms ≤2 times/week

- need for short-acting beta agonist (SABA) ≤2 times/week

- no nocturnal symptoms, or symptoms on waking up.

All asthmatic patients should have a SABA as a 'PRN' or as-needed reliever. A regular daily preventer (an inhaled corticosteroid, e.g. budesonide 100 mcg inhaled mane) should be commenced when symptoms exceed the description of a well-controlled asthmatic above, and all modifiable risk factors should be corrected (e.g. weight loss, smoking cessation, removal of triggers, medication review).

If the patient experiences symptoms more days than not, or is waking with symptoms more than once weekly, consider escalating the dose of daily inhaled corticosteroid or adding a regular long-acting beta agonist (e.g. salmeterol or indacaterol – a common combination formula is marketed as Symbicort® and contains 200 mcg budesonide and 6 mcg formoterol). These combination inhalers can be further escalated if necessary but, if a patient continues to have breakthrough symptoms, they should be seen by a specialist.

When a patient is started on an inhaler for the first time, try to facilitate a review with a pharmacist to help optimise their technique with a spacer. Consider down-titrating medications in patients with a period of ≥3 months optimal control to minimise the risk of side effects (e.g. cataracts, osteoporosis and reduced growth).

CHRONIC OBSTRUCTIVE PULMONARY DISEASE (COPD)

For the management of exacerbations of COPD requiring admission, please refer to the inpatient Respiratory chapter (Chapter 36).

COPD (sometimes annotated as chronic obstructive airways disease or 'COAD') is a very common (and preventable) respiratory disease characterised by airway limitation, symptom progression and chronicity of symptoms. COPD is an umbrella term that incorporates emphysema, chronic obstructive asthma and chronic bronchitis. COPD is responsible for a large number of hospital admissions, particularly in colder months. COPD is diagnosed on RFTs, with a post-bronchodilator FEV_1/FVC ratio of <0.70. Questions to consider for COPD patients include:

- When were they diagnosed with COPD? How was the diagnosis made? Was it confirmed with formal RFTs? Do they have a respiratory physician?

- Do they have a chronic cough? How often does it produce sputum? What is their effort tolerance on flat ground (in metres)? Have they had any symptoms suggestive of malignancy (e.g. weight loss >10% lean body mass in 3 months, fevers, rigors or anorexia)? If the patient is a new referral, try to exclude other differential diagnoses (e.g. congestive cardiac failure, bronchiectasis, asthma and tuberculosis).

- Have they ever been to pulmonary rehabilitation? There is good evidence for referral to pulmonary rehabilitation when patients experience dyspnoea when walking at their own pace on flat ground.

- What is their current medication regimen? Review for medications that can make airways disease worse, including aspirin, NSAIDs and beta-blockers. How often do they require breakthrough inhalers?

- Do they have home (a.k.a. domiciliary) supplemental oxygen? Has this been considered in the past?

- How often do they experience an infective exacerbation of their disease? Have they ever been admitted to hospital or ICU with an exacerbation before?

- Take a personal and passive smoking history. Enquire about their current and past occupations – have they been exposed to aerosols, dusts, asbestos and/or other fibres, smoke or gas and fumes? Outdoor air pollution, particularly in developing countries, is associated with an increased prevalence of COPD.

- Do they have a family history of lung disease or malignancy? If a patient is presenting with symptoms suggestive of advanced COPD at a young age, consider a serum alpha-1 anti-trypsin.

- Are their vaccinations up to date (i.e. Fluvax® annually and Pneumovax® every 5 years)? If not, try and arrange them with their local doctor.

- Have they had other screening tests completed? Those relevant for prognostication of COPD include a bone mineral density (BMD), 6-minute walk test (6MW) and arterial blood gases (ABGs) demonstrating hypercapnia.

Your examination should focus on the respiratory system, and excluding signs of concomitant illnesses (e.g. congestive cardiac failure, infection or malignancy). Similarly to asthma, consider documenting FVC, FEV_1 and DLCO on each outpatient appointment.

Due to the fact many patients developed COPD from tobacco smoking, enquire about constitutional symptoms and consider requesting a low-dose CT-chest to screen for malignancy. At the time of publishing, this had an adequate evidence base but had not yet entered Australian guidelines.

The COPD-X Australian and New Zealand guidelines suggest a step-wise escalation of therapy. Initially, patients with mild COPD (i.e. FEV_1 of 60–80% predicted) should be counselled about non-pharmaceutical management – i.e., cessation of smoking (with or without chemical assistance with nicotine replacement therapy), encouraging regular exercise, opportunistic vaccinations, nutritional optimisation and development of a GP management plan for exacerbations to prevent hospitalisation. It is vital to stress compliance with COPD medications – many patients are not aware they should take their preventers when well.

A SABA is typically commenced on diagnosis. Once the patient has progressed to moderate COPD (FEV_1 40–59% predicted) consider referral to pulmonary rehabilitation and escalating their pharmaceutical management to include a long-acting muscarinic agonist (LAMA) (e.g. tiotropium 18 mcg inhaled mane). LAMAs have been shown to prevent hospitalisation when used appropriately.

When the patient's COPD progresses further (i.e. <50% predicted FEV_1) commence inhaled corticosteroids and a LABA (e.g. Symbicort, outlined above, or Seretide®, which contains fluticasone and salmeterol). At this stage of illness, it is appropriate to discuss the need for home oxygen, surgical management (e.g. if criteria are met, lung reduction surgery or even transplant) and advanced care planning. With severe COPD (FEV_1 <40%) consider a low-dose theophylline (e.g. 100 mcg).

CYSTIC FIBROSIS

Cystic fibrosis (CF) is an autosomal recessive inherited disorder of complex chloride channels, resulting in dysfunctional transport of sodium, chloride and bicarbonate ions. It is the most common single-gene disease seen in Caucasian populations. Most CF is a result of a mutation in delta-F508, although other mutations exist.

Pulmonary disease is the most common presentation, but CF may also manifest as gastrointestinal, endocrine and gonadal dysfunction. For diagnosis, a patient must have two of the following clinical features:

- presence of typical clinical features
- a family history of a sibling with CF
- a positive newborn screening test.

in addition to one of the following laboratory features suggestive of dysfunction in the CF transmembrane regulator (CFTR) protein, responsible for sodium and chloride ion transportation:

- two elevated sweat chloride concentrations obtained on separate days
- CF mutations identified on genetic testing
- abnormal nasal potential difference.

Australian-born children are screened at birth, which has reduced the number of delayed diagnoses of cystic fibrosis. However, it is very occasionally diagnosed in adulthood when patients present with chronic respiratory infections, infertility or chronic sinusitis. Most cystic fibrosis patients have a good understanding of their illness and will be excellent historians. When reviewing a patient with cystic fibrosis, discuss:

- Were they diagnosed at birth? If so, which lab evidence was used to confirm the diagnosis (usually the sweat test)?

- Who is their respiratory physician? Most CF patients will have a paediatrician until age 18, when they transfer to an adult chest physician. They are typically reviewed quarterly.

- How often are they experiencing infective exacerbations? Do they experience chronic cough? Are they dyspnoeic? How often are they producing sputum, and what colour is it? Do they have haemoptysis? Are they wheezy? What is their current effort tolerance? Are they experiencing sinus symptoms (sinus pain, headaches, nasal congestion and pressure)?

- Do they have the results of their most recent RFTs? These should be performed quarterly, with a minimum of spirometry on each clinic visit. FEV_1 tends to decline on average at 2% per annum.

- How has their weight been changing? CF patients often suffer from malnutrition due to reduced caloric absorption. Are they seeing a nutritionist? How often do they pass a bowel motion – is it formed? Are they malodorous, do they contain oil or are they hard to flush (i.e. suggestive of steatorrhoea due to chronic pancreatitis)? What are their diet and appetite like?

- Have they been monitored for diabetes? Have they had polyuria, polydipsia, weight change or increasing fatigue? Pancreatic exocrine dysfunction is a classic feature of cystic fibrosis, with 20% of patients also experiencing pancreatic endocrine issues. Patients with cystic fibrosis-related diabetes mellitus should commence insulin and be reviewed by a diabetes educator.

- Have they experienced ascites, jaundice, melaena, haematochezia, abdominal pain or pruritus? Liver involvement is not uncommon in cystic fibrosis patients.

- Do any of their siblings have CF? Did their parents? Have they had trouble beginning a family? Are they planning on doing so in the future? Up to 98% of males with CF will be infertile, with the exact rates of infertility in women less well known but thought to be ˜20%. Female CF patients considering children should be counselled on the high incidence of spontaneous abortion, prematurity and maternal death. If a patient in clinic wishes to discuss fertility, they should be referred to a Genetics Clinic and/or an obstetrician with appropriate training.

- Have they had any fractures? Do they have regular osteoporosis screening?

- How is their mood? How do they feel they are coping with their illness? How does it affect their day-to-day life? Depression is common in patients with chronic disease, and cystic fibrosis is no exception (particularly as it impacts fertility and life expectancy). As patients enter adolescence and adulthood they should be screened for psychosocial issues and referred on if appropriate.

- What is their current medication regimen? Are they on enzymes with meals to assist nutrient absorption? Do they require regular aperients or prokinetic agents? Are they on prophylactic, weekly macrolide antibiotics? Are they on fat-soluble vitamin (i.e. K, A, D and E) replacement? Do they need a proton pump inhibitor for their reflux? Are they compliant with regular chest physiotherapy?

- Are they on the transplant list? If not, is it something they wish to pursue? CF does not recur in transplanted lungs, and 5-year post-transplant survival is 68%. See the section below for questions to ask transplant recipients.

- Are they aware of the Cystic Fibrosis Federation? If not, offer to put them in touch as they offer advocacy and peer support for both patients and their families.

- If a patient's illness is progressing – do they have an advanced care plan? The life expectancy of CF patients is currently 40 years.

Examination of patients with cystic fibrosis is broader than simply examining the respiratory system. Although clubbing, wheeze, crackles, chest inflation, respiratory rate, presence of nasal polyps and oxygen saturation are all very important, do not forget that cystic fibrosis affects almost every body system. Note cachexia, signs of chronic liver disease, diabetes, organomegaly, gastrointestinal abnormalities and cardiac illness (especially right ventricular failure from pulmonary hypertension). The patient should have a formal body mass index (BMI) evaluated on every visit, with the results tracked in comparison with previous measurements.

If possible, ask the patient to produce a sputum sample for culture on each clinic appointment to determine the choice of antibiotic agent if they were to experience a pulmonary exacerbation, and to retain a patient's eligibility on the transplant list as patients with *Burkholderia* may be excluded at some centres. The 'standard' progression of respiratory flora in CF patients ranges from *Staphylococcus* spp., to *Pseudomonas aeruginosa* colonisation, to *Burkholderia* and, eventually, opportunistic organisms such as *Mycobacterium avium* complex (MAC).

Chest X-rays are typically updated annually, or more regularly if the patient has been hospitalised. Patients should have an oral glucose tolerance test (OGTT) every year. CF patients should also have regular FBEs, UECs and LFTs. If an abnormality is detected on LFTs (e.g. low albumin or abnormal enzymes), an abdominal ultrasound should be considered.

BRONCHIECTASIS

Bronchiectasis is a syndrome involving the abnormal dilatation and breakdown of bronchial walls, manifesting clinically as chronic cough and daily sputum expectoration. Its aetiology is varied (see Table 57.1), including congenital and acquired causes, but in all cases there is disturbance in either the drainage of respiratory secretions, host defence or ability to ventilate thoroughly (in an obstructive pattern). It is more common in women, the elderly and the immuno-compromised. Bronchiectasis requires an infective insult.

TABLE 57.1 Selected causes of bronchiectasis

CAUSE	EXAMPLES	INVESTIGATIONS FOR DIAGNOSIS
Congenital anatomical defects	Bronchomalacia	CXR, bronchoscopy
Foreign body aspiration	Food, inhaled objects	CXR, bronchoscopy
Lymphadenopathy	May be due to sarcoid, TB or malignancy	CXR, bronchoscopy ± serum ACE ± QFG
COPD	–	RFTs, CXR
Connective tissue disease	Rheumatoid arthritis, lupus	RF, anti dsDNA, ANA
Immunodeficiency states	IgG or IgA deficiency, leucocyte dysfunction	Serum immunoglobulins with subclass, FBE
Abnormal secretion clearance	CF, other rare illnesses	Sweat test, genetic testing
Alpha-1 anti-trypsin deficiency	–	Serum alpha-1 anti-trypsin, CXR
Aspiration pneumonia	Delirium, alcohol, neurological conditions, any cause of decreased mental state	CXR
Inflammatory bowel disease	Crohn's, ulcerative colitis	Endoscopy with biopsy
Bacterial infections	*Staphylococcus, Klebsiella, Pseudomonas*	Sputum culture + CXR
Viral infections	Adenovirus, influenza, HSV	Nasopharyngeal airway swab for respiratory multiplex PCR, viral serology

Adapted from: Evaluation of bronchiectasis, 2016. In: UpToDate [Internet]. <http://www.uptodate.com/contents/image?imageKey=PULM%2F56821~PULM%2F69598~PULM%2F81561&topicKey=PULM%2F1444&rank=1~150&source=see_link&search=bronchiectasis&utdPopup=true>.

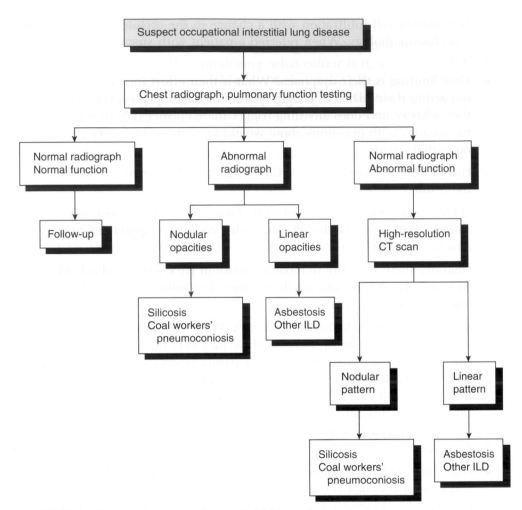

FIGURE 57.1 Diagnostic pathway for interstitial lung disease.

Reproduced from: Goldman, L. & Ausiello, D., 2008. In: Goldman, L. & Ausiello, D., eds., Goldman's Cecil Textbook of Medicine, 23rd ed., Philadelphia: Saunders.

bronchiectasis') or healed varicella pneumonia (diffuse, calcified and nodular interstitial opacites).

Fig. 57.1 shows the standard diagnostic pathway for ILD.

If a patient has never had an echocardiogram before, consider a transthoracic study to exclude pulmonary hypertension. Some consultants request a PET scan; however, there are no current guidelines suggesting this without evidence of disease progression or suspicion of malignancy. RFTs should be completed, with a restrictive pattern and reduced diffusing capacity of the lungs for carbon monoxide (DLCO) expected.

With careful patient selection, a bronchoscopy with bronchoalveolar lavage (BAL) and transbronchial biopsy may be useful for tissue diagnosis. Biochemistry should include FBE (reviewed for anaemia, polycythaemia, leucocytosis and thrombocytopenia), UEC (for baseline renal function), LFT, CK (for myositis), ANA, rheumatoid factor, ANCA and anti-topoisomerase (anti-Scl70). If ANA is positive, consider anti-dsDNA and extractible nuclear antigen antibodies (ENA).

The majority of cases of ILD are managed with oral steroids, dependent on their severity. Your role in clinic will be to identify patients who are experiencing regular decompensation of their illness, appear to be progressing or have optimal control of their disease, as these are the people who will most benefit from titration of their medication. Some may benefit from prophylactic antibiotics, such as a low dose of doxycycline (e.g. 50 mg PO daily). Medication changes should be discussed with the consultant or registrar. Patients with ILD are typically reviewed quarterly to twice per year, with HRCT-chests and RFTs regularly.

OBSTRUCTIVE SLEEP APNOEA

Obstructive sleep apnoea (OSA) is disordered breathing during sleep due to narrowing of the upper airway, be it due to the increasing peripharyngeal fat in obesity (big person), retrognathia (anatomical defect of the maxilla or mandible), adenotonsillar hypertrophy (big tonsils), macroglossia (big tongue) or neuromuscular weakness. The tongue, soft palate and pharyngeal walls are relaxed leading to a mechanical obstruction of the airway.

Apnoea is a complete cessation of breathing for >10 seconds, and hypopnoea is defined as a ≥50% reduction in airflow for >10 seconds. People at highest risk of OSA are men between 40 and 60 years who are obese and consume alcohol. Your history should cover:

- How many times do they wake during the night? Is their sleep refreshing? Are they experiencing daytime drowsiness (somnolence)? Are they having difficulty concentrating? Are they generally fatigued? Does their partner report loud or frequent snoring, or restlessness in bed? See Table 57.2 for the Epworth sleepiness scale, used to describe a patient's sleepiness. A score of ≥10 is considered excessive somnolence.

- Have they gained weight recently? Do they wake with a headache? Ask about mood and personality changes (collateral here can be useful). As OSA is an independent risk factor for cardiovascular health, screen for symptoms of cardiovascular illness.

- Take a brief medical, past and family history.

- Take a thorough medication history, concentrating on muscle relaxants and sedative agents.

- What is their occupation? Are their symptoms impacting upon their ADLs? A diagnosis of OSA has implications for people's occupations and ability to drive safely.

- Quantify their alcohol and tobacco consumption, and ask if it has changed recently. Ask about illicit drug use if relevant.

TABLE 57.2 Epworth sleepiness scale

ACTIVITY	SELF-REPORTED SCORE (0–3)
Sitting and reading	
Watching TV	
Sitting in public but inactive	
Passenger in a car >1 hour	
Lying to rest in the afternoon	
Sitting and talking to someone	
Sitting after lunch (without alcohol)	
In a car, stopped for a few minutes in traffic	

Adapted from: Johns, M.W., 1991. A new method for measuring daytime sleepiness: the Epworth sleepiness scale. Sleep 14(6), 540-545.

Physical examination in OSA is often unremarkable apart from obesity, but review for hypertension, narrowing of the upper airway and signs of pulmonary hypertension. The gold standard for diagnosis remains nocturnal polysomnography (i.e. a sleep study), with patients monitored for heart rate, oxygen saturation and respiratory rate in a special bedroom often containing infrared camera technology. Technicians take note regularly of the above observations in combination with the patient's position and quantity/quality of snoring. The key parameter is the apnoea–hypopnoea index (AHI), determined by the total number of apnoeic episodes divided by total sleep time. An AHI >5 is consistent with OSA, with >30 signifying severe disease.

Additional investigations to exclude other causes of symptoms include an ABG (obesity–hypoventilation syndrome or hypercapnoea), thyroid-stimulating hormone (hypothyroidism), FBE (anaemia), fasting glucose (due to the overlay with diabetes), ECG (cardiac illness), CXR (primary lung pathology) and possibly RFTs.

The first-line management of OSA is patient education and lifestyle modification, with increased exercise and weight loss advised. Patients should avoid caffeine and alcohol to improve the quality of their sleep. They should aim to limit activities in bed to sleep and sex, to maintain good 'sleep hygiene.' Sleeping in the prone position may also reduce obstruction. If these measures fail, continuous positive airway pressure (CPAP) is the mainstay of therapy. CPAP is set up initially by a respiratory physician and often maintained by chest physiotherapists or OTs.

Patients are unfortunately often non-compliant with the device as they can be quite noisy. Oral appliances, such as mandibular repositioning devices, may be trialled in mild-to-moderate OSA. Surgical management is indicated in a select group of patients with documented anatomical pathology. There are driving implications that come with a diagnosis of OSA – you should discuss these with a registrar or consultant as they vary from state to state.

LUNG TRANSPLANT MONITORING

Lung transplant recipients are usually only seen at four specialist centres around Australia and New Zealand, with transplants performed at The Alfred (Victoria), St Vincent's Hospital (NSW), Prince Charles Hospital (Queensland) and Royal Perth Hospital (WA). There is a complex protocol for determining who receives the next available donor lung, available from the Transplant Society of Australia and New Zealand's website. If referring a patient for consideration, include in your letter:

- Patient's demographics details, including age and gender. Candidates are eligible if aged between 5 and 65 years. A patient's height, weight and ethnicity are important with implications for donor lung volume.
- Patient's diagnosis, past treatment and current condition (with objective measurements such as HRCT, CXR and RFTs). Attach their full medical history.
- Patient's willingness to participate in ongoing medical care.
- Patient's social history with exposure to tobacco, marijuana and occupational irritants.
- A recent ABG, blood group, HLA typing, CXR *with lung field measurements*, bronchoscopy report (if performed) and viral serology.

Patients may be excluded for chronic and incurable infections, age >65 years, substance addiction, active malignancy and irreversible significant dysfunction of another bodily system (except the heart). When reviewing a lung transplant recipient in clinic, ask about:

- Which lung was donated? Did they receive a bilateral or unilateral transplant? Was their heart also transplanted?
- What respiratory symptoms are still present? How did they improve after the transplant? Did they experience an improvement in effort tolerance? Did they complete rehabilitation?
- What is their current immunosuppressant and other medication regimen?
- Who is their surgeon? When is their next review?
- Have they experienced any complications or infections since their transplant?
- What is their mood like? Screening for depression is advised.

Be wary with lung transplant patients – they can teach you a lot about a complex area of medicine, but their health care is a delicate balance. They should ideally be reviewed by an advanced trainee or consultant.

SECTION V

CHAPTER 58

GASTROENTEROLOGY OUTPATIENTS

Joseph M O'Brien

Gastroenterology Outpatients tends to be particularly busy. The majority of the patients you will see in smaller hospitals will be relatively straightforward, with the most common referrals being for endoscopy, opinions on deranged liver function tests (LFTs) or advice on the management of chronic liver disease. Before attending a 'Gastro' clinic you should either learn or have a copy of the guidelines for repeat scopes as this will help you approach your registrar or consultant with a solid plan.

PREPARATION FOR ENDOSCOPY

Both gastroscopy and colonoscopy are minimally invasive procedures; however, a patient still has to have a minimum physiological reserve to tolerate the sedation. Confirm with your parent hospital what their policy regarding interns consenting for gastroscopy and colonoscopy is – many hospitals will permit it, but some have documents stating you can only consent for procedures you can complete yourself. A double-balloon enteroscopy (DBE) for the small bowel should be consented by a registrar or a consultant.

While you are alone with the patient, explain the indication for the procedure. Common examples include altered bowel habit, unexplained weight loss, cryptogenic iron deficiency anaemia, positive faecal occult blood tests (FOBT), oesophageal dysmotility, early satiety with abdominal pain, characterisation of lesions identified on imaging, screening endoscopy (e.g. strong family history) or follow-up to previous endoscopy. See Table 58.1 for a more extensive list of indications. Consider the contraindications for the procedure and how they apply to the patient in front of you – will this change management? Do they have a known or suspected perforated viscus? What is their baseline level of function?

Outline the method of the procedure with the patient, from preparation to after-care. Explain that they are usually day cases (some frail patients may be brought in the night before for monitoring with bowel preparation), where they arrive to a Day Procedures Unit the morning of the endoscopy. Typically for

TABLE 58.1 Indications for endoscopy

GASTROSCOPY	COLONOSCOPY	BOTH
• Upper abdominal symptoms suggestive of malignancy (e.g. anorexia, weight loss) in a patient >45 years • Dysphagia, odynophagia • Melaena • Refractory reflux • Persistent vomiting without cause • Upper GI obstruction • Tissue confirmation of suspected malignancy, IBD or ulcer disease • To place a PEG tube • Assessing injury with caustic poison ingestion • EMR • Variceal banding • Management of bleeding lesions (e.g. portal hypertensive enteropathy or peptic ulcer disease) • Monitoring of Barrett's oesophagus	• Haematochezia • Lower abdominal symptoms and symptoms suggestive of malignancy in a patient >45 years • Abnormalities on barium enema • Malaena in the absence of an upper GI cause • Positive FOBT • Screening and surveillance for malignancy • 3–5-yearly after polypectomy • Second-yearly after age 25 years with family history of hereditary non-polyposis colorectal cancer with annual scopes >40 years • Monitoring for malignancy in ulcerative and Crohn's colitis 8 years after diagnosis • Annual scopes for UC with PSC, stricture, active disease, disease in >33% of their colon, or FHx of colon Ca <50 years • Clinically significant and unexplained diarrhoea • Polypectomy • Marking nondescript lesions for surgical excision	• Mixture of abdominal and bowel symptoms • Tissue confirmation of lesions identified on imaging • Familial polyposis syndromes • Removal of foreign bodies • Variceal monitoring (oesophageal and rectal) • Dilatation of stenosis • Palliative treatment of bleeding lesions • Investigation of iron deficiency anaemia

continued

SECTION V

TABLE 58.1 Indications for endoscopy—cont'd

GASTROSCOPY	COLONOSCOPY	BOTH
	• 5 years post-scope with 1–2 small (<10 mm) tubular adenomas, positive FOBT with no lesion found • 3-yearly for high-grade, tubulovillous, or multiple (≥3) adenomas • 12 months post-scope for multiple adenomas, or post-low grade dysplasia in IBD • 6 and 12 months post-scope after removal of sessile or large adenomas, or if polyps were found in someone with a known familial polyposis • 3 to 6 months post-surgical resection of colon cancer. If clear, then in 5 years	

Adapted from: Brown, G., 2012. Alfred Health referral guidelines: endoscopy. Melbourne: Alfred Health. <http://www.alfredhealth.org.au/Assets/Files/GP_Referral_Endoscopy.pdf>. National Health and Medical Research Council (NHMRC), 2011. Clinical practice guidelines for surveillance colonoscopy – in adenoma follow-up; following curative resection of colorectal cancer; and for cancer surveillance in inflammatory bowel disease. Canberra: NMMRC. <http://wiki.cancer.org.au/australiawiki/images/f/fe/Colonoscopy_Surveillance_Guidelines_FINAL_version_approved_Dec2011-boomarked2.pdf>.

gastroscopy they have been fasted for a minimum of 6 hours (longer is preferable; they are often fasted from midnight the night before).

A standard preparation regimen for a colonoscopy would be to limit the patient to clear fluids from after their evening meal 2 days before the scheduled scope, fasting completely from midnight the night prior. If a patient is otherwise well, they can have one sachet of bowel preparation (e.g. sodium picosulfate with magnesium and citric acid, sold as PicoPrep®) at 2 p.m. the day before their scope, with a second sachet at 6 p.m. the same day.

Optionally, if their bowels are still not clear at 6 a.m. the day of their procedure, they may have a third PicoPrep. Advise them to keep up their fluid intake (especially warm liquids), to avoid nuts and high-fibre foods, and that some cramping and vomiting is not unexpected but, if it persists, they should present to the hospital's Emergency Department. There is some variation in this protocol from unit to unit. Often there are handouts you can give to your patient to assist them in remembering their regimen. Patients are never keen for bowel preparation (would you be?), and the handout can help to explain it is vital, and an unclear endoscopy is a *wasted procedure* as lesions may be missed and they will usually be abandoned by the endoscopist.

Explain the procedure itself – how a 'camera with special tools attached' is passed either to the first part of the small bowel (gastroscopy) or up the 'back passage' to the junction of the large and small bowels. Any bleeding identified can be cauterised, and lesions discovered can be sampled with the tools at the end of the scope. Larger lesions may need a further surgical procedure for removal.

Convey that results are usually returned from Pathology within a week or two and they will need to return to Outpatients at this point. They will need someone to collect them from hospital after their procedure.

Explain the risks of the procedure – bleeding, infection, anaesthetic complications, lack of diagnosis, damage to underlying structures and perforation. The rate of perforation in endoscopy is operator-dependent, but usually stated as 1 in 2500 to 1 in 11,000. Patients may find it comforting to know that this is an air sufflation injury from inflating hollow viscus, and usually not because the endoscopist is too rough (i.e. mechanical injury)! It is thought to be less frequent with carbon dioxide sufflation when compared with air sufflation; however, solid data to confirm this hypothesis are still not available. After you have done this, the consultant or registrar will review the patient with you and answer any further questions.

Periendoscopy medication management

Deciding which medications to withhold and cease during preparation for endoscopy is often a confusing task for junior doctors, and to further complicate matters management varies from operator to operator. Note that many hospital departments *have their own protocol* for these medications in the periendoscopic period. Alpha-2 agonists, beta-blockers, calcium channel blockers, digoxin, H_2 antagonists, glucocorticoids and metformin can be continued. ACE inhibitors, sulfonylureas and NSAIDs can be withheld while fasting. Aspirin can usually be continued, unless it is a high-risk procedure (in which case they should be ceased 5–7 days prior). For high-risk procedures, clopidogrel or ticagrelor should be stopped at least 5 days prior. (Polypectomies, DBE and sphincterotomies are counted as high-risk procedures for bleeding). Anticoagulants and insulin therapy are outlined below – these patients may require an inpatient management to manage their preparation. The patient's other usual medications may be taken with sips without 'breaking their fast.'

Anticoagulants and endoscopy

In addition to warfarin, the novel oral anticoagulants (i.e. NOACs, including dabigatran, apixaban and rivaroxaban) are now in widespread use. These agents understandably increase the incidence of bleeding and reduce the ability to control perioperative blood loss. Careful consideration should be given as to the indication for anticoagulation and the complications of temporarily withholding it – do the benefits of the endoscopy outweigh the risks? Patients on anticoagulants for secondary prevention are usually safe to withhold for a few days prior to endoscopy to allow the INR to return to <1.5. As they are not currently chemically reversible, the NOACs should be withheld for a minimum of 48 hours for non-urgent, high-risk procedures.

Patients anticoagulated for mechanical heart valves (especially mitral valves, as they sit across a higher pressure gradient) or antiphospholipid syndrome should have bridging anticoagulation with a low molecular weight heparin, and will thus usually require admission for administration of this agent. You should *always* speak to your consultant or registrar before stopping someone's anticoagulation in the lead-up to a procedure. These medications can usually be recommenced the day after an endoscopy.

Insulin therapy and endoscopy

The aim with insulin-dependent diabetics in the periendoscopy period is to assist them in maintaining euglycaemia to prevent adverse outcomes. Patients with brittle diabetes should have the need and immediacy for their procedure reconsidered. If a patient needs an urgent endoscopy and has very difficult to control diabetes, you should consider an inpatient admission with preoperative anaesthetics review for consideration of a glucose/insulin infusion. It should be noted on all consent and booking forms if a patient is an insulin-dependent diabetic, so Inpatient Bookings can do their best to ensure they are on a morning list. If this is not possible, however, there are still simple strategies for adjusting a patient's insulin regimen on the day of the procedure and while fasting.

During bowel preparation, an insulin-dependent diabetic also on oral antihyperglycaemic therapy should have their oral medications withheld and should take half their usual short-acting insulin doses and one-third of their usual long-acting dose. Mixtures of long- and short-acting insulins can be halved. They should check their blood sugars regularly during the fasting period and consume a glucose-rich beverage if their BSL is <5.0 mmol/L. A patient's usual insulin dose should be halved the morning of their scope, and food should be re-introduced as soon as possible after the procedure.

Although the ability to titrate insulin in this fashion is at the level expected of an intern, if you are ever concerned do not hesitate to contact a senior doctor to ask for advice – particularly in the poorly-controlled diabetics!

INFLAMMATORY BOWEL DISEASES

Patients with inflammatory bowel diseases are living with chronic medical conditions of a relapsing/remitting nature, and thus will see their GP or gastroenterologist regularly. The aim when reviewing these patients in clinic is to monitor for and prevent complications from both their disease and medications. Questions to ask before reporting back to the consultant or registrar include:

- If this is the patient's first appointment – where is their disease located (e.g. terminal ileum)? When and how were they diagnosed? How did they initially present? Who were they previously known to? What treatment did they initially start, and how long did it hold them for? Did they have any complications of that treatment? Has their disease 'broken through' and required escalation of care – and if so, what? How often do they experience a flare requiring an inpatient stay? Are they (or have they ever been) on any biological agents?
- Have they had any flares since their last appointment? Was there bleeding, melaena or change in bowel habit? Are they anorectic?
- Has their weight changed? Briefly assess their nutritional intake (although at some specialist clinics there is a dietitian for this purpose!).
- Have they had any other illnesses since their last appointment? Have they needed to miss any infliximab infusions due to infection?
- When was their last set of bloods? When was their last magnetic resonance enterography (MRE)? When were their most recent scopes? You should try and review the reports and pathology, if possible. If they are due for more endoscopy, you could prepare their consent forms and paperwork to help your team.
- Do they have any other concerns not yet addressed?

LIVER DISEASE

Specialists will often be referred patients with deranged liver function tests (LFTs) for investigation. They will arrive with a varying degree of investigations already completed. In general, you should do the following:

- Take a detailed history including anorexia, weight change, ascites, pale stools, change in bowel habit, melaena or haematochezia, fevers, rigors, change in skin tone (pallor, jaundice), malaise, ankle oedema and darkened urine.
  - Ask if they have ever been investigated for liver disease before. When was it detected? Have they brought prior bloodwork?
- Take a detailed drug history – medications cause a large proportion of hepatic dysfunction.
- Take a family history of malignancy and liver disease.
- Take a past history, in particular biliary surgery (i.e. do they have a gallbladder?) and history of blood product transfusion.
- Take a social history, especially history of IV drug use, alcohol use, smoking and tattoos (parlour vs homemade).

- Perform a focused examination, concentrating on signs of chronic liver disease (e.g. palmar erythema, flap, fetor, spider naevi, jaundice, gynaecomastia, ascites, caputs medusae and ankle oedema).
- Complete the 'liver panel' serology (see Chapter 12, 'Investigations: serology').
- Request an abdominal ultrasound, if not performed in the last 6 months.
- Consider the need for an abdominal CT scan or FibroScan.

Even if you are unable to elicit a diagnosis based on the information garnered above, a consultant or registrar will be satisfied with the information you have collected. The patient will quite often have to leave the clinic to have these investigations completed, and return in 2–4 weeks with the results for further management.

When reviewing chronic liver disease patients, there are some further questions expected:

- How and when was their liver disease diagnosed? Do they have a specific diagnosis?
- Have they ever been confused (i.e. hepatic encephalopathy) due to their liver disease?
- Have they ever had to have an ascitic tap (i.e. paracentesis)? Have they ever had to have fluid drained from their lungs (i.e. hepatic hydrothorax)? If so, how recently and how long between regular taps? Do they weigh themselves regularly? What doses are their diuretics (e.g. frusemide and spironolactone)?
- How have their symptoms been trending? Have they been admitted for decompensation since their last review in clinic?
- Have they been seen by a dietitian to counsel them on a high protein/low salt diet and foods to avoid? Are they on thiamine, a multivitamin or late-night protein supplements?
- Have they ever had scopes for variceal monitoring? Did they require banding?
- Have they had their vaccinations, including annual influenza and 5-yearly pneumococcal shots?
- If relevant, are they still drinking or using IV drugs?
- Have they ever been considered for a liver transplant?
- Do they see their GP in between clinics for any other issues?

Review the blood work and imaging requested prior to their current appointment! Consultants will be particularly interested in changes in liver enzymes, coagulopathy, viral loads (for the viral hepatitises), AFP (performed annually as part of hepatocellular carcinoma monitoring) and abdominal ultrasound (6-monthly for HCC monitoring) and FibroScan reports. If a patient has hepatitis C, ensure they have been genotyped (it may be on the Pathology system) and investigate whether or not they have ever been considered for treatment. If a patient has haemochromatosis, enquire as to the frequency of their phlebotomy.

LIVER TRANSPLANT MONITORING

Although there are only six hospitals across Australia and New Zealand that offer adult liver transplants, you may encounter these patients for monitoring at smaller centres. These cases are understandably quite complex, and your consultant or registrar would not expect you to be making serious clinical decisions. Rather, they may want you to think about the long-term complications of the patient's liver disease, note any signs and symptoms of recurrence, interpret the biochemical changes on serology and ask about the side effects of the required immunosuppression. Taking a social and wider medical history are both essential to the management of transplant patients, so ensure you have done this before presenting back to the consultant.

If you are completing a work-up for someone being considered for a liver transplant, the required details by the transplant unit include:

- accurate height, weight, and abdominal circumference
- serology: FBE + UEC + CMP + LFT + blood group + viral serology (HIV + HCV + HAV + VZV + HSV + CMV + EBV + HBV surface AG and core AB) ± QFG, as well as the serology that confirmed the diagnosis insulting the liver (e.g. haemochromatosis genetics, serum copper or positive HCV viral load)
- imaging: abdominal USS, CT if already performed, FibroScan report
- endoscopy reports (i.e. variceal monitoring)
- if they have recently been performed, include any TTE or RFT reports as part of the preoperative assessment.

You may also dictate a formal referral letter on behalf of your consultant. Note that reasons for exclusion for receiving a liver include current alcohol/IV drug use, palliative indications, other life-threatening comorbidities, age >60 years (with some considerations), inability to participate in life-long medical supervision, severe neurological or intellectual development impairment.

CHAPTER 59

RENAL OUTPATIENTS

Joseph M O'Brien

Renal Outpatients Clinic is often dreaded, for fear of the ever-complicated dialysis patient. The most common referrals received are for patients with a rising creatinine, be it acute or chronic, from GPs or other inpatient units. Occasionally you will encounter patients with chronic renal impairment who are new to the area, were previously lost to follow-up or have suddenly decided to participate in their health care.

ACUTE KIDNEY INJURY

Acute kidney injury (AKI) is defined as a rapid deterioration in renal function with subsequent retention of renally-excreted substances and alteration of acid–base homeostasis over a period of <48 hours. There are multiple classification systems, but two of the more widely used are known as RIFLE (risk, injury, failure, loss of kidney function and end-stage kidney disease) and AKIN (acute kidney injury network), which are outlined in Table 59.1. Both systems use urine output as one parameter. However, RIFLE uses the estimated glomerular filtrate rate (eGFR) or serum creatinine as its second criterion to stratify the severity of renal injury, whereas AKIN uses changing serum creatinine. There is also evidence to suggest a worse RIFLE class is associated with a higher mortality. The greatest limitation with RIFLE is that it assumes the baseline creatinine is a known value, which in practice is often not the case.

The investigation of acute kidney injury is based on the principles of pre-renal, intrinsic renal and post-renal causes. Table 59.2 outlines in detail the many causes of deterioration in renal function. You could not possibly exclude all of these causes on the ward or in clinic, so instead your investigations are targeted at determining the instigating factors and excluding serious causes.

When taking a history from patients who have experienced acute kidney injury, ensure that you clarify:

- A history of events leading up to their presentation. Were they symptomatic? How was the change in renal function detected? Was any action taken at the time to try and improve their renal function (e.g. ceasing nephrotoxic medications, administering intravenous fluids or increasing oral intake)?

TABLE 59.1 AKIN and RIFLE classifications

RIFLE CLASSIFICATION		
	GFR criteria	Urine output criteria
Risk	GFR ↓25%; or 1.5× baseline Cr	<0.5 mL/kg/h for 6 hours
Injury	GFR ↓50%; or 2.0× baseline Cr	<0.5 mL/kg/h for 12 hours
Failure	GFR ↓75%; or 3.0× baseline Cr	<0.3 mL/kg/h for 24 hours; or anuria >12 hours
Loss of function	Persistent AKI >1 month	
End-stage renal disease	ESRD >3 months	
AKIN CLASSIFICATION		
Stage 1	Δ in Cr ≥0.3 mg/dl (30 μmol/L); or Cr 1.5–2.0× baseline	<0.5 mL/kg/h for 6 hours
Stage 2	Cr 2.1–3.0× baseline	<0.5 mL/kg/h for 12 hours
Stage 3	Cr >3.0× baseline; or need for RRT; or Cr ≥400 μmol/L with an acute rise of ≥50 μmol/L	<0.3 mL/kg/h for 24 hours; or anuria >12 hours

Cr, serum creatinine; ESRD, end-stage renal disease.

Adapted from: Ferri, F.F., 2015. Chapter: Acute kidney injury. In: Ferri, F.F., Ferri's Clinical Advisor. Philadelphia: Mosby, Table 1-14.

- The urgency of the referral. Has their renal function stabilised, begun to improve or continued to worsen? How frequently has this been monitored? Does the clinician making the referral have a working theory (e.g. a clear precipitant such as large contrast load 24 hours prior)?
- What medications are they currently taking? Had any medications been changed or commenced recently around the time of their change in renal function?
- Have they otherwise been unwell recently (e.g. an upper respiratory tract infection)?
- Do they have any other diseases that are known to affect renal function (e.g. anaemia, haematological malignancies [especially myeloma], diabetes, solid organ malignancy, connective tissue disorders and hypertension)?
- Were they still producing urine? If so, in what quantity, and was it discoloured? Did they have dysuria, frequency, nocturia, loin pain, haematuria, new incontinence, fevers, sweats, weight change or anorexia? If male, did they experience hesitancy, post-micturition dribbling or a change in urine stream?

TABLE 59.2 Causes of acute kidney injury

PRE-RENAL	INTRINSIC RENAL	POST-RENAL
Hypovolaemia due to dehydration, burns, renal losses – including diuretics and polyuria, gastrointestinal losses, haemorrhage or pancreatitis	**Glomerular injury** from Goodpasture's, ANCA-associated glomerulonephritis (Wegener's) or immune complex-mediated glomerulonephritis (SLE, post-infective cryoglobulinaemia, primary membranoproliferative glomerulonephritis)	**Ureteric obstruction** due to tumours (both inside and outside the renal tract), fibrosis, calculi or iatrogenic during surgery
Afferent vasoconstriction due to contrast nephropathy, hypercalcaemia, drugs (NSAIDs, noradrenaline, aminoglycosides and cyclosporine), or hepatorenal syndrome	**Vascular causes** including direct trauma, renal vein obstruction (e.g. clot), microangiopathy (e.g. TTP, HUS, DIC), malignant hypertension and severe atherosclerosis	**Bladder neck obstruction** due to prostatic hypertrophy, neurogenic bladder, blocked catheters, malignancy, calculi, clots, tricyclic antidepressants or ganglionic blockers
Decreased cardiac output from CCF, shock, anaphylaxis, sepsis, AMI, PE or anaesthetics	**Tubular disease** including ischaemia, cytotoxic chemotherapy, crystal nephropathies (e.g. gout, tumour lysis, MTX, acyclovir), excess haem (e.g. rhabdomyolysis or severe intravascular haemolysis) and drugs (aminoglycosides [again!], cisplatin, synthetic cannabinoids, lithium)	**Urethral obstructions** from malignancy, stricture, trauma, phimosis, retroperitoneal bleeding or renal calcinosis
Efferent arteriolar vasodilatation due to (for example) ACE inhibitors or aldosterone antagonists	**Interstitial nephritis** from infection (pyelonephritis) or drugs (including penicillins, cephalosporins, NSAIDs, PPIs, rifampicin, allopurinol and sulfonamides).	
	Systemic illnesses including Sjögren syndrome, sarcoidosis, SLE, haematological malignancies, tubulonephritis and uveitis	

Adapted from: Ferri, F.F., 2017. Chapter: Acute kidney injury. In: Ferri, F.F., Ferri's Clinical Advisor. Philadelphia: Mosby, Table 1A-12.

Perform a focused clinical examination, concentrating on their volume state (i.e. capillary refill, mucous membranes, jugular venous pressure, chest auscultation and peripheral fluid status). Most patients at Renal Clinic will have been weighed and had a set of observations completed prior to your assessment. Look for signs of chronicity of their renal disease – is this actually chronic illness that was previously missed? Do they appear to be anaemic or malnourished?

Investigations should begin with the basics – current basic bloods (FBE + UEC + CMP + LFT); a dipstick urine to look for protein, glucose, ketones and blood; and a formal urine with microscopy, culture and sensitivities (M/C/S), albumin-to-creatinine ratio (ACR) and protein-to-creatinine ratio (PCR). If indicated by prior pathology consider adding cast microscopy, urinary sodium and/or osmolality as well. If renal function has not recovered since your referral, consider an autoimmune screen (antinuclear antibodies, anti-glomerular basement membrane, anti-LKM, complement 3, complement 4, ANCA and possibly serum immunoglobulins) or myeloma screen (serum protein electrophoresis, lactate dehydrogenase, beta-2 microglobulin and free light chains).

A renal tract ultrasound is usually required, investigating renal size and post-renal pathology (e.g. obstruction). A renal biopsy may be indicated if there is still no diagnosis after these have been completed – patients will usually need a planned admission for this procedure. Check the pathology and radiology that has already been completed before you present to the consultant so that you both sound well-informed and don't waste money! Many investigations in the renal screen are costly.

After discussion with a senior doctor and before discharging the patient with their investigations, ensure there is a plan for follow-up and monitoring. Not every patient with an acute kidney injury will need to be followed up by the renal team indefinitely; many can be monitored by their GP. Those at highest risk for continuation on to chronic renal impairment include the elderly (>50 years), diabetics, smokers, hypertensives, Indigenous Australians, obese and those with a family history of kidney disease.

CHRONIC RENAL IMPAIRMENT AND DIALYSIS CLINICS

A terrifying prospect for many junior doctors is the management of the **chronic renally impaired**. Fortunately, you have this handy guide to make sure you don't knock off what little function is left in their feeble kidneys – especially as the incidence and prevalence of chronic renal insufficiency (CRI) continues to explode. Patients with previously documented CRI are reviewed regularly in clinic, usually 3- to 6-monthly. As is standard, start by taking a thorough history, covering the following issues:

- When was the patient diagnosed with renal impairment? How was this diagnosis made? What investigations did they have at the time (e.g. autoimmune screen, multiple urine samples, renal ultrasound, CT or even renal biopsy)?

- Was a cause for their renal impairment ever discovered?
- Are they currently on dialysis? What is their fluid restriction? If considering dialysis, have they had an assessment for access sites (e.g. ultrasound venous mapping)?
- What medications are they on? Have any of their doses been adjusted recently (e.g. prednisolone or erythropoietin)? Do they take any complementary or alternative medications?
- Do they have any ongoing blood transfusions or iron, intravenous immunoglobulin or zoledronic acid infusions? Do you need to help them book these? (NB: Blood transfusions are avoided as much as possible in patients who are likely candidates for transplant to minimise the risk of developing anti-red-cell antibodies.)
- Do they have any other medical issues, new or old?
- Have they experienced any neurological symptoms? Frequent infections? Bleeding tendency? Abdominal pain? Chest pain or proven ischaemic heart disease?
- Have they been increasingly fatigued or dyspnoeic (anaemia)?
- Have they had any fractures or new joint pains (osteomalacia and osteopenia)?
- Are they compliant with their 'renal diet' (i.e. one low in protein, potassium, sodium and phosphate)?

A complete social history is very important for a patient being considered for dialysis. Do you believe this person is able and willing to participate in their own health care? Can they make it to dialysis multiple times per week? Are they still smoking or drinking excess alcohol? Being a dialysis patient is a full-time commitment with many restrictions. If the patient is already on dialysis, ask:

- Are they on haemodialysis or peritoneal dialysis (PD)? Did they recently transition and, if so, why? Which centre do they dialyse at and how frequently?
- Do they know their 'dry weight' (i.e. their post-dialysis weight) or how much fluid they normally dialyse off? Alternatively, how much weight do they typically gain between runs?
- Do they take phosphate-binding drugs and when do they take them relative to meals (binders are most effective when taken with meals)?
- Do they still pass urine?
- Are they on the transplant list?

Complete a focused examination of the renal system, concentrating on signs of chronic disease including a change in skin pigmentation (including pallor signifying anaemia), cachexia, altered mental state or decreased attention, bony tenderness, nail changes, peripheral neuropathy, muscular fasciculation, excoriations from pruritus, multiple bruises suggestive of coagulopathy, fetor, dyspnoea, old surgical scars (especially access- or transplant-related, where they tend to be over one of the iliac fossas), abdominal tenderness, renal bruit or thrill and peripheral oedema. Of particular importance are the volume state, weight, blood pressure and condition of any fistulae they may have. If a patient displays multiple signs of worsening uraemia – anorexia, nausea, vomiting, neurological disturbance or rapidly increasing creatinine – they should be reviewed by a consultant.

The last thing to do before presenting is to review the investigations for this patient. Review their current UEC and CMP (particularly looking for hyperkalae-mia, which may require intervention ± admission via ED, changes in sodium, worsening creatinine and urea, hyperphosphataemia and hypercalcaemia), iron studies, parathyroid hormone (PTH), vitamin D, HbA$_{1c}$ and urine ACR. What is the size of their kidneys on a renal tract ultrasound? Have they had a CT-KUB (kidneys/ureters/bladder) to investigate malformations or structural abnormali-ties? If someone is approaching the need for dialysis, request venous mapping with ultrasound and discuss with a senior doctor whether the patient has reached the point of requiring a Tenckhoff catheter insertion (surgically-inserted, per-formed as a day case to allow for peritoneal dialysis). Once you have all of this information at hand, present it to the consultant or registrar with a potential plan for any issues you have identified. Remember, early preparation for access, even when dialysis may be years away, is best practice.

CRI is staged 1 through 5 dependent on the eGFR (see Table 59.3). A lower-case 'p' may be used to indicate significant proteinuria, an uppercase 'T' for a post-transplant patient and an uppercase 'D' for a patient already on dialysis. The most common causes for CRI include diabetes, glomerulonephritis (GN) and hypertension. Once a patient reaches stage 4, planning for dialysis should begin.

Initial management (typically seen in stages 1–3) aims to lower the risk factors for further kidney injury. The priority is to preserve as much renal function as possible, as such:

- Antihypertensives should be used to lower blood pressure, aiming for <130/80 mmHg.

TABLE 59.3 Stages of chronic renal impairment

STAGE	eGFR
1	>90 with proteinuria
2	60–89
3	30–59
4	15–29
5	<15; or on dialysis

Adapted from: [No Author], 2002. KDOQI Clinical Practice Guidelines for Chronic Kidney Disease: Evaluation, classification, and stratification. National Kidney Foundation. <http://www2.kidney.org/professionals/KDOQI/guidelines_ckd/p4_class_g1.htm> (accessed 3 Mar 2017).

- *Minimal change disease* – common in children. Noted association with NSAID use, atopy or Hodgkin's lymphoma, but is often idiopathic. Most patients have a relapse within 6 months. Managed with prednisolone for 4 weeks, with 10% not responding to steroids and requiring more intense immunosuppression.

Nephritic syndrome

- *Post streptococcal glomerulonephritis* – good prognosis, managed with supportive therapy. Typically appears anywhere between 1 and 3 weeks after exposure to group A beta-haemolytic *Streptococcus* species. The antigen from the Strep gets physically lodged in the glomeruli, inducing a form of proliferative glomerulonephritis.

- *IgA nephropathy* – most common cause worldwide, may involve the skin, liver, bowel (associated with inflammatory bowel disease and coeliac) and skeletal system (ankylosing spondylitis). Often diagnosed after a period of macroscopic haematuria. May also present as a nephrotic syndrome. Initial management is supportive and aims to reduce risk of progression with an ACE inhibitor or angiotensin-II receptor blocker (ARB). Corticosteroids were previously used if disease progressed; however, this is currently an area of controversy.

- *Rapidly progressive glomerulonephritis* – these have a poorer prognosis, and include anti-glomerular basement membrane glomerulonephritis (a.k.a. Goodpasture's if there is simultaneous lung involvement, seen in 70% of cases), anti-neutrophil cytoplasmic antibody (ANCA)-associated GN and idiopathic progressive glomerulonephritis.

If you encounter a patient with a suspected glomerulonephropathy on the wards or in clinic, they should have baseline UEC + CMP + LFTs (for the albumin) + urinary protein + a urine dipstick and formal M/C/S + blood sugar. If the history is suspicious, consider an antistreptolysin-O titre.

Other diagnostically useful (but expensive) tests include anti-glomerular basement membrane (anti-GBM), hepatitis B and C serology, HIV antibodies, cryoglobulins, anti-neutrophil cytoplasmic antibody (ANCA), antinuclear antibodies (ANA) and anti-double stranded DNA (anti-dsDNA). Ultimately, a renal biopsy remains gold standard for diagnosis of these conditions. See Chapter 38, 'Renal Medicine', for an outline of how to consent someone for a renal biopsy and care for them after the procedure.

CHAPTER 60

ENDOCRINOLOGY OUTPATIENTS

Joseph M O'Brien

The majority of endocrine conditions are of a chronic nature and, with a large focus on outpatient care, clinics will often be overflowing with referrals and reviews. Unless working in a smaller hospital, clinics will be subspecialised into subjects such as diabetes, thyroid (sometimes thyroid cancer has its own clinic with ENT Surgeons or Oncology present), electrolytes (for hyponatraemias, hypercalcaemias etc), metabolic nutrition (a.k.a. obesity), bone, reproductive endocrinology (in conjunction with Obstetrics and Gynaecology), growth (more common with Paediatric units) and general endocrine (encompassing pituitary, parathyroid and adrenal disease). Increasingly, diabetic clinics are further subdivided (e.g. type 1, type 2, latent autoimmune diabetes of adults [LADA], diabetic foot clinic and pump clinic [for type 1 diabetics with insulin pumps]).

DIABETES MELLITUS

Diabetes mellitus (DM) is a syndrome of hyperglycaemia of various aetiologies, and is currently the most rapidly growing chronic disease. Over 1.1 million diabetics currently reside in Australia, with this number expected to nearly triple to 3.1 million by 2030. In addition to its direct effect on morbidity, it also contributes to morbidity and mortality through its associated microvascular and macrovascular complications and propensity for infections.

Common annotations include type 1 diabetes mellitus (T1DM), type 2 diabetes mellitus (T2DM), latent autoimmune diabetes of adults (LADA), insulin-dependent diabetes mellitus (IDDM) and non-insulin-dependent diabetes mellitus (NIDDM). See Chapter 39, 'Endocrinology', for more detail about the pathophysiology of diabetes and its inpatient management.

Diabetes clinics can be frantic due to the sheer number of referrals. Diabetes educators (specially-trained nurses) are usually present, and are able to help the patient understand new management plans, explain commencing insulin in great depth and provide resources such as needles, new glucometers and glucose strips. Also present may be podiatrists, optometrists, dietitians and physiotherapists (depending on your hospital's resources). Before presenting to a consultant, discuss:

- When were they diagnosed with diabetes? Do they know what type of diabetes they have? Sometimes you will need to prompt with 'adult' or 'juvenile,' despite the fact these terms are no longer used by the medical community. How was their diagnosis confirmed? Do they still experience polydipsia, polyuria, fatigue or weight change? Do they ever have angina, dyspnoea or palpitations?

- Are they insulin-dependent, on oral hypoglycaemic (OHG) agents or 'diet-controlled'? If type 1, do they have or have they ever had an insulin pump? How long did they take to progress to the next level of diabetic control?

- Have they ever been admitted with hypoglycaemia? Have they ever experienced diabetic ketoacidosis (DKA)?

- Have they had macrovascular complications (ischaemic heart disease, cerebrovascular events, peripheral vascular disease)? Have they had microvascular complications (neuropathy, retinopathy, nephropathy)?

- Do they know their HbA_{1c} (some patients refer to it as their 'three-monthly sugar test')? Do they test their blood glucose levels (BGLs) at home? How often, and what are they like? Do they keep it in a diary or app? How often are they seeing their GP between clinic visits?

- Do they have a regular endocrinologist, optometrist or podiatrist? Does their GP complete diabetes management plans? If type 1, when did they transition from a paediatrician to an adult endocrinologist?

- If male (with appropriate rapport established), have they had issues with erectile dysfunction?

- If female, were they diabetic during any pregnancies? Gestational diabetes is associated with an increased incidence of type 2 diabetes.

- If insulin-dependent, do they keep Glucogel™ or a high glycaemic index (GI) snack on their person at all times? Are they storing their insulin correctly (in a dark, cool place – more relevant in Australia!)? Do they have sufficient needles? Is their glucometer working properly? Are they rotating their injection sites to prevent tissue necrosis?

- If type 1, have they been screened for other autoimmune conditions that often run parallel to diabetes, such as coeliac disease, thyroid dysfunction, Addison's and pernicious anaemia?

- Does their diabetes affect their activities of daily living (ADLs)? Have they missed school, university or work because of their condition?

- Quantify their alcohol (in grams/day) and tobacco consumption (in pack-years). Offer assistance with cessation if necessary.

- Is there a family history of diabetes or other endocrine dysfunction? If an adolescent, have their siblings been investigated? Do they have a positive family history for cardiovascular disease <55 years of age?

Examination of the diabetic patient should be thorough, reviewing for not only the signs of diabetes itself but its long-term sequelae and associated conditions (e.g. cardiovascular disease). Note body mass index (BMI), blood pressure (consider a postural BP), clubbing, palmar pallor, volume state, carotid bruit, striae, skin discolouration (e.g. acanthosis nigricans), heart sounds, chest fields, gynaecomastia, organomegaly, injection site necrosis, fine hair loss over the shins (sign of poor glycaemic control) and the nature of pedal pulses.

If confident, perform fundoscopy and a visual examination – however, this can be lengthy and is often best left to their ophthalmologist or optometrist. If they have an insulin pump, inspect the site for signs of infection or skin necrosis.

Investigations on first review of a diabetic patient should include basic blood work (FBE + UEC + CMP) with LFTs (non-alcoholic steatohepatitis and 'fatty liver' are very common in diabetics), thyroid-stimulating hormone (TSH), fasting lipids (second yearly) and a baseline glycated haemoglobin (HbA_{1c}). HbA_{1c} should be repeated quarterly, with a target of <7.0% in most patients (although <8.0% is not unreasonable in the elderly). If the diagnosis has not been confirmed, an oral glucose tolerance test (OGTT) should be performed. In adults who are diagnosed with diabetes and rapidly progress to insulin dependence, consider completing screening for LADA with anti-GAD antibodies and fasting serum insulin and C-peptide levels (see Chapter 12, 'Investigations: serology' for more information about interpreting these results). If the patient has hepatomegaly, request an abdominal ultrasound. Patients should have a baseline and annual urinalysis for albumin-to-creatinine ratio to monitor for nephropathy. Complete annual electrocardiograms (ECGs).

Management is truly multidisciplinary, with a focus on both pharmaceutical and non-pharmaceutical methods to achieve optimal glycaemic control and minimisation of cardiovascular risk factors. Dietary advice, weight loss and increase in physical activity are the first-line management for T2DM. Some patients may even be able to 'cure' their diabetes with weight loss. Cardiovascular risk factors should be minimised with antihypertensives (aim for a BP of <130/80 mmHg) and lipid-lowering agents. ACE inhibitors or angiotensin-II receptor antagonists are standard treatment for diabetic albuminuria. Consider opportunistic vaccination with influenza vaccine (annually) and polyvalent Pneumovax® 23 (5-yearly). Educate about nephrotoxic agents, especially those available over-the-counter (e.g. NSAIDs).

Current guidelines now suggest oral hypoglycaemics should be commenced when the diagnosis is confirmed, due to the low rate of success in improving glycaemic control with lifestyle modification alone. The typical first-line agent is metformin, an insulin sensitiser that will *not* cause hypoglycaemia. Its most common side effects are gastrointestinal upset (usually diarrhoea), so it is started at a low dose (e.g. 500 mg PO daily) and up-titrated as tolerated to a maximum of 1 g TDS. If metformin is contraindicated (e.g. poor renal function), not tolerated or insufficient, a sulfonylurea is typically commenced (e.g. gliclazide modified release 30–60 mg PO mane).

Alternatively, consider acarbose (a starch blocker) up to 25–100 mg PO TDS. If hypoglycaemia is a concern, a DPP-4 inhibitor such as sitagliptin could be used.

Lastly, a slow release injection of exenatide (sold as Byetta®), a GLP-1 agonist, could be considered in addition to dual therapy in a patient intolerant to multiple classes of OHG. The new kids on the block are sodium-glucose co-transporter 2 (SGLT-2 inhibitors – heavily simplified, these induce ˜7 g of glycosuria daily and have the additional benefit of weight loss. They should be avoided in those with regular UTIs or thrush. Discuss all medication changes with a registrar or consultant.

If all of these antidiabetic agents fail to achieve optimal glycaemic control (or if the patient has type 1 or LADA), insulin therapy must be commenced. A typical regimen would be a long-acting nocte (e.g. Lantus®) and if necessary, low-dose short-acting insulin (e.g. NovoRapid® or Actrapid®) with meals. A BGL diary is essential for titrating insulin therapy. Always discuss the issue with a consultant before making changes to a patient's regimen. Insulin-dependent patients experiencing frequent complications from their insulin therapy (e.g. multiple admissions for DKA) could be considered for an insulin pump. Although these can improve glycaemic control, they run the risk of site infections and DKA if the needle were to dislodge.

HYPERTHYROIDISM

The inpatient management, epidemiology and pathophysiology of thyroid disorders is covered in Chapter 39, 'Endocrinology.' In clinic, you may be required to try and identify the cause of someone's hyperthyroidism with a differential of Graves' disease, adenoma, multinodular goitre, thyroiditis, a thyroid carcinoma or a TSH-secreting paraneoplastic syndrome. Reviewing a hyperthyroid patient in clinic is mostly about ensuring adequate control of their illness with titration of therapy to minimise symptoms. Before reporting to the consultant, be sure to cover:

- When were they diagnosed with hyperthyroidism? Was it on a blood test? Do they know if they had antibody testing? Were they sick at diagnosis? Were they immediately started on anti-thyroid medication, or were they re-tested first? Did they have an ultrasound or nuclear scan of their neck?

- What symptoms were they experiencing at diagnosis? Did they have heat intolerance, insomnia, hyperactivity, tremor, muscle weakness, weight loss, hypertension, tachycardia, skin changes (hyperpigmentation, vitiligo), alopecia (i.e. hair thinning), palpitation (i.e. atrial fibrillation), tachypnoea, goitre, nausea/vomiting, diarrhoea, polydipsia, nocturia, pathological fracture, mood changes, psychosis or headaches? Have they experienced any of these since commencing therapy? If female, have they had disruption of their menstrual cycle?

  - Screening for malignancy on history-taking can be difficult as some patients with hyperthyroidism may experience anorexia, weight loss, fevers, rigors, and/or night sweats.

- Have they had medications, thyroid ablation with radioactive iodine or thyroid surgery? Were there any complications of this treatment?
- What medications do they take? Have they ever been on amiodarone or thyroxine?
- Do they have a family history of thyroid disease or malignancy?
- Quantify their alcohol or tobacco consumption. In particular, Graves' is closely associated with smoking.
- What do they do for a living? Have they needed time off due to their thyroid disorder?

As the wide-ranging list of signs and symptoms would suggest, thyroid examination must be very thorough and covers most bodily systems. A complete set of observations (with heart rate and blood pressure in particular) should be taken and body weight registered and compared with prior results. Note a wide pulse pressure, any skin changes (particularly alopecia, or patches of vitiligo or hyperpigmentation), tremor, ophthalmopathy (indicative of Graves'), lymphadenopathy, surgical scars and pretibial myxoedema. If a goitre is present, examine it thoroughly – examining from behind the patient with their neck extended slightly, look for tenderness, mobility or a thrill on palpation, and its movement when swallowing. Check for Pemberton's sign (a sign of SVC obstruction brought on by the patient raising their arms for >20 s).

Investigations in a newly diagnosed hyperthyroid patient will include basic blood work (FBE + UEC), CMP (some hyperthyroid patients have increased bone turnover and thus a high calcium – if elevated, consider a parathyroid hormone or 'PTH' level), LFTs (cirrhotic changes are sometimes seen with thyroid disease) and CRP (to exclude an inflammatory state). Consider BGL and fasting lipid profile.

The thyroid function tests (TFTs), including TSH, free T_3 and free T_4, should be regularly reviewed. Request an ECG to review for atrial fibrillation. Imaging should include a thyroid ultrasound (if goitre present), and a 24-hour radioactive iodine uptake (RAIU) scan. RAIU can help determine the cause of hyperthyroidism – overactive thyroid cells take up more radioactive iodine, and the pattern can suggest Graves' (homogeneous increased uptake), multinodular goitre (heterogeneous increased uptake) or a single hot nodule. RAIU can also be used for iodine ablation dosage.

Symptomatic hyperthyroidism is typically managed with propylthiouracil (PTU) or carbimazole (a pro-drug of methimazole, which prevents iodinisation of tyrosine). Carbimazole is more regularly used than PTU due to the risk of acute liver failure; however, carbimazole runs the risk of myelosuppression and agranulocytosis so FBE should be monitored when first commencing the drug. Radioactive iodine (^{131}I) is considered in symptomatic patients resistant to 12 months of treatment, achieving remission in 80% of patients. Hypothyroidism is a relatively common side effect of ^{131}I. In truly refractory cases, a surgical referral may be necessary for thyroidectomy.

If the patient is in AF, strongly consider anticoagulation to prevent stroke (be mindful that carbimazole affects warfarin metabolism). Propranolol may be considered at a low, frequent dose (e.g. 20 mg PO TDS or QID) for the beta-adrenergic manifestations of hyperthyroidism, up-titrated until effective. Patients with hyperthyroidism should be reviewed every 3 months with lifelong monitoring by either an endocrinologist or dedicated GP.

HYPOTHYROIDISM

Conversely, hypothyroidism is a deficiency in thyroid hormone. Myxoedema is hypothyroidism approaching a point of crisis. Similar to hyperthyroid patients, you may be asked to review a patient in clinic to assist in diagnosis of their condition or to monitor their disease. Hypothyroidism may be due to Hashimoto's, prior management of hyperthyroidism, altered homeostasis of iodine or idiopathic myxoedema. Review:

- When and how were they diagnosed with hypothyroidism? Were they symptomatic at presentation?
- Have they experienced weight gain, cold intolerance, weakness, fatigue, peripheral oedema, bradycardia, hypotension, skin changes (usually thin or dry), voice changes (bradyphonia or hoarseness of voice), memory loss or constipation? Have these symptoms improved or remained stable? If female, have they had disruption of their menstrual cycle?
- Were they immediately commenced on thyroid hormone supplementation with thyroxine? What dose? Has it worked? Has it needed up- or down-titration?
- What medications are they currently on? Have they ever been on lithium, amiodarone or sulfonamide antibiotics?
- Do they have a family history of thyroid or endocrine dysfunction/malignancy?
- Quantify their tobacco and alcohol exposure and advise about cessation if necessary.

Inspect for confusion, slow and nasal voice, dry or thin skin, areas of vitiligo, loss of the outer third of their eyebrows, peripheral sensory loss, periorbital oedema, goitre, pleural effusion and hyporeflexia. Hypothyroid patients' movements are commonly sluggish and require a great deal of effort.

Investigation is focused on excluding rare causes of hypothyroidism and differential diagnoses such as depression, dementia, nephrotic syndrome or congestive cardiac failure. Basic bloods (FBE + UEC) with CMP, LFT and TFTs are done at baseline. Imaging of the thyroid should also be performed. Hyponatraemia, anaemia and hyperlipidaemia are commonly associated with hypothyroidism. If autoimmune thyroiditis is suspected, request anti-microsomal and anti-thyroglobulin antibodies.

Treatment is supplementation of thyroid hormone with thyroxine. A standard starting dose in the elderly would be 25–50 mcg PO daily, up-titrated with TSH every 4–6 weeks. A younger patient might tolerate a higher initial dose of 100 mcg

PO daily. Patients with hypothyroidism can be reviewed 6-monthly by their GP, and do not necessarily need to return to Endocrinology Clinic on an ongoing basis.

HYPOPITUITARISM

Hypopituitarism (sometimes annotated as panhypopituitarism if all hormones are affected) is a state of deficiency of one or more of the anterior pituitary hormones. This can be due to a pituitary tumour, trauma, radiotherapy, intracranial surgery, a space-occupying lesion or, rarely, infarction. Discuss:

- When and how were you diagnosed with hypopituitarism? Did you start treatment straight away? Were there any issues with your dosage? Have you had any side effects from the steroid therapy?

- Prior to diagnosis, did you experience lethargy, weakness, fatigue (from adrenocorticoid deficiency), weight gain, cold intolerance, constipation, peripheral oedema (hypothyroid), loss of libido or erectile dysfunction in men and oligomenorrhoea in women (follicle-stimulating hormone deficiency), hair loss, reduced effort tolerance (growth hormone deficiency), infertility, or headache, visual changes or anosmia (potentially due to local expansion of a pituitary tumour)? If female, have you had difficulty with pregnancies?

  - Visual changes should be reviewed immediately by Neurosurgery with prior imaging.

- Is there a family history of endocrine disturbance or intracranial malignancy?

- What medications are you taking? Have there been any recent changes?

Examination should focus on the signs of thyroid dysfunction described above, in addition to inspection of secondary sexual characteristics (including hair distribution, body shape, nipple hypopigmentation and consideration of genitalia examination if appropriate), and visual fields. Patients may not present with any signs.

Investigation is broad, with basic blood work (FBE + UEC + CMP + LFT), HbA$_{1c}$ (diabetes can contribute to hypopituitarism), serum cortisol (± corticotrophin) and short Synacthen test (see Chapter 12, 'Investigations: serology', for interpretation), morning plasma cortisol, TSH, insulin-like growth factor (IGF-1, a substitute for growth hormone that fluctuates), luteinising and follicle-stimulating hormones (in men anytime, in women timed with menstrual cycle), serum testosterone levels in men and prolactin. Insulin tolerance test is sometimes indicated. Strongly consider neuroimaging with MRI.

Treatment is theoretically straightforward – simply supplement the affected hormones! However, getting the balance correct can be quite difficult. Thyroxine, cortisone and gonadal steroids can be administered and should have their doses titrated with serum monitoring. If the signs of hypoadrenalism have recently begun, mid-investigation supplementation of corticosteroids is appropriate. Any patient with symptoms or signs suggestive of mass effect should be referred to Neurosurgery without delay.

Any hypopituitary patient headed for surgery should have an increased dose of steroids in the perioperative period with a perioperative physician referral (or General Medicine/Endocrine if there is no perioperative service in your hospital). Patients will require a double dose of corticosteroid when acutely unwell. Patients who have not yet completed their family should be referred to an appropriate obstetrician. Cardiovascular health should be monitored as this patient group is of high susceptibility to cardiac illness. Panhypopituitary patients will require lifelong monitoring.

PAGET'S DISEASE OF THE BONE

Paget's disease of the bone (not to be confused with Paget's disease of the breast) is a focal, chaotic disease of bone remodelling with competing osteoclastic and osteoblastic cell behaviour. The result is poorly-formed, hypervascular, disorganised lamellar bone highly prone to fracture. Its exact aetiology is still not known, but it is hypothesised that viral exposure of people with a genetic susceptibility may be involved.

Paget's is reasonably common in the elderly, but is often asymptomatic and thus not requiring treatment. It is often detected incidentally on X-ray plain films. Initially lesions may be predominantly lytic, with sclerotic lesions evident after disease progression as osteoblasts are increasingly involved. Discuss:

- When were you diagnosed with Paget's? How did it first present – pathological fracture, incidental finding on imaging, pain (from bone overgrowth) or a bony lump? Did you have a bone biopsy to confirm the diagnosis? What treatment are you on, if any?
- Have they had any complications such as fracture, nerve impingement or osteoarthritis since diagnosis?
- Have they had any fevers, rigors, anorexia, weight loss or chills that may suggest a more sinister differential?
- Is there a family history of rheumatological or endocrine dysfunction or malignancy?
- Has their disease affected their ADLs? Do they require any gait aids or home modifications, and what do they already have in place?
- Quantify alcohol and tobacco consumption and advise cessation if necessary.

Examination is rather straightforward, focused on the musculoskeletal system. Note any signs that point to an alternative diagnosis such as osteoarthritis, fibrous dysplasia or malignancy. Investigation involves basic bloods (FBE + UEC), with a CMP (serum levels of calcium and phosphate, two components of bone, are important), LFTs (with a fractionated alkaline phosphatase to separate liver and bony source of the enzyme), vitamin D (25D) and serum protein electrophoresis

(SPEP) and free light chains (FLC) to exclude myeloma (although note that myeloma lesions or plasmacytomas in bone are usually lytic). Request a PTH if the patient is hypercalcaemic. An elevated urine NTx (N-terminal telopeptide)-to-creatinine ratio is indicative of high bone turnover.

Nuclear bone scintigraphy (a.k.a. a 'bone scan') with technetium-99m is the gold standard imaging, useful in combination with plain films of known Pagetic lesions. Diseased bone will have an increased uptake of the tracer. If a lesion is identifiable on imaging, bone biopsy could be considered to differentiate between Paget's and metastases or rare malignancies but is not always necessary.

Asymptomatic Paget's can be monitored without treatment, and does not necessarily need repeat Endocrine appointments. However, Paget's disease of the bone is usually progressive and patients with pain, fracture or deformity should be commenced on a bisphosphonate to attempt to normalise the ratio of bone turnover and stabilise the bone at a cellular level. Depending on physician and patient preference, the bisphosphonate may either be oral (e.g. weekly alendronate) or intravenous (e.g. 60 mg IV pamidronate as required, or 5 mg IV annual zoledronic acid). Patients should be counselled on the side effects of bisphosphonates (e.g. ulcerative oesophagitis and jaw avascular necrosis).

Alkaline phosphatase (ALP) may be used to monitor response. Paracetamol slow release or (if younger and without contraindications) NSAIDs can be used to relieve pain. Patients with Paget's of the bone who are symptomatic despite 2–3 months of treatment may be considered for surgical management, which is often complicated due to the hypervascular nature of Pagetic bone. If symptomatic, 3–6 monthly review is advisable.

CHAPTER 61

NEUROLOGY OUTPATIENTS

Joseph M O'Brien

Neurology Clinic is not often attended by residents or junior doctors due to the complex nature of cases present. However, in smaller or regional hospitals (or General Medical Clinics) you may encounter many of the following cases. Neurology is an excellent rotation for learning, and the senior doctors recognise the difficulty of the patient caseload and are usually very supportive. In larger centres, Neurology Outpatients may be divided into General Neurology, Epilepsy, First Seizure, Headache, Stroke, Dizziness, Movement Disorders and Memory Clinics. Depending on your home network, Memory Clinic may come under Geriatric Medicine or Neurology. The team members present at Neurology Clinic will usually be consultants, registrars, physiotherapists and occupational therapists (especially for movement disorders) and nurses.

EPILEPSY AND FIRST SEIZURE CLINIC

These are typically the busiest of the subtypes of Neurology Clinic, and also the kind you'll most likely be asked to attend. Many patients will have been referred from other inpatient units or doctors in the community having had an isolated seizure. Mixed amongst these patients will be long-term epileptics with varying degrees of control over their disease for their regular review. For inpatient management of epilepsy, see Chapter 40, 'Neurology'.

Epileptic seizures result from uncoordinated electrical activity in the cerebral cortex, and are generally classified into provoked (e.g. subsequent to infection, trauma, drugs, metabolic imbalance or malignancy) or unprovoked. When seeing a patient in clinic, ask the following:

- Do they have an established diagnosis of epilepsy? If so, how old were they when the diagnosis was made? How was it confirmed (did they have an EEG)? What has their control been like in the past?

- Have they had any breakthrough seizures? If so, what type of seizure was it? How often do they seize? Does the type of seizure ever change? Do they experience an 'aura' prior to symptoms? Did they have spontaneous resolution of their symptoms or were they administered an additional antiepileptic agent? Did they seize multiple times, and did they recover lucidity between seizures? Are they aware of triggers for their seizures, and what do they do to avoid them? Did they lose continence of urine, faeces or both? Did they bite their tongue? Did they injure themselves (if there was a fall)? Did they have a fever or any localising symptoms of infection at the time? The nature of seizures can reveal great detail about the location of the underlying pathology.

- What is their medication regimen? Has it been changed (up- or down-titrated) recently? Have they felt any adverse effects of this change? Drugs that can lower the seizure threshold include beta lactam antibiotics, antihistamines, cocaine, lithium, amphetamines, theophylline, tricyclic antidepressants and quinolones.

- Do they have any other medical conditions? Does epilepsy (or any other neurological condition, including Alzheimer's) run in their family? Have they ever had any trauma to their head or neck, a stroke, encephalitis or meningitis? Do they have an autoimmune condition (e.g. lupus or vasculitis)?

- What is their alcohol consumption like? Do they use any other substances? Did they formerly use these in an excessive fashion?

- Does the person usually drive? What is the patient's occupation? Does it involve driving or using machinery? Would a seizure at work put them or others in danger? Each state in Australia has a website where you can review the law for driving restrictions after a seizure.

Complete a neurological examination, looking for any residual focal deficits. Biochemical investigations should include FBE, UEC (particularly noting sodium), CMP (for hypocalcaemia or hypomagnesaemia), fasting glucose (diabetes), TSH and LFTs (hepatic failure). Patients on anti-epileptics should have regular LFTs due to the risk of cholestatic liver dysfunction.

If a patient has not already, they should be referred for electroencephalography (EEG), where electrodes are attached to a patient's scalp and electric impulses are recorded. Yield of abnormal findings can be increased with sleep deprivation and provocation measures (e.g. intermittent photic stimulation with flashing lights) – but understandably these are unpopular with patients. A normal EEG does not exclude epilepsy, and conversely not all abnormal EEGs confirm the diagnosis. You would not be expected by any reasonable consultant to be able to interpret the details of EEGs!

Similarly, all patients should have magnetic resonance imaging (MRI) of their brain for evaluation of new lesions or structural changes. If an MRI is contraindicated, a CT-brain could be used (preferably with contrast). Neuroimaging can exclude stroke, haemorrhage, signs of old trauma, mass lesions, vascular abnormalities and previously undiagnosed congenital malformations.

Commencing an anti-epileptic is not always necessary after an isolated seizure (especially if provoked); however, if multiple seizures have occurred, the patient has persistent neurological deficit or if there was a structural abnormality detected, anti-epileptic drug (AED) therapy may be warranted. First-line agent depends on the type of seizure (e.g. valproate or lamotrigine are popular for generalised epilepsy; carbamazepine, gabapentin, and topiramate are common agents in partial epilepsy) and the consultant's preference.

Compliance with AED therapy is very important and this should be stressed to the patient. Side effects common to most AEDs include fatigue, dizziness, diplopia and imbalance and patients should be consented to these complications of therapy. *All patients* beginning lamotrigine and carbamazepine should be warned to call their GP or the Neurology registrar if they experience a rash due to the serious nature of Stevens–Johnson syndrome, a life-threatening hypersensitivity reaction.

HEADACHE

Headache is a very common symptom (not a diagnosis) that can be due to a plethora of benign and serious aetiologies. However, more than 90% of benign headaches are categorised as migraines, tension or cluster headaches. Distinguishing features among these three are outlined in Table 61.1. More sinister causes of headaches include malignancy, raised intracranial pressure (ICP), arteriovenous malformations, hypertensive crisis, hydrocephalus, intracranial infection, stroke (although rarely), drug reactions and autoimmune conditions.

TABLE 61.1 Characteristics of common headache syndromes

MIGRAINE	CLUSTER	TENSION
• 60–70% are unilateral, with the other 30% global • Tends to gradually set in and pulse in a crescendo fashion • Exacerbated by light, exercise and noise • Lasts 4–72 hours • Associated with nausea and vomiting and a preceding aura. Rarely, may produce neurological deficit (e.g. weakness or dysarthria)	• 100% are unilateral, typically around the eye or temple • Rapid onset • Pain is continuous and severe • Lasts $\frac{1}{2}$ to 3 hours • Four times more likely in men than women • Not exacerbated by noise or light. Can often continue to remain active • Associated with same-sided lacrimation, rhinorrhoea, nasal congestion, diaphoresis and sensitivity to alcohol • Focal neurological deficit is rare	• Usually bilateral • Described as a fluctuating tightness • Variable in presentation, precipitating factors and duration • No other associated symptoms

Adapted from: Characteristics of migraine, tension-type, and cluster headache syndromes. Uptodate [Internet]. <http://www.uptodate.com/contents/image?imageKey=PC%2F68064&topicKey=NEURO%2F3349&rank=1~150&source=see_link&search=headache&utdPopup=true>.

Migraines are episodic, severe headaches typically associated with nausea, vomiting, photophobia (avoidance of light) and phonophobia (avoidance of noise) that are often preceded by an 'aura' (a period of focal visual or sensory disturbance).

Cluster headaches, seen far more commonly in men, are unilateral, episodic and often accompanied by ipsilateral sympathetic and congestive phenomena such as ptosis, miosis, diaphoresis and rhinorrhoea. As the name implies, they tend to occur in 'clusters' with up to eight experienced in one day. The side affected can switch between attacks.

Tension headaches (the most prevalent) are mild to moderate, bilateral and throbbing headaches not associated with any of the above symptoms. Tension headaches are classified by their frequency of occurrence into infrequent (less than monthly), frequent episodic (1–14/month), and chronic (≥15/month). When discussing headaches with a patient in Clinic, be sure to cover the following:

- How long have they been having headaches? What type of pain is their headache? On which side of their head is the pain? Is it associated with any other symptoms, including nausea, vomiting, tears, weakness, visual disturbance, sweating or difficulty speaking? Do they experience an 'aura' before their headache begins? How often are they getting headaches? Have they identified any triggers or exacerbating factors? Are the headaches worse at any time of the day? Do they ever get woken from sleep with a headache? Is there an association with their symptoms and alcohol? Have they found any method to improve symptoms (e.g. lying down in a dark room)? Do they ever lose consciousness? Are they ever told after their headache that they had a period of non-responsiveness? Do they ever lose continence?

- If female, have they recently changed their form of contraception? Is there any relationship between their headaches and their menstrual cycle?

- Do they have a history of head trauma, alcohol or other substance abuse, intracranial infection or malignancy (including skin cancers)?

- Do they have neck or back pain? Do they have a tremor? Have they noticed difficulty with their memory in recent months? Do they have difficulty swallowing or speaking?

- What medications are they currently taking?

- Have they lost weight or their appetite, or had fevers, rigors, sweats or chills?

- Is it affecting their ADLs?

- Is there a family history of migraines, epilepsy, aneurysms, polycystic kidney disease or neurological disorders?

Examination should attempt to determine if there is any persistent neurological defect, so a complete examination of the peripheral and central nervous system is necessary. Listen in particular for carotid bruit. If you have the capacity in clinic, fundoscopy should be performed (checking for papilloedema, a sign of raised intracranial pressure). Routine observations, particularly blood pressure, are also important.

Investigations for headache can be both expansive and expensive, and thus should be targeted based on the patient's history and your examination findings. Routine bloods (FBE, UEC, CMP, LFT) would be necessary, as well as ESR (for temporal arteritis, vasculitis and non-specific autoimmune conditions), TSH and urinalysis.

There are no strict guidelines for when imaging should be performed; however, neuroimaging with CT or MRI would be justified if any of the danger signs from Box 61.1 are present. While unlikely to be seen in clinic, the syndrome of severe headache, fever, photophobia and/or nuchal rigidity (i.e. neck stiffness) should prompt consideration of a lumbar puncture (LP) as it raises concern for meningitis.

Management will depend on the final diagnosis and underlying pathology. Migraines are often prevented with beta-blockers or triptans if severe or frequent enough. Cluster headaches are unfortunately often refractory to simple analgesia, and unusually seem to respond well to supplemental oxygen therapy. Tension headaches often respond to simple analgesia (i.e. paracetamol and NSAIDs). Some patients will benefit from non-pharmaceutical techniques, such as caffeine and alcohol reduction. Opiates should be avoided as ongoing analgesia as they often result in 'rebound' headaches.

Patients seen with headache in clinic can be difficult to manage due to the large number of possible aetiologies. Chronic headaches greatly affect a person's ability to live a fulfilling life and have even been linked with suicide (particularly

BOX 61.1 Danger signs of headaches

- Waking in pain
- Worse in the mornings
- Gradual worsening over time with increasing frequency
- Sudden onset, especially when described as 'thunderclap' or 'the worst headache in [their] life'
- Persistent, severe pain
- Focal neurological deficit (other than classic aura)
- Any decrease in alertness
- Headache with fever or rigors
- Change in personality
- Onset with exercise (especially lateral movement of the head)
- New headaches in patients <5 years or >50 years
- New headache in a patient with known malignancy or immunocompromise
- New headache during pregnancy

Adapted from: Digre, K.B., 2012. Chapter 405: Headaches and other head pain. In: Goldman, L. & Schafer, A.I., Goldman's Cecil Medicine, 24th ed. Philadelphia: Saunders.

cluster headaches). If you are ever concerned by a patient's symptoms, speak directly with your consultant or registrar.

MULTIPLE SCLEROSIS

Multiple sclerosis (MS) is a progressive, inflammatory, demyelinating condition of the central nervous system responsible for a significant quantity of disability in young adults. MS is heterogeneous in nature, with diverse presentations and a varied clinical course. MS in its later stages is debilitating, with patients requiring increasing assistance with progression (often culminating in residential care). Initial diagnosis can be difficult, but symptoms suggestive of multiple sclerosis include sudden deterioration (<24 hours), new incontinence or gait disturbance in a young person, peripheral paraesthesia (i.e. tingling and numbness), involuntary muscle spasms, optic neuritis, heat insensitivity, emotional lability and fatigue. It is classically taught that three neurological episodes separated in space and time should be considered MS until proven otherwise.

The classic pathological finding in MS is nerves with areas of focal demyelination, typically identified on MRI. Risk factors include female gender, viral infections, family history and (interestingly) birth and habitation far from the equator. The median age of onset is 28–31years. The most common cause of death with MS is pneumonia, followed by sepsis and myocardial infarction. There are three main subtypes described, classified depending on the presence and nature of 'relapses' (i.e. acute onset or worsening of neurological symptoms), as follows:

1   Relapsing-remitting multiple sclerosis (RRMS): the most common form, with relapses dispersed between periods of complete or near-complete recovery. The average remission between first and second attacks is 3.5 years.

2   Secondary progressive MS (SPMS): disability continues to progress, with minimal or no relapses.

3   Primary progressive MS (PPMS): seen in about one-fifth of cases, progression begins with the first presentation and typically continues without relapse.

The subtype of MS is useful for prognostication and patient education. When reviewing a patient with MS in clinic, cover the following:

- When were they diagnosed? How was the diagnosis confirmed (i.e. where was the MRI done)? Did they have a lumbar puncture at the time? Do they know what subtype of MS they have (if not, try to determine which subtype they have based on the nature of the disease's progression)? How often do they experience a relapse? How is their vision? Refer to an optometrist if necessary.

- Do they have a regular neurologist? How often do they have surveillance MRIs?

- Have they had difficulty ambulating, swallowing, speaking, maintaining continence or performing fine motor functions?

- Have they had any infections (e.g. pneumonia)? Any complications from their treatment?
- What is their current medication regimen? Has this changed recently?
- Do they have a family history of MS, epilepsy or other neurological conditions? Has their family been counselled on MS? Are they aware of the Multiple Sclerosis Foundation and their peer support program and advocacy?
- If the disease is progressing – do they have advanced care planning in place? Do they know their desired limitation of treatment? How has their mood been? Rates of depression are high in MS. Refer them to the appropriate psychological support programs if necessary.

Complete a focused neurological examination. Autonomic dysfunction is common, so postural blood pressures can be useful. If you are reviewing a patient with suspected MS, the gold standard of diagnosis lies with an MRI brain and whole spine. These are noisy, claustrophobic procedures requiring a patient to lie on an MRI table for up to 2 hours and some people will require sedation (e.g. with 5 mg oral diazepam). Typical findings in MS include 'Dawson's fingers' (lesions that originate around the ventricular veins of the brain) on T_1-weighted images and enhancing, concentric plaques on T_2-weighted images.

Also highly useful is a lumbar puncture with analysis for increased protein and oligoclonal banding, but it must be compared with serum electrophoresis (SPEP) taken at a similar time. Biochemistry should include FBE, UEC, CMP, LFT, TSH, ESR, ANA, vitamin B_{12} and vitamin D, with consideration given to angiotensin-converting enzyme (ACE), collagen vascular serum tests, neuromyelitis optica IgG antibody and anti-thyroglobulin antibody.

Acutely, relapse of MS is managed with high-dose intravenous (IV) methylprednisolone (e.g. 5 days of 1 g IV daily, or 15 mg/kg/day lean body mass) with a rapidly weaned course of oral corticosteroid (e.g. prednisolone). Long term, patients may receive interferon-based therapy and glatiramer. Typically given in the Medical Day Unit (and often written up but not understood by residents), the frequency and dose is dictated by a consultant.

Newer, oral disease-modifying agents include fingolimod, teriflunomide and dimethyl fumarate. These all have side effects including hepatotoxicity (all three), bradycardia (fingolimod), alopecia (teriflunomide) and abdominal pain and flushing (dimethyl fumarate). Natalizumab is a recombinant monoclonal antibody used for aggressive RRMS, but has the well-known but rare and potentially fatal side effect of causing progressive multifocal leucoencephalopathy (PML). Incidence of PML in natalizumab use is linked with previous exposure to the John Cunningham (JC) virus and extended natalizumab or immunosuppressant use.

Patients may be on long-term immunosuppression with steroid therapy; however, the risk of infections must be weighed up with delaying progression of the MS. Spasticity may be treated with oral baclofen, incontinence with muscarinic therapy (e.g. oxybutynin), tremor with beta-blockade (usually low-dose, regular propranolol) and neurological pain with gabapentin. Early referral should be made to physiotherapy and occupational therapy.

SECTION V

PARKINSON'S DISEASE AND PARKINSONISM

Parkinsonism is a syndrome of bradykinesia (i.e. slow movement), hypertonia (i.e. 'spasticity'), tremor and postural instability (usually with significance gait disturbance), of which Parkinson's *disease* is the most common cause. Parkinson's disease is a neurodegenerative disorder of the central nervous system, worsening as the dopamine-generating cells of the substantia nigra (a structure in the midbrain) atrophy or die. Parkinsonism may be due to drugs, toxins (e.g. pesticides, heavy metals, organic solvents), trauma, malignancy and subsequent structural changes in the brain, ischaemia, metabolic disorders (e.g. parathyroid dysfunction, hepatic failure, Wilson's) and infections (including HIV).

A common problem in the elderly, parkinsonism is particularly debilitating as, in addition to being a disorder of movement, it affects the person's ability to judge their position in space leading to an increased number of falls. Further compounding this is the autonomic dysfunction in later stages, leading to (amongst other symptoms) postural hypotension. You may encounter patients with parkinsonism for investigation, or for review of known disease in either Geriatric Medicine or Neurology Clinic. Be sure to discuss the following:

- When and how was their diagnosis of Parkinson's disease made? Has it progressed quickly, or stayed stable? Do they have a tremor? How is their swallow?

- Have they experienced incontinence? Are they 'socially continent' (i.e. able to achieve continence while out of their house)? How is their gait? Do they use any gait aids? Do they experience postural symptoms? Have they had any falls, either at home or in the community? Have they been constipated lately? Has their vision changed (particularly diplopia)? Have they had peripheral tingling or numbness?

- Have they noticed memory loss (a collateral is very useful – but not always accurate – for this part of the patient encounter)? Screen for a variation of dementia called dementia with Lewy bodies (DLB), a condition that overlaps with Parkinson's disease, by asking if they ever experience Lilliputian delusions (seeing small people or animals). Consider performing a mini-mental state examination if one has not been completed recently.

- What has their mood been like? How has their sleep been? Screen thoroughly for depression.

- Who is their regular neurologist or geriatrician, and how often do they meet with them?

- Are they still working? Are they able to complete their ADLs, or do they have assistance for meals, cleaning, managing finances or maintaining personal hygiene already in place? Which of their symptoms is the biggest factor?

- What is their current medication regimen? Review for anything that could exacerbate their symptoms (e.g. metoclopramide, antipsychotics, certain calcium channel blockers and stimulants – including amphetamines and caffeine).

- Do they have advanced care planning in place? Have they established a medical, financial and lifestyle power of attorney for decision making if they ever lose capacity? Are they aware of the Parkinson's Foundation?

If symptoms are progressing rapidly, or the patient is not responding to typical therapies, consider the 'Parkinson's plus' syndromes such as multisystem atrophy (MSA), corticobasilar degeneration (CBD) and progressive supranuclear palsy (PSP). Although levodopa does not have a typical effect in these patients, their additional symptoms may respond to alternate drug therapy.

Examination again focuses on the neurological system. Consider performing postural blood pressures. The diagnosis of Parkinson's disease is a clinical one, with essential features including bradykinesia and either rigidity or tremor. Further supporting evidence includes response to dopaminergic therapy, unilateral onset and tremor at rest.

Parkinson's patients are treated with levodopa (coupled with carbidopa to stop the levodopa from being entirely metabolised in the periphery, not the central nervous system where it is required) once their symptoms begin to impact upon their lives. Catechol-O-methyl transferase (COMT) inhibitors may also be given to prolong the central effects of levodopa.

Parkinson's patients may also benefit from the cholinesterase inhibitor donepezil, but in Australia this medication is tightly restricted by PBS. Parkinson's patients do not always require ongoing review in specialist clinics and are usually managed by their local GP. The aim of therapy is to maintain the patient's quality of life and independence as long as possible, avoid complications of drug therapy and prevent further disability (including falls).

DIZZINESS AND VERTIGO

Dizziness is a very common complaint from patients and, in the medical context, should be differentiated from the similar conditions vertigo (an illusory abnormality of movement), presyncope (a sensation of either light-headedness or being about to lose consciousness), disequilibrium (i.e. unsteadiness and imbalance) and non-specific dizziness (all others). Nearly half of patients who present to their GP or clinic with dizziness will be diagnosed with peripheral vestibular dysfunction, 15% will have a psychiatric component to their illness and ≤10% will have a central brainstem vestibular pathology. When taking a history from the dizzy patient, enquire about the following:

- How long have they been experiencing dizziness? How often does it occur? How long does it last? Is there any time of day it is worse? Have they noticed any exacerbating or relieving factors (e.g. does it get better if they sit still)? Is it worse on initially standing up? Does noise make it worse? Can it be reproduced by turning their head rapidly to the side?

- Do they have other signs of vestibular pathology, e.g. tilt illusions (where they feel they are tilted in relation to gravity), spatial disorientation, 'drop attacks' (acute loss of tone without loss of consciousness), imbalance or oscillopsia (illusion of environmental movement, worse when their head moves)?

- Are there any other associated neurological or cardiovascular symptoms (e.g. headache, seizures, tremor, dysarthria, dysphagia, altered sensation, peripheral neuropathy, incontinence, gait disturbance, syncope, chest pain or visual changes)? Are there multiple risk factors for stroke or transient ischaemic attacks (TIAs)? Concerning 'red flag' symptoms include recent-onset weakness, dysarthria, dysphagia, chest pain, dyspnoea or syncope.

- Is there a family history of neurological conditions?

- What is their current medication regimen? Has this changed recently (especially introduction of new antihypertensives and antidepressants)?

- What is their occupation? Have they been exposed to toxins at work or home? Do they need to drive for their work? Have they ever had symptoms while driving? Discuss these risks with the patient.

Examination should include a full neurological assessment, gait assessment, routine observations and postural blood pressures. Is nystagmus present at baseline? If it is available, use a tuning fork to assess hearing. Perform the Dix–Hallpike manoeuvre (lateral rotation of the head while sitting upright), with onset of nystagmus after 5–10 s suggestive of benign paraoxysmal positional vertigo (BPPV). An excellent guide for the investigation of the dizzy patient devised by David Newman-Toker of John Hopkins University is displayed in Fig. 61.1.

The treatment for the 'dizzy' patient depends on their final diagnosis (e.g. managing diabetes, thyroid dysfunction, anaemia or electrolyte disturbance). Once a reason for their dizziness is determined, they will not necessarily require ongoing review in Neurology Clinic unless a primary neurological pathology is diagnosed.

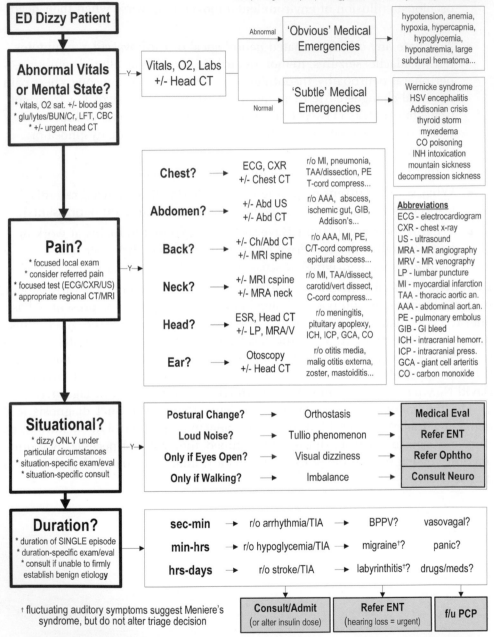

FIGURE 61.1 Triage approach to the evaluation of an Emergency Department dizzy patient.

Newman-toker, D., 2011. John Hopkins University: A new approach to the dizzy patient. NOVEL. Online image. Available from: <http://www.nanosweb.org/files/1_Newman-TokerApproachtotheDizzyPatient.pdf> (accessed 03.13.2015).

CHAPTER 62

MEDICAL ONCOLOGY OUTPATIENTS

Joseph M O'Brien

Medical Oncology is an incredibly busy rotation, both on the wards and in the clinics. As an intern, you will most likely end up managing the ward patients while the consultants, registrars and, occasionally, residents go to clinic. Bigger hospitals may even have a 'ward' registrar and an 'outpatient' registrar. Clinics are also attended by physiotherapists, occupational therapists and clinical nurse consultants (CNCs). CNCs are specially trained nurses who have done further training and subspecialised (e.g. the breast care nurses). They are an invaluable resource of information and support (for both you and the patient!).

Clinics tend to be centred around specific 'streams' of malignancy (e.g. breast, sarcoma, gastrointestinal, melanoma etc). In smaller hospitals they are combined, so clinic requires a bit more versatility. First appointment patients *must* be reviewed by a consultant or senior registrars, as often they will then present the patient's case at a multidisciplinary meeting (MDM) with surgeons, oncologists, radiation oncologists, pathologists and radiologists present. The principles of reviewing a patient with malignancy remain the same across streams:

- When was their cancer diagnosed? Did they present with symptoms, or was the malignancy detected through a screening program? How was tissue obtained? What was the stage at diagnosis, and was this completed with a computed tomography (CT) or positron-emitting tomography (PET) scan? Have they experienced any paraneoplastic syndromes (i.e. distant signs or symptoms caused by their primary malignancy, e.g. syndrome of inappropriate ADH secretion in lung cancer)?

- What regiment of chemotherapy have they had thus far? Document in the following format: 'Chemo Regiment Cycle x Day y', for example, 'FOLFOX Cycle 2 Day 12'. Note any plans for further chemotherapy.

- Have they had any surgical management of their malignancy? Who was their surgeon, and when are they due for follow-up? Was their procedure complicated? Did they require further surgeries (e.g. further resection for incomplete margins)? Are there any subsequent procedures planned?

- Have they had any radiotherapy, or is there a plan to commence it? Do they know the dose in grays (Gy)?
- If their therapy is complete – how often are they being monitored, and how? Regular PET scans? Blood work with tumour markers? Who is monitoring these? Don't forget specific tests (e.g. colonoscopies after colon cancer).
- How has their malignancy affected their activities of daily living (ADLs)? Have they required time off work, and how are they maintaining their income? Do they require any gait aids or home modifications? Try to determine the patient's (Eastern Cooperative Oncology Group (ECOG) status at present (Table 62.1), and compare it with the time of diagnosis.
- Do they continue to smoke or drink alcohol? Quantify their previous use of tobacco in pack-years (i.e. number of packs smoked per day × years spent smoking). Give advice on 'Quit' aids if necessary. If they feel they are continuing to lose weight or you suspect the patient is not otherwise meeting their nutritional needs, consider a dietitian referral.
- All cancers carry a significant psychiatric toll: give strong consideration to discussing the patient's mental wellbeing if appropriate rapport has been developed. Consider putting them in touch with appropriate peer-support networks (e.g. the Cancer Council).
- Take an extensive family history, considering a genogram. Many malignancies have a genetic component identified. If their particular malignancy is known to have a strong hereditary factor, discuss familial screening. Consider referral to Genetics Clinic if concerned.

TABLE 62.1 ECOG grading scale

GRADE	DESCRIPTION OF LEVEL OF FUNCTION
0	Completely active, with no effect on ADLs
1	Strenuous physical activity is limited by disease, but otherwise able to complete light work
2	Able to ambulate and maintain self hygiene, but unable to carry out work duties or housework
3	Only able to perform limited self care, and confined to rest (bed or chair) ≥50% waking hours
4	Completely disabled, with inability to perform self care and total confinement to rest
5	Dead

Adapted from: Oken, M.M., Creech, R.H., Tormey, D.C., et al., 1982. Toxicity and response criteria of the Eastern Cooperative Oncology Group. American Journal of Clinical Oncology 5, 649-655.

- Take a complete medical and past history. Other medical conditions will directly influence the treatment given (e.g. poor left ventricular ejection fraction [LVEF] prevents use of anthracyclines).

This chapter will outline specific history-taking questions and examination findings for some of the more common malignancies in Australia. For staging of these malignancies, please read the surgical counterpart to this chapter (e.g. colon cancer is outlined in Chapter 66, 'General Surgical Outpatients').

MELANOMA

Melanoma is the fourth most common cancer in Australia, and often associated with our previously outdoors-heavy lifestyle. Infamously aggressive and prone to metastasis, melanoma is principally managed by surgical excision. Metastatic melanoma ('met mel') carries an extremely poor prognosis, with few specific treatments available. In addition to the general oncology questions outlined above, discuss with the patient:

- What risk factors did they have? Did they spend large periods of time exposed to the sun, either for work or leisure? Did they frequent solariums? Were they exposed to the sun sporadically? Did they ever have severe sunburn?

- Do they know the 'Clark' grade of their tumour (please see Chapter 72, 'Plastic and reconstructive surgery' for melanoma staging)? Were there any lymph nodes involved? Had the cancer spread further?

- How often do they have skin checks?

- Were they exposed to petroleum, selenium, ionising radiation or polychlorinated biphenyls at work?

- Have they ever had a period of immunosuppression (e.g. infection, prior malignancy, prior chemoradiotherapy)?

Examination focuses on the primary skin lesion (if known) and signs of metastases. Note light skin, red or blonde hair, large amounts of freckling and light eye colour as these are all associated with higher risk of melanoma. If you feel confident, perform a complete skin check – many centres have tools (i.e. special forms with anatomical outlines) to assist in objectively tracking people's lesions over time. When describing potential melanomas, consider A – asymmetry, B – (irregular) border, C – colour change, D – diameter change or >6 mm and E – evolution of characteristics. Each of these factors could indicate a more serious lesion.

Investigations focus on both local and distant effects of malignancy. Complete basic bloods (FBE + UEC + CMP + LFT), lactate dehydrogenase (LDH) as a generic marker of cell turnover, a chest X-ray (CXR) for screening of metastases and review the histopathological staging of the cancer. You should also note the mitotic rate, and whether or not the tumour contained a *BRAF* mutation, as this is a potential target for therapy. Usually the patient will have had a PET scan well before review in clinic, and you should review the report. If a staging CT neck/chest/abdomen/pelvis has been performed, take note.

Treatment begins with surgical excision, with a wide surgical margin of 1–2 cm. Any affected lymph nodes are also excised. Metastatic melanoma is often not excised, with consideration of palliative chemotherapy and/or radiotherapy. Management will always be a consultant-level decision. Medical therapy includes interferon and/or high dose interleukin-2 (IL-2) in metastatic melanoma, ipilimumab (a monoclonal antibody against CTLA-4) and, if *BRAF* positive, the *BRAF* inhibitors vemurafenib and dabrafenib This is an area of rapid advancement, with new drugs such as the PD-1 inhibitors entering the market.

Palliative local radiotherapy may also be used if the patient is symptomatic. Ongoing surveillance in patients with melanoma is *vital*. Stages I and II should have annual skin checks with the above bloods. Stage III+ should have these investigations with strong consideration given to annual CXR and PET or CT scans.

BREAST CANCER

Breast cancer affects 1 in 8 Australian women (and 1 in 688 men), and is discussed frequently in the media. Although the exact mechanism of breast cancer is unknown, it is associated with advanced age, certain genetic mutations (including *BRCA1, BRCA2* and *p53*), excess alcohol consumption, obesity and prolonged exposure to oestrogen. When discussing breast cancer with a patient, cover:

- Do they know the type of breast cancer they had? Do they know the receptor status of their cancer? If not, review the pathology on the system for oestrogen receptor (ER), progesterone receptor (PR) and HER2 status.

- Was their malignancy detected by mammography screening? Was the diagnosis confirmed on fine needle aspirate (FNA) or core biopsy?

- What type of surgery did they have? Did they have any complications of their procedure? Have they experienced lymphoedema on that side? Did they have an axillary clearance?

  - Wide local excision (WLE) is the correct term for 'lumpectomy'.

  - Mastectomy refers to the removal of breast tissue.

  - Radical mastectomy involves removal of all underlying tissue down to the pectoralis muscle and also the ipsilateral axillary chain, and is now rarely necessary.

- Has the affected breast ever undergone trauma or been exposed to ionising radiation?

- Have they been on hormone replacement therapy? Did they use the oral contraceptive pill for a prolonged period? Were they on oestrogen for any other reason (e.g. IVF)?

- Take a full obstetric history. Have they completed their family?

- If there is a strong family history, have they had (or considered) genetic testing?
- Are they taking hormonal or trastuzumab (Herceptin®) therapy?
- Have they had osteoporosis screening?
- When did they experience menarche ± menopause?
- What do they do for a living? Have they led a sedentary lifestyle?

Examination should involve palpation of the breast and axillary chain (noting skin or nipple retraction or erythema, ulceration or discharge), as well as auscultation of the chest, review of the supraclavicular nodes and palpation of the abdomen (particularly right upper quadrant). Consider checking for spinal tenderness. Note pallor or cachexia. Tumours are often palpable if >10 mm in size.

Initial investigations should include basic bloodwork (FBE + UEC + CMP + LFT) as well as LDH. Imaging should include breast sonography, a mammogram and CXR. If anything is detected on CXR have a low threshold to order a CT-chest. If bony metastases are suspected, request a nuclear bone scan. If not already completed, tissue diagnosis should be confirmed with a core biopsy (or FNA if the lesion is unamenable to core). Take note of the hormone receptor status and Ki67 (pronounced kcy-67; higher number indicates higher degree of cell reproduction).

Treatment depends on the stage and receptor status of the malignancy. Surgical management is covered in Chapter 72, 'Plastic and reconstructive surgery'. Selective oestrogen receptor modulators (SERMs) such as tamoxifen and aromatase inhibitors (e.g. anastrozole) are used to 'starve' oestrogen-dependent tumours in addition to standard regimens of chemotherapy.

Trastuzumab is a monoclonal antibody against the HER2 receptor that down-regulates cell turnover. Radiotherapy is also often used for localised disease with 1–3 positive nodes in the ipsilateral axilla. See Fig. 62.1 for a standard flow chart of progression of therapy in breast cancer.

Surveillance is again necessary, with annual blood work and mammograms or breast MRI suggested. Patients should be taught to self-examine for lumps. Some patients will ask about bilateral mastectomy for prophylaxis against recurrence - this reduces risk for invasive neoplasia of the breast by 90%.

COLON CANCER

Colon cancer (colloquially known as 'bowel' cancer) is common, accounting for 12.7% of cancers in Australia (excluding non-melanoma skin cancers). It may present acutely, with altered bowel habit, haematochezia (blood mixed with stool) and/or melaena, or in a more subtle fashion with weight loss, anorexia or low-grade fevers. There is a screening program in Australia whereby people aged >55 years are requested to complete a faecal occult blood test (FOBT) to investigate microscopic haematochezia. Colon cancer is largely covered in Chapter 45, 'General Surgery'. However, patients are occasionally reviewed in Medical Oncology clinics when preparing to or currently receiving adjuvant chemotherapy. Discuss:

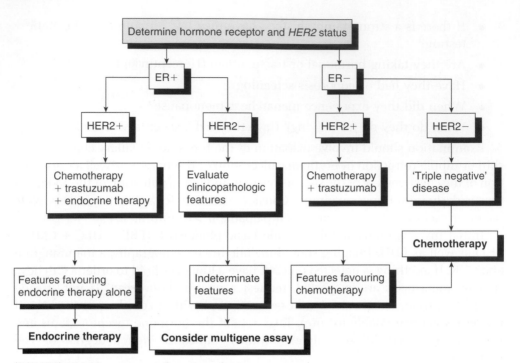

FIGURE 62.1 Management flow chart for breast cancer.

Reproduced from: Ferri, F.F., 2015. Breast cancer. In: Ferri, F.F., Ferri's Clinical Advisor. Philadelphia: Mosby.

- How was their malignancy detected?
- Who is their surgeon? Did they have a hemicolectomy (surgical resection of half the large bowel), targeted resection or polypectomy? Was their bowel reconnected immediately (i.e. joined by primary anastomosis) or did they temporarily have a stoma? If they currently have a stoma, is there a plan to reverse it? Do they see a stoma nurse?
- Does their diet contain a lot of red meat? Do they eat much fibre? How much alcohol do they consume?
- Do they have a history of inflammatory bowel disease? Do they have a family history of inflammatory bowel disease, polyps or bowel cancer?
- How often have they been advised to have surveillance colonoscopies? Who is performing these, and when is their next one due? What was their tumour marker and LDH at baseline?

Examination concentrates on the gastrointestinal system, with consideration of auscultation of the chest and heart sounds, palpation of the supraclavicular node and any sites of known metastases. Strongly consider performing a digital rectal examination (DRE), but **never** perform a DRE on a neutropenic patient due to risk of causing septicaemia.

Investigations include monitoring of basic bloods (FBE + UEC + CMP), as well as LFTs (in the case of liver metastases or hepatotoxicity from treatment), LDH and the colon cancer tumour marker carcinoembryonic antigen (CEA). Review the initial tissue pathology for description of the histological type of the tumour (e.g. adenocarcinoma, mucinous carcinoma, medullary carcinoma or poorly differentiated), surgical margins and presence of associated lymphadenopathy or genetic abnormalities (e.g. 18q deletion) or oncogenes (e.g. K-RAS, c-myc). The patient should have also had an initial staging CT-chest/abdomen/pelvis (±brain, if clinically indicated) and many will also have had a PET scan, and you should have these results on hand before presenting to the senior doctor.

First-line treatment of potentially resectable tumours will always be surgery, unless contraindicated (e.g. multiple medical comorbidities). Local colorectal cancer is usually presented at an MDM with a planned operation at a later date. If possible, tissue should be obtained by endoscopy with biopsy prior to scheduling large surgeries.

Adjuvant chemotherapy is considered for patients with stage II+ colorectal cancer – the usual combination is nicknamed FOLFOX and contains **fol**inic acid (a.k.a. 'leucovorin'), 5-fluorouracil (annotated as 5-FU, a pyrimidine analogue that disrupts synthesis of thymidine, necessary for DNA replication) and **ox**aliplatin (a platinum-based agent) An alternative course is capecitabine (a 5-FU pro drug), used either as a single agent or in combination with oxaliplatin, 5-fluorouracil and folinic acid. Raltirexed is an antimetabolite drug that may be used in the unusual circumstance of 5-FU and folinic acid intolerance.

A biological agent known as cetuximab may be used for metastatic colorectal cancer if strict criteria are met (primary tumour resected or inoperable; metastases limited to liver; patient fit for theatre if these lesions become amenable to surgery; and contraindication to oxaliplatin). They should continue to take the maximum dose of FOLFOX tolerable. Radiotherapy is considered by Radiation Oncology on a case-by-case basis.

Monitoring should continue after treatment, with CEA twice yearly for 3 years, surveillance colonoscopy at 12 months and (if clear) 5 years and a minimum of two CT-chest/abdomen/pelvis scans in the first 3 years post-op. Reinvestigation should be completed with a low threshold.

PROSTATE CANCER

Globally, prostate cancer is the second most diagnosed cancer in males. This figure is increasing due to the trend among some doctors of screening prostate-specific antigen (PSA). Risk factors include older age (with up to 73% of men over 80 years having prostate cancer noted on autopsy), positive family history, *BRCA1* and 2, obesity, tobacco smoking and occupational exposure to certain chemicals (including Agent Orange and possibly biphenyl A, used in the production of plastics).

Prostate cancer is a carcinoma, and should not be confused with benign prostatic hyperplasia (BPH), which as the name suggests is not malignant and requires treatment only when symptomatic. The surgical management of prostate cancer is outlined in Chapter 52, 'Urology'. If reviewing a patient in clinic:

SECTION V

- How did they present? Were they experiencing hesitation, post-micturition dribbling, an intermittent stream, nocturia, urinary frequency, incontinence, a sensation of incomplete voiding, suprapubic pain or complete urinary obstruction? Was their prostate enlarged on physical examination?

- Was their disease confined to the prostate, or had it spread locally or distally? The classic pattern of spread with prostate cancer is to bone and locally up the urinary tract.

- Who is their treating urologist and what surgical management have they had thus far? Did they have a trans-rectal ultrasound (TRUS) biopsy to confirm the diagnosis? Have they had a transurethral resection of the prostate (TURP), or a subtotal or radical prostatectomy?

- Were they detected on PSA screening? Do they know the value of their PSA at diagnosis? Is it currently being monitored?

- If appropriate rapport has been established – do they maintain an active sex life? Although difficult for junior doctors to discuss with their patients, many therapies for prostate cancer can cause erectile or sexual dysfunction, and the importance the patient places upon this should be understood.

- Do they have a family history of prostatic malignancy?

Examination requires a DRE (noting abnormalities in texture, consistency or size) and a general 'physical' to look for signs of metastases and chronic renal impairment. Take particular note of any sites where the patient complains of bony pain. A patient with an elevated PSA and an abnormal DRE should be referred to Urology for TRUS biopsy. Other blood work should include an FBE, UEC (for renal impairment), CMP (for hypercalcaemia with bony involvement) and LFTs (again for potential metastatic involvement).

If marrow involvement is suspected (e.g. hypercalcaemia, pancytopenia, anaemia or sclerotic lesions seen on plain X-ray) consider a CT-chest/abdomen/pelvis. CT of the pelvis does not provide optimal views and, as such, urologists often prefer MRI of this region to assess local disease. If tissue diagnosis cannot be reached from a primary prostatic biopsy and bony lesions are visible on imaging, consider a CT-guided bone biopsy.

Management of localised prostate cancer depends on the histological nature and anatomy of the malignancy, serum PSA and the patient's medical comorbidities. Treatment varies from 'wait and watch' (i.e. observational with monitoring of PSA) to immediate surgery. Adjuvant chemotherapy with androgen suppression may be of limited survival benefit but carries side effects including hot flushes, gynaecomastia, muscle loss and osteopenia. Additional forms of chemotherapy are available, but should be discussed with a multidisciplinary team and the patient before commencing treatment. Prostate cancer with local invasion is often managed with a radical prostatectomy, with consideration given to radiotherapy.

Radiotherapy for prostate cancer is either given as external beams ('normal' radiotherapy) or brachytherapy, where sources of radiation (tiny capsules or 'seeds') are placed into the body in a space close to the site of malignancy to slowly release radiation. In the case of the prostate, the seeds are inserted directly into the prostate under the guidance of ultrasound via the perineum.

With widespread metastatic disease, a referral should be made to Palliative Care. As with all malignancy, excess tobacco and alcohol consumption should be strongly discouraged. Side effects of treatment should be treated as they occur (e.g. bisphosphonates for osteopenia). Ongoing monitoring is typically done by the Urology team after surgical management.

LUNG CANCER

The fifth most common cancer in Australia, lung cancer is a significant cause of both morbidity and mortality. Neoplasia of the lung are broadly classified into small cell carcinoma and non-small cell lung cancer (NSCLC) depending on their histology. NSCLC (comprising 85% of lung cancers) can be further broken down into adenocarcinoma, squamous cell carcinoma and large cell carcinoma. Rarely, lymphoma may also present as a solitary lung mass. Some unique features of the various kinds of lung cancer are outlined in Table 62.2.

Lung cancers may present overtly, with symptoms such as non-productive cough, dyspnoea, hyperphonia (i.e. hoarse voice), haemoptysis or chest pain, in a more subtle fashion with low-grade fevers, anorexia, weight loss or, in more rare cases, Horner's syndrome or paraneoplastic syndromes. When reviewing a patient in clinic with either suspected or confirmed lung cancer, cover:

- When were they diagnosed? Do they know the subtype? How was the diagnosis confirmed?

- Have they had surgery? Was it 'keyhole' (i.e. video-assisted thoracoscopic surgery or VATS) or did they have an open procedure? Did they have chemotherapy or radiotherapy before or after the procedure?

- Have they had baseline respiratory function tests (RFTs)? How often are these performed and has there been a change?

- How is their breathing? Are they dyspnoeic? What is their effort tolerance? Are they using domiciliary oxygen (or do they require it now)? Do they have a cough – and, if present, is it productive or blood-stained?

- Do they have any other medical illnesses (especially respiratory or viral illnesses that cause immunosuppression, e.g. HIV)?

- A thorough tobacco history should be taken, including passive exposures. If still smoking, offer assistance with 'Quit' aids.

- Take a complete occupational history, including exposure to asbestos, beryllium, radon, vinyl chloride, smoke, fumes, sawdust and aerosolised substances (e.g. paints).

TABLE 62.2 Selected features of lung neoplasia

| SMALL CELL | NON-SMALL CELL | | |
	Adenocarcinoma	Squamous cell	Large cell
• Highly aggressive and generally carries poor prognosis • Seen centrally in the lungs on CXR • May excrete ectopic ACTH causing a paraneoplastic syndrome of SIADH or hypercalcaemia from PTH-related protein (PTHrP)	• Most common lung cancer in non-smokers, thus comparative incidence increasing • Typically seen peripherally in the lungs on CXR • Less responsive to radiotherapy • Managed surgically where possible • Stains positive for both mucin and TTF-1 (an adenocarcinoma cell marker) • Common genetic mutations include EGFR and HER2 • Two chromosomal rearrangements – ALK and ROS1 – can be targeted for therapy	• Seen centrally in the lungs on CXR • Male predominance • Most closely associated with smoking • Often spreads locally to hilar nodes, with later distant metastases	• Less frequent (5–10% lung cancers) • Rare in never-smokers • A diagnosis of exclusion when the histology doesn't correlate to another subtype

Adapted from: Horn, L., Eisenberg, R., Gius, D., et al., 2014. Cancer of the lung. In: Niederhuber, J.E., Armitage, J.O., Doroshow, J.H., et al., eds. Abeloff's Clinical Oncology, 5th ed. Philadelphia: Saunders.

Examine the patient for signs of respiratory illness and metastases. Note in particular cachexia, pallor, hypoxia, respiratory rate, signs of respiratory distress (e.g. use of accessory muscles of respiration), clubbing, asterixis, nicotine staining, hypothenar wasting (sign of brachial plexus compression), ptosis (droopy eyelid), miosis (constricted pupil), anhidrosis (lack of sweating), lymphadenopathy, altered respiratory sounds on auscultation or signs of right ventricular failure. Consider examining for superior vena cava obstruction with Pemberton's sign.

Investigations on initial work-up should include FBE (looking for anaemia or pancytopenia), UEC (renal impairment), LFTs (metastases), CMP (hypercalcaemia from paraneoplastic syndrome) and CRP (to exclude concurrent infection). Request a parathyroid hormone (PTH) level if hypercalcaemic – it should be 'appropriately suppressed.' Ask the patient to try and produce a sputum sample for M/C/S (more sensitive for central masses). Baseline RFTs and an echocardiogram (TTE) should be performed, both for assessment of baseline function and to see if the malignancy is affecting their respiratory state. Staging with CT-chest/abdomen/pelvis ± brain or PET should also be completed, depending on service availability.

If a tissue diagnosis has not yet been obtained, strongly consider referral to Interventional Radiology for percutaneous CT-guided biopsy, or to a respiratory physician or thoracic surgeon for bronchoscopy with biopsy and bronchoalveolar lavage (BAL). Plain CXR should be performed frequently. Biopsies should have histopathology + *EGFR* (epidermal growth factor receptor) + *K-RAS* + *ALK* (anaplastic lymphoma kinase) requested, as these particular cellular and genetic abnormalities are relevant for prognosis and as potential treatment targets.

Treatment depends on staging, the histological subtype of lung cancer and presence of *EGFR*, *KRAS* or *ALK* mutation. Most patients will be presented at a thoracics MDM prior to commencing treatment. Surgical resection ± radiotherapy is gold standard for potentially resectable NSCLC (but is often limited by comorbidity). Adjuvant chemotherapy is offered for more advanced disease, or malignancy involving the mediastinal nodes. Patients with a single metastatic location are still occasionally offered surgical resection.

Patients with widespread disease or multiple comorbidities should have an early referral to Palliative Care and strongly considered for domiciliary (i.e. home) oxygen. Unfortunately, small cell has often metastasised prior to diagnosis. As such chemotherapy is standard treatment. Prophylactic whole brain radiotherapy is used in some circumstances to prevent brain metastases.

EGFR is an extracellular protein that can be targeted by drugs (e.g. erlotinib and gefitinib). *KRAS*-positive malignancies do not respond to erlotinib or gefitinib. *ALK* may be targeted directly with an ALK inhibitor known as crizotinib. The decision to use these targeted treatments is made by a consultant (or MDM) due to their high cost.

CANCER OF UNKNOWN PRIMARY

Cancers of unknown primary ('CUP') are malignancies that by definition are stage IV (i.e. metastatic or disseminated), with primary site unidentifiable despite comprehensive investigation. They are not uncommon, comprising 8% of malignancies in Australia and causing 5% of cancer-related deaths. Prior to modern imaging, 85% were diagnosed on autopsy. They have a poor prognosis, with a 5-year progression-free survival (PFS_5) of only 16%.

CUP may present in many ways, but the most common are 'B symptoms' (weight loss, anorexia, rigors, fevers, night sweats, chills), unexplained pain, jaundice or lymphadenopathy or obstructive symptoms as a mass compresses an important structure. They may be discovered incidentally. History-taking must be broad, with an attempt to further narrow down the possible site of primary. Consider discussing:

- When did they first have their malignancy identified? How did they present?
- Did they have any localising symptoms (e.g. other masses, skin changes, regional lymphadenopathy, cough, haemoptysis, dyspnoea, chest pain, confusion, seizures, focal neurology, abdominal pain, jaundice, ascites, hormonal changes, haematemesis, melaena, haematochezia, goitre, bony pain, pathological fracture, urinary obstruction, haematuria or renal impairment)?

Similar to the history, examination in patients with a CUP must be incredibly detailed and thorough as the smallest of signs may provide a likely primary. Do not forget examination of skin and nails, breasts, testicles and rectum. Investigation of a CUP will also be broad, with basic bloods (FBE + UEC + CMP + LFT + CRP), TSH, LDH, myeloma screen (SPEP + FLC + B2M + urinary Bence-Jones protein), consideration of tumour markers (CEA + Ca19.9 + CgA + αFP + βHCG + thyroglobulin ± ALK genes, CA15-3, CA125 or PSA) and a determined effort to obtain tissue from any abnormalities. Imaging should include a CXR, mammogram in women, CT brain/neck/chest/abdomen/pelvis and consideration of whole body MRI or PET.

If indicated by symptoms or bloods, consider bone marrow for potential haematological malignancy. Consider GI endoscopy. On histological examination under light microscopy, 60% will be shown to be adenocarcinomas, 25% poorly differentiated carcinomas, 10% squamous and 5% remain indistinguishable.

Management depends on further classification of the malignancy. Poor prognostic markers include involvement of brain, pleura, lung, liver or adrenal glands. Empirical chemotherapy (for ECOG 0–2 patients) will be determined by the closest histological match for the cancer, and these patients will **always** be discussed by multiple consultants at an MDM. Radiotherapy is indicated for larger masses or those impinging upon other structures. Early Palliative Care referral is often of value, especially for ECOG 3–4 patients who are unlikely to be offered chemotherapy.

REVIEWING CHEMOTHERAPY DAY UNIT PATIENTS

A common task for a senior resident on an Oncology rotation will be to review patients in the Chemotherapy Day Unit (CDU). As there is a trend to manage patients in the community, people with stable disease will come into the hospital for a few hours to have their chemotherapy administered. They may also attend the CDU for other procedures (e.g. bone marrow aspiration and trephine, iron infusions or planned/regular blood product transfusion). Occasionally, a patient being managed at home will be sent to CDU by the Hospital in the Home (HITH) nurses if they have a medical concern.

Although the indication and type of review will differ, the key question remains the same – do you think you need to admit the patient? Ask yourself what you would do with the patient if you were a GP and this patient were in your rooms. Would you send them to the Emergency Department, keeping in mind whether or not they are immunocompromised? If concerned, contact the Outpatients registrar for assistance but be prepared with a thorough history, examination and a basic plan outline.

Have a low propensity for admission – it is easier for the inpatient team to grumble and send your patient home early, than for an Emergency Department to resuscitate a sick patient they do not know in the middle of the night. Always notify the home team of their new patient. For more assistance with Oncology emergencies, see Chapter 42, 'Medical Oncology'.

CHAPTER 63

HAEMATOLOGY OUTPATIENTS

Joseph M O'Brien

Haematology is a very busy ward rotation, involving the management of both very complex and very sick patients. As such, it will be rare that you find yourself with sufficient time to use it to assist your registrars and consultants in Haematology Clinic. However, knowledge of what is done and investigated in clinic can be useful for planning the ongoing management of inpatients.

Haematology Clinics in larger centres are broken down into subspecialties such as Blood (for investigation and management of splenomegaly, and benign and malignant anaemias, white cell disorders and platelet pathologies), Thrombosis and Haemostasis, Stem Cell Transplant, Myeloma, Skin Lymphomas (with Dermatology and Plastic Surgeons present), and 'Late Effects' (to monitor patients >2 years from transplants for long-term complications).

Smaller hospital networks may contrarily combine Haematology and Medical Oncology Clinics, depending on their patient load and available consultants. Some of the most commonly seen issues are discussed below. See Chapter 62, 'Medical Oncology outpatients' for advice on managing patients in the Chemotherapy Day Unit.

ANAEMIA

Anaemia is defined as a reduced number of circulating erythrocytes available for physiological use. In Australia, this is typically reported as <135 g/L for males and <115 g/L for females but may differ between laboratories. (NB: Your consultant may use the older units, g/dL, which would be 13.5 and 11.5, respectively.)

Diagnosing the cause of anaemia requires an understanding of both the mean corpuscular volume (MCV, or average red cell size) and iron studies (as covered in Chapter 12, 'Investigations: serology'). The MCV, measured in femtolitres (fL), is used to classify anaemias into macrocytic (>95 fL), normocytic (85–94 fL), or microcytic (<85 fL). The MCV is a clue as to the cause of the anaemia, with some causes of anaemia listed below in Table 63.1.

TABLE 63.1 Differential diagnosis of anaemia

MICROCYTIC	NORMOCYTIC	MACROCYTIC
Iron deficiency	Acute haemorrhage	Alcoholism
Anaemia of chronic disease	Haemolysis: • Valvular disease • Splenomegaly • Hereditary (e.g. spherocytosis or G6PD deficiency) • Autoimmune • Drug reaction • Burns	Megaloblastic anaemia: • Folate deficiency • Pernicious anaemia • B12 deficiency
Thalassaemia	Pregnancy	Hepatic disease
	Bone marrow failure or myelosuppression	Marrow infiltration, from malignancy or infiltrative diseases
	Anaemia secondary to liver or renal failure	Hyper- or hypothyroidism
	Mixed deficiencies	Addison's disease
		Drugs

Adapted from: Raftery, A.T., Lim, E.K.S. & Östör, A.J.K., 2014. Anaemia. In: Raftery, A.T., Lim, E.K.S. & Östör, A.J.K., Churchill's Pocketbook of Differential Diagnosis, 4th ed. Edinburgh: Churchill Livingstone, p. 543, Table 1.

Anaemia is a very common presenting complaint, particularly in the critically ill patient. People may present with lethargy, dyspnoea and worsening of vascular disease (angina or claudication). Mild-to-moderate anaemia is much better tolerated in younger populations, and may be asymptomatic and incidentally detected on routine bloodwork.

Anaemia of the elderly should not be 'normalised' and still requires investigation. When reviewing a patient for anaemia, you need to determine whether you believe it is due to a serious or benign cause and decide what action will be taken. Before talking to a registrar or consultant, ask:

- Have they experienced lethargy, dyspnoea, fatigue, claudication or chest pain? Do they feel these symptoms have been gradually getting worse, or were they quite sudden onset?

- Have they had haemoptysis, haematemesis, haematuria, haematochezia or melaena? Any lacerations or other trauma? Most patients will not have, but if you don't ask you won't know. Occult gastrointestinal (GI) bleeding is common.

- Have they had any symptoms suggestive of pancytopenia (diminished red cells, white cells and platelets), such as easy or spontaneous bruising (usually when platelets are <20,000) or recurrent infections? Have they had fevers, rigors, night sweats, chills, anorexia or weight loss that could suggest malignancy?

- What is their diet like? Do they eat sufficient green, leafy vegetables and red meat? If vegetarian or vegan, are they on regular supplements or are they tested routinely?

- Have they ever had GI surgery, particularly on the stomach? The body's only source of intrinsic factor (for absorption of vitamin B12) is located in the stomach.

- How much alcohol do they drink? Has this changed recently?

- What drugs are they on? Have they recently been on any other medications or complementary substances?

- Take a complete medical history. Ask specifically about a liver disease, renal disease or a past history of malignancy, radiotherapy and chemotherapy.

- Has anyone in their family had any bleeding, clotting or other blood diseases?

Examination focuses on signs of haematological illness (petechiae, pallor, jaundice, racial origin, palmar pallor, arthralgia, lymphadenopathy, splenomegaly, atrophic glossitis, angular stomatitis, hepatomegaly, bony tenderness, leg ulcers near the malleoli and peripheral neuropathy), and potential sources of blood loss (respiratory, GI or urinary tracts). In men, consider a testicular examination (for malignancy). Perform a digital rectal examination if indicated. Consider a full ward test to review for microscopic haematuria.

Investigations, if not already completed, should include a *current* FBE (drastic changes should be repeated for confirmation), UEC, LFT, B12, folate, iron studies, thyroid-stimulating hormone (TSH) and coagulation studies, with consideration given to myeloma screen – serum protein electrophoresis (SPEP), free light chains (FLC), beta-2 microglobulin (B2M) – and a 'haemolytic screen' – fractionated bilirubin, direct antibody test (DAT), blood film with spherocyte and reticulocyte count and lactate dehydrogenase (LDH) – based on your history.

A faecal occult blood test (FOBT) may also be of value. In certain ethnic groups, consider haemoglobin electrophoresis for detection of sickle cell and thalassaemia. If B12 deficiency is noted, request anti-parietal cell antibodies and anti-intrinsic factor antibodies to look for true pernicious anaemia (with antibodies against stomach cells leading to decreased B12 absorption). If none of the above investigations provides a satisfactory diagnosis, consider gastroscopy and colonoscopy, and/or bone marrow aspirate and trephine (BMAT).

Treatment will depend on the underlying cause of anaemia. Admission from clinic may be required if the patient is severely anaemic, with consideration of blood transfusion for a Hb <80 (or symptomatic disease).

NEUTROPENIA

White blood cells are classified morphologically and functionally, with neutrophils being the workhorse of the immune system's front line. When deplete, a person is at high risk of life-threatening infection. Neutropenia is defined by the World Health Organization (WHO) as $<1.8 \times 10^9$ cells/L, but be mindful other institutions may have other definitions (1.5×10^9/L is common). It is commonly encountered in the setting of malignancy – both from the malignant process itself, and in its treatment with chemoradiotherapy.

Febrile neutropenia is an emergency condition and covered in Chapter 42, 'Medical Oncology'. Chronic neutropenia is a reduced neutrophil count persistent ≥ 3 months. A less common referral from community doctors, referrals for investigation of neutropenia should always be discussed with a senior doctor. Ask about:

- The patient's infectious history. Are they getting regular or recurrent infections? Do they have any sick contacts? Have they travelled recently? (If appropriate) have they ever used IV drugs? Have they had any risky sexual encounters? Viruses of many species can cause myelosuppression, from minor viral pneumoniae to the viral hepatitises and human immunodeficiency virus (HIV).

- Have they had fevers, rigors, night sweats, chills, anorexia or weight loss that could suggest malignancy? Do they have bony pain, kidney stones, episodes of confusion or polydipsia suggestive of hypercalcaemia (which is common in malignancy)?

- Has the patient ever had a malignancy or infiltrative disease process, and how was it managed? Do they have a history of autoimmune illness or atopy?

- How much alcohol do they drink?

- What medications do they take regularly? Have these changed recently? Some of the drugs implicated in neutropenia include chemotherapy, trimethoprim with sulfamethoxazole, NSAIDs, clozapine, carbimazole, flecainide, digoxin, spironolactone, amphotericin B, quinine, macrolides, chloramphenicol, vancomycin and sulfasalazine.

- Is there a family history of malignancy or haematological disorder? What is the patient's ethnicity (some diseases are more common in certain population groups)?

Examination again covers haematological signs, but must also include review for signs of autoimmune disease (e.g. arthralgias and bony pain), infection and non-haematological malignancy. A thorough examination of the spleen and lymph nodes is a necessity.

Serology should include: a current FBE (with differential counts, and compared with older studies if available); UEC and LFT (for possible infiltrate and signs of alcoholic or viral liver disease); a nutritional panel including folate, B12 and copper; consideration of an autoimmune screen (antinuclear antibodies, anti-neutrophil cytoplasmic antibodies, complement 3 and 4 levels and anti-double-stranded DNA); screening for subclinical infection with ESR and CRP; a myeloma screen (SPEP + FLC + B2M); and a chest X-ray (both to exclude malignancy or granulomatous disease, and subclinical infection). A BMAT may be indicated if no cause is found on less invasive tests, or the suspicion of malignancy is high.

If asymptomatic, neutropenia could be investigated and monitored (e.g. initially fortnightly, then less frequently if they remain well). If a patient seen in clinic has an active infection and a neutropenia, they should be admitted for antibiotics and investigation. Appropriateness of granulocyte colony-stimulating factor (GCS-F, a protein that promotes production of granulocytes in the marrow) is determined by a consultant.

THROMBOSIS AND HAEMOSTASIS

Thrombosis Clinics are very busy. Recall how many deep vein thromboses (DVTs) you've seen on the ward – then add to those the community-based referrals! The majority of patients in Thrombosis and Haemostasis Clinic will have already been started on an anticoagulant therapy for a DVT or pulmonary embolism (PE). In this circumstance, your role is to determine the need for a thrombophilia screen (i.e. was the DVT provoked or unprovoked?) and the length of duration for the anticoagulation.

Ideally, if making a referral to one of these services you should at least request an FBE, UEC and coagulation studies. Also reviewed by consultants in these clinics are thrombophilias (patients with a tendency to clot), polycythaemia (too many red blood cells) and other bleeding disorders. When taking a history, discuss:

- What were the circumstances of the patient's clot? Was it 'provoked' (i.e. do they currently have cancer, or had they had surgery, suffered a traumatic injury, received hormone therapy or been significantly immobile within 3 months) or unprovoked? Do they still have a swollen or tender limb?
  - If they are able to provide you with one, an ultrasound report of the initial clot is very useful. Note the location and length of the clot (particularly in lower limbs whether or not it is above the knee), and the degree of occlusion. Larger and more proximal vessel thromboses are considered more important.
  - Occasionally, due to a lack of understanding, you will see a patient with a superficial vein thrombosis who has been inappropriately anticoagulated and referred to Haematology. These are often provoked by IV lines or trauma and need anticoagulation only if extensive or causing significant discomfort to the patient.
- If a patient with PE, do they have ongoing dyspnoea, chest pain, cough or haemoptysis? Did they also have peripheral clot screening to search for DVT?
- Do they have any symptoms suggestive of malignancy (see above)?

- Is there a family history of clotting disorders (e.g. PE, DVT, strokes, acute coronary syndromes or known thrombophilias)?
- What is their current medication list and medical history?
- Quantify their smoking history.

Examine for bruising, swollen, tender or erythematous limbs (especially important with a single swollen limb) and signs of malignancy (e.g. cachexia, lymphadenopathy). If the patient had a PE, auscultate their chest. Investigation is determined by the history and examination findings. A single episode of provoked DVT does not require a thrombophilia screen; however, you might consider doing so in a person who has had two provoked clots.

The standard thrombophilia screen would be requested in a patient with an unprovoked clot. As outlined in Chapter 12, 'Investigations: serology', this includes FBE + UEC + CRP + ESR + factor V Leiden + proteins C and S + antithrombin III + ANA + anti-dsDNA + anti-cardiolipin + anti-b2 glycoprotein 1 ± prothrombin gene. DVTs should be re-imaged with ultrasound at 6 weeks to check for clot resolution.

If the patient has had a provoked DVT or PE, the usual period of anticoagulation is 3 months (with the exception of malignancy, which is a persistent risk factor and thus managed like an unprovoked event). Unprovoked and proximal clots are typically anticoagulated for life. Unprovoked, distal DVTs may be anticoagulated for 3–6 months then reviewed.

Anticoagulation may be performed with warfarin (requiring ongoing monitoring of INRs and co-administration of low-molecular-weight heparin until therapeutic) or one of the novel oral anticoagulants (NOACs), rivaroxaban, apixaban or dabigatran. Rivaroxaban requires a loading dose of 15 mg PO BD for 3 weeks, which is a good time to bring a patient back to Haematology Clinic and convert them to the ongoing dose of 20 mg PO daily.

Before stopping someone's anticoagulation ensure their level of mobility has improved sufficiently, and discuss their case with the consultant or registrar. Inferior vena cava (IVC) filters may be used in patients who remain at high risk with an absolute contraindication to, or failure of, anticoagulation therapy.

THROMBOCYTOPENIA

Thrombocytopenia is defined as a decrease in platelets to $<150 \times 10^9/L$, being considered a moderate reduction if <100 and severe if <50. The causes are many, and the action taken usually depends on the patient's risk factors. The obvious concern with a low platelet count is bleeding, but there are rare cases (such as disseminated intravascular coagulation or DIC, antiphospholipid syndrome, thrombotic microangiopathies and heparin-induced thrombocytopenia syndrome or HITS) where the danger is thrombosis.

There is no clear consensus regarding 'safe' levels of platelets for people in the community. Some guidelines suggest a count of <10 is high risk for spontaneous bleeding, <50 is a contraindication for smaller surgical cases and minor procedures and <100 for orthopaedic, cranial or thoracic surgeries.

In thrombocytopenia, there is insufficient megakaryocyte production in the marrow, increased destruction by antibodies or consumption as clots, or pooling in the spleen. The life expectancy of a platelet is 8–10 days. Ask:

- Has the patient experienced spontaneous or minimal trauma bleeding (e.g. gums when brushing teeth)? Common sites of bleeding include joints (haemarthrosis), GI tract (melaena or haematochezia), urinary tract (haematuria), nose (epistaxis) and respiratory tract (haemoptysis). If they do bleed, does it take a long time to stop?
- Conversely, have they had a VTE (see above for questions to ask about clots)?
- Have they got focal symptoms of infection? Have they been generally unwell, suggesting a viral illness?
- Do they have any symptoms suggestive of malignancy?
- If of reproductive age and female – is there the possibility of pregnancy? Up to 5% of women develop an idiopathic thrombocytopenia of pregnancy.
- Have they ever had chemo- or radiotherapy in the past?
- Do they have any mechanical valves or vascular grafts that may be mechanically destroying circulating platelets?
- Is there a family history of platelet disorders?
- What is their current medication list and medical history? Many medications can cause thrombocytopenia and common ones to look out for include diuretics, vancomycin, quinines, phenytoin, NSAIDs and aspirin.
- Do they have an obvious dietary insufficiency (suggestive of B12 deficiency)?
- Quantify their smoking history.
- How much alcohol do they consume? Not only can alcohol suppress platelet production, but the portal hypertension of chronic liver disease can lead to platelet sequestration in the spleen.

On examination, look for signs of recent or past bleeding, petechial rash and lymphadenopathy. Investigations should include FBE, UEC, LFTs, coags and consideration of B12, a blood film, TSH and viral serology (including HIV, EBV, CMV and VZV – if indicated). Patients with concurrent renal failure should be urgently reviewed.

Treatment depends on the underlying aetiology of thrombocytopenia. Corticosteroids (e.g. prednisolone) are given first line for immune thrombocytopenia purpura (ITP) when the platelets reach <50. Pregnant patients are normally monitored closely for the development of either preeclampsia or HELLP (haemolysis, elevated liver enzymes and low platelets), but the majority with gestational thrombocytopenia go on to have normal deliveries. Drug-induced thrombocytopenia should be discussed with a consultant and the patient – while some can be easily ceased (e.g. NSAIDs), others such as anti-epileptics may require crossover to another agent. Patients with a high suspicion of malignancy should be considered for further evaluation, and must be reviewed by a consultant.

MONITORING OF HAEMATOLOGICAL MALIGNANCIES

As much as possible, patients with haematological malignancies are managed as outpatients. They are admitted for administration of initial chemotherapy, monitoring with high-risk treatment (e.g. when having mobilisation for CD_{34} cell collection) and when experiencing disease progression, infections or complications of their treatment. The following is a template for discussion with a patient you review in clinic; however, keep in mind all management decisions should be conveyed to the treating haematologist.

- What is their diagnosis? How was it initially detected? How was the diagnosis confirmed? Have they had a BMAT? Did they have a staging CT or PET, and where was it done?

- Have they had any therapy yet? If so, document in the following format: 'Chemo Regimen Cycle *x* Day *y*'; for example, 'R-CHOP Cycle 4 Day 12.' Note any plans for further chemotherapy or radiotherapy. If known, radiotherapy is expressed as Grays (Gy) with total dose over the dose delivered per cycle (e.g. 75 Gy/5).

- Were these treatments marred by any complications? Did they require change of therapy (e.g. substitution of another agent)?

- Have they had any infective symptoms? Signs of marrow failure (e.g. dyspnoea and fatigue from anaemia, bruising from thrombocytopenia or opportunistic infection from neutropenia)? Have they been to their local doctor with any other complaints?

- Who is their treating haematologist? Do they have ongoing monitoring blood tests and, if so, at what frequency (e.g. a common plan is Mon/ Wed/Fri bloods)?

- What is their current medication regimen? Are they on antibacterial, antiviral, antifungal, or *Pneumocystis jirovecii* pneumonia (PJP) prophylaxis? Are they still on tumour lysis prophylaxis and, if so, can this be stopped?

- Go through their complete medical, past, family and social history.

Examination should focus on progression of disease, signs of infection and complications of treatment (which are regimen-specific). Review any investigations completed prior to the appointment, and trends in the FBE and UEC. Read any correspondence from Radiation Oncology, Pathology and/or Radiology. Haematology patients can get sick very quickly, and you should have a low propensity for admission if they are unwell. Discuss all cases with a consultant.

SECTION V

CHAPTER 64

RHEUMATOLOGY OUTPATIENTS

Joseph M O'Brien

Rheumatology is not a common rotation for junior doctors per se; however, rheumatological presentations are common amongst the general population. With few inpatients under their bed card, the Rheumatology teams often share their residents with another speciality. Common subspecialty 'Rheum' clinics include Joint Clinic, Connective Tissue, Rheumatism, Osteoporosis and Metabolic Bone (sometimes a service provided by Endocrinology), Chronic Pain and Rehabilitation. Some highly specialised centres have disease-specific clinics (e.g. lupus or scleroderma). Clinics are also attended by physiotherapists, occupational therapists (OTs) and often social workers to help optimise the patient's home situation.

RHEUMATOID ARTHRITIS AND ANKYLOSING SPONDYLITIS

Rheumatoid arthritis (RA) is a polyarthritis (i.e. many joints) that is typically symmetrical, inflammatory and initially peripheral (often in the hands and feet). Ankylosing spondylitis is also an inflammatory, systemic joint condition, but is limited to the axial skeleton and sacroiliac joints. Although they are quite separate illnesses, the principles of their management are similar.

A person with suspected disease (i.e. someone with symmetrical small joint involvement in more than three locations) should be referred to a specialist clinic early, with prompt investigation, early implementation of disease-modifying antirheumatic drugs (DMARDs), close monitoring of disease activity and use of additional agents (e.g. NSAIDs or corticosteroids) as breakthrough relief when required. Much of the damage caused (including commencement of joint erosion) happens in the early stages of disease. When reviewing a patient in clinic, discuss:

- When were they diagnosed with RA? How was it confirmed? Do they have a regular rheumatologist? Have they had the 'initial' blood work? Have their arthralgias been better or worse since then? Have they had joint swelling, heat or tenderness? Is their joint pain worse in the morning, and does it last >30 minutes? Have their symptoms persisted >4 weeks?

- What treatment was started initially? Did it work – and, if so, for how long? What was the next step in management? Did they experience any complications from their treatment? How often do they experience a flare requiring breakthrough medication (or even admission) for analgesia?

- Have they experienced any extraarticular complications of RA – i.e. pulmonary disease, splenomegaly or fracture? Do they have osteoporosis screening? How is their cardiac health? Has their vision changed? Patients with RA have an increased incidence of cardiovascular events.

- How does their RA affect their activities of daily living (ADLs)? Are they still able to work? If not, where do they get their income (e.g. disability support pension or 'DSP')? Are they requiring gait aids? Do they feel they are coping? A brief screen for depression is advisable, with implementation of psychosocial aids if necessary.

- Do they have any other medical conditions? Have they had any surgery before (especially orthopaedic)?

- If on DMARDs – have they had any signs of myelosuppression (such as recurrent infections, spontaneous bruising, ulcers, fatigue or dyspnoea), liver disease (fatigue, jaundice), pulmonary deterioration (e.g. 'methotrexate lung'), renal impairment, new rashes or gastrointestinal upset (nausea, vomiting, melaena, PR bleeding)
  - If female – do they plan on becoming pregnant? RA often remits during pregnancy, but their immunosuppression should be reviewed by a consultant as it can have significant implications.

- Do they smoke? Smoking increases the activity of disease and is associated with an increased frequency of flares. Provide assistance with smoking cessation if amenable.

Examination in RA patients should be thorough, examining not only their joints but more systemically to detect any potential complications of their disease and side effects of treatment (including ischaemic heart disease, osteoporosis, interstitial pneumonitis, liver disease, renal disease, splenomegaly and hypertension). Do not exclude gait examination if the lower limbs are involved. If assessing a patient with ankylosing spondylitis, perform Schober's test to objectively measure their back flexion.

Consider a baseline grip strength and plain film X-rays of affected joints. If there is an effusion in any joint, strongly consider aspiration. Baseline serology should include a 'rheumatoid screen' with FBE, UEC, LFT, CRP, erythrocyte sedimentation rate (ESR), anti-citrullinated protein antibody (anti-CCP), rheumatoid factor (RF), complement 3 and 4 levels and ANA (if the diagnosis is not already clear, ANA could be used for alternative diagnoses). It is possible to have RF negative disease.

Prior to commencing DMARDs, a serological screen should be completed (above investigations + HBV + HCV + chest X-ray ± QuantiFeron® Gold) to assess baseline renal and liver function, obtain a value of baseline inflammatory markers and prevent reactivation of latent disease.

The choice of DMARD will ultimately be the consultant's, as will any change in therapy or progression to biological agents. DMARDs are all immunosuppressants and require close monitoring (see Table 64.1). Typically, one or two agents are started simultaneously (e.g. methotrexate with short-term glucocorticoids) with progression to addition of TNF-alpha inhibitors (e.g. adalimumab, etanercept and infliximab) after 6 months without response, then consideration of rituximab, and ultimately a combination of all of the above therapies. Ongoing monitoring of both disease activity (with CRP preferably to ESR) and for complications of treatment is necessary as outlined below with regard to specific treatments. Before commencing DMARDs, it is important to consider a patient's family planning.

Non-pharmaceutical optimisation should be completed concurrently whenever starting DMARD therapy, including advice for the patient on their condition,

TABLE 64.1 Monitoring of DMARD therapy

DRUG	SIDE EFFECTS	MONITORING
Gold-based	Hepatic failure Renal failure Myelosuppression	FBE + UEC + LFT + urinalysis with each injection
Penicillamine	Renal impairment Anorexia GI upset	FBE + UEC ± urinalysis fortnightly for 3 months, then monthly
Methotrexate	Interstitial pulmonitis Liver disease Myelosuppression Ulcerative gastritis Fatigue Fever	FBE + UEC + LFT ± folate each review, more frequently when initiating. FBE initially fortnightly, more frequently after dose increases
Chloroquinines	GI upset Alopecia or hair bleaching Visual loss	Annual optometry
Infliximab	Hypersensitivity Reactivation of latent illness Immunosuppression Lymphoma Drug lupus Hepatic derangement Vitiligo Psoriasis Solid tissue cancers	FBE + UEC+ LFT + ESR monthly

TABLE 64.1 Monitoring of DMARD therapy—cont'd

DRUG	SIDE EFFECTS	MONITORING
Cyclosporine	GI upset Gingival hyperplasia Pancreatitis Delirium Peripheral neuropathy Nephrotoxicity Hepatotoxicity Hypertension Dyspnoea	FBE + LFT monthly for 6 months then once every 2 months. UECs fortnightly until stable for 3 months
Leflunomide		FBE + UEC + LFT monthly
Sulfasalazine	Depression Temporary infertility Thrombocytopenia Hepatic failure Haemolytic anaemia	FBE + UEC + LFT fortnightly for 3 months, then gradually weaned out to quarterly. Consider quarterly sulfasalazine levels
Etanercept	Hypersensitivity Reactivation of latent illness Immunosuppression Lymphoma Drug lupus Hepatic derangement Vitiligo Psoriasis Solid tissue cancers	FBE + UEC + LFT monthly

Adapted from: Knott, L., 2009. Disease-modifying antirheumatic drugs (DMARDs). In: Patient.co.uk [Internet]. <http://www.patient.co.uk/doctor/disease-modifying-antirheumatic-drugs-dmards-pro>.

weight loss, diet, exercise, appropriate levels of rest and a plan for breakthrough pain. Consider opportunistic vaccination. A referral to hand surgeons should be considered with resistant synovitis of ≥3 months. RA patients are typically reviewed annually in a specialist clinic with regular GP appointments between.

OSTEOARTHRITIS

Osteoarthritis (OA; a.k.a. osteoarthrosis) is a degenerative joint disease resulting from multiple factors including 'wear and tear' mechanical force, genetics and inflammation, resulting in breakdown of the bone and cartilage. It is a significant cause of disability and pain for the general populace, with few management options having a legitimate effect on mobility. Osteoarthritis is discussed in detail in Chapter 67, 'Orthopaedic outpatients'.

GOUT AND PSEUDOGOUT

Gout is an inflammatory arthritis caused by the build-up of urate that causes severe, debilitating pain. Pseudogout – known as calcium pyrophosphate deposition disease – causes similar symptoms to gout, but is due to precipitation of calcium pyrophosphate dihydrate (CPPD) crystals in connective tissues rather than urate.

Gout is often described by patients as, 'The worst pain I've ever felt'. Patients with severe enough pain may need admission for analgesia. Gout is typically monoarticular (i.e. one joint), but can affect multiple joints and cause a significant increase in biochemical markers of inflammation (e.g. ESR and CRP), fevers and joint effusions. When discussing gout with a patient in clinic, discuss:

- When was their first attack of gout? How was it confirmed (e.g. joint aspiration, or assumed from a high serum uric acid level)? Which joint(s) were affected? What treatment did they receive? Did they go on 'prophylaxis' with allopurinol (sold as Progout)? Have they had a recurrent attack since their first episode? Do they know what precipitates their attacks?

- Take a dietary history, especially consumption of alcohol, meat and seafood. Do they drink much free water? Have they recently increased the amount of meat they eat (e.g. a long-term vegetarian moving back to eating meat)?

- Do they have a family history of rheumatological disease?

- Take a complete medical and past history.

Examine all of the person's joints, concentrating on the affected area. Be mindful if inflamed; it will be principally tender. Note any tophi (i.e. periarticular protrusions caused by uric acid crystal deposition). Investigations should include basic blood work (FBE + UEC + CMP), LFT (in the case of liver damage from alcohol, which precipitates gout), serum uric acid (to support diagnosis) and fasting lipid profile (hypertriacylglyceridaemia is associated with gout) and glucose (diabetes is also of higher incidence amongst people with gout).

Consider joint aspiration if there is an effusion (remember to request polarised microscopy, Gram stain, cell count and culture on the slip). Gout crystals have strongly negative birefringence, and pseudogout has weakly positive. A plain film X-ray of the joint could be considered. Consider a 24-hour urinary uric acid, to determine if a patient is an 'over-excreter' of uric acid (and thus will require ongoing attack prophylaxis).

Pseudogout is managed supportively with analgesia and rest of the affected joint. An acute episode of gout is managed with NSAIDs and colchicine. The dose of colchicine recommended by the *Australian Medicines Handbook* is 1 mg PO stat, followed by 0.5 mg 1 hour later with no further colchicine administered for 72 hours. Colchicine may cause abdominal pain and diarrhoea. Pain is managed with NSAIDs (unless contraindicated by peptic ulcer disease; renal, heart, or liver failure; or poorly controlled hypertension) with consideration of adjunct prednisolone for severe attacks.

Rasburicase is an enzyme that metabolises uric acid, and a recombinant version sold as Respirakase is available on the Australian market (at great cost). It is only used in emergencies, as it is only currently supplied on PBS for patients undergoing chemotherapy with tumour lysis syndrome. Allopurinol should not be given in the acute phase as it can make a gout attack worse – if considered for prophylaxis, it should be commenced 2–4 weeks later by their local doctor. Allopurinol prophylaxis would be indicated with severe gout, regular recurrence, soft tissue tophi, confirmed high urinary uric acid excretion or gout in the setting of renal impairment. Allopurinol requires dose-adjustment for renal patients.

Non-pharmaceutical management should also be discussed with the patient, including transition to a low purine or 'gout diet'. Consider providing the patient with a handout from the internet. Advise weight loss if overweight, reduction in alcohol consumption (especially beer) and smoking cessation if necessary. If the patient is on a hydrochlorothiazide diuretic, consider switching to an alternative antihypertensive. Explain to the patient that gout is a relapsing/remitting condition, and to expect further episodes in the future despite best adherence to their management plan.

CONNECTIVE TISSUE DISORDERS

'Connective tissue disorders' is a very broad term, used here to refer to systemic lupus erythematosus (SLE), scleroderma (denoted as Scl, and as systemic sclerosis when widespread), polymyositis, mixed connective tissue disease and the undifferentiated diseases that make up 25% of this category. Rheumatoid arthritis and isolated Sjögren's syndrome (a constellation of symptoms incorporating dry eyes, dry mouth and a rheumatic component) are included by some texts in this category of illness.

Diagnosis can be difficult, as there is significant overlap between these conditions. Patients often present with non-specific signs and symptoms such as myalgias, weakness, fatigue, arthralgias and low-grade fevers. Referrals are often made to Rheumatology Clinic for follow-up of positive antibody titres (e.g. ANA, ENA or ANCA), with request for ongoing management. When reviewing these patients in clinic, try to gather as much of the following information as possible prior to reporting back to the consultant or registrar:

- What is their diagnosis? When was it made? How was it confirmed? Who is their regular rheumatologist? Was treatment initiated straightaway? If so, what doses? Has it needed to be escalated or decreased due to side effects? Have they required addition of any further agents? Have they ever used any biological agents (e.g. infliximab)?

- If as yet undiagnosed, have they had any symptoms that could suggest a specific diagnosis? Examples include pleurisy, pericarditis, alopecia, malar rash or photosensitivity in SLE; Raynaud's, dysphagia or patches of tightened skin in scleroderma; tremors or proximal weakness in polymyositis; or dry eyes and dry mouth in Sjögren's.

- o Side effects of steroid use: hyperglycaemia, weight gain, GI upset, insomnia, metallic taste, mood changes, weakness (especially in proximal muscles), Cushing's syndrome, osteoporosis, cataracts, glaucoma, hypertension, thin skin and delayed wound healing.
- Do they have any other medical conditions? Have they required surgery?
- How is their disease affecting their home situation, employment and hobbies? Do they need gait aids or home modification? Consider OT and physiotherapy review.
- Are their vaccinations current?
- Do they smoke? Advise smoking cessation and provide access to 'Quit' aids if necessary.
- Have they had osteoporosis screening? Have they had their cardiovascular health optimised?
- Is their renal function and thyroid state being monitored?
- Enquire about their mental health. Connective tissue diseases can be difficult to live with and often have a significant psychiatric toll associated. In men, ask about sexual dysfunction if appropriate rapport has been established.

Examination must be thorough, and covers all major systems. Aside from examining joints, also examine the head and neck, auscultate the heart sounds and lung fields and palpate the abdomen. Skin check in many connective tissue diseases is a necessity. If not done by the clinic nurse prior to the appointment, take the blood pressure. Note particularly signs of progressive disease, pathognomonic signs (e.g. malar rash in SLE) and indications of side effects of treatment (e.g. Cushing's syndrome or signs of diabetes).

Investigations should be targeted. A current FBE + UEC + LFT is useful, and TSH and fasting glucose and lipids should be monitored for side effects of treatment. ESR or CRP are commonly used as substitute markers of disease activity, with CK if muscle damage is suspected. Imaging of the chest with plain film is suggested if signs of pulmonary disease are present, with consideration of high resolution CT (HRCT)-chest if positive. Respiratory function (RFTs) should be done at baseline and every 1–2 years. If renal function deteriorates, urinalysis should be performed with cast microscopy. A transthoracic echocardiogram should be considered for evaluation of pulmonary hypertension. Refractory reflux should be considered for endoscopy.

Treatment of the connective tissue diseases is primarily with DMARDs and corticosteroids initially, progressing to more powerful agents (such as biological agents and immunosuppressants) only if required. Acute flares may be managed with simple analgesia and NSAIDs (if there are no contraindications such as ulcerative disease or renal impairment). Plasmaphoresis may be of use if circulating immune complexes are involved in the disease process. Monitoring and patient education are essential.

OSTEOPOROSIS AND OSTEOPENIA

Osteoporosis (OP) is a progressive disease involving reduced bone mineral density and increased bone fragility, resulting in greatly increased risk of fracture. It is rigorously defined as a bone mineral density (BMD) with a T-score of −2.5 or lower, typically measured at the pelvis and/or femur. Osteopenia is lower than normal bone mineral density, not yet meeting the required degree of bone loss to constitute osteoporosis, with a T-score of between −1 (normal) and −2.5.

Osteoporosis is common, and most infamously affects post-menopausal women (although it does also affect men and pre-menopausal women). Other risk factors include progressive age, family history, physical inactivity, inadequate nutrition (especially a diet low in calcium), persistent use of steroids, anti-epileptic agents or proton pump inhibitors, and many chronic illnesses (including but not limited to inflammatory bowel, rheumatism, liver disease, renal disease and solid tumour and haematological malignancies).

Subsequently, osteoporosis can be divided into primary (subsequent to genetic factors or nutritional deficiency) or secondary (due to another identifiable cause [e.g. endocrine disturbance]). As such, history should encompass:

- How and when they were diagnosed with osteoporosis? Did they require a BMD scan, or did they have a pathological or low impact fracture? Have they had regular bone densitometry performed?

- Do they have any other medical conditions? Is there osteoporosis related to another illness?

- What medications are they on? Take particular note of long-term steroids, aromatase inhibitors, proton pump inhibitors, selective serotonin reuptake inhibitors and anti-epileptics.

- What is their current level of activity? What is their effort tolerance? Do they have any gait aids or home modifications in place? Do they require any?

- Do they have a family history of osteoporosis, multiple fractures, low impact trauma or other rheumatological conditions?

- Take a dietary history, and recommend minimisation of alcohol if required.

- Similarly, advise to quit smoking if necessary.

Examination may not demonstrate any abnormalities. Review for signs of systemic illness and causes of secondary osteoporosis, as is the case in 20% of patients. Investigation initially can be quite broad, with baseline bloods (FBE + UEC + LFT), CMP, TSH, parathyroid hormone (PTH), vitamin D and testosterone in men. If alkaline phosphate (ALP) is elevated, consider requesting a fractionated ALP that will differentiate biliary from bone source. If not already completed, bone densitometry should be performed. Repeat bone densitometry is advised in 10–15 years for women with a normal T-score, in 3–5 years with osteopenia and annually with osteoporosis. If fracture is suspected, plain films should be requested.

Some units have clinics that are specifically designed to address busy acute patient workloads, and serve as an avenue for early review for emergency and trauma that present to primary care facilities and the ED:

- Fracture clinics
  - These clinics form the majority of the acute outpatient workload for the Orthopaedic Unit. New referrals come from the Emergency Department, GPs and other peripheral hospitals without an orthopaedic service. Some review patients from previous fracture clinics are also booked appointments during these clinics for surveillance of conservatively managed fractures. Patients are nearly always required to have recent imaging for a complete assessment, which should be organised prior to the appointment.
- Wound clinics
  - Wound (or dressing) clinics are commonly associated with Plastic Surgery units; however, large volume General Surgery and Orthopaedic clinics will often use nurse-led clinics for reviews of wounds and dressings.
  - Plastic Surgery patients with healing skin grafts, minor hand wounds and stable chronic wounds can be reviewed by nurse-led wound clinics. Patients will initially be referred to the doctor-led clinic for initial assessment, but can be diverted to the wound clinic.

Booking post-discharge appointments

The junior doctor should ensure that each patient has a clear and appropriate follow-up plan booked. Typically, the treating team will document the preferred review timeframe in the patient's progress notes on the ward, and the nursing staff will liaise with the ward clerks to book the appointment. For patients who require time sensitive reviews, it's best to specify the clinic date and reviewing clinician in the progress notes and confirm the appointment time directly with the ward clerks. In any case the name of the clinic should be specified as documenting follow-up for 'wound review' can often lead to patients having incorrectly booked appointments in the Plastic Surgery wound clinics.

ELECTIVE THEATRE BOOKINGS

Almost all elective cases are booked through outpatient clinics. The process involves the completion of:

- notice of future admission form (for theatre bookings), indicating the proposed procedure, the treating clinician/unit and urgency category
- written informed consent
- a health questionnaire for the patient to complete.

Most busy metropolitan surgical units employ a 'liaison nurse' who is responsible for coordinating with the consultant surgeons and theatre bookings staff to

TABLE 65.1 National standard elective waiting list urgency categories

URGENCY CATEGORY	TIMELINE FOR ADMISSION
Category 1	Within 30 days as condition has the potential to deteriorate quickly to become an emergency
Category 2	Within 90 days as condition causes pain, dysfunction or other disability. Not likely to deteriorate quickly or become an emergency
Category 3	Admission at some point in the future for a condition having minimal clinical impact and does not have the potential to become an emergency. Some states list this urgency category as less than 365 days

Australian Institute of Health and Welfare, 2012. National definitions for elective surgery categories. Canberra: Australian Institute of Health and Welfare. <http://www.aihw.gov.au/WorkArea/DownloadAsset.aspx?id=10737421533>.

plan the scheduled theatre lists. An essential aspect of planning these lists is designating a clinical priority for any proposed procedure (see Table 65.1).

Another aspect of the waiting list categories relates to whether a patient is 'ready for care', that is, is currently suitable to undergo a procedure. Some states list these patients as 'category 4', typically reserved for those patients who are to have staged operations with a recommended minimum waiting time between procedures. Other patients with low acuity surgical issues can also elect to be declared 'not ready for care' due to work or personal issues.

Once the patient's procedure and clinical urgency category have been determined, the patient can be placed on the waiting list. If the unit does not have a liaison nurse to help book elective cases, often the junior doctors are required to submit these forms to the bookings office.

There will be situations in which GPs or patients themselves will call the hospital and the treating team to report deterioration in their clinical symptoms. These patients should have been seen in a clinic appointment to determine whether they require a change in their clinical priority.

DOCUMENTATION

As with any patient encounter, accurate and complete documentation is essential for continuity of care. Most hospital networks use dictation software to create formal letters to GPs and other referring clinicians (Chapter 55).

For patients who have had imaging or pathology investigations, it's important to include the results in correspondence so that the referring clinician is made aware of the clinical progress of the patient and to confirm that these investigations have indeed been reviewed and noted. For results (such as incomplete or unsatisfactory excisions) that require further discussion with the unit regarding

SECTION V

ongoing surgical management, there should be documentation that outlines a plan for when this discussion will take place and in what forum (unit meeting, MDM) so that everyone is aware of the next step in management.

Surgical clinics can be quite busy, but a priority should be given to clear documentation to avoid confusion when the patient presents for their following appointment. This also ensures that clinical issues are not missed if a different member of the inpatient team sees the patient in a following appointment.

CHAPTER 66

GENERAL SURGERY OUTPATIENTS

Paul Watson

BREAST LUMPS

Evaluation of a breast lump is a common outpatient referral for patients in both younger and older age groups.

The key is to determine whether there is a discrete palpable mass and ascertain the risk of malignancy.

History and examination

- The consultation begins with the standard history and examination:
  - How long has the lump been present? Has it grown in size? Have you noticed any change in the skin overlying the breast? Have you noticed any nipple discharge (bilateral)? Have you had any previous breast lumps?
  - Ask about associated symptoms including:
    - nipple discharge, which is most commonly benign and spontaneous, though blood-stained secretions can be suggestive of duct papilloma or tumour
    - breast pain, which is common and can be a cyclical benign process that has presented multiple times.
  - Get a full account of any previous breast lumps and subsequent management.
  - Examination should begin with inspection, checking for best symmetry, pigment changes, obvious mass lesions and skin tethering.
  - Palpation in a systematic fashion examining each quadrant of the breast including the axillary tail and lymph nodes.
- Common causes of breast lumps are given in Table 66.1.

TABLE 66.1 Common causes of breast lumps

Fibroadenoma	Benign breast tumour that is particularly common in younger women. The classic presentation is a small, painless mass, often missed on examination, only to be noticed on routine imaging (see Fig. 66.1). These lesions can grow in size, requiring excision for local discomfort
Fibrocystic changes	Large fibrocystic changes in the breast tissue are part of a benign process that can result in the development of discrete cysts. These lesions can be managed with surveillance or image-guided aspiration if not particularly bothersome to the patient. Cysts with a solid component may need formal tissue diagnosis
Duct ectasia	Common in older patients (pre-menopause). There is a hard, firm and often painful lump on the edge of the areola. Patients with significant symptoms may benefit from ductal excision
Breast carcinoma	See the following section

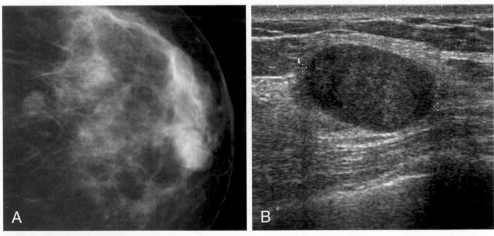

FIGURE 66.1 Fibroadenoma on mammogram (A) and demonstrated as a smooth well-defined lesion on U/S (B).

Reproduced from: Phelps, K. & Hassed, C., 2011. Chapter 51: Breast disease. In: Hassed, C., General Practice: The Integrative Approach. Elsevier Australia, pp. 719–727, Fig. 51.2.

Investigations

- Imaging is a useful initial investigation to help differentiate between the causes of breast lumps.
- Mammograms provide an overview of the margins of a breast lump and can visualise features of suspicious breast lesions including irregular margins and microcalcifications.

- Targeted ultrasound is useful in the diagnosis of cystic vs solid lesions. This may be the ideal first approach in young patients (<30 years) who present with breast lumps unlikely to be breast carcinoma.
- MRI scans are occasionally used for complex lesions without clear diagnosis.
- **Fine needle aspiration (FNA)** can provide definitive diagnosis and guide management.
    - Samples of cells are sent to pathology for cytological studies.
- Lesions that are suspicious for malignancy should have core biopsies taken, allowing for identification of carcinoma type for surgical planning.

BREAST CANCER

Breast cancer is the most common type of cancer for women (affecting 1 in 8 by the age of 85 years) and is ranked second among all deaths resulting from cancer. Though breast cancer can affect men, it is very uncommon.

Due to the high incidence and impact of breast cancer on the community BreastScreen Australia sends invitations for women aged between 50 and 74 years to undergo surveillance mammograms every 2 years.

Risk factors for developing breast cancer include:

- genetic factors – strong family history and genetic mutations involving the BRCA2, BRCA1 and CHEK2 genes
- patient factors – obesity, alcohol consumption and hormone therapy.

Clinical presentation is classically a single painless lump. Some breast cancers are found after imaging and are not clinically detectable:

- Associated features of breast cancer such as pain, skin pigment changes, tethering and nipple discharge are uncommon.
- Some patients may present with locally advanced breast cancer; check the patient's axilla for prominent lymph nodes.

Investigations

- Investigations should include biopsy for tissue diagnosis once there is suspicion of breast cancer.
- All breast cancer cases are typically discussed at MDMs to gain consensus regarding management.

Classification and staging of breast cancer

- Ductal carcinoma in-situ (DCIS)
    - Represent around 25% of all breast cancer diagnoses.

SECTION V

- o Malignant epithelial cells within the ductal system do not involve the surrounding breast tissue (non-invasive).
- o Without treatment these tumours can progress to invasive tumours.
- o Dependent on the position of the tumour, patients may be suited to wide local excision with breast tissue conservation, which can be supplemented with radiotherapy.
- o Early and appropriate treatment confers good prognosis with recurrence <6% at 20 years.
- o Recurrence may require mastectomy.
- Invasive breast cancer
    - o Infiltrating ductal carcinoma (IDC) accounts for up to 80% of all invasive breast tumours.
    - o Infiltrating lobular cancer (ILC) represents around 10% of invasive tumours.
- For staging of breast cancer refer to Table 66.2.

Management

- For surgical management of breast cancer, see Chapter 45.
- Systemic therapy for breast cancer
    - o There are a wide variety of treatment options available from medical and radiation oncology services; the junior doctor should be loosely familiar with patients who are likely to need referral to these services to expedite treatment.

TABLE 66.2 TNM breast cancer staging

T	N	M
Tis (DCIS), carcinoma in situ	N0: no lymph node (LN) involvement	M0: no metastasis
T1: tumour <20 mm	N1mi: micrometastasis, <2.0 mm	M1: metastasis present
T2: >20 mm, <50 mm	N1: 1–3 axillary (LN) involved	
T3: >50 mm	N2: 4–9 axillary LN involved	
T4: adherence to chest wall, skin and muscle	N3: >10 axillary LN involved	

Adapted from: Edge, S.B., Byrd, D.R., Compton, C.C., et al., eds., 2010. AJCC Cancer Staging Manual, 7th ed. New York, Springer-Verlag.

- o Following the excision of breast tissue, testing is performed on the receptor status: oestrogen receptor (ER), progesterone receptor (PR) and human epidermal growth factor receptor 2 (HER2).
    - These patients may benefit from endocrine (hormone) therapy.
- o Chemotherapy
    - Offered in early stage breast cancers with high risk morphological features (high grade) or lymph node involvement.
    - Patients with tumours >50 mm (T3) have an increased risk of metastasis and should be referred for consideration of chemotherapy.
- o Radiotherapy
    - Recommended in patients with breast conservation surgery (Chapter 45) to aid in preventing loco-regional recurrence.
    - Patients with positive lymph nodes with any intervention should be referred to radiation oncology for discussion of treatment.

Prognosis

- Overall earlier detection of breast cancer has led to improved 5-year survival rates with 96% survival in disease localised to the breast.
- Overall 80% survival rate for those with lymph node involvement.

UPPER GI CANCER

Oesophageal cancer

An uncommon form of cancer, it accounts for 1.4% of all cancers in males and 0.8% in females.

Risk factors include a history of GORD and Barrett's oesophagus (see Chapter 37), smoking and a family history.

Oesophageal cancer has an insidious onset due to the slow growing nature of the tumours. Symptomatic oesophageal cancer (dysphagia, haematemesis) is often not present until the disease is locally advanced. Early detection may occur as a result of endoscopic investigation of persistent GORD or surveillance for Barrett's.

The vast majority are either SCC or adenocarcinoma, with adenocarcinoma becoming more common.

Investigations

- Initial investigation for GORD, Barrett's and dysphagia (Chapter 37) (can include barium swallow, see Fig. 66.2).
- Once malignancy is suspected or confirmed the patient should have full staging CT with a PET scan.

- Endoscopic U/S (Chapter 45) is used to fully characterise the lesion and can visualise nearby lymph nodes.

Staging of oesophageal cancer

- Evolution of staging criteria has led to the separation of tumours into two main entities:
  - superficial oesophageal cancer, no deeper than the submucosa (T1)
  - locally advanced oesophageal cancer (T2–T4)
    - further delineated into resectable and non-resectable tumours.

Management

- Superficial cancers that involve the top layer of the submucosa may be amenable to endoscopic mucosal resection (EMR) provided they are small. Larger superficial tumours may still require oesophagectomy.
- Locally invasive tumours that are suited to resection include T1 and T2 without lymph node involvement. Patients with T3 tumours may undergo neoadjuvant chemotherapy before resection.
- Patients with diffuse locally spread tumours, metastatic disease and the elderly may not be suited for definitive surgical management, but can receive palliative chemoradiotherapy with dysphagia symptoms managed by oesophageal stenting.
- Oesophageal surgery (see Chapter 45).

Prognosis

- Largely influenced by the lateness of detection, prognosis is poor with 49% survival rate at 1 year for local tumours and 12% for metastatic disease.

Gastric cancer

Tumours affect the stomach, and are similarly characterised by the development of symptoms at advanced stages of disease, with nearly half of patients demonstrating loco-regional spread. Gastric cancer represents 2% of all cancers in men and 1.4% in women.

Risk factors include *Helicobacter pylori* infection, smoking, family history, dietary factors.

Adenocarcinoma is by far the most common histological subtype.

Clinical presentation is varied. Some patients have incidental findings during biopsy for endoscopic work-up of reflux or non-specific abdominal pain, while others present with dysphagia, loss of weight and vomiting.

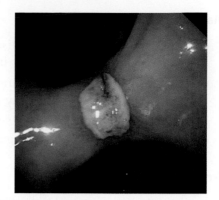

FIGURE 66.3 Malignant gastric ulcer on endoscopy.

Reproduced from: Liao, Z., Hou, X., Lin-Hu, E.Q., et al., 2016. Accuracy of magnetically controlled capsule endoscopy, compared with conventional gastroscopy, in detection of gastric diseases. Clinical Gastroenterology and Hepatology 14(9), 1266-1273, Fig. 2D.

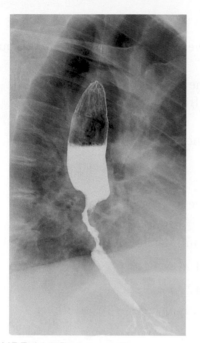

FIGURE 66.2 Barium swallow demonstrating locally advanced oesophageal cancer.

Reproduced from: Spicer, J., Dhupar, R., Kim, J., et al., 2017. Chapter 41: Esophagus. In: Townsend, C., Sabiston Textbook of Surgery, 20th ed. Saunders, pp. 1013–1042, Fig. 41-12.

Investigations

- Endoscopy allowing biopsy is the gold standard for establishing diagnosis (see Fig. 66.3).
- Barium contrast meals may help identify suspicious lesions, but lack sensitivity.
- There is increasing research regarding the role of microRNA markers for detecting gastric cancer.
- Patients require full staging scans with CT and PET for management planning.

Gastric cancer staging

- Gastric cancer staging via the TNM criteria focuses on the depth of tumour invasion and the number of affected lymph nodes.
  - The depth of tumour can be assessed directly via EUS.
  - Peritoneal deposits can occur via intra-abdominal dissemination. A staging laparoscopy may be required.

SECTION V

Management

- Patients without metastatic disease have a potentially resectable tumour, unless there is gross vascular invasion.
- Patients with tumours invading into the subserosal layer (T3) or with lymph node involvement may benefit from neoadjuvant chemoradiotherapy prior to resection.
- For surgical management of gastric cancer see Chapter 45.

Prognosis

- Patients with mucosal only disease have a 5-year survival rate of 85–100%.
- Locally invasive tumours have significantly worse outcomes:
  - invading through mucosa (52–61%)
  - invading through muscle wall (44–47%).
- Involvement of lymph nodes significantly decreases survivability (5–17%).

LIVER MASSES

Most patients present with no symptoms, with lesions detected incidentally during imaging.

Can be largely divided into cystic and solid masses, though a mixed appearance is common. Types of liver lesions are presented in Table 66.3.

Imaging plays an important role in diagnosis:

- Targeted ultrasound can provide an overview of the lesion and determine whether it is solid or cystic.
- MRI provides excellent resolution of liver masses; the use of contrast to provide arterial and portal phases allows for easier diagnosis.
- Tissue diagnosis can be obtained via image-guided core biopsy to guide management.

Primary liver cancer

Around 1600 cases are diagnosed in Australia per year, though much high numbers occur overseas particularly in Asia. Hepatocellular carcinoma (HCC) is the predominant type with a close association with chronic hepatitis B and C infections (75–80% of cases) and liver cirrhosis (see Chapter 37). As such the clinical features of HCC are often masked by the patient's chronic liver disease (CLD).

Investigations

Investigations should include dedicated imaging to help identify the size and position of the tumour(s).

SECTION V

TABLE 66.3 Types of benign liver lesions

Simple liver cysts	An incidental finding in up to 5% of adults. Typically not symptomatic and can be left alone without intervention. Haematoma can occur but are not significant. Symptomatic cysts should be formally excised
Adenoma	Adenomas are benign lesions, more commonly affecting women. The two common issues affecting adenomas are the low probability of transformation into HCC and severe haemorrhaging from rupture. Where possible they are typically excised
Haemangioma	Common tumour of the liver with low risk of spontaneous rupture. When large may require intervention via enucleation where possible. Kasabach–Merritt syndrome is coagulopathy resulting from large, cavernous lesions
Focal nodular hyperplasia	Benign nodules of normal liver tissue; intervention only required when patients develop pain
Mucinous cystic neoplasms	Uncommon tumours with malignant potential (10–15% of cases). Previously termed cystoadenocarcinoma

- CT or MRI is the modality of choice, with contrast scans used to demonstrate vascularity of the tumour (Fig. 66.4).
  - Dedicated angiography is often required for management planning.
- PET is used for staging.
- Tumour markers such as AFP can suggest the presence of HCC but lack sensitivity and specificity.
- If diagnosis is not certain, core biopsy is indicated.
- Staging laparoscopies are often used to determine suitability for resection.

Management of HCC

These patients often present a management challenge, as surgical resection is not always possible due to their underlying CLD.

- Multiple systems exist for staging of HCC, including the TNM staging (Table 66.4).
- Surgical resection of HCC (Chapter 45) is the ideal treatment choice for patients with sufficient hepatic reserve (cirrhosis is generally a contraindication) and suitable tumour characteristics.
  - Tumours <5 cm are considered resectable.
  - Only 10–20% of patients fit this criterion.

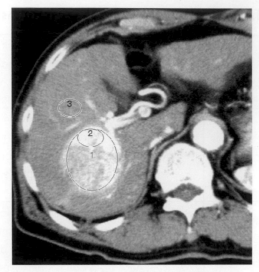

FIGURE 66.4 Arterial phase scan clearly demonstrates HCC.

Reproduced from: Kanata, N., Yoshikawa, T., Ohno, Y., et al., 2013. HCC-to-liver contrast on arterial-dominant phase images of EOB-enhanced MRI: comparison with dynamic CT. Magnetic Resonance Imaging 31(1), 17–22, Fig. 1.

TABLE 66.4 Staging of HCC

T	N	M
T1: solitary tumour, no vascular invasion	N0: no lymph node involvement	M0: no distant metastasis
T2: solitary tumour with vascular invasion or multiple tumours <5 cm	N1: regional lymph node involvement	M1: distant metastasis present
T3a: multiple tumours >5 cm		
T3b: single or multiple tumours invading a major branch of the portal or hepatic vein		
T4: direct invasion of adjacent viscera or peritoneum		

Adapted from: Edge, S.B., Byrd, D.R., Compton, C.C., et al., eds., 2010. AJCC Cancer Staging Manual, 7th ed. New York, Springer-Verlag.

- ○ Select patients may undergo complete hepatectomy with liver transplant.
- Other treatment modalities include arterial therapies:
  - ○ direct hepatic vessel embolisation
  - ○ transarterial chemoembolisation (TACE) – chemotherapy infused directly into a tumour-feeding vessel
  - ○ selective internal radiation therapy (SIRT) – radioisotopes used for embolisation.

Prognosis

- Although there is no single system accurate for predicting prognosis, survivability is poor due to the late detection and low hepatic reserve of affected patients, with 16% surviving at 5 years.

Metastatic liver disease

Much more common than primary liver cancer with 28,000 cases in Australia every year. Predominantly arise from the GIT via portal drainage (colorectal, gastric). Other primary sites include breast, skin (melanoma) and prostate.

Typically detected during routine staging for primary cancer.

Colorectal liver metastases are by far the most common and can be considered for surgical resection. Around 50% of patients with colorectal cancer develop liver metastases.

Management

- The classical rationale was patients with fewer than four deposits that can be excised with >1 cm margin were considered to have resectable tumours.
  - ○ Some surgeons use an expanded set of inclusion criteria based on anatomical distribution of the tumours and the patient's functional reserve.
  - ○ Intraoperative ultrasound helps determine if there are any smaller metastatic deposits not detected on imaging that rule out resection.

Prognosis

- Only 1 in 5 patients has clinically resectable colorectal liver metastasis at time of diagnosis.
- Outcomes for patients with resected liver lesions are improving, with current 5-year survival rates at 25–58%.
- Median survival for patients with a non-resected tumour is 16 months.

SECTION V

PANCREATIC CANCER

Pancreatic cancer is ranked the 9th most common cancer in men, 10th in women.

Risk factors are not completely understood but are thought to include smoking, alcohol consumption, diabetes, family history and chronic pancreatitis.

Clinical presentation typically occurs at advanced stages of disease with signs of obstruction: jaundice, nausea, pain. Patients may report a history of unintended weight loss. Some tumours are detected incidentally during imaging.

90% of tumours are ductal adenocarcinoma, with 75% of tumours found in the head of the pancreas.

Investigations

- Dedicated CT of the pancreas helps characterise the appearance and extent of the tumour.
- EUS is useful for gaining tissue diagnosis to confirm the presence of pancreatic cancer.
- Serum markers such as Ca19.9 lack the sensitivity to screen for pancreatic cancer, but can be used to monitor the progression of disease.
- Full staging scans should be ordered including PET.
  - Staging laparoscopy is commonly performed prior to consideration of resection.
- For staging of pancreatic cancer see Table 66.5.

TABLE 66.5 Staging of pancreatic cancer

T	N	N
Tis: carcinoma in situ	N0: no lymph node involvement	M0: no distant metastasis
T1: tumour <2 cm, within pancreas	N1: regional lymph node involvement	M1: distant metastasis present
T2: tumour >2 cm, within pancreas		
T3: tumour extends beyond pancreas, without involvement of coeliac axis or SMA		
T4: involves coeliac axis or SMA (unresectable)		

Adapted from: Edge, S.B., Byrd, D.R., Compton, C.C., et al., eds., 2010. AJCC Cancer Staging Manual, 7th ed. New York, Springer-Verlag.

Management

- Surgical resection of the tumour is undertaken in patients considered to have suitable tumour characteristics (limited involvement or encasement of major vessels and no metastasis).
  - Pancreatic head tumours require pancreaticoduodenectomy (Whipple's procedure – see Chapter 46).
- More than 80% of patients present with locally advanced disease and should be referred for consideration of chemotherapy.

Prognosis

- Very poor with a 5-year survival rate of <7%. These deaths account for around 5% of all cancer deaths in Australia.

GALLSTONE DISEASE

Cholelithiasis is very common, found in around 10–15% of all adults, more commonly affecting females and patients with obesity. Gallstones are primarily formed as a combination of cholesterol and bilirubin.

The clinical presentation of these patients is largely dependent on the positon of the gallstone within the biliary system (see Table 66.6).

Most outpatient referrals are for patients with gallstones related to intermittent but often severe episodes of pain and nausea termed biliary colic:

- The classic history is RUQ pain associated with fatty meals, with the pain subsiding after a period of time.
- Patients may report tenderness in RUQ during examination.

Investigations

- Abdominal ultrasound is the gold standard for detecting cholelithiasis and will also give information regarding the number and sizes of stones, thickness of the gallbladder wall and the diameter of the bile duct.
  - It is sometimes possible to visualise gallstones within the duct, though not always.

TABLE 66.6 Clinical manifestations of gallstone disease

GALLBLADDER (CHOLELITHIASIS)	BILIARY TREE (CHOLEDOCOLITHIASIS)
Acute cholecystitis	Cholangitis
Empyema	Pancreatitis
Mucocoele	
Biliary colic	

SECTION V

- LFTs should be performed routinely as obstruction of the bile duct from stones can be represented by increased liver enzymes (ALP, GGT) and bilirubin.

Management

- Patients with symptomatic cholelithiasis should be offered cholecystectomy (Chapter 46) unless they have significant medical comorbidities.
- Patients with suspected choledocolithiasis should be referred for ERCP to remove the stones; due to the likelihood of developing pancreatitis or cholangitis, patients should also undergo cholecystectomy.

PERIANAL CONDITIONS

Perianal pain and lumps represent a distinct group of conditions affecting the anal canal and surrounding skin.

These common conditions are typically easily identifiable from the history and examination with little need for formal investigation.

Haemorrhoids

- Abnormal dilations of the rectal venous vessels with a varying degrees of severity.
- Can be external, internal or a mix of both.
- Commonly associated with straining when defecating due to hard stools or constipation.
- Typically present as a painless swelling associated with bleeding, noticed during defecation.
  - Some patients may develop thrombosis, which can cause significant pain.
- Examination with proctoscopy in the outpatient setting can lead to accurate diagnosis and grading of internal haemorrhoids:
  - grade I: internal, do not prolapse below the dentate line
  - grade II: prolapse from the anal canal but spontaneously reduce
  - grade III: prolapse from the anal canal requiring manual reduction
  - grade IV: prolapsed and irreducible.
- Haemorrhoids should be distinguished from skin tags that are present at the edge of the rectum.

Management

See also Chapter 45.

- Grade I haemorrhoids do not necessarily require treatment; patients should be encouraged to develop normal stool habits with increased water intake and observed.
- Grades II and III haemorrhoids may be suited to rubber band ligation.
- Grade IV and some grade III haemorrhoids are typically managed by haemorrhoidectomy.

Anal fissure

- Tear or ulcerations within the rectum leading to painful defecation and sometimes mild bleeding.
- Associated with Crohn's disease and other localised infections (herpes simplex).
- The primary issue relates to hypertonicity and spasm of the internal sphincter.
- Physical examination can be difficult as the patient is often apprehensive and tender.
  - Fissures typically occur on the posterior midline with a palpable lump.

Management

- Patients should be booked for an examination under anaesthetic (EUA).
  - These procedures are combined with either a lateral sphincterotomy or injection of Botox to reduce tonicity.

Anal fistula

- Following perianal abscess, fistula tracts may develop as the abscess cavity migrates in multiple directions.
- Patients may report ongoing pain and swelling following a recent infection, with small amounts of pus sometimes noticeable from the rectum or from external skin openings.
- Fistulas are largely categorised as either intersphincteric (medial to external sphincter) or transsphincteric (extending through the external sphincter).

Management

- Definitive treatment requires obliteration of the fistula to prevent ongoing sepsis.
  - EUA allows for probing of the fistula tract and appropriate management (Chapter 45).

SECTION V

Pilonidal sinus

Refer to Chapter 45.

COLORECTAL POLYPS AND COLORECTAL CANCER

As colorectal cancer (CRC) is the second most pravelent cancer in both men and women there is a substantial focus on screening and early detection. The National Bowel Screen service seeks to provide faecal occult blood testing (FOBT) to everyone aged 50–74 years every 2 years by 2020. Positive FOBT tests are an indication for screening colonoscopy.

Risk factors for CRC include:

- genetic syndromes including hereditary nonpolyposis colorectal cancer (HPNCC) and familial adenomatous polyposis
- family history
- inflammatory bowel disease, age, male gender, obesity, dietary factors and previous polyps.

Due to the increased usage of screening, a number of CRCs are detected in asymptomatic patients (up to 80%).

Symptomatic presentations are therefore suggestive of more advanced tumours:

- rectal bleeding
- abdominal pain
- large bowel obstruction and/or perforation
- altered bowel habit, which may include sensation of incomplete rectal emptying

Examination must include a rectal examination looking for palpable tumour.

Investigations

- Colonoscopy is often one of the first investigations allowing for inspection of the mucosal lining of the colon.
  - Patients who are not suited to have endoscopy may undergo CT colonography.
- In patients with suspected CRC full staging scans should be undertaken including CT and PET.
  - MRI for rectal cancer.
- Tumour markers – CEA is used as a marker of disease progression but is not considered diagnostic.

Polyps

- During colonoscopy polyps are often visualised and biopsied for tissue diagnosis.

- Largely split into benign and neoplastic polyps (see Table 66.7).
- Adenomas account for around 67% of all colonic polyps.
  - They are further classified as tubular, villous or a mixture of the two.
- Polyps themselves may be asymptomatic but have the potential to develop malignancy and thus require close observation following biopsy or polypectomy (Fig. 66.5).

Colorectal cancer staging

- 90% of CRC are adenocarcinomas.
- For staging of CRC see Fig. 66.6.

Management

See also Chapter 45.

- Majority of cases are localised to the colon and are curable via surgical resection.

TABLE 66.7 Different types of colonic polyps

BENIGN	NEOPLASTIC
Mucosal polyps Hyperplastic polyps Submucosal polyps	Adenomatous polyps (adenomas) Serrated polyps

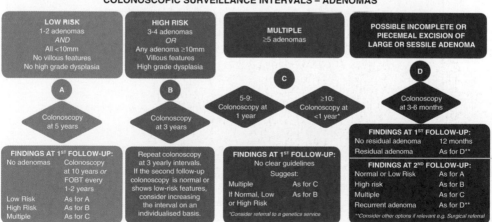

FIGURE 66.5 Recommended ongoing surveillance for bowel adenoma.

Image from: Barclay, K., Cancer Council of Australia Surveillance Colonoscopy Guidelines Working Party, 2013. Algorithm for Colonoscopic Surveillance Intervals – Adenomas.

SECTION V

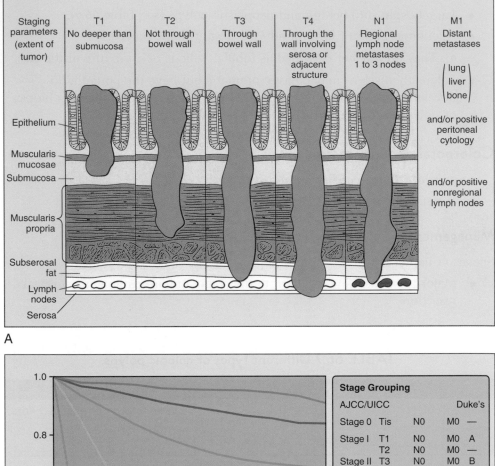

A

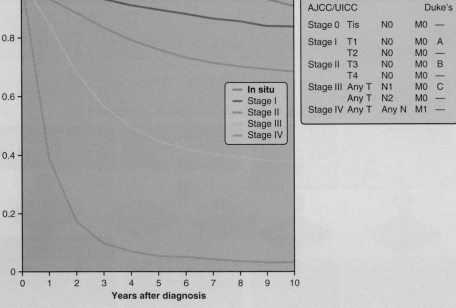

B

FIGURE 66.6 Staging and 10-year survival rates for colon cancer.

Reproduced from: Van Schaeybroek, S., Lawler, M., Johnston, B., et al., 2014. Chapter 77: Colorectal cancer. In: Niderhuber, J., Abeloff's Clinical Oncology. Churchill Livingstone, pp. 1278-1335, Fig. 77-5A and B.

- T4 tumours may be suited to resection following a period of neoadjuvant chemoradiotherapy.
- Patients with liver metastasis can still undergo primary resection as the metastasis may be excised.
  - All patients with node positive disease should undergo adjuvant chemotherapy.

HERNIAS

A hernia is an abnormal protrusion of tissue beyond its normal anatomical boundaries. They most commonly affect the abdominal cavity, relating to two main processes: weakness of the overlying abdominal wall (congenital or due to previous surgery) and increased abdominal pressure from heavy lifting or excessive coughing.

Contents of hernias vary, but can include fat, peritoneum and bowel. A key process of examination is determining whether the hernia is reducible. Hernias with a narrow neck and large herniated sac are at risk of incarceration (see Chapter 46).

The classification of hernias is dependent on the anatomical location.

Inguinal hernias

- Account for around 80% of external abdominal wall hernias. 20 times more common in men.
- Natural history is of an increasing pain and palpable lump (can occur bilaterally):
  - Patient may note a more prominent lump on straining.
  - Examination may detect a lump with obvious cough impulse.
- The diagnosis is clinical with little role for imaging studies.

Management

- Surgical repair should be offered in fit, symptomatic patients (Chapter 45).
- Hernias containing bowel should be repaired to prevent risk of strangulation.

Incisional hernias

- Defined as a hernia through a surgical scar.
- Account for 10% of all hernias.
- Size and position of the hernia are largely dependent on the defect from the surgical site.
  - Large and multiple hernias are not uncommon and present a management challenge.
  - Patients often have bulky hernias, which may contain bowel.

- Imaging can play a role in complicated cases with multiple previous surgeries. CT can give an overview of the clinical picture.

Management

- Management is either by open or laparoscopic repair (Chapter 45).

Femoral hernias

- 7% of all hernias, predominantly affecting females.
- Develop as the hernia sac passes through the saphenous opening, tending to migrate superiorly from the opening to the lower groin.
- Cough impulse may be present.
- Can be difficult to distinguish from inguinal hernia repair, though most commonly occurs in older women due to laxity of ligamentous structures.

Management

- Management is via open repair.

Umbilical hernias

- Represent about 3% of all hernias.
- Present as an inversion of the umbilicus.

Management

- Management is usually open repair as a day case (Chapter 45).

Epigastric hernias

- Around 1% of all hernias.
- Occur superiorly to the umbilicus where the linea alba is wider; gradual weakness with age may slowly lead to hernia development.
- Often asymptomatic with a palpable lump, though some patients report pain.

Management

- Symptomatic hernias should be repaired.

CHAPTER 67

ORTHOPAEDIC OUTPATIENTS

Paul Watson and Lachlan Wight

FRACTURE CLINIC

Patients with low acuity closed fractures that present to the Emergency Department or their local GP can be reviewed in the outpatient setting provided that their pain can be adequately controlled and there is no neurovascular injury or wound requiring review.

Orthopaedic fracture clinics deal with a wide variety of fracture referrals. The following section covers fracture assessment and management accounting for around 98% of all outpatient fracture clinic presentations. A large majority of simple, common fractures can be managed by a GP; consider speaking to the registrar or consultant, as discharge planning can never occur too early!

General approach to the fracture clinic

History and examination findings in combination with the available imaging provide the necessary information to present a fracture case. History should include:

- demographic information of the patient (age, gender, occupation and dominant hand for upper limb injuries)
- date and mechanism of injury
- previous injury to the same site
- general medical history (past medical history, medications, smoking status)
- impact of the current injury on function.

Examination should focus on:

- general appearance of the affected fracture site (i.e. deformity; check for skin breaches that may have been missed prior to referral)
- assessment of the neurovascular status of the injury site (distal pulses, muscle power, sensation)

- swelling and tenderness around fracture site
- function (i.e. able to weight bear, range of motion).

Describing fractures

A large part of communicating well in Orthopaedics is learning how to describe a fracture presentation in an accurate and concise manner. Imaging should be recent and clearly display the fracture pattern. For plain films taken through bulky plaster that obscures visualisation, the patient should be taken to X-ray with a removable backslab. This is particularly important for fractures that may extend into articular surfaces.

There are key descriptive terms that are universally used to convey information regarding fracture patterns. State the location of the fracture, both name of bone and which anatomical part is affected by the fracture. The terms in Table 67.1 can aid in giving a complete assessment of the fracture.

Verbal case presenting of fractures should follow a clear structure (as for Fig. 67.1):

1. State the patient demographics: 'Mr F is 45-year-old right-handed carpenter... '.

2. Briefly outline the mechanism and date of injury: '... who presents after a mechanical fall onto an outstretched right hand 6 days ago... '.

3. Use the terms in Table 67.1 to describe the fracture pattern: '... sustaining a transverse fracture of the right distal radius. There is around 45 degrees of dorsal angulation with minimal displacement and no shortening'.

4. Then further relevant history and examination findings should be discussed, including initial steps of management taken by the referring clinician (i.e. closed reduction and splinting).

TABLE 67.1 Descriptive terms for fracture patterns

DESCRIPTIVE TERM	USAGE
Transverse, spiral, oblique and comminuted	These terms give an impression of the basic shape of the fracture pattern
Displacement and angulation	Describe the distance between the fracture fragment and the rest of the bone. Similarly, angulation describes the deviation of the axis of the bone compared to normal. Can be quantified in degrees
Shortening	Impaction or overlap of fractures may result in a shortened appearance of the bone
Rotation	Fracture fragment has lost correct anatomical position. Typically, describe the rotation of the distal fragment in relation to the proximal fragment

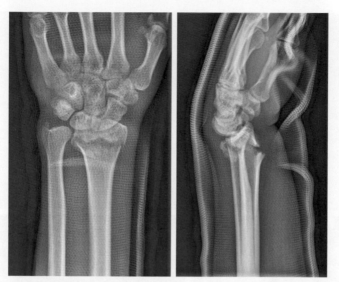

FIGURE 67.1 Distal radius fracture.

Reproduced from: Kim, J. & Tae, S., 2014. Percutaneous distal radius: ulna pinning of distal radius fractures to prevent settling. Journal of Hand Surgery 39(10), 1921–1925, Fig. 2.

The greatest use of this skill is for describing X-ray pathology over the phone, such as when making referrals from the ED.

DISTAL RADIUS (DR) FRACTURES

Accounting for around 3% of upper limb injuries seen in the ED, distal radius fractures are classically related to falls in the elderly patient and high-energy impacts in the younger population. The younger patient with a distal radius fracture following a low-energy fall should be investigated for osteoporosis.

Examination

- Examination reveals swollen, tender wrist with decreased ROM. There may be obvious deformity. Check median nerve.

Investigations

- Initial investigations include plain X-ray films (specify a lateral to evaluate angulation). Intraarticular fractures are further evaluated by CT (Fig. 67.2).
- Multiple classification systems, but there are two common eponymous fractures:
  - Colles' fracture:
    - Extraarticular distal radius fracture with dorsal displacement. Typically seen in elderly patients.
    - Can be stable enough to undergo closed reduction and plaster

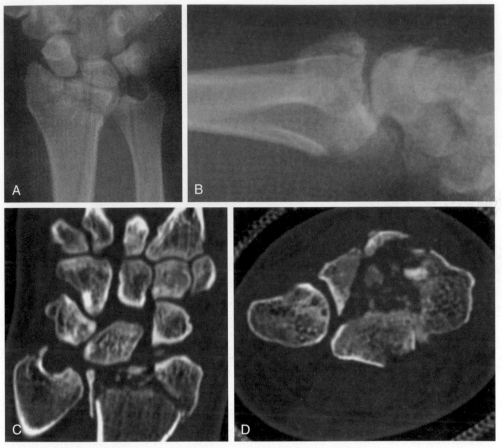

FIGURE 67.2 Assessment of intraarticular fracture on CT scanning.

Reproduced from: Wolfe, S., 2011. Chapter 17: Distal radius fractures. In: Wolfe, S., Green's Operative Hand Surgery. Churchill Livingstone, pp. 561-638, Fig. 17.11.

- o Smith's fracture:
    - – Extraarticular distal radius fracture with volar displacement.
    - – Amount of displacement renders these fractures unstable.

Management

- Extraarticular fractures can be managed by closed reduction if good anatomical alignment can be achieved with plaster cast.
- Intraarticular fractures and shortening typically require ORIF due to the associated instability (Fig. 67.3).
    - o Surgical treatment is recommended in fractures that display:
        - – articular displacement of >2 mm
        - – radial shortening of >5 mm
        - – dorsal angulation of >20°.

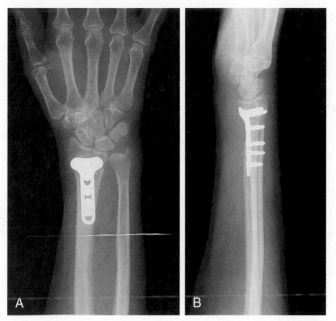

FIGURE 67.3 Typical postoperative film demonstrates plate and screw ORIF.

Reproduced from: Wulf, C. & Ackerman, D., 2007. Contemporary evaluation and treatment of distal radius fractures. Hand Clinics 23(2),209-226, Fig. 9 H and I.

- Patients undergo 4–6 weeks of cast immobilisation in both operative and conservative cases.
- Patients with distal radius fractures have been shown to be at risk (10–37%) of developing complex regional pain syndrome CRPS; ensure the patient has sufficient analgesia on discharge.
  - Use of vitamin C post injury is associated with a lower incidence of developing CRPS.
- Complications can include non-union, median nerve neuropathy (particularly in high impact injuries) and long-term arthritis.

Distal radial ulnar joint (DRUJ) injuries

DRUJ injuries are a disruption of the normal anatomy between the head of the radius and ulna. Soft tissue components include radioulnar ligaments and the triangular fibrocartilage complex (TFCC). These provide the primary stabilisation of the DRUJ. As the DRUJ is involved in load distribution of the wrist, the mechanism of injury is similar to that of distal radius fracture. Therefore, there is a common association with fractures.

Examination

- Presentation includes a swollen, painful wrist with decreased ROM.
- DRUJ can be examined via direct view or arthroscopy allowing visualisation of the TFCC.

SECTION V

Investigations

- Plain films can demonstrate widening of the radius and ulna.
- MRI can help diagnose tears in the TFCC.

Management

- Isolated DRUJ injuries with no fractures can be treated conservatively with 4 weeks of immobilisation.
  - Anatomical reduction of the wrist is key to restoration of DRUJ position.
- Operative management is recommended in patients with highly unstable DRUJ injuries and associated fractures, including distal radius and ulna styloid fractures.
- Complications include chronic DRUJ instability and progression to arthritis.

SCAPHOID FRACTURE

This is the most common carpal fracture. The mechanism of injury is typically a fall on an outstretched hand (FOOSH). Scaphoid fracture is difficult to assess and treat with patient and injury factors influencing management. Fractures can lead to long-term chronic arthritis regardless of treatment due to non-union of the fracture.

Examination

- Upon general inspection of the wrist it typically appears normal with no obvious swelling.
- Closer examination may reveal snuffbox (classical sign) tenderness.
- Patient may report pain when attempting to pronate against resistance.

Investigations

- Initial investigation includes X-ray. Specify 'scaphoid view' on request form to obtain appropriate angled film to view scaphoid.
  - X-ray may not reveal signs of fracture; up to 25% are not visible on initial imaging.
  - CT or MRI allows for superior visualisation of scaphoid (Fig. 67.4).
  - If clinical suspicion is high for fracture, patients can be immobilised and reviewed with repeat X-ray films in 1–2 weeks.

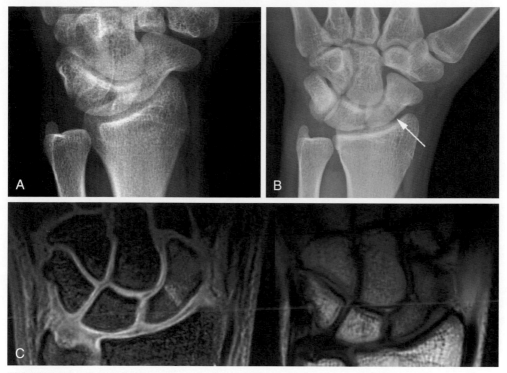

FIGURE 67.4 Scaphoid fracture. **A** is the initially normal appearing X-ray with **B** a month later finding the waist fracture. Confirmed on MRI (**C**).

Reproduced from: Fowler, J.R. & Hughes, T.B., 2015. Scaphoid fractures. Clinics in Sports Medicine 34(1), 37-50, Fig. 3A.

Management

- Anatomy of bone relevant for management:
  - majority of surface covered by articular cartilage
  - around 70–80% blood supply from retrograde branch of dorsal carpal artery
  - fracture carries risk of avascular necrosis
  - around two-thirds of scaphoid fractures occur at the waist.
- Management of scaphoid fractures: see Table 67.2.
- Complications include non-union, which can progress to long-term scaphoid non-union advanced collapse (SNAC) manifesting as localised pain and decreased function.
  - Management will depend on severity of arthritic changes and features of collapse.

CLAVICULAR FRACTURE

Clavicular fracture is common in younger patients, particularly those engaging in contact sports. The mechanism is typically contact to the anterolateral shoulder

TABLE 67.2 Summary of management for scaphoid fractures

TYPE OF FRACTURE	TREATMENT
Stable fractures, non-displaced	
Tubercle fracture	Short arm cast for 6–8 weeks
Distal third fracture/incomplete fracture	
Waist fracture	Long arm thumb spica cast for 6 weeks, short arm cast for 6 weeks or until CT confirms healing
	ORIF or K-wire for selected patients: • active, young, manual worker • athlete, high-demand occupation • preference for early range of motion
Proximal pole fracture, non-displaced	ORIF or K-wire
Unstable fractures	
Displacement >1 mm Lateral intra-scaphoid angle >35° Bone loss or comminution Perilunate fracture/dislocation	ORIF (Fig. 67.5) or K-wire

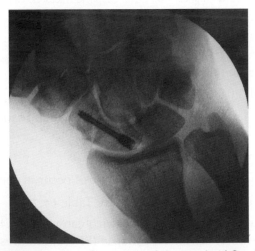

FIGURE 67.5 An intraoperative view of insertion of the scaphoid fixation screw. The approach is via the dorsum of the wrist.

Reproduced from: Chung, K., Haase, S., et al., 2013. Fractures and dislocations of the wrist and distal radius. In: Neligan, P.C., Plastic Surgery, 3rd ed. Saunders, pp. 161-177, Fig. 8.12D.

from a fall or from a direct blow. Around 70–80% occur in the middle third of the clavicle. Influencing forces of the sternocleidomastoid and the arm on the pectoral girdle can cause displacement.

History confirms the mechanism.

Examination

- Examination often reveals an obvious clavicular deformity and a limited range of motion on the affected side.

Investigations

- Chest X-ray and shoulder X-ray focusing on the clavicle are appropriate initial investigations (Fig. 67.6).
  - In high energy collisions obtain a formal CXR due to the risk of pneumothorax from displaced fragments.
  - Patients with confirmed significant posterior displacement have a risk of injury to subclavian vessels.

Management

- Initial management involves a 'cuff and collar' sling.
  - If not available, a triangular bandage sling supporting the weight of the arm is a useful temporary measure.
- Management depends on appearance and location of fracture (medial, middle or lateral third of clavicle).
  - Conservative management involves sling immobilisation for 4 weeks, followed by physiotherapy for range of motions exercises.
  - Lateral clavicle
    - Operative management is considered in fractures in close relation to the coracoclavicular ligament or extensive fracture comminution, causing instability in the fracture, as these fractures are associated with higher rates of non-union.
    - Fractures on the lateral side of the ligament are considered stable.
  - Middle clavicle
    - Management is typically conservative unless significant displacement (>100%), then ORIF (Fig. 67.7).
    - Intervention is considered in fractures that threaten the overlying skin.
  - Medial clavicle
    - Anterior displacement is generally treated conservatively.
    - Posterior displacement of the fracture risks injury to underlying vessels.

SECTION V

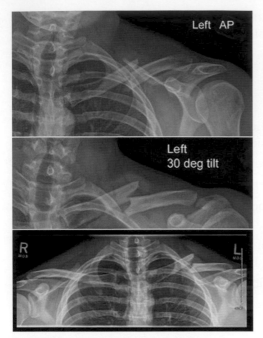

FIGURE 67.6 L middle third clavicular fracture. The tilt X-ray allows for clearer visualisation of the fracture.

Reproduced from: Rubright, J., Bushnell, B., Taft, T., 2010. Chapter 51: Clavicle fractures. In: Miller, M., Essential Orthopaedics. Saunders, pp. 212-216, Fig. 51.2.

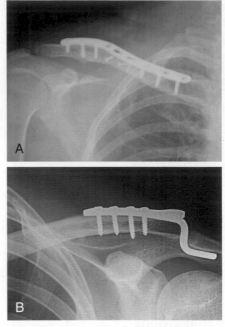

FIGURE 67.7 Plate and screw ORIF and hook plate operative approaches for treatment of clavicular fracture.

Reproduced from: Jiang, H. & Qu, W., 2012. Operative treatment of clavicle midshaft fractures using a locking compression plate: comparison between mini-invasive plate osteosynthesis (MIPPO) technique and conventional open reduction. Orthopaedics and Traumatology: Surgery and Research 98(6), 666-671, Fig. 2B. Boström Windhamre, H.A., von Heideken, J.P., Une-Larsson, V.E., et al., 2010, Surgical treatment of chronic acromioclavicular dislocations: a comparative study of Weaver-Dunn augmented with PDS-braid or hook plate. Journal of Shoulder and Elbow Surgery 19(7), 1040-1048, Fig. 2.

PROXIMAL HUMERUS FRACTURES

Injuries to the proximal humerus include a variety of fractures affecting the humeral head, neck and tuberosities. These fractures occur most commonly in the elderly, typically after falls. Mean age at injury is around 78 years, with osteoporosis highlighted as an important risk factor.

Multiple methods are used for describing these fractures, with the Neer classification commonly used (see Fig. 67.8):

- Categorised by the fracture pattern of the 'parts' of the proximal humerus: shaft (surgical neck), articular aspect of the humeral head (anatomical head) and the greater and lesser tuberosities.

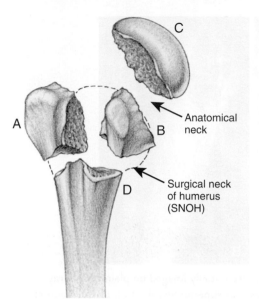

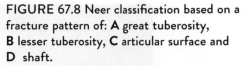

FIGURE 67.8 Neer classification based on a fracture pattern of: A great tuberosity, B lesser tuberosity, C articular surface and D shaft.

Scolaro, J. & Taylor, R., 2015. Chapter 11: Orthopedic trauma. In: Namdari, S., Orthopedic Secrets. Elsevier, pp. 381-442, Fig. 11.9.

- A displacement of one component by 45° or >1 cm is considered a 'separate part'.
- Fractures with no displaced parts are termed one-part fractures.
    - Displacement of one part creates a 'two-part' fracture.
    - Displacement of two parts creates a 'three-part' fracture.
    - Dislocation of the humeral head is also classified as a separate part, resulting in a 'four-part' fracture (Fig. 67.9).

History generally involves a fall, with sudden onset pain and pain when moving the affected limb.

Examination

- Examination may reveal obvious deformity with extensive bruising around the shoulder and chest.
    - The fractured arm will be most comfortable when the weight is supported.
    - Assess for power in the lower limb and sensation, particularly over the axillary nerve distribution.

Investigations

- Initial investigations include shoulder X-ray, with lateral views essential for adequately assessing fracture and potential dislocation.

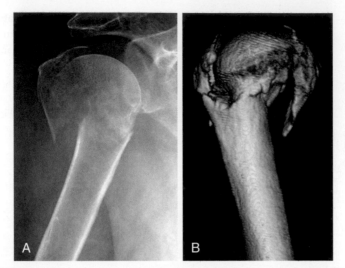

FIGURE 67.9 Four-part proximal humerus fracture initially imaged on plain film X-ray.
A, subsequent CT with 3D reconstructions allows for superior visualisation of the fracture
fragments **(B).**

Reproduced from: Hinds, R.M., Garner, M.R., Tran, W.H., et al., 2015. Geriatric proximal humeral fracture
patients show similar clinical outcomes to non-geriatric patients after osteosynthesis with endosteal fibular
strut allograft augmentation. Journal of Shoulder and Elbow Surgery 24(4), 889-896, Fig. 1.

Management

- Treatment is dependent on the degree of fracture displacement.
  - Minimally displaced proximal humerus fractures can be managed
    conservatively with good functional outcome in around 80% of
    presentations (Fig. 67.10). This includes:
    - Neer classification fractures minimally displaced with no
      glenohumeral dislocation
    - <5 mm greater tuberosity displacement.
  - ORIF (Fig. 67.11) indicated in:
    - >5 mm displacement of greater tuberosity fractures
    - younger patients with high energy multi-fragment humeral head
      fractures.
    - IM Nails are suitable for patients with SNOH fractures, particularly
      in younger patients.
    - Elderly patients with comminuted fractures can be considered for
      treatment of the fracture by arthroplasty.
      - Patients with a healthy glenoid surface may be suitable for
        hemiathroplasty of the humeral head, particularly those with
        extensive damage to the articular surface. This is also indicated in
        patients with avascular necrosis of the humeral head following
        disruption of the blood supply around the surgical neck.

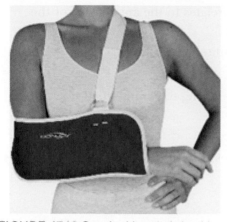

FIGURE 67.10 Standard hospital shoulder-based sling.

Reproduced from: Rizzone, K. & Gregory, A., 2013. Using casts, splints, and braces in the Emergency Department. Clinical Pediatric Emergency Medicine 14(4), 340-318, Fig. 5.

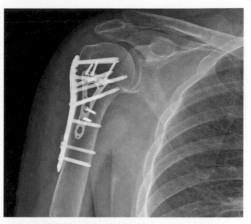

FIGURE 67.11 ORIF of a proximal humerus fracture.

Reproduced from: Choi, S. & Kang, H., 2014. Technical tips: dual plate fixation technique for comminuted proximal humerus fractures. Injury 45(8), 1280-1282, Fig. 2C.

> An arthritic glenohumeral joint may require a total shoulder replacement, provided the patient has adequate shoulder function.

MIDSHAFT HUMERAL FRACTURE

These fractures are associated with bimodal presentation with high energy trauma in younger patients and low impact fractures related to osteoporosis in older patients.

Examination

- There may be obvious deformity of the limb with bruising around the arm and elbow.
- These fractures can be associated with neurovascular injuries, necessitating careful examination of the lower limb, particularly the radial nerve, which lies in close proximity to the midshaft of the humerus.
  - Radial nerve palsy is a common postoperative complication, even in closed fractures (10%).
  - Will require monitoring in the outpatient setting.

Investigations

- As the mechanism is often similar to proximal humerus fractures, a shoulder X-ray is recommended to ensure the humeral head is enlocated.
- Initial investigations should include AP and lateral plain X-ray films.

SECTION V

- The AO trauma classification system relates to the appearance of the fracture (A, B and C):
  - A – simple fractures (transverse, spiral and oblique)
  - B – wedge fractures
  - C – complex fractures, typically referring to comminuted fractures.

Management

- Much like proximal humerus fractures, around 80% of humeral fractures can be managed conservatively.
  - Indications include:
    - <3 cm of shortening
    - <20° of anterior or posterior angulation
    - <30° of varus angulation.
  - Management includes splinting and a functional brace (Fig. 67.12), applying traction to maintain length of the fracture.
- Operative management is indicated in patients with open fractures and obvious radial nerve or vascular injury requiring exploration of the fracture site.
  - Oblique and transverse fractures can be managed by ORIF with plates and screws (Fig. 67.13).
  - Segmental fractures may be amenable to intramedullary (IM) nails.
- Complications of midshaft humeral fractures include:
  - Non-union of fracture:
    - similar rates for operative and non-operative interventions (5–10%)
    - affected by fracture factors such as the displacement of fragments and presence of segmental fractures
    - patient factors such as nutritional status and presence of osteoporosis.
  - Radial nerve palsy as above.

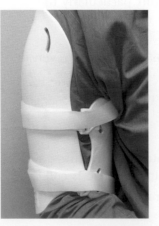

FIGURE 67.12 Brace used in the conservative management of humerus fracture.

Reproduced from: Scolaro, J. & Taylor, R., 2015. Chapter 11: Orthopedic trauma. In: Namdari, S., Orthopedic Secrets. Elsevier, pp. 381-442, Fig. 11.11.

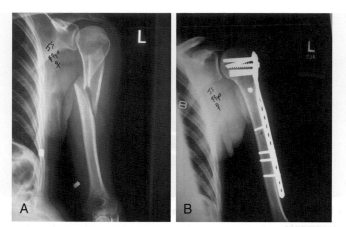

FIGURE 67.13 Displaced spiral left humerus fracture managed with plate and screw ORIF. A segmental fracture could undergo an IM nail.

Reproduced from: Infante, A. & Lindvall, E., 2008. Chapter 6: Fractures of the humeral shaft. In: Sanders, R., Core Knowledge in Orthopaedics: Trauma. Mosby, pp. 79-88, Figs 6-6 & 6-7.

RADIAL HEAD FRACTURE

This is the most common fracture affecting the elbow. The mechanism is typically a fall onto an outstretched hand while the arm is pronated. Injury can be associated with other soft tissue injuries. The history should include wrist pain, which may indicate a separate injury at the DRUJ.

The Mason classification system is commonly used:

- type I – non-displaced fractures (displacement ≤2 mm)
- type II – displaced fractures >2 m
- type III – comminuted fractures
- type IV – radial head fracture with dislocation.

Examination

- On examination patients demonstrate a tender lateral elbow with decreased ROM.
- A full assessment of ROM, as allowed by the patient's pain, should be undertaken to determine if there is a mechanical block of the elbow joint from fracture fragments or haemarthrosis.
  - Due to its close proximity to the radial head, there should be assessment of the posterior interosseous nerve (PIN) by asking the patient to extend their thumb.

Investigations

- Plain films can identify fractures and positions of fragments with AP and lateral films (Fig. 67.14).
  - In the acute setting the position of the radial head must be checked to ensure a dislocation requiring urgent reduction.

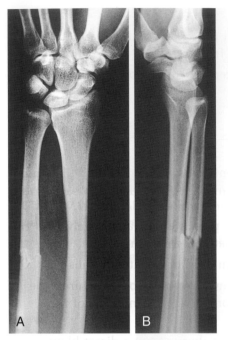

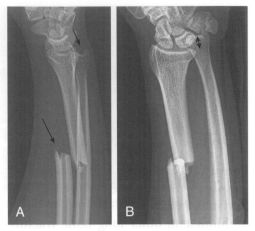

FIGURE 67.17 Galeazzi fracture. B more clearly demonstrates a DRUJ injury, highlighting the importance of obtaining clear imaging of the nearby joints.

Reproduced from: Singh, A. & Kaewlai, R., 2009. Chapter 4: Extremity trauma. In: Soto, J., Emergency Radiology: The requisites, 2nd ed. Elsevier, pp. 112-161, Fig. 4.14.

FIGURE 67.16 Minimally displaced nightstick fracture amenable to conservative management.

Reproduced from: Prawer, A., 2012. Chapter 6: Radius and ulna fractures. In: Eiff, P., Fracture Management for Primary Care. Saunders, pp. 102-112, Fig. 6.24.

Management

- Management of isolated ulna fracture can be conservative with plaster immobilisation, provided:
  - fracture involves distal two-thirds of ulna (higher rates of mal-union are seen in non-operatively managed proximal third fractures)
  - <50% overlap of the fracture fragments (displacement)
  - <10% angulation.
- ORIF is indicated in virtually all fractures of the radius due to the instability caused by the rotation of the radius (Fig. 67.18). Position of the fracture cannot be reliably maintained by plaster cast alone.
  - Also suggested for patients with isolated ulna fractures that do not meet the above criteria for conservative management.
  - Evidence of bone loss in the fracture site may necessitate the use of bone graft in addition to ORIF, which might otherwise result in non-union.

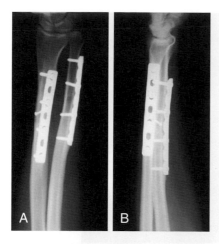

FIGURE 67.18 Plate and screw ORIF of a radius and ulna fracture.

Reproduced from: Moss, J. & Bynum, D., 2007. Diphyseal fractures of the radius and ulna in adults. Hand Clinics 23(2), 143-151, Fig. 9.

- Complications
  - Non-union:
    - associated with high energy comminuted fractures
    - may require further intervention with bone grafting.
  - PIN palsy:
    - results from proximal forearm fractures, particularly those involving the ulna.
- Postoperative care involves a period of immobilisation for 6–8 weeks with no heavy lifting for 3 months.

PATELLA FRACTURE

The patella is a sesamoid bone serving as the insertion of the quadriceps and contributing to the knee extension mechanism. Patella fractures account for around 1% of all fractures. Two of the most common mechanisms involve either: 1) direct blow to the patella, typically while the knee is flexed or 2) sudden and forceful extension of the quadriceps.

History typically reveals anterior knee pain after the above-described mechanism with pain on palpation and weight bearing.

Examination

- Assessment of the patient should include a straight leg raise test involving the patient demonstrating the ability to lift the leg off the bed.
  - A swollen and particularly tender knee may be suggestive of a haemarthrosis.

SECTION V

ANKLE FRACTURE

Ankle fractures refer to bony injuries to the distal tibia and fibula, in particular the medial, lateral and posterior malleolus.

Ankle injuries are common presentations to the Emergency Department, with a range of severity. Mechanisms vary from high energy trauma, which can result in open fracture/dislocations (Chapter 46), to low energy falls and sports injuries.

For low energy, closed injuries presenting to the ED, the key is to establish whether the patient has sustained a fracture or a soft tissue injury (sprain):

- The clinical likelihood of a fracture will determine whether a patient should have imaging.

- The 'Ottawa ankle rules' are a commonly used aid in this decision-making process, stipulating that imaging should be ordered for patients who meet set criteria:

  ○ aged >55 years

  ○ inability to weight bear immediately following injury (If the patient is able to weight bear initially then develops pain and swelling, it is more suggestive of sprain.)

  ○ tenderness over bony prominences (lateral, medial malleolus).

High energy ankle injuries associated with MVAs can result in severe open fracture dislocations with significant soft tissue and neurovascular damage.

History should focus on establishing the mechanism of injury, with inversion, eversion and external rotation commonly described movements.

Examination

- Examination may reveal a generally swollen joint with decreased ROM and possible instability.

Investigations

- Initial investigation should include:
  ○ AP and lateral views of the ankle
  ○ external rotation stress/weight bear views of the mortise (allows for visualisation of widening of any joint space – widening is associated with disruption to ligamentous structures, in particular the syndesmosis).

- Fracture/dislocations of the ankle require urgent reduction, following X-ray.

- Due to the complex nature of ankle injury multiple classification systems are used based on a variety of injury factors such as the mechanism and/or location of injury.

Management

Management of ankle fracture is dependent on the location of the fracture(s).

- For isolated fractures:
  - Medial malleolus fracture
    - Undisplaced fractures can be managed conservatively with a below knee cast for 4–6 weeks.
    - Displacement of the fracture (>2 mm) or evidence of talar shift are indications for ORIF.
  - Lateral malleolus (fibula) fracture
    - See Table 67.3 for classification and management according to the Weber classification system.
  - Posterior malleolus fracture
    - Conservative management can be offered to patients with minimally displaced fractures (<2 mm) involving <25% of the articular surface.
- Multiple sites of injury are common:
  - Around 15–20% of ankle fractures are bi-malleolar.

TABLE 67.3 Weber classification of ankle fibula fractures

Weber A
- Injury below the level of the syndesmosis
- Intact
- Mechanism typically an inversion injury
- Fracture is usually considered stable
- Managed conservatively with cast immobilisation unless significant displacement of fracture fragment

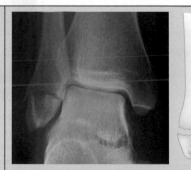

FIGURE 67.22 Weber A fracture.

Reproduced from: Raby, N. & Hughes, P., 2015. Chapter 52: Appendicular and pelvic trauma. In: Grant, L. & Griffin, N., Grainger and Allison's Diagnostic Radiology Essentials. London: Churchill Livingstone, pp. 1211-1240, Fig. 52.65. Abu-Laban, R. & Rose, N., 2014. Chapter 58: Ankle and foot. In: Marx, J., Hockberger, R. & Walls, R,, Rosen's Emergency Medicine, 8th ed. Philadelphia: Saunders, pp. 723-750, Fig. 58.8.

continued

Management

Calcaneal fractures are largely categorised as extraarticular (25% of fractures) and intraarticular (75%).

- Extraarticular fractures
  - Can be managed conservatively if fragments displaced <1 mm with a below knee cast for 10–12 weeks
  - Fragments displaced > 1 mm are managed dependent on their size:
    - Large fracture fragments (>1 cm) might be amenable to percutaneous K-wiring.
    - Smaller displaced fragments will require ORIF.
- Intraarticular fractures
  - Non-displaced fractures can be managed conservatively, with same immobilisation as above.
  - Displaced fractures in multiple sizeable fragments will require ORIF.
    - Some patients may require subtalar joint fusion.
- Postoperatively these patients may develop long-term pain associated with degenerative changes in the sub-talar joint.
- Soft tissue swelling can persist leading to difficulties with wound healing and impingement.

ACUTE SOFT TISSUE INJURIES

Referred to as 'sports medicine', soft tissue injuries affecting the joints can have a large impact on function.

Knee

Anterior cruciate ligament (ACL) injuries

These are more common in younger patients.

The mechanism is typically from either a torsion force through the knee while the foot is planted or a direct blow.

Examination

- Examination of the knee focuses on the presence of ligament instability. Lachman's test (Fig. 67.25) will assess laxity of the ACL by observing for translation of the tibia.
- Can be associated with other knee injuries, particularly meniscal tears.

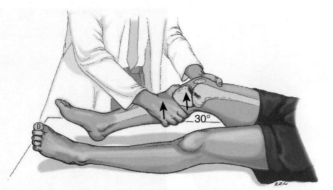

FIGURE 67.25 Lachman's test for assessing ACL laxity.

Reproduced from: Miller, M. & Sanders, T., 2012. Chapter 79: Anterior cruciate ligament. In: Miller, M., Presentation, Imaging and Treatment of Common Musculoskeletal Conditions. Saunders, pp. 419-430, Fig. 79.2.

Investigations

- Plain X-rays are typically normal, though a small tibial avulsion fragment may be visualised.
- MRI is the gold standard to assess ligament integrity.

Management

- Management can be conservative with physiotherapy and activity modification.
  - Patients may report symptoms of instability, including the knee giving way.
- Operative management techniques vary around the world but the common approach is the use of a tendon graft (hamstring/quadriceps/patellar/allograft) to replace the function of the damaged ligament.
  - Initial debridement of damaged tissue and preparation for graft are done arthroscopically.
  - The graft is threaded through carefully selected femoral and tibial 'tunnels'(Fig. 67.26).
    - The 'button' secures the graft at the proximal end of the femoral tunnel.
    - Metal screws or 'anchors' secure the graft distally.
  - Positions of these components can be confirmed with postoperative film.
- Procedure is performed as an overnight stay.
  - Patients are often given strengthening exercises prior to the operation date.

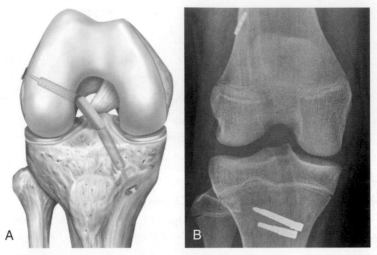

FIGURE 67.26 ACL reconstruction with graft demonstrating femoral and tibial tunnels with postoperative film confirming the position of the metalware.

Reproduced from: Lubowitz, J. & Amhad, C., 2011. All-inside anterior cruciate ligament graft-link technique: second-generation, no-incision anterior cruciate ligament reconstruction. Arthroscopy: The Journal of Arthroscopic and Related Surgery 27(5), 717-727, Fig. 10. Wall, E.J., Myer, G.D. & May, M.M., 2011. Anterior cruciate ligament reconstruction timing in children with open growth plates: new surgical techniques including all-epiphyseal. Clinics in Sports Medicine 30(4), 789-800, Fig. 2C.

- Postoperatively patients are able to weight bear immediately with a focus on early physiotherapy.
  - Recovery time to full activity is influenced by the site of graft selection.

Meniscal injury

Acute meniscal tears mostly originate from twisting injuries.

Examination

- Patients present with generalised swelling and joint line tenderness. Close examination of the knee may reveal an effusion.
  - Observing the patient's gait and asking the patient to squat and rise allows for an assessment of the patient's functional status.
  - McMurray's test assesses for impingement of the meniscal tears in the fully extended knee.
    - The knee is flexed with internal or external rotation of the tibia.
    - The test is positive if the patient experiences pain or experiences a popping sensation.
  - The patient may have difficulty with mobility in the initial injury phase, though will improve once swelling and pain subside.

Management

- In the acute setting patients may improve with symptomatic management (analgesia, ice, elevation), though the tears will not.
- Symptoms may persist, however, leading to chronic pain and disability requiring further investigation and management (see below).

Ankle ligament injuries

Ankle 'sprains' refer to injuries to the ankle ligaments. Most common ligamentous injuries result from a combination of dorsi/plantar flexion and inversion forcers.

There are three main areas of injuries:

1 lateral ligament complex:
   ○ accounts for 85% of all ankle sprains
   ○ more commonly associated with high grade injuries
2 medial ligament (deltoid)
   ○ strong, thick ligament less frequently injured
   ○ can be associated with avulsion fractures
3 syndesmosis injuries resulting from high energy dorsiflexion of the foot
   ○ high grade injury can lead to long-term instability of the ankle
   ○ external rotation stress test will produce pain in the area of the syndesmosis
   ○ may require surgical fixation.

Examination

- Physical examination findings correlate to the grade of ligament injury (see Table 67.4).

TABLE 67.4 Grades of ankle ligament sprains

GRADE OF SPRAIN	LIGAMENT INJURY	EXAMINATION FINDINGS
1	Stretching of ligament with no macroscopic tears	Minor swelling. No instability
2	Partial tearing of ligament	Moderate swelling with some instability
3	Complete tear of ligament	Severe swelling with inability to weight bear

Adapted from: Ferri, F.F., 2015. Ankle sprain. In: Ferri, F.F., Ferri's Clinical Advisor. Philadelphia: Mosby.

Investigation

- Imaging has a limited role in the initial injury phase, as most ligamentous injuries only require symptomatic management.
- For ongoing symptoms or suspicion of syndesmosis disruption an MRI can be useful.

Management

- Most sprains will resolve within 4–6 weeks.
- Analgesia and ankle support such as strapping and braces can assist patients to ambulate.
- Patients with grade 3 fractures can require a plaster cast.

THE CHRONIC JOINT

Painful hip

Careful evaluation of the presenting signs and symptoms can aid with diagnosis of the patient presenting with chronic hip pain.

History

Joint pain, stiffness, decreased mobility are common symptoms. Lateral hip pain typically represents non-joint pathology, typically associated with trochanteric bursitis.

The consultation should also establish how the patient's symptoms impact upon their function:

- Particularly with respect to their activities of daily living (ADLs), including self-grooming and household chores.
- Enquire about the use of analgesia medication.
- Ask the patient if they use gait aids.
- Get a timeline of the patient's previous management by their GP.
- These factors are important in determining whether to proceed with operative intervention.

Examination

The examination should similarly focus on an assessment of the patient's function:

- Observe the gait and ability of the patient to rise from a sitting position.
- The patient may report tenderness over the medial thigh and groin.
- Loss of active and passive ROM, particularly internal rotation (easiest to examine with the patient in a lying position).

Investigations

- Investigations will include plain X-rays of the affected hip and a whole pelvis view to allow comparison to the other hip joint.
- Patients planned for surgery will need hard copy films taken with magnification markers ('mag markers') to allow the templates for the prosthesis size to be used on the pelvis X-ray.

Avascular necrosis (AVN)

Osteonecrosis of the femoral head is related to the use of steroid therapy and excessive alcohol intake in over 80% of cases. Patients can be largely asymptomatic in the early stages of disease; as symptoms progress they manifest similarly to OA.

Investigations

- Plain X-rays may reveal subchondral lucency with progressive subchondral loss and collapse of the femoral head.
- MRI can provide a definitive diagnosis.

Management

- Early stage disease with small lesions can potentially be managed with osteotomy or core decompression, potentially supplemented with a bone graft or flap, though patients typically present with advanced disease.
- Advanced disease can be managed with joint replacement arthroplasty, particularly younger patients.

Osteoarthritis (OA) of the hip

The most common form of arthritis, with around 10% of males and 18% of females affected by symptomatic osteoarthritis. Risk factors include age, female gender, high level physical labour and sporting activities and obesity.

Patient's symptoms can progress over the course of several months to years:

- joint pain and stiffness, particularly in the morning
- pain that is associated with the hip joint tends to be medial
- decreased ROM, which can influence the patient's ability to mobilise.

Investigations

- Look for radiographic evidence of osteoarthritis: joint space narrowing, subchondral sclerosis and cysts, osteophytes (Fig. 67.27).

SECTION V

- OA confined to one compartment can potentially be managed with a unicompartmental joint arthroplasty (Fig. 67.30).

- Multicompartmental or severe disease is typically managed with a total knee replacement (TKR) arthroplasty (see Figs 67.31 and 67.32) (Chapter 46).

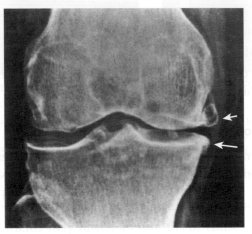

FIGURE 67.29 Knee X-ray showing features of OA. Arrows demonstrate osteophytes.

Reproduced from: Sein, M., Wilkins A. & Phillips, E., 2015. Chapter 70: Knee osteoarthritis. In: Frontera, W., Essentials of Physical Medicine and Rehabilitation: Musculoskeletal disorders, pain, and rehabilitation. Saunders, pp. 361-368, Fig. 70.1.

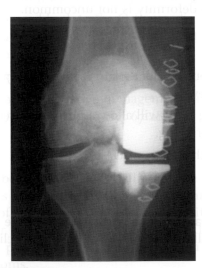

FIGURE 67.30 Unicompartmental knee arthroplasty.

Reproduced from: McKinely, J. & Ahmed, L., 2012. Chapter 27: Orthopaedic surgery. In: Garden, O.J., Bradbury, A.W., Forsythe, J.L.R., et al., Principles and Practice of Surgery, 6th ed. Edinburgh: Churchill Livingstone, pp. 476-490, Fig. 27.14.

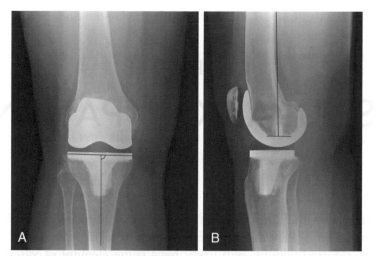

FIGURE 67.31 Postoperative films of a TKR.

Reproduced from: Brooks, M., Palestro, C. & Weissmann, B., 2012. Chapter 10: Imaging of total knee arthroplasty. In: Scott, N., Insall & Scott Surgery of the Knee. Churchill Livingstone, pp. 125-139, Fig. 10.1.

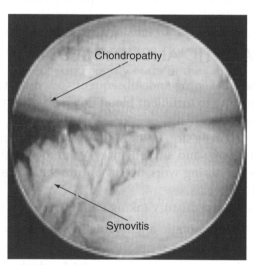

FIGURE 67.32 Arthroscopy of the knee showing degenerative changes.

Reproduced from: Di Cesare, P.E., Haudenschild, D.R., Samuels, J., et al., 2013. Chapter 98: Pathogenesis of osteoarthritis. In: Firestein, G.S., Budd, R.C., Gabriel, S.E., et al., Kelley and Firestein's Textbook of Rheumatology, 10th ed. Philadelphia: Saunders, pp. 1685-1704, Fig. 98.4.

TABLE 68.1 Annual risk of AAA rupture based on the diameter of the aneurysm

ANNUAL RISK OF RUPTURE	DIAMETER OF ANEURYSM
0%	<4.0 cm
0.5–5%	4.0–4.9 cm
3–15%	5.0–5.9 cm
10–20%	6.0–6.9 cm
20–40%	7.0–7.9 cm
30–50%	>8.0 cm

Adapted from: Brewster D.C., Cronenwett J.L., Hallett, J.W. Jr., et al., 2003 Guidelines for the treatment of abdominal aortic aneurysms. Report of a subcommittee of the Joint Council of the American Association for Vascular Surgery and Society for Vascular Surgery. Journal of Vascular Surgery 37(5), 1106.

- Patients with suitable anatomical features might be candidates for endovascular stenting (EVAR).
- Patients will require a full pre-admission work-up including an anaesthetics appointment, and an HDU/ICU bed should be booked for the day of surgery.

PERIPHERAL ANEURYSM

Peripheral aneurysm is defined as an increase in arterial diameter >1.5 × normal. It is considered a true aneurysm if all layers of the artery are involved, a false (or pseudo)aneurysm if only some layers are involved. True aneurysms are typically the product of chronic vascular disease related to atherosclerosis whereas false aneurysms are more commonly associated with complications of arterial punctures.

Aneurysms can present in a huge variety of sizes and some are large enough to be continuous with aneurysms from other anatomical sites.

Though the process of working up these patients remains largely the same, the exact surgical approach is dictated by patient and disease factors.

Iliac artery aneurysm (IAA)

IAAs are strongly associated with AAAs, with up to 40% of AAA patients presenting with an iliac aneurysm at time of diagnosis. Some IAAs are continuations of AAAs. Nearly three-quarters of IAAs involve the common iliac artery.

Presentations are varied, with patients often asymptomatic unless the aneurysm has become sufficiently large to compress surrounding tissue. Ruptured IAAs may present with localised or abdominal pain with haemodynamic instability requiring urgent exploration and repair.

TABLE 68.2 Indications for repair of peripheral arterial aneurysms

ILIAC ARTERY ANEURYSM	COMMON FEMORAL ARTERY ANEURYSM	POPLITEAL ARTERY ANEURYSM
• Symptomatic/ruptured • Asymptomatic, but >3 cm diameter or >1 cm growth in 12 months • As part of a dual repair with an AAA if diameter >2 cm	• Symptomatic/ruptured true or false aneurysm • Asymptomatic true aneurysm >3 cm • False aneurysm > 2 cm with failed non-operative management or on anticoagulant therapy	• Symptomatic/ ruptured • Symptomatic >2 cm in diameter

Adapted from: Hirsch, A.T., Haskal, Z.J., Hertzer, N.R., et al., 2006. ACC/AHA 2005 guidelines for the management of patients with peripheral arterial disease. Journal of the American College of Cardiology 47, 1239-1312.

Examination

- Outpatient monitoring should include regular physical examination and serial imaging to determine the diameter of the aneurysm.
- Examination should include looking for evidence of distal embolus suggesting thrombosis of the aneurysm, a risk factor for limb ischaemia.
- Document all pulses, present or otherwise.
- Look for evidence of distal peripheral vascular disease.

Management

- Current recommendations for surgical repair are listed in Table 68.2.
- Options include endovascular or open surgical repair: the decision between the two is dependent on the indication for intervention and the anatomical factors of the aneurysm.
- Conservatively managed aneurysms need interval follow-up with imaging.

Common femoral artery aneurysm

The common femoral artery is routinely accessed for endovascular procedures, with 1% of all access-based procedures complicated by a **false aneurysm** (see Fig. 68.1). The history will include a recent femoral arterial puncture with pain and swelling present in larger aneurysm. Examination can reveal a pulsatile mass in the groin.

True aneurysms are a product of peripheral vascular disease and may present with gradual onset of symptoms (localised pain/swelling). Note the patient's risk factors for vascular disease and pay close attention to other features of distal peripheral vascular disease (claudication, rest pain).

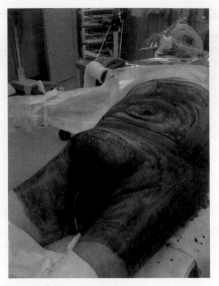

FIGURE 68.1 Large right femoral false aneurysm.

Reproduced from: Wyatt, M. & Rose, J., 2015. Chapter 13: Peripheral and abdominal aortic aneurysms. In: Beard, J., Vascular and Endovascular Surgery: A companion to specialist surgical practice, 5th ed. Elsevier, pp. 226-245, Fig. 13.10.

Investigation

- The key is to determine whether the aneurysm is true or false:
  - Duplex ultrasound can confirm the presence of either type.
  - CT provides clear imaging of the entirety of the aneurysm for patients who may undergo repair.

Management

- True aneurysm
  - If intervention is indicated (see Table 68.2), open surgical repair is considered the gold standard. Endovascular repair is not considered suitable due to the flexion forces through the hip.
- False aneurysm
  - Non-operative options include ultrasound-guided manual compression or thrombin injection. The vast majority that are <2 cm will spontaneously resolve.
  - Patients who fail medical therapy or who have a sufficiently large aneurysm should undergo open repair.

Popliteal artery aneurysm (PAA)

PPA is the most common peripheral aneurysm, accounting for over 70% of those found in the lower limb. Almost always a true aneurysm, PPAs are associated with atherosclerosis and, as such, frequently associated with other aneurysmal disease. The 50% rule is: up to 50% are bilateral; 50% of patients will also have AAA.

Up to 40% of patients will be asymptomatic at the time of diagnosis. Detection often occurs in these circumstances as an incidental imaging finding.

History of symptomatic aneurysm can include:

- localised pain and swelling
- evidence of ischaemia such as claudication or rest pain.

Examination

- Routine physical examination may often reveal the presence of aneurysm, leading to investigation and confirmed diagnosis.
- A subset of presentations include acute limb ischaemia secondary to embolus from aneurysm thrombus, requiring urgent assessment and intervention.

Investigations

- Investigation includes duplex ultrasound ± CT to confirm diagnosis.
  - Due to the strong association with peripheral vascular disease a full blood work-up of cardiovascular risk factors is worthwhile.
  - Screening for AAA with U/S is often appropriate.

Management

- Non-operative management includes a strong emphasis on reducing risk factors for peripheral vascular disease.
- Small diameter (<2 cm) aneurysms can be observed with regular follow-up.
  - Increasing thrombus build-up should be carefully monitored.
- It has been shown that larger popliteal aneurysms (>2 cm) present a higher risk of distal limb ischaemia and should undergo elective repair (Table 68.2).
- Repair by either open surgical repair or endovascular stenting (Fig. 68.2).
  - Open repair is still the more common repair method, though stenting is often considered in patients considered not suitable for open repair.

PERIPHERAL ARTERIAL DISEASE (PAD)

Peripheral vascular disease (PVD) has a large impact on the health of Australians, ranked as the 12th and 14th leading cause of death for men and women, respectively. There is a clear correlation with age, smoking, diabetes and other established peripheral vascular disease. Although patients can experience chronic vascular disease of the upper limb, peripheral arterial disease is much more common in the lower limb.

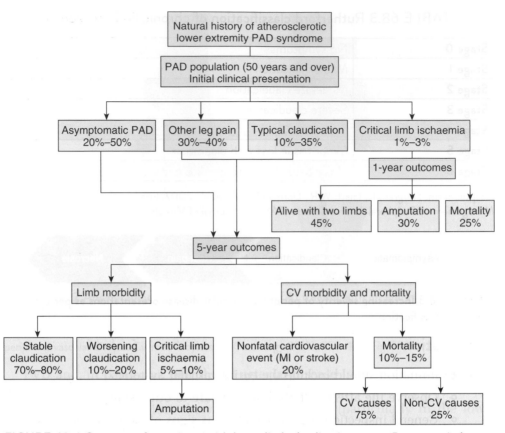

FIGURE 68.4 Outcomes for patients with lower limb claudication over a 5-year period.

Simons, J. & Schazner, A., 2014. Chapter 109: Lower extremity arterial disease. In: Cronenwett, J.L. & Johnston, K.W., Rutherford's Vascular Surgery. Philadelphia: Saunders, pp. 1675-1700, Fig. 109.2.

- The presence of rest pain and necrosis are highly suggestive of critical limb ischaemia, requiring urgent investigation and management.
- Peripheral vascular disease is present in around 20–40% of patients with a diabetic foot wound.
  - Patients with diabetes have a lifetime risk of 15–20% of developing a foot ulcer.
  - Patients are often referred to Vascular Outpatients for opinion regarding revascularisation options.
  - Patients with infected diabetic foot ulcers will need admission for antibiotics and/or debridement.
- The ABI is a useful bedside test in determining the presence of lower limb peripheral vascular disease. It is the ratio of the ankle systolic blood pressure to the brachial systolic blood pressure, recorded by inflating a blood pressure cuff and noting the reading where the Doppler signal disappears (Fig. 68.5).

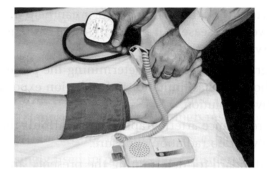

FIGURE 68.5 ABI performed using a handheld Doppler.

Reproduced from: Ko, S.H. & Bandyk, D.F., 2013. Interpretation and significance of ankle-brachial systolic pressure index. Seminars in Vascular Surgery 26(2-3), 86-94, Fig. 1.

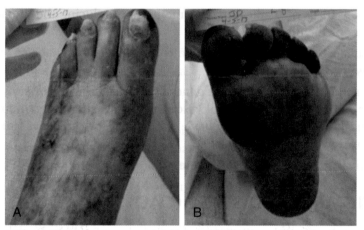

FIGURE 68.6 Widespread toe necrosis, a finding of severe peripheral vascular disease requiring amputation.

Reproduced from: Issa, A. & Newman, M., 2014. Toe necrosis, etiologies and management, a case series. Journal of the American College of Clinical Wound Specialists 5(2), 26-35, Fig. 4.

- o Normal is considered to be between 0.9 and 1.3.

- o Low ABI is <0.9, and is diagnostic of PVD in patients who present with symptoms of disease.

- o High ABI (>1.3) is typically due to calcification of the arteries secondary to chronic renal disease or diabetes (toe pressure readings are recommended in these patients).

- o This reading can be compared to a reading post treadmill (exercise ABI) to confirm the presence of claudication.

Investigations

- As PVD is predominantly a clinical diagnosis and ABI provides a sensitive bedside test, routine imaging is not used for further investigation unless the patient has critical limb ischaemia (Fig. 68.6).

SECTION V

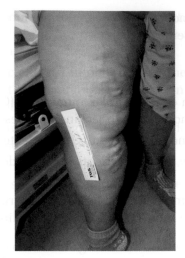

FIGURE 68.7 Prominent varicose veins.

Reproduced from: Freischlag, J. & Heller, J., 2017. Chapter 64: Venous disease. In: Townsend, C., Sabiston Textbook of Surgery, 20th ed. Elsevier, pp. 1827-1847, Fig. 64-5.

Investigation

- Venous Doppler U/S can help further map the extent of varicosity and presence of DVT.

Management

- Management is largely dependent on patient expectations and medical morbidities.
- Non-operative options such as weight loss and exercise modification can be recommended in patients not suitable for intervention or with low-grade disease.
- Ultrasound-guided sclerotherapy can be beneficial to patients with localised disease
  - This is a process of chemical ablation of the varicosities.
  - Can be performed as an outpatient procedure.
- Varicose vein surgery, see Chapter 47.

CHAPTER 69

CARDIOTHORACIC OUTPATIENTS

Paul Watson

CORONARY ARTERY HEART DISEASE

Coronary artery related heart disease is a leading cause of mortality and morbidity in Australia with a prevalence of 4% of adult males and 2% of adult females. This increases to 17% in adults >75 years. It is considered the leading single cause of death in adults.

The natural history of coronary heart disease and early investigation and management including angiography are covered in Chapters 35 and 56.

In the early stage of cardiac disease patients will predominantly be managed by their GP with input from Cardiology for patients who have experienced or are at risk of ischaemic heart disease. Patients who remain symptomatic or have progression of disease with medical management may benefit from an assessment regarding the need for coronary revascularisation. Some patients may only have heart disease diagnosed after an acute ischaemic event.

Coronary revascularisation

There are two main methods of revascularisation (see Chapter 35):

- Coronary artery percutaneous intervention (PCI)
  - An endovascular approach in which stents are used to maintain vessel patency.
  - Has a varied role in both acute and chronic coronary disease.
- Coronary artery bypass graft (CABG)
  - Open surgical access to the coronary arteries with bypassing of the diseased artery with vessel grafts.
- Indications
  - There are a number of specific disease factors that influence whether:
    - the patient should undergo coronary revascularisation
    - the type of revascularisation (PCI vs CABG; see Table 69.1).

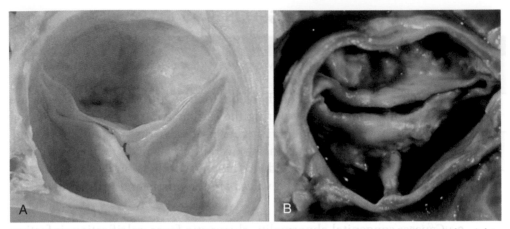

FIGURE 69.1 Normal trileaflet aortic valve on the left, a stenotic bicuspid valve on the right.
Reproduced from: Carabello, B., 2016. Chapter 75: Valvular heart disease. In: Goldman, L. & Schafer, A.I., Goldman Cecil Medicine. Saunders, pp. 461-473, Fig. 75.1.

- Aortic regurgitation (AR)
  - Causes: bicuspid aortic valve, aortic root disease, inflammatory changes from infection.
  - Symptoms: largely asymptomatic, but chronic or severe may manifest as an effect of left ventricular failure: orthopnoea (shortness of breath).
  - Signs: auscultation reveals an elongated diastolic murmur. The patient may also demonstrate a wide pulse pressure. Evidence of cardiac failure in chronic cases.
  - Investigations: CXR, ECG may reveal evidence of LVH.
  - Echocardiogram
    - Essential for evaluating the need for intervention.
    - The anatomy and retrograde velocity of the valve provide useful information for the classification of severity.
  - Role of surgery
    - Patients with symptomatic AR are generally recommended to have surgery.
    - Asymptomatic AR with TTE features of severe AR (residual volume [rVol] >60 mL per beat, LVEV <50% and LV end systolic dimension [LVESD] of >60 mm).
    - Aortic valve replacement (see Chapter 48).
- Mitral stenosis (MS)
  - Causes: rheumatic heart disease is the most common, though only around 50% will report a history of rheumatic fever. Calcification of the mitral valve (MV) is common in the elderly.

- Symptoms: progression of MS leads to increased left atrial pressure, causing s**hortness of breath**. Dilatation of the atria may result in the development of AF and increased risk of cardiac embolism.

- Signs: auscultation may reveal an 'opening snap' murmur due to restricted movement of the valve leaflets. P2 can be loud in patients with RHF.
  - Look for signs of decreased cardiac output (cutaneous vasoconstriction of the cheeks, decreased arterial pulse intensity, irregular pulse).

- Investigations: CXR, ECG may demonstrate LA hypertrophy (elongated P wave) or RV hypertrophy.

- Echocardiogram
  - Visualise mitral valve leaflet thickening (Fig. 69.2), evidence of rheumatic heart disease.
  - Measure the mitral valve area, with severe MS classified at <1.5 cm².

- Role of surgery
  - Surgery is usually reserved for patients who present with symptoms or have echocardiogram-confirmed severe MS.
  - Mitral valve replacement, repair mitral valvotomy (Chapter 48).

- Mitral regurgitation (MR)
  - Causes:
    - Primary (due to disruption of the valve itself): mitral valve prolapse, valve calcification, infection, rupture of chordae tendinae.

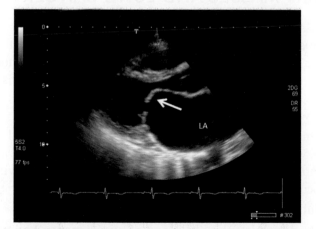

FIGURE 69.2 Echocardiogram allows for direct visualisation of the valves: this image demonstrates thickening of the mitral valve.

Reproduced from: Natale, L. & Meduri, A., 2015. Chapter 21: Non-ischaemic acquired heart disease. In: Belli, A.-M., Lee, M.J. & Adam, A., Grainger & Allison's Diagnostic Radiology, 6th ed. Elsevier, pp. 447-500, Fig. 21.37.

SECTION V

- – Secondary (systemic causes): cardiac hypertrophy, ischaemic heart disease, dilated left ventricle.

o Symptoms: most remain asymptomatic in early disease, though exertional dyspnoea is common as patients begin to develop LV failure. Patients may complain of other symptoms of heart failure as symptoms progress.

o Signs: the classic ausculatory sign is a holosystolic murmur, though the pattern is highly variable. Patients may have added heart sounds (S3), and a decrease in S1 intensity with splitting of the first heart sound in severe MR. AF is common in advanced MR.

o Investigations: CXR, ECG, BNP sometimes used in patients with LVF.

o Echocardiogram

- – Inspects the valve for evidence of calcification of flailing leaflets.
- – Examines the valve regurgitant orifice area, with >40 mm considered a key indicator for the need for surgery.
- – Determines the overall LV function. A failing LV with decreased LVEF is another important determinant for intervention.

o Role of surgery

- – Surgery is generally considered in symptomatic patients and asymptomatic patients with evidence of severe MS and LV dysfunction.
- – Mitral valve replacement (Chapter 48).

PULMONARY MASSES AND LUNG CANCER

Pulmonary masses represent one of the most common reasons for referrals to thoracic outpatient clinics. Due to the widespread use of chest X-rays and CT scans, a number of these masses are found incidentally in asymptomatic patients. Other patients may have had imaging ordered due to persistent cough or haemoptysis.

There are a wide number of benign and malignant causes:

- Benign: infectious granulomas account for over 75% of all benign tumours, with haematomas accounting for another 10%; vascular, autoimmune and other infectious processes (including cavitating staphylococcal infections).

- Malignant: primary lung cancer, pulmonary metastasis.

The key is to determine the likelihood of a malignancy and whether further investigation is warranted. The presence of risk factors for lung cancer (see below) increases the index of suspicion as do characteristics of the mass itself (size, shape, sub solid appearance).

Further investigations may include the following:

- PET scans can help distinguish highly metabolic lesions (potential malignancies) from low metabolic lesions (fibrosis, inflammation) (see Figure 69.3).
- If the lesion is suspicious for malignancy tissue diagnosis may be required:
  - bronchoscopy (±U/S) if the lesion is close to the bronchus (see Figure 69.4)
  - peripheral lesions may be amenable to percutaneous sampling
  - VATS with wedge resection (Chapter 48).

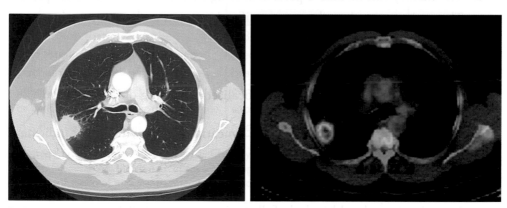

FIGURE 69.3 Solitary mass on CT demonstrates high metabolic activity on PET scan.

Reproduced from: Hu, X., Yi, E.S., Ryu, J.H., et al., 2015. Solitary lung masses due to occult aspiration. American Journal of Medicine 128(6), 655–658, Figs 3 and 4.

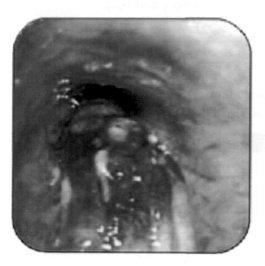

FIGURE 69.4 Bronchoscopy revealing obstructive tumour.

Reproduced from: Ferri, F.F., 2009. Chapter 132: Lung neoplasms. In: Ferri, F.F., Ferri's Color Atlas and Text of Clinical Medicine, 1st ed. Saunders, pp. 494–499, Fig. 132-4D.

SECTION V

Management

- Discussion regarding treatment is largely split into non-small cell lung cancer (NSCLC) and small cell lung cancer (SCLC).
- NSCLC
  - Stage I and II tumours should be initially treated with surgical resection (Chapter 48), followed by consideration of adjuvant chemoradiotherapy once the final pathology has been established.
  - Locally advanced NSCLC (stage III) is typically treated with chemoradiotherapy and surgery may be used in select circumstances.
- SCLC
  - No real role for surgical management.
  - Chemoradiotherapy is the mainstay of treatment.
- Prognosis
  - Patients with smaller, completely excised tumours have up to an 80% 5-year survival rate.
  - Once regional spread has occurred this drops to 25–30%.

CHAPTER 70

EAR, NOSE AND THROAT AND HEAD AND NECK OUTPATIENTS

Paul Watson

OBSTRUCTION

There are a variety of conditions leading to an obstruction of the upper airway. Careful history and examination supplemented by bedside investigations can help narrow the list of potential causes and expedite treatment.

It is common for symptoms to have lasted for months, and patients and their GPs may report multiple attempts at medication management with little relief of symptoms or frequent recurrence.

The two major broad categories of obstruction include inflammatory and structural abnormalities.

Chronic rhinitis and sinusitis

The causes of rhinitis are split into allergic and non-allergic. Allergic rhinitis affects up to 30% of adults and is a leading cause of chronic disease. Nasal irritation or itching distinguishes allergic rhinitis from non-allergic.

Chronic sinusitis can be defined by the presence of two or more of the following symptoms, for a period lasting more than 12 weeks:

- discoloured rhinorrhoea
- postnasal drip
- nasal obstruction
- facial pressure or sensation of pain
- anosmia.

Risk factors include: asthma, smoking, immunodeficiency and allergies and irritants.

The retention of mucus and debris from chronic inflammation fosters the colonisation of bacteria within the sinus. An abnormal position of the middle turbinate can lead to impaired sinus drainage. Enlargement of the inferior turbinate is commonly associated with chronic sinusitis. Patients with mucosal disease may undergo initial treatment with intranasal steroids.

- Examination can reveal the presences of nasal polyps and, for those patients with obstructive symptoms, a CT or MRI can aid in evaluating the extent of polyps and sinus inflammation.
- Patients should be given antibiotic therapy based on the presence of organisms from culture samples.
  - A longer course of antibiotics is usually indicated due to issues regarding tissue penetration.
  - Persistent chronic sinusitis should be investigated for potential fungal aetiology.
- Complications of chronic sinusitis can include acute superimposed infections that may lead to overlying cellulitis and osteomyelitis.
  - Unchecked fronto-ethmoidal and maxillary sinusitis may lead to periorbital infection.

Nasal polyps

Although the aetiology is not fully understood, there is a strong association between asthma and cystic fibrosis with polyps.

Relapsing episodes of acute rhinitis and sinusitis lead to mucus-filled growths, which develop into the observable nasal polyps. Patients who experience chronic sinusitis are especially at risk. The characteristics are benign pale, mobile, non-tender and avascular growths that typically become noticeable to the patient if they are visible or lead to progressive nasal obstruction.

Small polyps (see Fig. 70.1) can be treated with topical steroids; larger polyps respond to a combination of systemic and topical steroids.

Neoplastic polyps

These appear as unilateral, tender growths that bleed on palpation.

Nasal endoscopy along with imaging are essential for diagnosis (see Fig. 70.2).

In advanced cases neoplastic polyps present with foul-smelling discharge and can include septal perforation, There has also been a noted association with regional pain. The polyps can arise from the nasal lining or the paranasal sinuses.

On histology benign polyps tend to be papillomas whereas neoplastic lesions tend to be of epithelial origin (squamous cell carcinoma and basal cell carcinoma).

Nasal septum

Deviation of the septum is particularly common with a prevalence of around 80% in the general population.

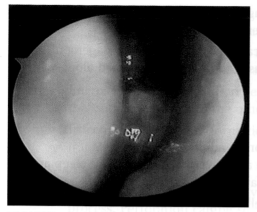

FIGURE 70.1 Simple nasal polyp viewed on nasal endoscopy.

Reproduced from: Bachert, C., Calus, L. & Gevaert, P., 2014. Rhinosinusitis and nasal polyps. In: Adkinson, F., Middleton's Allergy: Principles and practice. Saunders, pp. 686-699, Fig. 43.4.

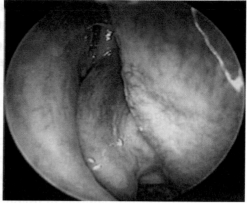

FIGURE 70.2 Paranasal neoplastic polyp.

Reproduced from: Jégoux, F. & Métreau, A., 2013. Paranasal sinus cancer. European Annals of Otorhinolaryngology, Head and Neck Diseases 130(6), 327-335, Fig. 1.

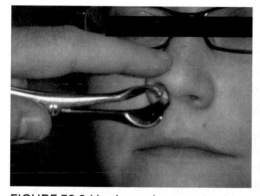

FIGURE 70.3 Nasal speculum examination.

Reproduced from: Manes, P., 2010. Evaluating and managing the patient with nosebleeds. Medical Clinics of North America 94(5), 903-912, Fig. 2.

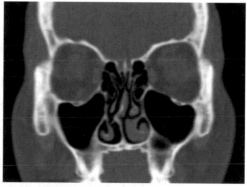

FIGURE 70.4 Septal deviation with left inferior turbinate hypertrophy.

Reproduced from: Fattahi, T. & Quereshy, F., 2011. Septoplasty: thoughts and considerations. Journal of Oral and Maxillofacial Surgery 69(12), e528-e532, Fig. 4.

SECTION V

Significant obstructive symptoms can be present even in patients with seemingly minor cartilage abnormalities.

Septal deformity can be associated with acute nasal injuries (see Chapter 49).

- Examination may reveal associated bony deformity suggesting previous injury; a nasal speculum allows for inspection of the septum directly (Fig. 70.3).
- Chronic septal deviation can lead to inferior turbinate hypertrophy (Fig. 70.4).

Oesophageal (Chapter 66) and neurological (Chapter 61) causes of dysphagia are discussed elsewhere.

Dysphonia

Often termed 'hoarseness', dysphonia refers to either an increased effort in phonation (weakness, tremor) or a change in the character of the voice (pitch, quality).

Transient dysphonia is common with acute infections of the throat (laryngitis), resolving when the illness passes. 'Straining' of the larynx from excessive shouting and coughing can have a similar presentation.

- Chronic laryngitis or dysphonia lasting more than 2 weeks should be investigated for the underlying cause.
  - Reflux is a particularly common cause of laryngeal irritation.
  - Smoking and other industrial-based fumes lead to chronic irritation of the larynx.
  - Chronic infection of the larynx may be fungal.
- Vocal polyps can develop secondary to chronic laryngeal irritation.
  - Smoking tends to produces multiple cord polyps known as Reinke's oedema.
  - Smoking cessation is a key first step.
  - Other vocal polyps similarly result from chronic inflammation of the larynx due to irritants or trauma (overuse or coughing).
- Neurological disorders affecting the muscles of phonation include Parkinson's, myasthenia gravis and motor neuron disease. Nerve injury, particularly involving the recurrent laryngeal nerve, can be another cause.
- Laryngeal cancer is associated with dysphonia.

Management

- **Microlaryngoscopy** allows for direct visualisation of the larynx and biopsy of suspicious lesions (see Figs 70.6 and 70.7).
  - Performed as a day procedure, a scope is passed down the laryngoscope.
  - Direct visualisation of the larynx allows for inspection of the vocal cords, biopsy of lesions and/or laser ablation.
  - Potential complications include: damage to teeth, laryngeal oedema, bleeding and aspiration.

SALIVARY GLAND STONES (SIALOLITHIASIS)

Stone disease primarily affects the submandibular gland (80%) with parotid disease accounting for around 15%.

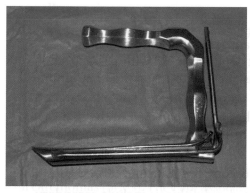

FIGURE 70.6 Laryngoscope.

Reproduced from: Schindler, J., Ossoff, R., Rosen, C.A., et al., 2011. Chapter 3: Operative pharyngoscopy and laryngoscopy. In: Cohen, J., Atlas of Head and Neck Surgery. Saunders, pp. 11-26, Fig. 3.2.

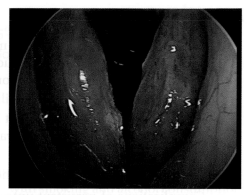

FIGURE 70.7 Suspicious lesion on laryngoscopy.

Reproduced from: Hoffman, H., Gailey, M., et al., 2015. Chapter 107: Management of early glottic cancer. In: Flint, P., Cummings Otolaryngology, 6th ed. Saunders, pp. 1634-1654, Fig. 107.15.

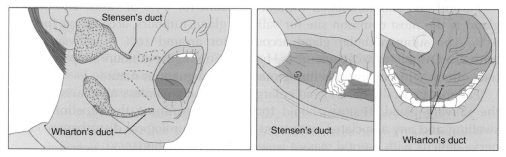

FIGURE 70.8 Diagrams demonstrating parotid and submandibular gland ducts with their terminal orifices.

Buttaravoli, P. & Leffler S., 2012. Chapter 57: Sialolithiasis. In: Buttaravoli, P., Minor Emergencies, 3rd ed. Saunders, pp. 207-209, Fig. 57.1.

Early stone formation is asymptomatic. The classically described periprandial colicky pain is due to large stone formation and impaction near the ducts (Fig. 70.8).

Examination

- Examination findings may reveal a non-tender unilateral swelling; further palpation round the duct orifice may reveal calculi sitting superficially. Stones within the submandibular (Wharton's) duct can be noticeable to the patient during meals as a lump below the jaw.

Investigations

- Investigations include high resolution CT to detect the position of the calculi. Larger stones may be visible on plain films or ultrasound.

- The typical approach for advanced laryngeal tumours is for total laryngectomy and bilateral neck dissection to account for nodal disease with postoperative RTx.

- However, some laryngeal tumours, such as T3 glottic tumours, have a lower incidence of nodal spread and may be amenable to less radical management. As such, these cases, as with all head and neck cancers, are discussed at MDM meetings.

Figs 70.9 to 70.12 illustrate various types of neck and throat abnormalities.

THYROID MASSES

Evaluation of a thyroid mass includes an endocrine history screening for the potential systemic effects of abnormal thyroid function (Chapter 59).

Examination

- Examination of the thyroid gland involves palpation of the neck from behind; the normal thyroid gland should not be clinically detectable.

- Enlarged thyroid tissue can present a uniform enlargement known as a goitre or discrete nodules.

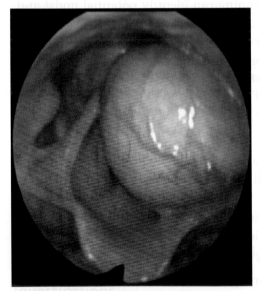

FIGURE 70.9 Endoscopic view of a large supraglottic mass.

Reproduced from: Morvan, J.-B. & Veyrières, J.-B., 2011. Solitary fibrous tumour of the larynx: a case report. European Annals of Otorhinolaryngology, Head and Neck Diseases 128(5), 262–265, Fig. 1.

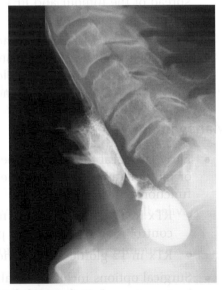

FIGURE 70.10 Pharyngeal pouch demonstrated on barium swallow.

Reproduced from: Kanagalingam, J. & Shaida, A., 2007. Diseases of the ear, nose and throat. In: Lim, E., Medicine and Surgery: An integrated textbook. Elsevier, pp. 175–227, Fig. 3.61.

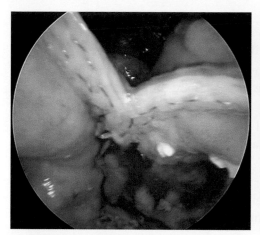

FIGURE 70.11 Endoscopic division of muscular septum with stapling to treat a pharyngeal pouch.

Reproduced from: Kanagalingam, J. & Shaida, A., 2007. Chapter 3: Diseases of the ear, nose and throat. In: Lim, E., Medicine and Surgery: An integrated textbook. Elsevier, pp. 175-227, Fig. 3.76.

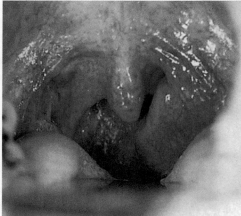

FIGURE 70.12 Uncommon oropharyngeal tumours include tonsillar non-Hodgkins lymphoma.

Reproduced from: Dhillon, R. & East C., 2013. Chapter 4: Head and neck neoplasia. In: Dhillon, R., Ear Nose and Throat and Head and Neck Surgery, 4th ed. Elsevier, pp. 87-117, Fig. 4.47.

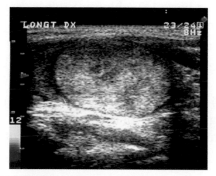

FIGURE 70.13 Benign thyroid nodule. Smooth and rounded.

Reproduced from: Kim, E.H., Potretzke, A.M., Figenshau, R.S., et al., 2015. Metastatic renal cell carcinoma presenting as a thyroid mass. Journal of Urology 193(2), 677-678.

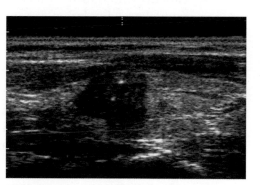

FIGURE 70.14 Malignant Thyroid nodule, irregular borders and micro calcifications.

Reproduced from: Kim, E.H., Potretzke, A.M., Figenshau, R.S., et al., 2015. Metastatic renal cell carcinoma presenting as a thyroid mass. Journal of Urology 193(2), 677-678.

- Goitres (Fig. 70.13) tend to occur as a result of abnormal levels of thyroid-related hormones, managed with medications or radiation ablative therapy.
- Thyroid malignancies (Fig. 70.14) typically present as nodules and are detected clinically or revealed on imaging.

SECTION V

Investigations

- Once a suspicious nodule is identified:
  - Sample by fine need aspiration (FNA), which will give an indication if a lesion is benign, inconclusive or malignant, but does not provide definitive tissue diagnosis.
  - Staging via CT imaging should be used, as some thyroid cancers readily metastasise, such as anaplastic thyroid, a particularly aggressive subtype.
  - CT scanning will also allow for evaluation of any intrathoracic extension of the thyroid, as well as appreciation of the impact of the thyroid on surrounding structures.

Management

- Clearly benign lesions can be managed with close ultrasound serial surveillance.
  - However, if the patient reports discomfort from the size of a nodule or if it is particularly bulky and rapidly growing, the patient may benefit from surgical management.
  - Patients who return an inconclusive FNA result despite a suspicious or rapidly growing lesion can undergo a bore tissue biopsy, progressing to a diagnostic lobectomy if required.
- The surgical approach to some of the thyroid cancer subtypes involves confirming diagnosis (see Tables 70.2 and 70.3) before proceeding to total thyroidectomy.
  - Papillary carcinoma on FNA is an indication to proceed for lobectomy with frozen section to confirm diagnosis, with total thyroidectomy once confirmed. Recurrence rates are high if total thyroidectomy not performed.

TABLE 70.2 Thyroid cancer overview

TYPE OF THYROID CANCER	PERCENTAGE OF ALL CASES	10-YEAR SURVIVAL RATE
Papillary	80%	>90%
Follicular	11%	85–92%
Hürthle	3–4%	75%
Medullary	5–10%	70–90%
Anaplastic	1–2%	5–10% (at 5 years)
Lymphoma	1–5%	50–70%

TABLE 70.3 TNM staging of thyroid cancer

T	N	M
Tx: primary tumour cannot be assessed	Nx: Regional lymph nodes cannot be assessed	Mx: Distant metastasis cannot be assessed
T0: No evidence of primary tumour	N0: No regional lymph node metastasis	M0: No distant metastasis
T1: Tumour <2 cm	N1: Regional lymph node metastasis	M1: Distant metastasis
T2: Tumour >2 cm but <4 cm Limited to the thyroid	N1a: Metastasis to level VI pretracheal, paratracheal nodes	
T3: Tumour >4 cm Limited to the thyroid or any tumour with minimal extrathyroid extension	N1b: Metastasis to unilateral or bilateral cervical lymph nodes or superior mediastinal nodes	
T4a: Tumour of any size extending beyond the thyroid capsule into soft tissue		
T4b: Tumour invades prevertebral fascia or encases vessels		
All anaplastic tumours are considered T4 tumours		
T4a: Intrathyroidal: resectable T4b: Extrathyroidal: unresectable		

- FNA results that are suggestive of follicular or Hürthle cell carcinoma are an indication for a hemithyroidectomy.
- An intraoperative frozen section provides an unreliable diagnosis of these cancers.
- Single stage progression to total thyroidectomy is not feasible. Around 20% of patients require the second stage total thyroidectomy.
- A suggestion of medullary carcinoma on FNA requires further work-up for genetic testing, which can influence the likelihood of unilateral disease.
- Anaplastic thyroid cancer is associated with advanced disease at detection, if there is presence of metastatic disease.

Refer to Chapter 49 for further details of thyroid surgery.

CHAPTER 71

NEUROSURGERY OUTPATIENTS

Paul Watson and Rami Shenouda

INTRACRANIAL TUMOURS

Intracranial tumours represent only 2% of all cancer diagnoses, yet are implicated in the greatest loss of potential years of life (12 years on average).

There are a number of tumour subtypes, though lesions are largely split into two categories: primary tumours arising from the central nervous system (CNS) and secondary metastasis. Primary CNS tumour incidence is associated with age, with a noticeable increase from age 55. Meningioma in particular is more common in elderly patients.

Primary tumours are described by their histopathological subtypes (see Table 71.1). Due to the large variance in tumour types, the classification of tumours is based on their malignancy potential (Table 71.2). Gliomas and meningiomas account for over 66% of adult intracranial tumours. Metastatic deposits may develop from gastrointestinal, breast, prostate, skin and lung and are more common than primary tumours.

Clinical presentations of brain tumours are characterised by a *large* variety of generalised and focal symptoms:

- Generalised symptoms include: seizures, headaches, nausea and vomiting, cognitive impairment, dizziness and syncope.
  - These symptoms may have an insidious and progressive onset, developing over months.
- Focal symptoms include: sensory disturbances, motor weakness and aphasia.
  - The pattern of symptoms is dependent on the tumour location.
- The signs and symptoms can be related to direct tumour invasion or can be the result of a mass effect and surrounding oedema.

Investigations

- Imaging plays an important role in localising and identifying tumours.

TABLE 71.1 Common primary intracranial tumours and their malignancy potential across all age groups

HISTOPATHOLOGY	EXAMPLES	WHO MALIGNANCY GRADING
Meninges (37%)	Meningioma	I
	Atypical meningioma	II
	Malignant meningioma	III
Gliomas (neuroepithelial) (30%)	Astrocytoma (6.8%)	I–III
	Glioblastoma (16.3%)	IV
	Oligodendroglioma	II–IV
	Ependymoma	I–III
Tumours of the sellar region (16%)	Pituitary (15%)	I
Cranial nerve and paraspinal tumours (8%)	Vestibular schwannoma (acoustic neuroma)	I
Lymphomas (2%)		
Unclassified tumours (5.5%)	Haemangioma	

Adapted from: Dorsey, J.F., Hollander, A.B., Alonso-Basanta, M., et al., 2014. Chapter 66: Cancer of the central nervous system. In: Niederhuber, J.E., Armitage, J.O., Doroshow, J.H., et al., Abeloff's Clinical Oncology, 5th ed. Philadelphia: Saunders, pp. 938-1001. Louis, D.N., Ohgaki, H., Wiestler, O.D., et al., 2007. World Health Organization histological classification of tumours of the central nervous system. Lyon: International Agency for Research on Cancer. Ostrom, Q., Gittleman, H., Fulop, J., et al., 2015. CBTRUS statistical report: primary brain and central nervous system tumors diagnosed in the United States in 2008–2012. Neuro-Oncology 17(Suppl 4), iv.

TABLE 71.2 Who malignancy grading and description of CNS tumours

GRADE	DESCRIPTION
I	Low proliferative potential, possible cure with surgical resection
II	Infiltrative, low proliferative potential; tendency for local recurrence
III	Pathological evidence of malignancy, some mitotic activity
IV	Cytologically malignant, rapid disease

Adapted from: Louis, D.N., Ohgaki, H., Wiestler, O.D., et al., 2007 The 2007 WHO classification of tumours of the central nervous system. Acta Neuropathologica 114(2), 97–109.

- CT imaging may indicate the presence or mass effects of a tumour; however, MRI is the standard, allowing for detection of tumours as well as associated oedema, tumour enhancement, infiltration and calcifications (see e.g. Fig. 71.1).
- PET scans can help identify potentially malignant lesions, further aiding diagnosis.

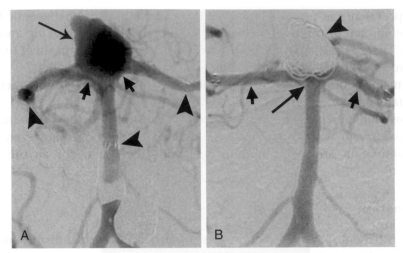

FIGURE 71.2 Cerebral aneurysm before (A) and after (B) embolisation therapy.

Reproduced from: Miller, J.C., Hirsch, J.A., Colen, R.R., et al., 2010. Cerebral aneurysms. Journal of the American College of Radiology 7(1) 73-76, Fig. 2.

HYDROCEPHALUS

Hydrocephalus results from an imbalance of the production, flow and absorption of cerebrospinal fluid (CSF). It is far more common in children, though there are presentations specific to adults. Specific causes include the following:

- Obstruction (non-communicating) of the flow due to narrowing in the ventricular system is the most common cause of hydrocephalus.
    - The passages between the 3rd and 4th ventricle are typical sites of obstruction.
    - Imaging will reveal dilation of the system proximal to the area of obstruction, allowing for localisation of the lesion (see Fig. 71.3).
    - Intracranial tumours are usually implicated in obstructive hydrocephalus.
- Reduced absorption of CSF (communicating) is the next most common cause of hydrocephalus.
    - Results from decreased absorption at the subarachnoid villi.
    - Imaging will reveal dilatation of the entire ventricular system.
    - Infection and haemorrhage result in inflammation of the villi and fibrosis of the absorption mechanism.
        - This results in a common adult form known as *normal pressure hydrocephalus* (see Fig. 71.4).
- Increased production of CSF is due to neoplasia of the choroid plexus (paediatric).

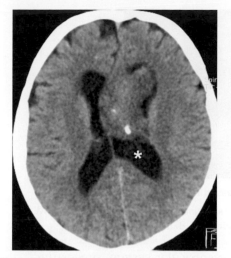

FIGURE 71.3 Hydrocephalus resulting from an obstructive tumour.

Reproduced from: Fenchel, M., 2012. Primarily solid intraventricular brain tumors. European Journal of Radiology 81(4), e688-e696, Fig. 3.

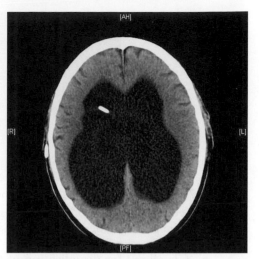

FIGURE 71.4 CT demonstrating large normal pressure hydrocephalus.

Reproduced from: Keong, N., 2011. Clinical evaluation of adult hydrocephalus. In: Winn, H.R., Youmans Neurological Surgery, 6th ed. Philadelphia: Saunders, pp. 494-504, Fig. 34.12.

Patients with a slow development of hydrocephalus may report no symptoms in the early stages of disease. However, symptoms may be observed in more advanced cases:

- Rapid expansion may lead to headaches, nausea and vomiting, particularly in the morning.
- Severe hydrocephalus can have a wide-ranging effect: compression of the vital brainstem functions can lead to drowsiness, cranial nerve palsies and visual disturbances.
- Normal pressure hydrocephalus is associated with a classic triad of dementia, gait disturbances and urinary incontinence.

Examination

- Examination should include full cranial nerve examination, and fundoscopy.
- Look for signs of eye movement and gaze palsies.
- Fundoscopy may reveal papilloedema (Fig. 71.5).

Investigations

- Lumbar puncture with a manometer can reveal increased pressure.
- Definitive imaging is required to confirm diagnosis.

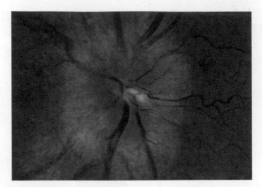

FIGURE 71.5 Papilloedema, a classic sign of increased ICP.

Reproduced from: Sadun, A.A., 2014. Papilledema and raised intracranial pressure. In: Yanoff, M. & Duker, J.S., Ophthalmology, 4th ed. Philadelphia: Saunders, pp. 875-878.

- ○ CT: allows for visualisation of the ventricular system, suggesting potential aetiology based on the degree of dilation.
- ○ MRI: provides higher resolution images and superior detail of the CSF system, allowing for identification of pathology in the subarachnoid villi and detection of small lesions obstructing flow.

Management

Management of hydrocephalus will usually necessitate intervention to prevent worsening of symptoms.

- Non-operative techniques such as diuretics and serial lumbar punctures have been shown to be less effective than surgical intervention.
- Choice of treatment is dependent on the cause of hydrocephalus (Chapter 50).
  - ○ CSF production/absorption imbalances are typically managed with *shunts.*
  - ○ Obstructive hydrocephalus may require relief with ventriculostomy.

THE CHRONIC SPINE

Chronic back pain with spinal degeneration is a common referral to both Orthopaedic and Neurosurgery Outpatients. Patients present across a wide range of age groups, with a mix of localised pain and lower limb neurological symptoms. Mechanical back pain is particularly prevalent in the community, accounting for around 1% of all GP visits. The lumbar–sacral region is most commonly affected with mechanical back pain the typical mechanism.

The history can be long and complex, often involving previous interventions with varying improvement and worsening of symptoms:

- Determine the onset of symptoms and potential cause (i.e. trauma).
- Establish the severity of symptoms and enquire about the presence of lower limb symptoms and urinary/bowel incontinence.

- Ask the patient about the impact of their symptoms on their ability to complete normal daily activities.
- List all previous interventions and the patient's current medication regimen.

Examination

- Examination should include inspection of the back to determine if there is localised tenderness.
- Lower limb neurological examination and PR examination (if indicated by history) should be performed with mapping of power and sensation.

Investigations

- Patients who are referred for surgical opinion will typically have undergone investigations including plain X-ray and/or CT/MR imaging.
- This can reveal elements of chronic disease:
  - intervertebral discs – herniation or degeneration
  - osteoarthritis, particularly of the facet joints
  - spinal canal stenosis
  - old fractures.
  - MRI can determine the extent of nerve impingement.
- The presence of spinal disease on imaging must be correlated with clinical findings as MRI of asymptomatic patients can reveal evidence of degeneration.

Management

- Management is determined by the severity of symptoms and a discussion with the patient about their preference for treatment options.
  - Physiotherapy for exercises may help improve posture and identify opportunities for activity modification.
  - Extradural steroid injections, which typically requires imaging guidance, can help the patient with confirmed mechanical back pain from disc-related pathology.
- Surgical intervention (Chapter 50) is reserved for patients with confirmed pathology and an established history of debilitating symptoms.
  - Options for surgery are dependent on pathology:
    - herniated lumbar discs – open discectomy, microdiscectomy
    - degenerative disease – spinal fusion
    - spinal stenosis – laminectomy.

SECTION V

CHAPTER 72

PLASTIC AND RECONSTRUCTIVE SURGERY OUTPATIENTS

Paul Watson

HAND FRACTURES

The management of hand fractures falls within the practice of either Plastics or Orthopaedics dependent on the location of the health service (which varies between states). Referrals from ED for simple closed hand fractures are fast-tracked to the outpatient clinic for urgent review.

When reviewing these patients, establish basic demographical information such as age, occupation and hand dominance. History should include the exact mechanism of injury and the exact date of injury, as some fractures have a 2-week window for operative intervention.

Examination

- Examine the hands on a flat surface while facing the patient, allowing for both hands to be examined simultaneously if need be (Fig. 72.1).
- The examination should focus on the gross appearance of the hand or fingers (swelling, erythema, deformity).
  - Note that certain fracture patterns will affect the appearance of the digit at rest.
  - The site of the deformity is not always the site of fracture.
  - An accurate mapping of where the patient is tender is useful.
- Check the patient's active range of motion (ROM) of the affected area, then passive as tolerated.
  - Observe for differences between the hands that indicate rotation of the digit due to fracture, and 'scissoring' when making a fist.

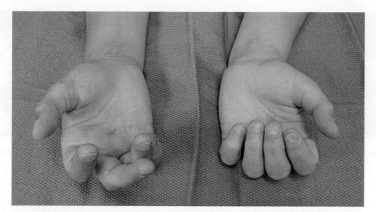

FIGURE 72.1 Bilateral hand examination demonstrates obvious rotational deformity of the right middle finger.

Reproduced from: Hammert, W.C., 2011. Treatment of nonunion and malunion following hand fractures. Clinics in Plastic Surgery 38(4), 683-695.

- ○ The extremes of ROM are of clinical importance:
    - – extensor lag for patients with metacarpal and distal phalangeal fractures
    - – ability to achieve power grip with ulna-sided metacarpal fracture.
- Examine stability of the joints – particularly the thumb (fractures and ligament tears).

Investigations

- All patients will require recent X-rays for evaluation.
- After completing an examination the junior doctor should ensure the imaging is on hand to discuss the case with a senior. See Chapter 67 for tips on how to describe X-rays.

Locations and types of hand injury

Distal phalanx

- Tuft fractures
    - ○ Usually sustained from crush injuries; can involve disruption of the nail bed.
    - ○ Repair of the nail bed: usually sufficient to splint fracture.
- Mallet injuries (Fig. 72.2)
    - ○ Typically result from a direct blow to the finger.
    - ○ Injuries older than 4 weeks classified as 'chronic'.
    - ○ An avulsion fracture involves the extension tendon.

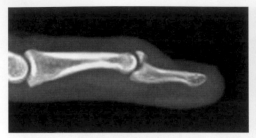

FIGURE 72.2 X-ray of mallet injury.

Reproduced from: Earp, B. & Blazar, P., 2012. Chapter 32: Extensor tendon injuries: primary management. In: Tang, J.B., Tendon Surgery of the Hand. Saunders, pp. 347–354, Fig. 32.2.

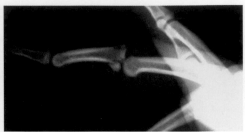

FIGURE 72.3 Middle phalanx fracture with dorsal dislocation.

Reproduced from: Hammert, W., 2013. Hand fractures and joint injuries. In: Neligan, P., Plastic Surgery. Elsevier, pp. 138-160.

- o If undisplaced with no volar subluxation, can be managed conservatively; mallet finger injury requires splinting for 2–3 weeks with hand therapy input.

Middle phalanx

- Shaft fractures
  - o Often result from direct trauma.
  - o The angle of fracture determines stability.
  - o Undisplaced transverse fractures can be splinted then buddy-strapped for 2–3 weeks.
  - o Oblique fractures are unstable and may cause shortening of the digit with impact on function; fixation with K-wire is indicated in unstable fractures.
- Base of middle phalanx fractures
  - o Result from direct force when the finger is slightly flexed.
  - o Commonly present as fracture–dislocations (Fig. 72.3).
  - o If they involve over 30% of the articular surface of the proximal interphalangeal (PIP) joint, they are considered unstable.
  - o Extensor tendon injury may result in entrapment within the joint, preventing reduction.
  - o If especially comminuted (as with pilon fractures), the fracture can be reduced and held with external fixation (Fig. 72.4).

Proximal phalanx

- Shaft and base fractures
  - o Tend to be oblique or transverse; are prone to instability.

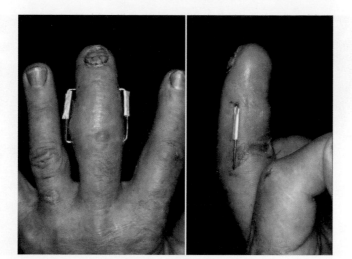

FIGURE 72.4 Modified external fixation for middle phalanx fracture.

Reproduced from: Calandruccio, J., 2013. Chapter 67: Fractures, dislocations, and ligamentous injuries. In: Canale, S.T., Campbell's Operative Orthopaedics. Elsevier, pp. 3305-3365, Fig. 67.53.

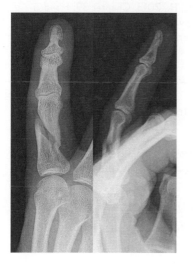

FIGURE 72.5 Spiral proximal phalanx fracture.

Reproduced from: Franz, T., von Wartburg, U., Schibli-Beer, S., et al., 2012. Extra-articular fractures of the proximal phalanges of the fingers: a comparison of 2 methods of functional, conservative treatment. Journal of Hand Surgery 37(5), 889-898, Fig. 6.

- o Shortening can occur and affects function.
- o K-wires can be used for fixation.
- o With spiral fractures (Fig. 72.5) the risk of rotation may lead to consideration of ORIF.

5th metacarpal

- Injury typically sustained by punching a hard object.
- Commonly fracture around the neck, but it is important to distinguish neck from head fractures.

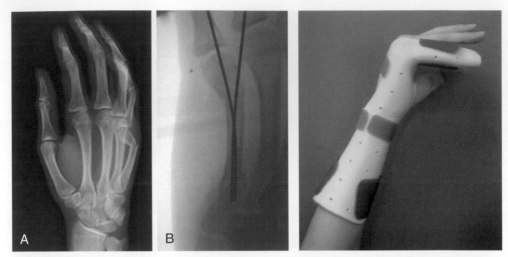

FIGURE 72.6 5th metacarpal fracture (left) undergoing percutaneous K-wiring.

Reproduced from: Cotterell, I.H. & Richard, M.J., 2015. Metacarpal and phalangeal fractures in athletes. Clinics in Sports Medicine 34(1), 69-98, Fig. 12.

FIGURE 72.7 Typical thermoplastic splint for conservative management of a 5th metacarpal fracture.

Reproduced from: Novak, C. & von der Heyde, R., 2013. Chapter 39: Hand therapy. In: Neligan, P., Plastic Surgery. Elsevier, pp. 855-869, Fig. 39.13.

- Fractures along the shaft and base are prone to shortening and will likely require reduction.
- Degree of angulation, extensor lag and rotation are important for consideration of operative intervention; up to 45° of angulation are acceptable (see Fig. 72.6).
- Otherwise managed conservatively with splinting (Fig. 72.7).
- Spiral fractures of metacarpals are also likely to have rotational deformity and may require ORIF.

1st metacarpal

- Injury typically results from direct blows or falls on the end of the thumb.
- The majority of fractures occur at the base of the 1st metacarpal.
- These fractures, particularly if intraarticular, are classically unstable due to the opposing forces of stabilising ligaments and tendon insertions (Fig. 72.8).
- Dedicated thumb X-rays include careful positioning of the thumb to obtain a true AP (Robert's) view combined with lateral and oblique (particularly to evaluate articular surface involvement).

and physical characteristics of a skin lesion can assist in identifying the type of lesion.

Clinical point: any chronic, non-healing wound should have a biopsy to rule out skin malignancy.

Important history includes:

- How long has the lesion been there? Is this a new skin lesion?
- Has it changed in size, colour (specifically enquire about rate of growth)?
- Has there been any bleeding/pus/scabbing/itchiness?
- Have you had other skin lesions?
- Do you have regular skin checks?
- Are you on any immunosuppressive medications?
- Do you have any wounds that have not healed fully?

Examination

Examination should be focused on:

- Identifying the boundaries of the lesion, determining the size, colour and shape.
- Examining other sun-exposed areas including the back. Local and regional lymph nodes should be examined for lesions on the limbs and head and neck.
- Differentiating skin lesions from subcutaneous growths such as cysts and lipomas. Sebaceous cysts may appear fixed to the skin, though a punctum is characteristic, aiding in diagnosis.

Investigations

Skin biopsy

- Skin biopsy is the gold standard for identifying suspicious lesions.
- Some units will routinely perform 'punch' skin biopsies in clinic using local anaesthetic.
  - Larger units may book these patients to 'local-only' theatre lists for biopsy to reduce the workload on the clinic.
  - If routinely performed in clinic, the junior doctor is often required to perform these biopsies.
- The technique is outlined in Fig. 72.14.
  - With an aseptic approach the lesion is infiltrated with local anaesthetic. It's sometimes advisable to use a marking pen so the biopsy target is not obscured by blanching of the skin following infiltration of the local.

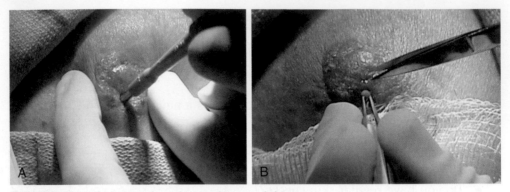

FIGURE 72.14 Technique for taking a skin punch biopsy.
Reproduced from: Tuggy, M. & Garcia, J., 2011. Chapter 1: Punch biopsy. In: Tuggy, M. & Garcia, J., Atlas of Essential Procedures. Philadelphia: Saunders, pp. 3-5, Figs 1.5 and 1.6.

- o The punch biopsy has a sharp leading edge; piercing the skin is achieved by rotating the instrument until it is through to the underlying subcutaneous fat.
- • Alternatives to punch biopsies include:
  - o Excisional biopsies – for small, well circumscribed lesions, histology can identify the lesion and adequacy of the excision.
  - o Shave biopsies – scaly lesions or those mostly contained within the epidermis can be removed by scraping the lesion with a sharp blade.
- • Where multiple biopsies are taken, the individual specimens should be clearly labelled in separate pathology containers with a diagram recorded in the notes to allow clear determination of where the biopsy was taken.

Benign and premalignant lesions

There are many subtypes of benign and premalignant lesions (Table 72.1), with some differences in the initial management stages. Seborrhoeic and actinic keratosis (particularly those with a scaly plaque appearance) will often undergo treatment with a GP, offering cryotherapy or simple local excision. Some lesions, however, will be referred for specialist management:

- • lesions on the face, head and neck or hands
- • lesions that are large or rapidly growing
- • potential local recurrence of previous malignancy.

MALIGNANT SKIN LESIONS

Non-melanoma skin cancer (NMSC) predominantly refers to basal cell carcinoma and squamous cell carcinoma. These conditions are particularly common with an estimated 2% of the Australian population undergoing treatment per year. The lesions are especially common in immunosuppressed patients, with 43% of solid organ transplant recipients developing NMSC within 10 years.

TABLE 72.1 Examples of benign and premalignant lesions

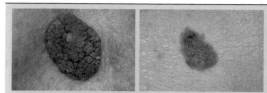

FIGURE 72.15 Seborrhoeic keratosis.

Reproduced from: Brinster, N. & Liu, V., 2011. Seborrheic keratosis. In: Brinster, N., Dermatopathology: High-yield pathology. Saunders, pp. 365-366, Figs 1 and 2.

Seborrhoeic keratosis

Arises as a skin-coloured, yellow or tan-brown plaque-like lesion that is classically described as having a 'stuck-on' appearance. Can range up to a few centimetres in length. Due to pigmentation can be difficult to distinguish from melanoma

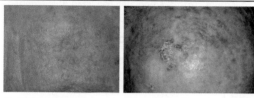

FIGURE 72.16 Actinic keratosis. On the left is a red flat lesion and on the right a scaly raised plaque.

Reproduced from: Soyer, P., Rigel, S. & Wurm, E., 2012. Actinic keratosis, basal cell carcinoma and squamous cell carcinoma. In: Bolognia, J.L., Dermatology, 3rd ed. Elsevier, pp. 1773-1793, Fig. 108.3 B and C.

Actinic (solar) keratosis (AK)

Commonly found on sun-exposed areas of skin, AK is considered premalignant due to the potential transformation to SCC. Appearances range from a tan or red rough flat lesion to crusted plaques. These lesions are also known as solar or senile keratosis. They are found in over 50% of patients >40 years

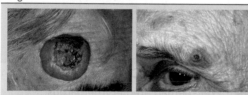

FIGURE 72.17 Keratoacanthoma.

Reproduced from: Brinster, N. & Liu, V., 2011. Keratoacanthoma. In: Brinster, N., Dermatopathology: High-yield pathology. Saunders, pp. 380-381, Fig. 1. Owen, C. & Telfer, N., 2014. Chapter 117: Keratoacanthoma. In: Lebwohl, M., Treatment of Skin Disease: Comprehensive therapeutic strategies, 4th ed. Elsevier, pp. 358-360, Fig. 1.

Keratoacanthoma (KA)

A rounded, firm nodule with a rapid proliferative phase. Though considered a separate histological entity, it shares features with SCC and should be excised early for diagnosis. These lesions can be large and locally invasive

SECTION V

TABLE 72.4 Application of the generic TNM staging to SCCs

T STAGE	FIVE-YEAR DISEASE-FREE SURVIVAL OF TREATED PRIMARY SCC
T1	95–99%
T2	85–60%
T3	60–75%
T4	<40%

Cancer Council Australia and Australian Cancer Network, 2008. Basal cell carcinoma, squamous cell carcinoma (and related lesions) – a guide to clinical management in Australia. Sydney: Cancer Council Australia and Australian Cancer Network, Table 5.2. <www.cancer.org.au>.

TABLE 72.5 Presence of nodal metastasis and five-year survival

NO. OF NODES INVOLVED	FIVE-YEAR SURVIVAL
1	49%
2	30%
>3	13%
Extracapsular extension	
Absent	47%
Present	23%

Cancer Council Australia and Australian Cancer Network, 2008. Basal cell carcinoma, squamous cell carcinoma (and related lesions) – a guide to clinical management in Australia. Sydney: Cancer Council Australia and Australian Cancer Network, Table 5.3. <www.cancer.org.au>.

- Tumour size – five-year recurrence rates based on tumour size:
  - <2 cm 7.4%
  - >2 cm 15.2%.
- Recurrent or previously inadequately treated SCC (incomplete excision). Patients with invasive SCC T3 and T4 have lower rates of recurrence following adjuvant radiotherapy.
- Patients with head and neck SCC who have confirmed nodal or metastatic spread will require multidisciplinary discussion with input regarding chemo- and radiotherapy.
  - Lesions are often large and require soft tissue coverage, which can include free flap coverage.
  - Patients with suspected nodal disease can also undergo a neck dissection involving removal of the locoregional node group (i.e. neck – cervical). Refer to Fig. 72.25.

MELANOMA

Melanoma is a skin neoplasia that develops from the abnormal proliferation of melanocytes. Strongly associated with exposure to UV sunlight, the incidence of

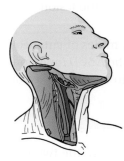

Radical neck dissection

A

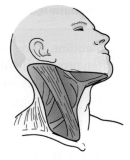

Modified radical neck dissection: one or more of the nonlymphatic structures are preserved

B

Supraomohyoid neck dissection

C

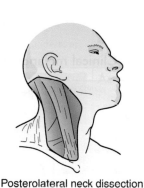

Lateral neck dissection

D

Posterolateral neck dissection

E

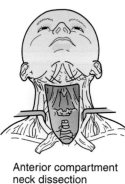

Anterior compartment neck dissection

F

FIGURE 72.25 Types of neck dissections, which can be modified dependent on the location and characteristics of the lesion.

Romesser, P. & Riaz, N., 2014. Chapter 68: Cancer of the head and neck. In: Niederhuber, J.E., Armitage, J.O., Doroshow, J.H., et al., Abeloff's Clinical Oncology, 5th ed. Saunders, pp. 1037-1070, Fig. 68.1.

melanoma is increasing in Australia and is the second most prevalent cancer in Australia.

When reviewing the patient with a suspicious skin lesion, history should focus on previous sunburn exposure, previous skin cancer, history of melanocytic naevi and family history of melanoma. Individual lesions may give a presenting history of evolution over months with increasing pigmentation, itchiness and bleeding.

Examination

Clinical examination of the lesion can be aided by the ABCD(E) mnemonic:

A – **A**symmetry

B – **B**order irregularity

C – **C**olour, heterogeneous pigmentation

D – **D**iameter >6 mm

TABLE 72.7 TNM staging of melanoma

TUMOUR: ASSESSED AS TUMOUR (OR BRESLOW) THICKNESS	NODES: NO. OF METASTATIC NODES	METASTASIS: PRESENCE OF DISTANT METASTASIS AND LOCATION
T1: <1.0 mm	N0: No nodes	M0: No metastasis
T2: 1.01–2.0 mm	N1: 1 node	M1a: Distant skin, subcutaneous or distant node metastasis
T3: 2.01–4.0 mm	N2: 2–3 nodes	M1b: Lung metastasis
T4: >4 mm	N3: 4 or more metastatic nodes	M1c: All other visceral metastasis
Ulceration: T stage given suffix (a) absence of ulceration or (b) presence of ulceration		

Adapted from: Australian Cancer Network Melanoma Guidelines Revision Working Party, 2008. Clinical Practice Guidelines for the Management of Melanoma in Australia and New Zealand. Sydney: Cancer Council Australia and Australian Cancer Network, and Wellington: New Zealand Guidelines Group. Ferri, F.F., 2015. Melanoma. In: Ferri, F.F., Ferri's Clinical Advisor. Philadelphia: Mosby. Soltani-Arabshahi, R. & Sweeney, C., 2015. Predictive value of biopsy specimens suspicious for melanoma: support for 6-mm criterion in the ABCD rule. Journal of the American Academy of Dermatology 73(3), 412-418.

TABLE 72.8 Breslow thickness and five-year survival

<0.76 mm	99%
0.6–1.49 mm	85%
1.5–2.49 mm	84%
2.5–3.9 mm	70%
>4 mm	44%

Adapted from: Ferri, F.F., 2015. Melanoma. In: Ferri, F.F., Ferri's Clinical Advisor. Philadelphia: Mosby. Balch, C.M., Soong, S.-J., Atkins, M.B., et al., 2004. An evidence-based staging system for cutaneous melanoma. CA: A Cancer Journal for Clinicians 54, 131–149.

- Melanoma in situ
  - Refers primarily to three in situ, non-invasive entities:
    - lentigo maligna
    - superficial spreading melanoma
    - acral lentiginous melanoma in situ.
  - Should be excised with a margin of 5 mm.
- Primary melanoma
  - Excision margin is guided by the thickness of the lesion:
    - (pT1) melanoma <1.0 mm: margin 1 cm
    - (pT2) melanoma 1.0–2.0 mm: margin 1–2 cm

- – (pT3) melanoma 2.0–4.0 mm: margin 1–2 cm
- – (pT4) melanoma >4.0 mm: margin 2 cm.
- Lymph node disease
  - ○ Imaging for staging: CT/PET can help identify suspicious nodes.
  - ○ Distant nodes may be amenable to fine needle aspiration (FNA).
  - ○ Patients will typically undergo lymphoscintigraphy to accurately map the sentinel node, allowing excisional sentinel lymph node biopsy (SLNB) in conjunction with wide local excision of the lesion.
  - ○ SLNB is typically offered to patients with locally deep tumours or the presence of ulceration, high mitotic rate and other poor prognostic factors.
- Patients with positive SLNB can then be considered for lymph node dissection.
- Patients with metastatic disease have a particularly poor prognosis (5–10% is the 5-year survival rate).
- Follow-up of these patients is dependent on the stage of disease with further management including the potential use of adjuvant therapy for discussion at MDM meetings.
- Patients who present with melanoma will often require rapid imaging assessment, biopsy of suspicious nodes and collection of information regarding previous treatment in preparation for prompt MDM discussion and surgical intervention.
  - ○ The junior doctor should regularly discuss these patients with the registrars and consultants to ensure there are no delays in the work-up.

THE 'CHRONIC HAND'

Carpal tunnel syndrome (CTS)

CTS refers to symptoms related to the compression of the median nerve as it passes through the carpal tunnel. The aetiology is not completely understood. It affects around 3% of the population (though estimates vary in the literature), and is more common in females with the typical patient aged between 30 and 60 years.

History will reveal pain and paraesthesia in the hand over the median nerve distribution, with the symptoms classically worse at night. Pain may involve the wrist and forearm.

Examination

- Examination of the hand may reveal altered sensation in the median nerve distribution, thenar muscle wasting but sparing of the sensation of

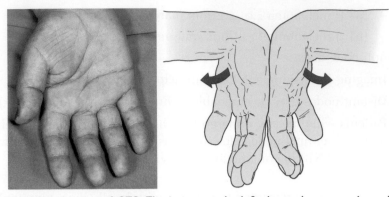

FIGURE 72.31 Assessment of CTS. The image on the left shows thenar wasting, with Phalen's test on the right utilised to reproduce symptoms.

Reproduced from: Hoffbrand, A.V., Pettit, J. & Vyas, P., 2010. Chapter 22: Myeloma and related conditions. In: Hoffbrand, A.V., Pettit, J.E. & Vyas, P., Color Atlas of Clinical Hematology, 4th ed. Elsevier, pp. 395-412, Fig. 22.39. Magee, D. & Sueki, D., 2011. Forearm, wrist and hand. In: Magee, D., Orthopedic Physical Assessment: Atlas and video. Elsevier, pp. 183-214, Image 6-11.

the thenar eminence; these are typically indicative of long-standing, severe CTS.

○ Specialised tests seek to reproduce compression to elicit symptoms:
  – Phalen's test (Fig. 72.31) – wrist flexion at 90°, with the dorsum of each wrist pushed against the other to provide further compression of the median nerve. Considered positive if symptoms occur within 60 seconds.
  – Tinel's test – percussion over the median nerve to reproduce symptoms (less sensitive than Phalen's).

Investigations

- Nerve conduction studies (NCS) are routinely performed to assess the severity of the neuropathy.
  ○ Though the sensitivity varies for NCS (56–85%), it has more reliable specificity (94–99%).

Management

- The decision for intervention is based largely on the severity of the patient's symptoms.
  ○ Mild or moderate discomfort with mostly nocturnal symptoms may be adequately treated by hand therapists via night splinting and exercises. Steroid injections may also offer benefit to these patients.

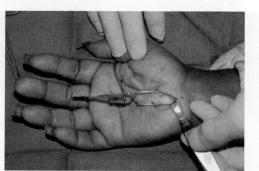

FIGURE 72.32 Open CTR via minimal access.

Reproduced from: Lee, M., Biafora, S. & Zelouf, D., 2011. Chapter 41: Management of hand and wrist tendinopathies. In: Skirven, T., Rehabilitation of the Hand and Upper Extremity. Mosby, pp. 569-588, Fig. 41.23.

- ○ Carpal tunnel release (CTR)
  - – Definitive treatment of long-term symptoms that have failed conservative treatment or cause moderate-to-severe discomfort.
  - – Open carpal tunnel release is the most common approach (Fig. 72.32). Can be performed as a day case under local anaesthetic. Percutaneous, ultrasound-guided and arthroscopic approaches are also utilised.
  - – Patients will typically report an improvement in symptoms within 24 hours. Those who present with ongoing pain may have an incomplete release, warranting further exploration.
  - ○ Postoperative input can be provided by Hand Therapy for scar management and exercises.

de Quervains tendonitis

This is a common cause of wrist pain affecting younger adults (30–50 years), particularly females. There are a number of potential differential diagnoses including osteoarthritis of the 1st carpometacarpal joint. X-rays can help exclude a degenerative cause.

The pain arises from the tendinopathy of the first extensor compartment (adductor pollicis longus and extensor pollicis brevis). There is a thickening of the tendons as they pass through the fibrous tunnel close to the radial styloid.

History should include questions regarding the location and severity of pain and functional impact. Pain can be generalised, affecting the wrist and distal forearm.

Examination

- • Examination may reveal swelling near the affected site with localised tenderness over the radial styloid.

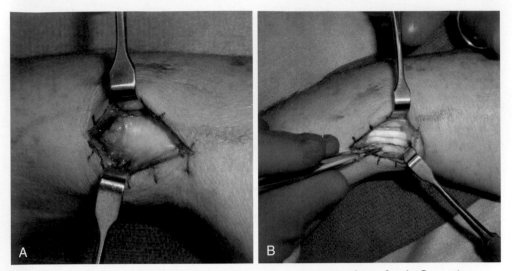

FIGURE 72.33 Open approach to a 1st extensor compartment release for de Quervains tendonitis. Note the thickened retinaculum in A.

Reproduced from: Lee, M., Biafora, S. & Zelouf, D., 2011. Chapter 41: Management of hand and wrist tendinopathies. In: Skirven, T., Rehabilitation of the Hand and Upper Extremity. Mosby, pp. 569-588, Fig. 41.23.

Management

- Conservative management is initially adopted through Hand Therapy with an immobilisation spica splint and regular simple analgesia; steroid injections can be offered to those patients who do not improve after 4–6 weeks of splinting.
- Surgical release of the 1st extensor compartment can be offered to patients who do not progress with conservative management; release can be performed via an endoscopic or open approach (Fig. 72.33).

Dupuytren's contracture

Dupuytren's is a genetic disorder resulting in the contracture of the longitudinal palmar fascia, which eventually leads to inflexion deformity of the digits.

Contractures form nodular bands of tissue called 'cords'. Early signs of disease include puckering of the skin. The disease progression is typically painless though individual nodules can be tender. It most commonly affects the little and ring finger, though all fingers can be affected.

Risk factors include family history, Caucasian ancestry, age >50 years and smoking.

Examination

- Examination of patients with advanced disease may reveal severe flexion deformity, with palpable cords affecting beyond the PIP joint. Assess the range of motion of all joints.

Management

- Mild disease can be referred to Hand Therapy for stretching exercises and advice regarding activity modification.
- Patients with persistent symptoms may initially benefit from collagenase injections into the diseased cord, with a recurrence rate of 35%.
- Surgical interventions are typically reserved for advanced disease (MCP flexion deformity >30°) and include:
  - Percutaneous needle fasciotomy:
    - transection of diseased cord through the skin
    - can also be performed as an open procedure.
  - Open fasciectomy (Fig. 72.34):
    - diseased tissue is excised, sometimes with the overlying skin
    - closed using Z-plasty to avoid scar contracture (Fig. 72.34).
  - These patients have extensive Hand Therapy input in the postoperative period.

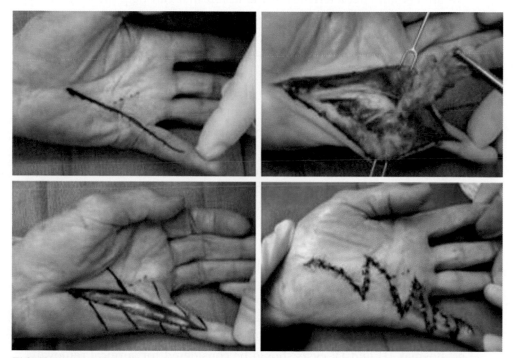

FIGURE 72.34 Open fasciectomy for advanced Dupuytren's contracture. The wound is closed using a Z-plasty technique.

Reproduced from: Calandruccio, J., 2016. Technique 77: Subcutaneous fasciotomy, partial fasciectomy for Dupuytren contracture. In: Canale, T., Campbell's Core Orthopaedic Procedures. Elsevier, pp. 328-332, Figs 77.5 to 77.8.

CHAPTER 73

UROLOGY OUTPATIENTS

Paul Watson and Todd Galvin Manning

RENAL MASSES

Renal cysts

Renal cysts are particularly common, with an estimated 50% prevalence in patients over 50.

There are certain characteristics of the lesion that can help identify the type of lesion:

- Definitive imaging including CT can help visualise the walls and whether the lesion is cystic or solid.
- Renal cysts are classified as either simple (see Figs 73.1 and 73.2) or complex (Fig. 73.3).
- The Bosniak classification system (Table 73.1) allows for further classification and assessment of malignancy risk based on their appearance on contrast enhanced CT.
- Management of the cyst is determined by the Bosniak classification, influenced by the patient's medical comorbidities.
  - Bosniak I and II cysts do not typically require further urological input. The patient can return to their GP with 6- or 12-monthly imaging for surveillance.
  - Bosniak IIF cysts will need to be satisfactorily distinguished from a class III. Further characterisation with ultrasound (usually) or the addition of MRI can help; if confirmed as a IIF, the patient should have regular follow-up with the Urology Clinic with repeat imaging (typically 3-, 6- and then 12-monthly).
  - Bosniak III and IV cysts should be considered for surgical removal either via partial or total nephrectomy with each option dependant on the location, character and size of the lesion.
  - For patients who might not be ideal surgical candidates, percutaneous biopsy can play a role in establishing the diagnosis and prognosis and

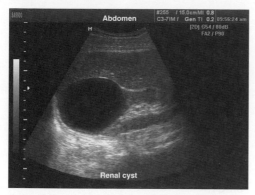

FIGURE 73.1 Simple renal cyst on U/S.

Reproduced from: Popo, J., 2012. Chapter 118: Renal dysgenesis and cystic disease of the kidney. In: Wein, A., Campbell-Walsh Urology. Elsevier, pp. 3161-3196, Fig. 118-22.

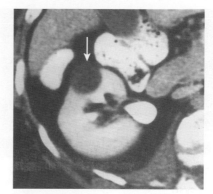

FIGURE 73.2 Simple renal cyst on CT.

Reproduced from: Bhatt, S. & Dogra, V., 2009. Chapter 41: Kidney. In: Haaga, J., CT and MRI of the whole body. Elsevier, pp. 1863-1953, Fig. 41-20.

TABLE 73.1 Bosniak classification of renal cysts

BOSNIAK CATEGORY	DESCRIPTION	RISK OF MALIGNANCY
I	• Simple cyst with a hairline thin wall. No calcifications, septa	1.7%
II	• Walls of lesion may contain few hairline septa, occasional calcifications • <3 cm in diameter with no CT enhancement	18.5%
IIF	• Multiple hairline septa and potential thickening of wall • >3 cm in diameter, intrarenal, no enhancement on CT	18.5%
III	• 'Cystic mass' with prominent, thick and irregular septa • Enhancement present on CT	33%
IV	• Thick-walled, irregular lesions with a clear malignant appearance • CT enhancement, including surrounding soft tissue	>80%

Adapted from: Margulis, V., Karam, J., Matin, S., et al., 2016. Chapter 56: Benign renal tumours. In: Wein, A., Campbell-Walsh Urology. Elsevier, pp. 1300-1313, Table 56-1.

SECTION V

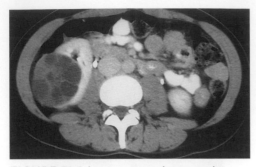

FIGURE 73.3 Large septated or complex renal cyst.

Reproduced from: Guay-Woodford, L., 2015. Chapter 47: Other cystic kidney diseases. In: Johnson, R., Comprehensive Clinical Nephrology. Saunders, pp. 549-564, Fig. 47-11.

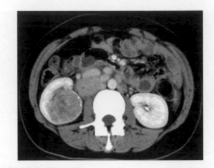

FIGURE 73.4 Renal cell carcinoma shown on CT.

Reproduced from: He, J. & Huan, Y., 2014. Renal carcinomas associated with Xp11.2 translocations: are CT findings suggestive of the diagnosis? Clinical Radiology 69(1), 45-51, Fig. 2c.

ablative therapies may be considered; however, surgical excision remains the gold standard.

Renal neoplasms

Renal cell carcinoma (RCC) is the most common primary renal cancer (90%). It arises from the proximal renal tubular epithelium. RCCs account for 2–3% of all cancers.

The classically associated symptoms of haematuria, flank pain are indicative of late stage disease with around 50% of tumours detected incidentally. As such, around 25% of patients have local nodal disease or metastasis at time of presentation.

Risk factors for RCC include cigarette smoking, obesity, diabetes, established renal disease and viral hepatitis.

Subtypes of RCC include clear cell (75–80%) and papillary (15%).

- Initial investigations should include:
  - Bloods: FBE, UEC, CMP, LFTs (screen for paraneoplastic syndrome).
  - Urinalysis: haematuria/ensure no WCC rise.
  - Imaging is essential for staging the lesion:
    - Usually renal tract ultrasound and CT-KUB + staging if appropriate are utilised in the first instance (see Fig. 73.4).
    - Biopsy of indeterminate lesions also has a role but remains controversial as tissue analysis and operative control can be achieved via partial or total nephrectomy.
    - MRI may be required to assess local invasion of the tumour, particularly regarding vascular structures.
    - Bone scan to assess for metastasis in patients with bony pain or elevated ALP. Certain hospitals may use PET scanning instead.

- Newer modalities are being utilised more recently, including 3D reconstruction technology and 3D printing to assist surgeons with anatomy conceptualisation.
- RCC is staged using the TNM criteria and has significant implications for mortality rates (see Table 73.2).
- Five-year survival rates can be calculated using this classification.
  - Stage I (T1 No Mo) – >90%
  - Stage II (T2 No Mo) – 75–95%
  - Stage III (T1–2 N1 Mo) or (T3 No–1 Mo) – 59–70%
    - Invasion into the urinary collection system is a poor prognostic sign (30–34% 5-year survival).
  - Stage IV (T4 or M1) – <10%.
- Definitive management of RCC is surgical excision.
  - Small confined tumours (T1) can be managed by partial nephrectomy.
  - Larger tumours (T2–T4) require total nephrectomy.

TABLE 73.2 TNM staging of renal cell carcinoma

TUMOUR	NODES	METASTASIS
T1: <7 cm, confined to renal parenchyma • T1a: <4 cm • T1b: 4–7 cm	N0: No regional nodes	M0: No metastasis
	N1: Spread to a single node	M1: Presence of distant metastasis
T2: >7 cm, confined to renal parenchyma • T2a: 7–10 cm • T2b: >10 cm	N2: Spread to a single node between 2 and 5 cm or multiple nodules <2 cm	
T3: tumour extends into major veins or adrenal, but not Gerota's fascia • T3a: into adrenal or sinus fat • T3b: into renal vein or infradiaphragmatic IVC • T3c: into supradiaphragmatic IVC	N3: node >5 cm	
T4: Tumour extends beyond Gerota's fascia		

Adapted from: Edge, S.B. & Compton, C.C., 2010. The American Joint Committee on Cancer: the 7th edition of the AJCC cancer staging manual and the future of TNM. Annals of Surgical Oncology 17(6),1471-1474. Icarra, V., Galfano, A., Mancini, M., et al., 2007. TNM staging system for renal-cell carcinoma: current status and future perspectives. Lancet Oncology 8, 554–558.

- ○ Adequate preoperative imaging is essential to determine the location and local extension of the tumour.
- ○ Lymph node dissection (LND) is performed when there is evidence of disease or for staging (in some rarer cases RPLND [see testicular mass section]).
- ○ Once histological diagnosis is established the patient's case should be re-discussed at an MDM meeting.
- ○ Note: There is no role for chemotherapy in RCC, but patients may benefit from adjuvant immunotherapy such as interferon or interleukin-2.

BLADDER CANCER

The second most common urological malignancy after RCC, bladder cancer accounts for around 2% of all cancers. The vast majority are transitional cell carcinoma (TCC) (90–95%). Bladder SCC is strongly associated with *Schistosoma haematobium* infection in patients of African origin.

Risk factors include: **smoking**, males, age, use of cyclophosphamide and industrial exposure to chemicals such as rubbers, leather and arsenic. One in 43 males >85 years will develop bladder cancer vs 1 in 166 females.

The most common presenting symptoms include haematuria (typically painless), abdominal discomfort and dysuria.

- Examination findings may reveal a palpable mass or lymphadenopathy in advanced cases.
- Investigations should include urinalysis to confirm the presence of haematuria and urine cytology if possible (usually three separate urine samples) to attempt to confirm the presence of malignant cells.
  - ○ Haematuria is a non-specific feature of bladder tumours as the source can be any part of the urinary tract.
  - ○ CT IVP is a useful tool for visualising the entire tract, particularly with respect to the upper urinary tract.
  - ○ Ultrasound can also be useful but invasive tumours can be further evaluated with MRI.
  - ○ Patients are then often booked for cystoscopy (see Fig. 73.5).
    - – Flexible cystoscopy is helpful for investigating haematuria undifferentiated patients as it can be confirmed rapidly without the need of anaesthetic.
    - – Patients may also be booked for rigid cystoscopy ± transurethral resection of bladder tumour (TURBT), allowing subsequent surgical removal of superficial tumours (see below).

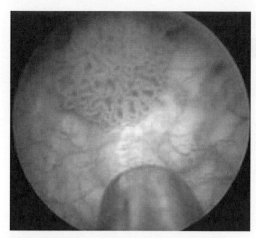

FIGURE 73.5 Cystoscopy demonstrating bladder tumour.

Reproduced from: Schäfauer, C. & Ettori, D., 2013. Detection of bladder urothelial carcinoma using in vivo noncontact, ultraviolet excited autofluorescence measurements converted into simple color coded images: a feasibility study. Journal of Urology 190(1), 271-277, Fig. 7.

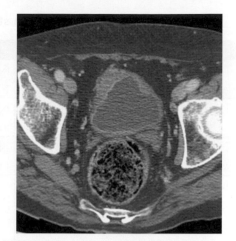

FIGURE 73.6 CT demonstrating bladder wall carcinoma.

Reproduced from: Cowan, N., et al., 2015. Chapter 38: Urothelial cell cancer, upper tract and lower tract. In: Adam, A., Grainger and Allison's Diagnostic Radiology. Elsevier, pp. 905-930, Fig. 38-3.

- The depth of the tumour is the key prognostic factor, which may be either:
  - 'Superficial' tumours (75% of tumours) with a papillary appearance at low risk of progression
    - There are three grades of superficial tumours that will influence the extent of adjuvant therapy when the patient is discussed at the MDM.
    - Higher grade tumours have a higher risk of tumour recurrence and progression.
  - 'Deep' tumours (25%) that invade the muscle wall and beyond. These are solid tumours with high risk of disease progression (see Fig. 73.6).
  - Deep tumours cannot be fully staged until the entire specimen has been removed. These patients will always require full staging imaging (CT/PET) (refer to Table 73.3 for TNM staging).

Management

(See Chapter 52.)

- Superficial tumours
  - TURBT, which should be followed up with repeat cystoscopy.
  - The grade of tumour will dictate the extent of adjuvant therapy and possible repeat TURBT.

SECTION V

TABLE 73.3 TNM staging of bladder cancer

T	N	M
T1: Tumour invades submucosa or lamina propria	N1: Single node in true pelvis	M0: No metastases
T2: Tumour extends into muscle wall	N2: Multiple nodes in true pelvis	M1: Metastases present
T3: Tumour extends beyond muscle wall into perivesical fat and tissue	N3: Common iliac nodes involved	
T4: Tumour invades into adjacent structures and organs • T4a: Prostatic stroma, uterus, vagina • T4b: Pelvic or abdominal wall		

- Invasive tumours
  - Invasive muscle tumours are an indication for cystectomy with urinary diversion unless the patient is unfit for surgery (Chapter 52).
    - Prostatectomy should be performed if involved in the invasive tumour.
  - Some patients may be suited to bladder sparing surgery, which can involve:
    - partial cystectomy, and/or
    - TURBT combined with chemotherapy and radiotherapy.
    - Note: This treatment option should be extensively discussed with the patient and the MDM team due to the high risk of recurrence.
  - Metastatic disease: adjuvant therapy with input from Medical and Radiation Oncology.
- Follow-up
  - Superficial tumours that undergo TURBT should have regular flexible cystoscopy follow-up (3/12 for the first 2 years, then 6/12 ongoing).
  - Invasive tumours post cystectomy should have at least 6–12/12 CT IVPs with inspection of the neobladder or conduit.

PROSTATE CANCER

Prostate cancer accounts for nearly a third of all cancer diagnoses in men. Incidence for patients over 85 is 20%.

- Around 60% of prostate cancer in asymptomatic patients is detected due to biopsy following elevated PSA levels.

- Though the use of serum PSA levels results in the detection of more cases, the test is not specific to prostate cancer and can also represent benign prostate hyperplasia (BPH) or infection.
- PSA test results should be correlated with findings from digital rectal examinations (DRE), which alone can lead to detection in 20% of cases.
    - Suspicious features of prostate cancer on DRE include unilateral, irregular nodular growths.
    - In contrast, BPH often presents with loss of the central sulcus or reduction in its apparentness on DRE.
- Presenting symptoms can include disruptions to the lower urinary tract including haematuria, difficulty voiding, poor urinary stream with dribbling towards the end of urination.
    - Some patients may present with late stage disease.
- Patients with a suspicion of prostate cancer should undergo biopsy, either via:
    - transperineal biopsy ± targeted guidance (i.e. with MRI)
    - transrectal ultrasound (TRUS) guided biopsy.
- Staging of prostate cancer is done using the TNM staging criteria by a combination of clinical and pathological features (see Table 73.4).

TABLE 73.4 TNM clinical staging systems for prostate cancer (1997 and 1992)

T	N	M
TX: Primary tumour cannot be assessed	N(+): Involvement of regional lymph nodes	M(+): Distant metastatic spread
T0: No evidence of primary tumour	NX: Regional lymph nodes cannot be assessed	MX: Distant metastases cannot be assessed
T1: Non-palpable tumour – not evident by imaging • T1a: Tumour found in tissue removed at transurethral resection; ≤5% is cancerous and histological grade <7 • T1b: Tumour found in tissue removed at transurethral resection; ≥5% is cancerous or histological grade >7 • T1c: Tumour identified by prostate needle biopsy due to elevation in PSA	N0: No regional lymph node metastases	M0: No evidence of distant metastases

continued

TABLE 73.4 TNM clinical staging systems for prostate cancer (1997 and 1992)—cont'd

T	N	M
T2: Palpable tumour confined to the prostate • T2a (1997): Tumour involves one lobe or less • T2a (1992): Tumour involves less than half of one lobe by normal tissue on all sides • T2b (1997): Tumour involves more than one lobe • T2b (1992): Tumour involves more than half of one lobe but not both lobes • T2c (1992): Tumour involves more than one lobe	N1: Metastases in single regional lymph node, ≤2 cm in dimension	M1: Distant metastases • M1a: Involvement of non-regional lymph nodes • M1b: Involvement of bones • M1c: Involvement of other distant sites
T3: Palpable tumour beyond the prostate • T3a: Unilateral extracapsular extension • T3b: Bilateral extracapsular extension • T3c: Tumour invades seminal vesicle(s)	N2: Metastases in single lymph node (>2 cm but ≤5 cm) or in multiple lymph nodes with none >5 cm	
T4: Tumour is fixed or invades adjacent structures (not seminal vesicles) • T4a: Tumour invades bladder neck, external sphincter and/or rectum • T4b: Tumour invades levator muscle and/or is fixed to pelvic wall	N3: Metastases in regional lymph node >5 cm	

Adapted from: Loeb, S. & Eastham, J., 2016. Chapter 111: Diagnosis and staging of prostate cancer. In: Wein, A., Campbell-Walsh Urology. Elsevier, pp. 2601-2608, Table 111-2.

- >95% of tumours are adenocarcinoma.
- Further pathological testing determines whether the cancer is high or low grade using the Gleason score (see Table 73.5).
  - The appearance of the prostate cells is grouped into patterns from 1–5 based on the level of differentiation (from well to poorly differentiated).
  - The numbers of the two most common patterns identified are combined to give the Gleason score (i.e. 3+3 or 3+4), where the first

TABLE 73.5 Risk stratification of prostate cancer

RISK OF DISEASE PROGRESSION	(T)	PSA	GLEASON
Very low	T1a–c	PSA <10	Gleason ≥6
Low	T2a	PSA <10	Gleason ≤6
Intermediate	T1a–c	PSA <20	Gleason 7
	T1a–c	PSA ≥10<20	Gleason ≤6
	T2a	PSA ≥10<20	Gleason ≤6
	T2a	PSA <20	Gleason 7
	T2b	PSA <20	Gleason ≤7
	T2c	Any PSA	Any Gleason
High	T1–2	PSA ≥20	Any Gleason
	T1–2	Any PSA	Gleason ≥8
	T3a	Any PSA	Any Gleason
Very high	T3b	Any PSA	Any Gleason
	T4	Any PSA	Any Gleason

Positive nodes or metastasis is termed disseminated or metastatic prostate cancer

number represents the most common level of differentiation and the second represents the second most common.

○ The combination of these clinical and pathological factors with the patient's PSA level is used to develop their overall stage.

○ Patient comorbidities influence the management plan, typically discussed during the MDM.

Management

- Management of localised disease: it should be noted that there is much debate amongst urologists and oncologists about the management of lower grade disease, with some considering Gleason 6 prostate 'cancer' as non-malignant change.

  ○ Very low/low risk

    – Active surveillance as long as 2 or less TRUS biopsy cores are positive.

    – Patients should have regular 3/12 PSAs with a repeat of the TRUS biopsy within 12/12.

    – Patients can be considered for more active management such as brachytherapy with input from the MDM team.

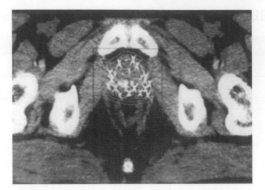

FIGURE 73.7 CT demonstrating radioactive seeds for brachytherapy.

Reproduced from: Nelson, W., Carter, H., DeWeese, T., et al., 2014. Chapter 84: Prostate cancer. In: Niederhuber, J., Abeloff's Clinical Oncology. Churchill-Livingstone, pp. 1463-1496, Fig. 84-14B.

- Intermediate risk
  - Should be considered for prostatectomy (Chapter 52) with lymph node dissection. Note: dependent on final staging, patients should have Medical and Radiation Oncology input for opinion on adjuvant therapy.
  - Patients with significant medical comorbidities and/or poor life expectancy can be considered for active surveillance; if suited these patients may also be considered for radiotherapy (see Fig. 73.7).
- High risk/very high risk
  - Radical prostatectomy with pelvic lymph node dissection.
  - Patients should undergo long-term androgen deprivation therapy (ADT).
  - Essential opinion from Radiation Oncology; referral is routine.
- Management of metastatic prostate cancer
  - Once confirmed, these patients should be considered for commencement of ADT.
    - Patients resistant to ADT are classified as having castration resistant prostate cancer.
    - Patients may also be suited to further hormone and anti-androgen therapy.
  - Bone metastasis associated with metastatic disease can be investigated with bone scan and plain X-ray imaging.
  - Patients should be referred for Oncology input for opinion on chemotherapy regimens and radiotherapy.

- Follow-up
  - Low risk and intermediate risk patients require regular Urology outpatient review with relevant investigations; it's worthwhile reminding the patient each time.
  - All postoperative patients should have PSAs to ensure there are no remnant diseased cells.
  - Adjuvant therapy may be required for months to years; early involvement with the MDM team can help speed up the process in setting appointments and pretreatment work-up.
- Prognosis
  - 10-year survival rates:
    - Low risk: 70–80%
    - Intermediate risk: 50–70%
    - High risk: 30%.
  - Mean survival rate for ADT treated metastatic disease is 2–6 years, <3 years if castration resistant.

TESTICULAR MASSES

There are multiple causes for testicular mass but one must always consider (and ultimately rule out) the diagnosis of testicular cancer (especially in young men). Despite this, other causes are more common and can be broadly divided into intrascrotal and extrascrotal causes as well as benign and malignant causes (see list of differentials in Table 73.6).

Testicular cancer

This is the second most common cancer after skin cancers in men aged between 18 and 39 years. Almost 800 new diagnoses are made each year.

TABLE 73.6 Breakdown of testicular masses

INTRASCROTAL		EXTRASCROTAL
Benign	Malignant	Benign
Hydrocele	Testicular cancer	Indirect inguinal hernia
Epididymal cyst	Lymphoma	Ascites
Varicocoele		Generalised oedema
Benign tumours		
Idiopathic scrotal oedema		

SECTION V

There are two common types:

- Seminomatous germ cell tumour (SGCT)
  - Diagnosis made by:
    - presence of normal AFP AND histology revealing only seminoma
    - despite this, still remains most common germ cell tumour (65%).
  - Usually confined to testis and rarely metastatic.
  - Chemotherapy and radiotherapy sensitive.
  - 95% classic or typical (10% of these express beta-HCG).
  - 5% spermatocytic (more common in older men, especially >50 years).
- Non-seminomatous germ cell tumour (NSGCT)
  - 'Mixed' GCT: mixture of seminoma and non-seminoma.
  - Treated as per SGCT.
  - Aside from 'mixed' GCT there are four broad categories: embryonal carcinoma, yolk sac tumour, choriocarcinoma, teratoma.

A summary of the various characteristics is shown in Table 73.7.

Management

- The management is dependent on tumour type and stage and can include any combination of:
  - active surveillance
  - chemotherapy/radiotherapy

TABLE 73.7 Testicular tumours

TUMOUR TYPE	USUAL AGE RANGE	RAISED AFP	RAISED BETA-HCG	METASTASIS
True seminoma (SGCT)	30–40 years	No	Possible (10%)	Rare
Embryonal carcinoma	25–35 years	Possible	Possible	Dependent on time to diagnosis
Yolk sac tumour	<10 years	Possible	Possible	Dependent on time to diagnosis: usually haematogenous spread
Choriocarcinoma	20–30 years	No	Yes (100%)	Early, common in lung and often bizarre locales
Teratoma	24–35 years	No	No	Dependent on time to diagnosis

- surgery.
  - Usually in the case of retroperitoneal mass or LN that has not responded to chemotherapy and tumour markers are not elevated.
  - Retroperitoneal LN dissection (RPLND): involves meticulous dissection of all para-aortic lymph nodes via various 'template' resections.
- Follow-up
  - Is dependent on a multitude of factors and usually decided with input from MDM.
  - Often includes repeat imaging (especially if RPLND is performed).
- Prognosis
  - Generally good – even with high grade disease.
    - This is often attributed to the young age and relative health of patients who are able to undergo significant operative management and chemotherapy.
  - Differs between SGCT and NSGCT in the more advanced stages.
  - Both stage 1 SGCT and NSGCT: >98% 5-year survival.
  - Both stage 2 SGCT and NSGCT: >95% 5-year survival.
  - Stage 3:
    - SGCT: ˜70–85% 5-year survival
    - NSGCT: ˜70–95% 5-year survival.

BENIGN PROSTATE HYPERPLASIA (BPH)

A process of gradual growth of the transitional zone of the prostate leading to lower urinary tract symptoms (LUTS) (see Fig. 73.7).

BPH is particularly common in older patients, and histologically present in 90% of patients aged >85 years.

- Careful history with the aid of a 'symptom score' known as the IPSS (international prostate symptom score) questionnaire can assist in gauging the severity of symptoms.
  - Incomplete emptying, increased frequency, intermittent or weak stream, straining and nocturia.
  - The questionnaire ultimately seeks to determine how bothersome the symptoms are to the patient.
  - Bladder diary is a critical tool.
- Examination must include a DRE to assess the prostate; in established BPH the prostate will generally feel uniformly enlarged and smooth (Fig. 73.8).

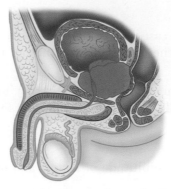

FIGURE 73.8 Illustration demonstrating abnormal growth of the prostate pushing on the rectum.

Reproduced from: Ball, J. & Dains, J., 2014. Chapter 20: Anus, rectum, and prostate. In: Ball, J., Seidel's Guide to Physical Examination. Mosby, pp. 485-500, Fig. 20-15.

Investigations

- Investigations should include PSA (if symptomatic LUTS); the percentage of free PSA is useful for determining the potential risk of prostate carcinoma.
  - If significantly elevated, the patient should be considered for a TRUS biopsy.
    - If the patient's symptoms are particularly bothersome, they may elect operative intervention in any case, allowing for diagnosis.
  - Urine flow via a Uroflow machine which measures:
    - post void residual (PVR)
    - peak flow rate
    - average flow rate
    - total void volume.

Management

- Management can begin with medical therapy.
  - Alpha-blockers such as tamsulosin and prazosin can help relax the urinary sphincter, easing the flow of urine.
  - Hormone therapies such as dutasteride can help decrease the size of the prostate.
  - It is worth noting that recent evidence cautions use of hormonal treatment for BPH, especially by GPs, given a select group of patients who present with a delayed diagnosis of high grade cancers, which are often metastatic.
- If patient symptoms are not improved by a trial of medical therapy, the next set of options are surgical and include most commonly TURP (via

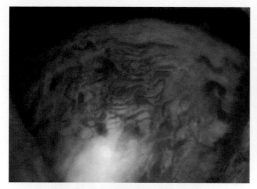

FIGURE 73.9 Transurethral view of a uniformly enlarged prostate lobe causing bladder outlet obstruction.

Reproduced from: Milam, D., 2012. Chapter 71: Transurethral resection of the prostate. In: Smith, J., Hinman's Atlas of Urologic Surgery. Saunders, pp. 449-458, Fig. 71-1.

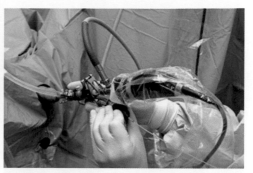

FIGURE 73.10 Laser-based TURP.

Reproduced from: Andrés, G., Arance, I., Gimbernat, H., et al., 2015. Laser transurethral resection of the prostate: safety study of a novel system of photoselective vaporization with high power diode laser in prostates larger than 80 ml. Spanish Urology (Actas Urológicas Españolas, English Edition). 39(6), 375-382, Fig. 2.

traditional electrocautery or, more recently, laser [Figs 73.9 and 73.10]) for symptom relief, but also sling procedures such as 'Urolift'.

RENAL TRACT CALCULI

This refers to a build-up of material into 'stones' that can be found in the kidney, ureters and bladder.

Referral to the 'stones' clinic can come from:

- ED or a GP after an acute ureteric calculi episode (Chapter 52)
- post discharge review from the Urology unit
- incidentally detected calculi on imaging.

The composition of renal tract calculi includes:

- calcium oxalate (>50%)
- calcium phosphate (10–20%)
- uric acid (7%), struvite (7%), cysteine (3%).

Risk factors for developing calculi include: previous calculi, obesity, T2DM, poor fluid intake, sedentary lifestyle (those with spinal injuries are particularly at risk) and hypercalcaemia.

- Uric acid stones are associated with decreased urinary pH.
    - They are not radio-opaque and are amenable to alkalisation therapy.
- Struvite stones are classically associated with Proteus and Klebsiella urinary tract infections (see Fig. 73.11).

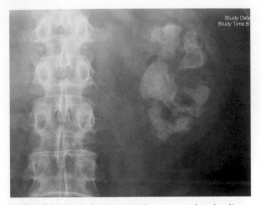

FIGURE 73.11 Large staghorn renal calculi consistent with a struvite stone.

Reproduced from: Miller, N. & Matlaga, B., 2007. Techniques for fluoroscopic percutaneous renal access. Journal of Urology 178(1), 15-23, Fig. 9.

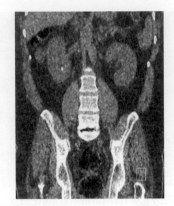

FIGURE 73.12 Ultra low dose CT for demonstrating renal calculi.

Reproduced from: Chew, B. & McLaughlin, P., 2015. MP38-06 ultra low dose CT-KUB to detect kidney stones with 44% less radiation: is the plain radiograph obsolete? Journal of Urology 193(4), e448-e448.

- Cysteine stones result from a genetic disorder resulting in cystinuria.
  - Stones tend to form at a younger age compared to other types.
  - Patients must remain well hydrated with good urinary output to prevent stone formation.

Patients may complain of flank pain although apart from acute ureteric stone episodes, they tend to be asymptomatic, and often flank pain is indicative of stone movement through the ureter.

Investigations

- Ongoing serial imaging is useful for surveillance. Typically, plain film KUB is sufficient as almost 80% of stones contain calcium, although low dose plain CT-KUB may be required and is becoming increasingly more common as a primary investigative tool (see Fig. 73.12). This may be attributable to diagnostic uncertainty.
  - Even if the patient has had only a single attack, the recurrence rate is 50% at 5 years, warranting close follow-up.
- On initial review patients should have urinalysis to check for chemical traces of stones, the presence of haematuria, pH and elevated specific gravity indicative of dehydration.
  - It's key to establish the composition of the patient's stone for ongoing management.

- Patients should initially have 6–12/12 imaging and review depending on the size of the stone, and symptoms and previous history with renal calculi.
  - Reviews can be lengthened beyond yearly if calculi display a stable appearance.

Management

- Asymptomatic small stones that are not obstructing the kidney can be conservatively managed with advice to maintain hydration and report for earlier review if symptoms persist.
- Management of symptomatic calculi can be achieved by three 'procedural' approaches (see Chapter 52).

URINARY INCONTINENCE

Urinary incontinence refers to the involuntary voiding of urine, even small amounts. Women are twice as likely to experience urinary incontinence, affecting around 11% of women in the community.

There are many types of incontinence with a range of potential causes (see Table 73.8).

History should include determining the pattern of incontinence and associated symptoms:

- Look for potential risk factors: elderly, obesity, pregnancy, UTI, cognitive impairment and diabetes.
- Medication history and fluid intake chart can be helpful.
- Bladder diaries are often used to create a timeline.

A focused examination should look for:

- vaginal abnormalities: cystocoele, prolapse, urethral diverticula

TABLE 73.8 Causes of the different types of urinary incontinence

STRESS INCONTINENCE	URGENCY INCONTINENCE	OTHER
Loss of urine associated with increased abdominal pressure 'sneezing/ coughing/exercise'	Patient has sudden onset need to void associated with loss of urine	
• Pelvic floor weakness • Sphincter weakness	• Detrusor overactivity • CNS disturbances • Neurogenic bladder	• Chronic urinary retention • Functional/cognitive • Medications

Brauer, S., 2014. Urinary incontinence. Journal of Physiotherapy 60(3), 169-169.

- rectal examination: stool impaction, prostate size, anal tone (may suggest underlying neurological disturbance)
- a palpable bladder that may suggest urinary retention and overflow incontinence.

Investigations

- Urodynamic studies
  - Can help determine the type of incontinence while determining the severity and overall bladder function.
  - Catheterisation of the bladder allows for filling and observation of flow. The patient can be instructed to cough to simulate stress incontinence.
  - Cystometry with transducers allows for recording of bladder wall activity (urgency).

Management

- See Table 73.9.
- Catheterisation is a treatment of last resort due to the associated complications.

TABLE 73.9 Management of urinary incontinence

GENERAL	STRESS	URGENCY
Dietary changes Weight loss Bladder education	Pelvic floor exercises Pessaries **Surgical**: Repair of vaginal wall/prolapse Bladder slings	Medications – antimuscarinics Botox injections

Thüroff, J.W., Abrams, P., Andersson, K.E., et al., 2010. EAU guidelines on urinary incontinence. European Urology 59(3), 387-400.

SECTION VI
APPENDICES

APPENDIX I

COMMON MEDICATIONS

Please note that all of these dosages are intended as a guide – each patient has individual needs and requirements. Some will need dose reduction for renal, cardiac or liver impairment. If you are ever unsure of a medication you are prescribing, check with the *Australian Medicines Handbook* or MIMS. Alternatively, confirm the administration with your registrar or consultant. Senior clinicians prefer safe practice!

If you require further information, good resources include your friendly neighbourhood pharmacist (especially some of the sub-specialised teams such as Infectious Disease or Oncology Pharmacists), the Pharmaceutical Benefits Scheme website and Therapeutic Guidelines.

TABLE I.2 Antimicrobials—cont'd

MEDICATION	DOSAGE	NOTES
Chloramphenicol	1–2 cm topical affected eye BD *or* 2 drops topical each affected eye BD	Comes in ointment or drops. The usual course is 5–7 days
Ciprofloxacin (Cipro)	500 mg PO BD (usual dose) 750 mg PO BD (severe infection)	Restricted access in Australia – must call PBS for authority. IV mixture also available
Clindamycin (Cleocin)	150–300 mg PO QID	
Doxycycline (Doxy, Alodox)	100 mg PO BD (treatment dose) 50 mg PO daily (prophylactic dose) 100 mg PO D (malaria prophylaxis)	Don't lie down afterwards – it causes painful oesophageal erosion!
Erythromycin	400 mg PO QID	Can also be used as a GI pro-kinetic
Famciclovir (Ezovir, Famvir)	250–500 mg PO TDS	Must be renally adjusted when eGFR <30
Flucloxacillin (Fluclox, Staphlex)	1–2 g IV QID (acute) 500 mg–1 g PO QID (step-down, or less severe infections)	Standard for most skin-related infections. Beware liver dysfunction
Fluconazole (Diflucan)	200 mg PO daily (prophylaxis) 400 mg PO daily (systemic fungal infection)	Beware liver dysfunction
Gentamicin (Gent)	4–6 mg/kg IV daily	Gentamicin levels should be done after the third dose, and then after every subsequent dose. Should not be given indefinitely due to risk of nephro- and ototoxicity
Meropenem	1 g IV TDS	

TABLE I.2 Antimicrobials—cont'd

MEDICATION	DOSAGE	NOTES
Metronidazole (Flagyl, Metro)	500 mg PO TDS (*C. difficile*) 400 mg IV BD (triple anti's)	More effective orally for *C. difficile* infections
Moxifloxacin	400 mg IV daily 400 mg PO daily	Used commonly in pneumonia with penicillin allergies. Often requires approval from antibiotic stewardship
Piperacillin/tazobactam (Tazocin)	4.5 g IV TDS	QID in febrile neutropenia
Trimethoprim (Triprim)	300 mg PO nocte	Given nocte as it stays in the bladder longer overnight. Avoid in pregnancy
Trimethoprim and sulfamethoxazole (Resprim Forte, Bactrim DS)	800/160 mg PO daily (prophylaxis) 1.6 g/320 mg PO BD (treatment dose) 800/160 mg PO BD twice weekly (respiratory prophylaxis)	Patients will usually know how they take their Bactrim, it is important to clarify due to the many different regimens. Can be myelosuppressive
Valacyclovir (Valtrex)	400 mg PO daily (prophylaxis)	Can be escalated to BD or even TDS for treatment of minor viral infections in the immunocompromised
Vancomycin (Vancocin)	1.5 g IV TDS	Vancomycin levels should be performed after the third dose, usually every second day (more frequently in the setting of renal impairment)

TABLE I.3 Aperients

MEDICATION	DOSAGE	NOTES
'Shaw's cocktail'	1 PO daily PRN = 2–4 teaspoons senna granules 30 mL liquid paraffin (Agarol) Mixed in warm milk ± Milo	Favourite of geriatricians and palliative care physicians for patents with constipation resistant to other interventions
Docusate with senna (Coloxyl + Senna)	100/16 mg (2 tabs) PO BD	Sometimes just given as a single nocte dose depending on requirements. Docusate can be prescribed without senna at the same dose Coloxyl = softener, senna = stimulant
Fleet enema	1–2 enemas PR daily PRN	Avoid multiple enemas in a 24-h period if possible Avoid in AKI/CKD due to phosphate content
Lactulose (Actilax, Dulose, Genlac)	20 mL PO BD (constipation) 30 mL PO up to Q1H (hepatic encephalopathy)	Down-titrate the Lactulose in hepatic encephalopathy once patient begins to open their bowels and their conscious state improves
Microlax enema	1 enema PR daily PRN	Safe in renal patients as it doesn't contain phosphate
Movicol	1 sachet PO daily 1–2 sachets PO Q10H PRN	
PicoPrep	2 PO usually at 1600 and 1800 day prior to endoscopy, with a third PRN at 0600 day of scope	Safe to use in renal patients

TABLE I.4 Antiemetics

MEDICATION	DOSAGE	NOTES
Cyclizine	50 mg PO or IV Q8H PRN	Good for post-op nausea
Domperidone (Motilium)	10 mg PO TDS/QID pre-meals	Alternative to metoclopramide for intractable nausea and vomiting, diabetic gastroparesis
Metoclopramide (Maxolon)	10 mg PO/IV/IM Q8H PRN (up to maximum of 80 mg in palliative)	Monitor for dystonic reactions Contraindicated in bowel obstruction, Parkinson's disease
Ondansetron (Zofran)	4–8 mg PO/SL/IV Q8H PRN	Can be constipating
Prochlorperazine (Stemetil)	5–10 mg PO Q8H or Q6H PRN 12.5 mg IV/IM Q8H or Q6H	Central dopaminergic effects, nausea with migraines or vertigo

TABLE I.5 Resuscitation medications

MEDICATION	DOSAGE	NOTES
Adenosine	6 mg rapid IV, then if needed 12 mg after 1–2 min, and then 18 mg after another 1–2 min	SVT
Adrenaline	1 mg rapid IV every 3–5 min (cardiac arrest) 0.1 to 0.5 mg IM stat (anaphylaxis)	Use for cardiac arrest in ALS pathway Note, adrenaline can also be used in infusion for shock but discuss with senior/ICU prior to commencing
Amiodarone	300 mg IV stat (cardiac arrest) 150–300 mg in 100 mL 5% dextrose IV over 30–60 min (loading dose rate control AF/flutter) then 900–1200 mg in 500 mL dextrose over 24 h (maintenance)	Use for cardiac arrest in ALS pathway
Atropine	0.4–1 mg IV every 5 min (max 2 mg)	Use for bradyarrhythmias
Calcium chloride 10%	10 mL rapid IV every 3 to 5 min	Use for cardiac arrest with hyperkalaemia, stabilises cardiac membrane
Lignocaine	100 mg rapid IV every 3 to 5 min	Cardiac arrest in refractory VF/PVT if amiodarone unavailable
Noradrenaline	2 mg in 500 mL NaCl 0.9% IV infusion at 15 mL/h	Vasopressor support in shock

TABLE I.6 Cardiology

MEDICATION	DOSAGE	NOTES
Amiodarone (Cordarone)	100 mg PO mane (maintenance) 300–400 mg PO stat (loading dose)	Long washout period (3 months!), typically started at high doses (e.g. 400 mg PO daily) and stepped down by 100 mg/day weekly, as tolerated. Many people remain on 200 mg/daily. Requires monitoring of thyroid function
Amlodipine (Norvasc)	5 mg PO daily (standard)	
Aspirin (Astrix, Cartia)	100 mg PO mane 300 mg PO stat (ACS loading dose)	
Atenolol (Noten)	25–50 mg PO daily	
Atorvastatin (Lipitor)	40 mg PO daily (standard) 20 mg PO daily (liver reduced) 80 mg PO daily (post-ACS)	All statins may be dose-reduced in people with liver dysfunction, or those who have had a true myalgia associated with it
Bisoprolol (Bicor)	2.5–10 mg PO daily	Standard starting dose is 5 mg PO daily
Carvedilol (Dicarz)	6.25 mg PO daily	Can go up to 25 mg/day
Clopidogrel (Plavix)	75 mg PO mane 600 mg (ACS loading dose)	Also available mixed with 100 mg of aspirin as 'CoPlavix' Restricted on PBS to post-ACS, stent or stroke
Digoxin (Sigmaxin, Lanoxin)	62.5 mcg PO mane 500 mcg PO stat with 250 mcg 6 hours later, and 250 mcg another 6 h later (loading dose)	If ineffective, 62.5 mcg/day may be increased. Serum levels may be needed to ensure the drug is in the therapeutic window
Diltiazem SR (Cardizem)	180 mg PO daily	Increased in quantities of 60 mg as required
Frusemide (Lasix, Uremide)	40 mg PO mane (starting) 40 mg PO mane + midi (actively diuresing)	Wide variance in dosage. Usually increased in units of 40 mg
Glyceryl trinitrate (Anginine, Nitrolingual)	300–600 mcg PO PRN (Anginine tabs) 400 mcg sublingual PRN (Nitrolingual spray)	One Anginine tablet is 600 mcg. People are usually advised to start with ½ tablet and take the other half if chest pain persists

TABLE I.6 Cardiology—cont'd

MEDICATION	DOSAGE	NOTES
Indapamide (Natrilix)	1.5–2.5 mg PO daily	
Irbesartan (Avapro)	150 mg PO daily (standard)	Can be 75–300 mg PO daily
Isosorbide mononitrate SR (ISMN, Imdur)	30–60 mg PO mane (Imdur)	Better for small vessel ischaemia, not used for acute angina. The doses vary with brand; Imdur is most common in Australia
Metoprolol (Minax)	25 mg PO BD (standard)	Can be up to 100 mg PO BD
Metoprolol XR (Toprol)	47.5–90 mg PO daily	
Nebivolol (Nebilet)	1.25–10 mg PO daily	Standard starting dose is 5 mg PO daily if BP non-prohibitive
Nicorandil (Ikorel)	10 mg PO daily	
Olmesartan (Olmetec)	20–40 mg PO daily	Commonly found in combination tablets with other antihypertensives
Perindopril (Coversyl)	2.5–10 mg PO daily	Some versions are in units of 4 mg (i.e. 5 mg = 4 mg, 8 mg = 10 mg) and you will need to make the change depending on what is available in the hospital pharmacy
Prazosin (Minipress)	5 mg PO BD	
Ramipril (Tritace, Altace)	5–10 mg PO daily	5 mg standard starting dose
Rosuvastatin (Crestor)	5 mg PO daily (standard) Up to 20 mg PO daily (post-ACS)	
Simvastatin (Zocor, Simva)	20–40 mg PO daily	
Sotalol (Betaloc)	80 mg PO BD	
Spironolactone (Spiro, Aldactone)	12.5–25 mg PO mane	In chronic liver patients can be up to 100 mg PO daily
Telmisartan (Micardis)	40–80 mg PO daily	40 mg is the standard starting dose
Ticagrelor (Brilinta)	90 mg PO BD 180 mg PO stat (loading dose)	PBS-restricted for treatment of ACS with aspirin
Verapamil XR (Isoptin)	180–240 mg PO daily	

TABLE I.7 Respiratory

MEDICATION	DOSAGE	NOTES
Budesonide (Pulmicort)	200 mcg inhaled BD	
Budesonide + eformoterol (Symbicort)	200/6 mcg inhaled daily to BD	Note there are other strengths of Symbicort available
Cetirizine (Zyrtec)	10 mg PO daily	Used in allergy prophylaxis (e.g. pre-meds)
Fluticasone + salmeterol (Seretide)	250/25 two puffs inhaled BD (standard)	Note there are other strengths of Seretide available
Hydrocortisone	100 mg IV QID	Converted to prednisolone
Ipratropium (Atrovent)	500 mcg nebulised QID	Converted to tiotropium on discharge, unless the patient has a home nebuliser. Can stop tiotropium while on Atrovent
Montelukast (Singulair)	5–10 mg PO daily	
Prednisolone (Prednisone)	Up to 50 mg PO daily	Weaned on cessation if used >72 h
Promethazine (Phenergan)	25 mg PO daily or stat	Sedating, use loratadine 10 mg instead if wanting non-sedating
Salbutamol MDI (Ventolin)	100–200 mcg inhaled PRN 5 mg neb QID (while inpatient)	Stepped down to PRN inhaler. Ensure patient knows how to use a spacer properly!
Tiotropium (Spiriva)	18 mcg PO daily	

TABLE I.8 Gastroenterology

MEDICATION	DOSAGE	NOTES
"Pink lady" or Gastrogel	20–30 mL PO stat	120 mL/day maximum
Azathioprine (Imuran)	50 mg PO daily (starting dose, up-titrated to 1.5 mg/kg)	Beware leukopenia
Esomeprazole (Nexium)	20–40 mg PO daily	
Hydrocortisone (Hydrocort)	100 mg IV QID (flare of IBD)	Stepped down to prednisolone, usually starting a weaning dose at 50 mg/day
Lactulose	30 mL PO up to Q1H (hepatic encephalopathy [HE])	Continue until HE resolving, then slowly down-titrate
Lansoprazole	30 mg ('1 sachet') PEG daily	Available as granules for PEG tubes
Methotrexate	12.5–25 mg PO weekly	5 mg folic acid every other day
Omeprazole (Maxor)	20 mg PO daily	
Pantoprazole (Somac)	40 mg PO mane (GORD) 40 mg IV in 100 mL N/saline over 5 h (GI bleed) 40 mg PO BD (step-down for one month post-GI bleed)	
Predsol enemas	20 mg PR mane	
Predsol suppositories	5 mg PO nocte	
Propranolol (Deralin)	20 mg PO TDS	For portal hypertension
Rifaximin (Rifamax)	550 mg PO BD (HE)	Lifelong, but for PBS must remain on Lactulose
Sulfasalazine	1 g PO BD	Up to 4 g/day
Terlipressin	0.85 mg IV QID (hepatorenal syndrome)	Very specialised medicine. Must be weaned

TABLE I.11 Endocrine

MEDICATION	DOSAGE	NOTES
Cortisone	12.5–50 mg PO daily	Useful in several endocrine conditions including panhypopituitarism and adrenal insufficiency
Exenatide (Byetta)	5 mcg subcut BD before meals	Can be up-titrated to 10 mcg BD after 1 month of therapy
Gliclazide MR (Diamicron)	60–120 mg PO mane (standard) Sometimes additional 30–60 mg introduced nocte	Beware hypoglycaemia when up-titrating
Metformin (Glucophage)	500 mg PO mane (starting) Up to 1 g PO TDS	Start low, go slow. Often complicated by GI upset. Won't cause hypos!
Sitagliptin (Januvia)	25–100 mg PO daily	Available with metformin as 'Janumet'
Thyroxine (Synthroid)	50–100 mcg PO mane	Start low, go slow. Monitor response after 1 month with serum TSH

TABLE I.12 Rheumatology

MEDICATION	DOSAGE	NOTES
Allopurinol	300 mg PO daily (standard) 100 mg PO daily (renal dose)	Requires renal adjustment. Can also be used at 300 mg/day for tumour lysis
Colchicine	500 mcg PO daily	Can be uptitrated higher
Folic acid	5 mg PO daily (except day of MTX)	
Hydroxychloroquine (Plaquenil)	200 mg PO daily	May be escalated to 400 mg/day
Iloprost	As per hospital protocol	
Leflunomide		
Methotrexate (MTX)	12.5–25 mg PO weekly	
Mycophenolate	Variable; typically 1 g PO BD in transplant patients	Always confirm with a more senior doctor
Prednisolone	25–50 mg PO daily	Weaned if used for more than 72 h
Zoledronic acid (Aclasta)	5 mg IV annually for osteoporosis	Avoid in people with a CrCl <35 mL/min

TABLE I.13 Haematology

MEDICATION	DOSAGE	NOTES
Apixaban (Eliquis)	5 mg PO BD (standard) 2.5 mg PO BD (renally-adjusted)	Not advised or dose reduction required with 2/3 present: older age (>85 y), renally-impaired (eGFR <30) or weight <60 kg
Dabigatran (Pradaxa)	150 mg PO BD (AF, Tx of DVT/PE) 75 mg PO BD (renally-adjusted)	Needs renal adjustment when GFR <30
Dalteparin (Fragmin)	5000 units subcut daily (prophylaxis)	Less frequently used alternative to Clexane. 2500 units <50 kg or eGFR <30
Enoxaparin (Clexane)	40 mg subcut daily (DVT prophylaxis) 1 mg/kg subcut BD or 1.5 mg/kg subcut daily (treatment dose)	Renal adjustment
Heparin	5000 units subcut daily (DVT prophylaxis)	Heparin infusions are typically 5000 units in a bag of normal saline, titrated as per the hospital policy using the APTT
Rivaroxaban (Xarelto)	15 mg PO BD (loading dose) 20 mg PO daily	Load for 3 weeks then continue on maintenance dose. Not advised or dose reduction required with 2/3 present: older age (>85 y), renally-impaired (eGFR <30) or weight <60 kg
Warfarin (Coumadin, Marevan)	5 mg PO 1600 daily (usual starting dose)	Start at this dose for 3 days then up- and down-titrate with INR

APPENDIX II

NORMAL LABORATORY VALUES

Please note there are variations between laboratories. These values are provided for a 40-year-old male/non-pregnant female and act as a guide only; local reference intervals should be confirmed with your hospital's own Pathology Department.

TABLE II.1 Normal laboratory values

TEST	MEASUREMENT	RANGE	UNITS
Full blood examination (FBE)	Hb	130–180 (M)	g/L
	WCC	4.0–11.0	10^9/L
	Platelets	150–400	10^9/L
	MCV	80–96	fL
	RCC	4.5–6.5	10^{12}/L
	Hct	40–54	%
	MCH	27–32	pg
	MCHC	320–360	g/L
	Neutrophils	2.0–7.5	10^9/L
	Lymphocytes	1.0–4.0	10^9/L
	Monocytes	0.1–0.8	10^9/L
	Eosinophils	0.0–0.4	10^9/L
	Basophils	0.0–0.2	10^9/L
Urea, electrolytes and creatinine (UEC)	Sodium	135–145	mmol/L
	Potassium	3.5–5.2	mmol/L
	Chloride	95–110	mmol/L
	Bicarbonate	22–32	mmol/L
	Urea	F: 2.5–7.2; M: 3.0–9.2	mmol/L
	Serum creatinine	F: 45–90; M: 60–110	micromol/L
	eGFR	>90	mL/min/1.73 m^2

continued

TABLE II.1 Normal laboratory values—cont'd

TEST	MEASUREMENT	RANGE	UNITS
Calcium, magnesium and phosphate	Calcium	2.10–2.60	mmol/L
	Magnesium	0.7–1.1	mmol/L
	Phosphorous	0.75–1.50	mmol/L
General chemistry	CRP	<5	mg/L
	Glucose	3.3–7.7	mmol/L
	Cholesterol	<4	mmol/L
	Triglycerides	<2.0	mmol/L
	Amylase	22–100	U/L
	Lipase	<60	U/L
	Digoxin	0.5–0.8	mg/L
	Uric acid	F: 0.15–0.35; M: 0.21–0.42	mmol/L
Cerebrospinal fluid (CSF)	Protein	0.60–0.80	g/L
	Glucose	2.2–3.9	mmol/L
	Cells	<5 WBC; <1RBC	–
Cardiac enzymes	AST	F: <32; M: <40	U/L
	LDH	120–250	U/L
	CK	F: 20–170; M: 20–200	U/L
	hs Troponin I	<15	ng/L
Liver function tests (LFTs)	Bilirubin	<21	micromol/L
	AST	F: <32; M: <40	U/L
	ALT	F: 5–35; M: 5–40	U/L
	Alkaline phosphatase	30–110	U/L
	Gamma GT	F: <40; M: <60	U/L
	Total protein	60–80	g/L
	Albumin	35–50	g/L
Arterial blood gas (ABG)	pH	7.35–7.45	–
	pCO_2	35–45	mmHg
	pO_2	80–100	mmHg
	Bicarbonate	22–30	mmol/L
	Base excess	−3–+3	–
	O_2 saturation	95–100	%

continued

TABLE II.1 Normal laboratory values—cont'd

TEST	MEASUREMENT	RANGE	UNITS
Thyroid function tests (TFTs)	TSH	0.27–4.20	mIU/L
	Free T$_3$	3.1–6.8	pmol/L
	Free T$_4$	12–22	pmol/L
Coagulation	PT (INR) normal	0.9–1.4	–
	Therapeutic	1.5–4.0	
	APTT normal	22–38	s
	Therapeutic	50–100	
	Fibrinogen	2.0–4.0	g/L
	D-dimer	<0.5	mg/L

F = female; M = male.
Reference intervals supplied by Austin Pathology, Melbourne Australia.

APPENDIX III

MICROBIOLOGY

Kelsey Broom

INTRODUCTION

Out of the varied, vast and dense population of microorganisms that exist, only the most common and important relating human flora and disease are captured in this appendix. The series of initial diagrams outline the classification and structure of organisms before focusing on the normal human flora, infections of various anatomical distributions and their main causes. The addition of a simple 'coordinates' system aims to make it easy to find which organisms are associated with a particular disease.

BACTERIA 'FAMILY TREE'

This flowchart-style diagram (Fig. III.1) contains a select number of important **bacteria** in human disease and also normal flora. It splits the bacteria into their most popular classifications:

- Gram stain – this classification is based on what colour of 'dye' the bacteria take up using the gram stain technique in a laboratory, dependent on the composition of the cell wall. Gram positive (+ve) bacteria stain purple due to their thick layer of peptidoglycan in their cell wall. Gram negative (−ve) bacteria only have a thin layer of peptidoglycan and therefore they do not take up the purple 'dye', remaining red in colour.

- Microscopy – after culture (growing) and gram stain, bacteria colonies can be observed under a microscope. Most bacteria are either cocci (round shape) or bacilli (rod). Some bacteria are variable shapes such as spirochete (spiral).

- Growth requirements aka aerobic or anaerobic – some bacteria require oxygen in order to replicate and grow (aerobic), whereas others require carbon dioxide and oxygen is poison to them (anaerobic). Some bacteria can survive under both conditions (e.g. facultative anaerobes use oxygen if it is present but do not require it).

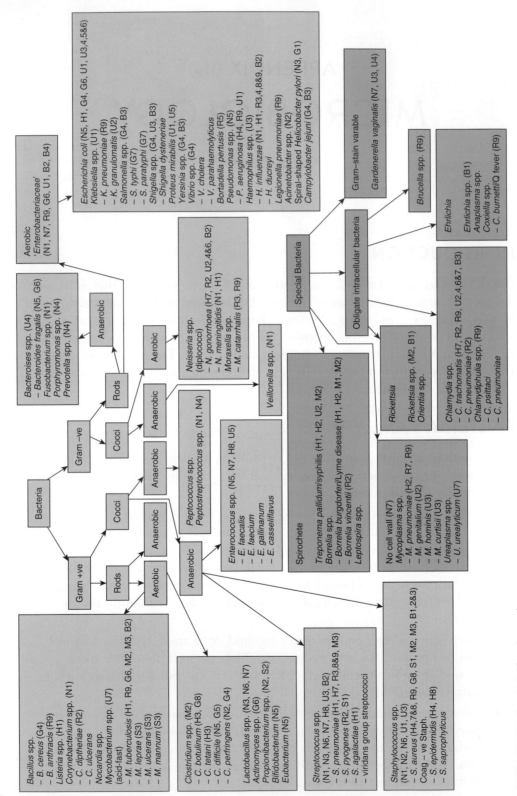

FIGURE III.1 Bacteria 'family tree'.

VIRUS 'FAMILY TREE'

As for bacteria, this section is a small capture of important viruses. The flowchart (Fig. III.2) is organised by whether the virus' genome consists of DNA or RNA, which is important for replication styles within a host cell.

FUNGI 'FAMILY TREE'

Unlike the other flowcharts, fungi are classified in this one (Fig. III.3) based on the site of infection/colonisation. This is because there are various different fungi that cause 'tinea'. However, their specific species names are not as commonly used in practice.

PARASITES 'FAMILY TREE'

Parasites reproduce and sustain their life cycle by causing damage to their host. In humans, parasites can cause disease via mechanisms such as mechanical damage, using host resources (e.g. iron), cytotoxicity, hypersensitivity reactions, cytokine-mediated response, autoimmune disease or forming an immune complex. Parasites often have detailed life cycles that can include a number of different hosts.

Parasites are split up into protozoa, which are unicellular, and helminths aka worms, which are multicellular (see Fig. III.4). They are also then further divided into shape. Of the various different worms, very few species are listed (only the ones mentioned in the disease tables to follow).

NORMAL FLORA

This is a diagram (Fig. III.5) of the important organisms that make up the normal flora of the human body. Normal flora are an essential aspect of the healthy human. Microorganisms (mostly bacteria) colonise selected anatomical sites. There are approximately 10^4 normal flora in/on the human body. They have various roles including the formation of normal intestinal anatomy and function, competition with pathogens, building the host's natural immunity, digestion, metabolism and vitamin and enzyme production.

INFECTIOUS DISEASES

These pages list common causes (and also rare but important causes) of infections at various anatomical sites (Figs III.6 to III.11). It is important to note that infection is not the only cause of disease for some sites and other causes also include autoimmune, injury, allergy etc and, in some clinical settings, these causes are *more common* than infection.

Bolded organisms are the most common cause/s.

SECTION VI

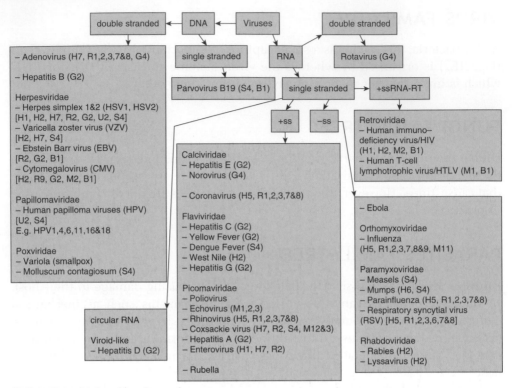

FIGURE III.2 Virus 'family tree'.

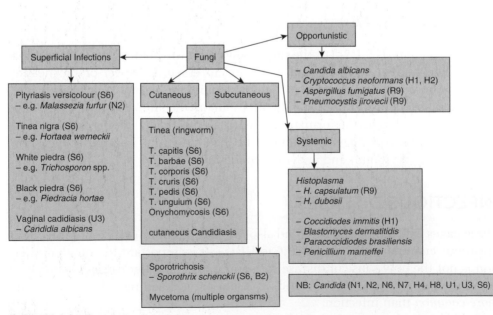

FIGURE III.3 Fungi 'family tree'.

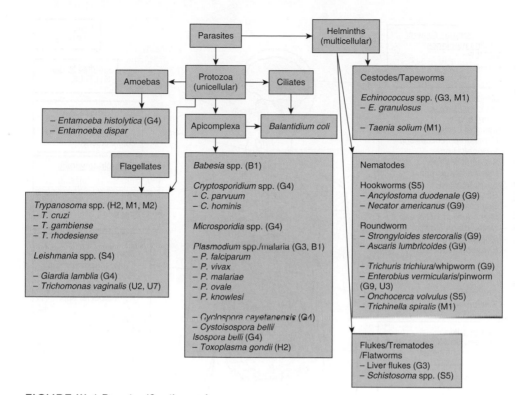

FIGURE III.4 Parasite 'family tree'.

Each page and section of the appendix is given a 'coordinate' (e.g. 'Normal flora of the upper respiratory tract' is N1 and 'Pneumoniae' is R9).

Therefore, if an organism has N1 next to its name in the 'family tree' then you can turn to this section and find it labelled there as part of the normal flora of the upper respiratory tract.

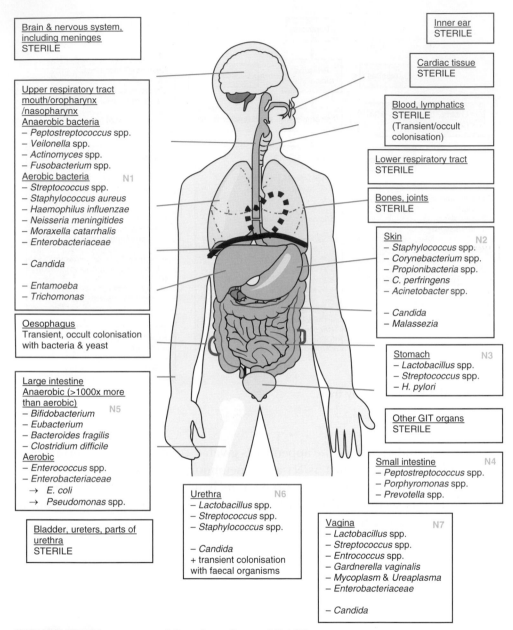

Brain & nervous system,
including meninges
STERILE

Inner ear
STERILE

Cardiac tissue
STERILE

Upper respiratory tract
mouth/oropharynx
/nasopharynx
Anaerobic bacteria
 – *Peptostreptococcus* spp.
 – *Veilonella* spp.
 – *Actinomyces* spp.
 – *Fusobacterium* spp.
Aerobic bacteria   N1
 – *Streptococcus* spp.
 – *Staphylococcus aureus*
 – *Haemophilus influenzae*
 – *Neisseria meningitides*
 – *Moraxella catarrhalis*
 – *Enterobacteriaceae*

 – *Candida*

 – *Entamoeba*
 – *Trichomonas*

Blood, lymphatics
STERILE
(Transient/occult
colonisation)

Lower respiratory tract
STERILE

Bones, joints
STERILE

Skin   N2
 – *Staphylococcus* spp.
 – *Corynebacterium* spp.
 – *Propionibacteria* spp.
 – *C. perfringens*
 – *Acinetobacter* spp.

 – *Candida*
 – *Malassezia*

Oesophagus
Transient, occult colonisation
with bacteria & yeast

Stomach   N3
 – *Lactobacillus* spp.
 – *Streptococcus* spp.
 – *H. pylori*

Large intestine
Anaerobic (>1000x more
than aerobic)   N5
 – *Bifidobacterium*
 – *Eubacterium*
 – *Bacteroides fragilis*
 – *Clostridium difficile*
Aerobic
 – *Enterococcus* spp.
 – *Enterobacteriaceae*
   → *E. coli*
   → *Pseudomonas* spp.

Other GIT organs
STERILE

Small intestine   N4
 – *Peptostreptococcus* spp.
 – *Porphyromonas* spp.
 – *Prevotella* spp.

Bladder, ureters, parts of
urethra
STERILE

Urethra   N6
 – *Lactobacillus* spp.
 – *Streptococcus* spp.
 – *Staphylococcus* spp.

 – *Candida*
+ transient colonisation
with faecal organisms

Vagina   N7
 – *Lactobacillus* spp.
 – *Streptococcus* spp.
 – *Entrococcus* spp.
 – *Gardnerella vaginalis*
 – *Mycoplasm* & *Ureaplasma*
 – *Enterobacteriaceae*

 – *Candida*

FIGURE III.5 Human normal flora (coordinates N1-N7).

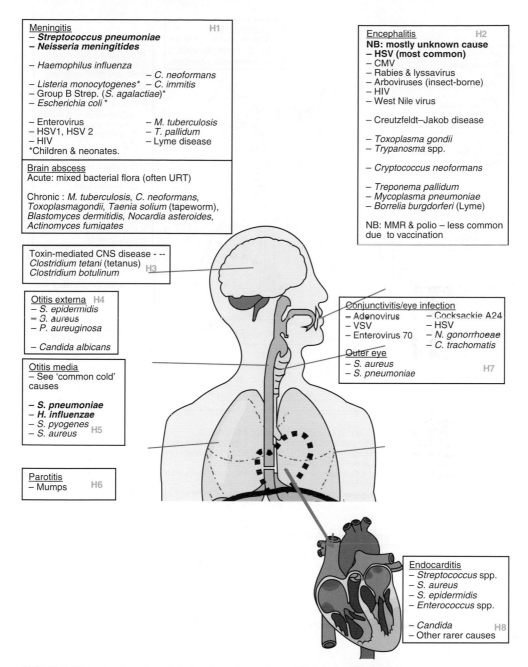

Meningitis H1
– **Streptococcus pneumoniae**
– **Neisseria meningitides**

– *Haemophilus influenza*
                              – *C. neoformans*
– *Listeria monocytogenes* * – *C. immitis*
– Group B Strep. (*S. agalactiae*)*
– *Escherichia coli* *

– Enterovirus   – *M. tuberculosis*
– HSV1, HSV 2   – *T. pallidum*
– HIV   – Lyme disease
*Children & neonates.

Brain abscess
Acute: mixed bacterial flora (often URT)

Chronic : *M. tuberculosis, C. neoformans,
Toxoplasmagondii, Taenia solium* (tapeworm),
*Blastomyces dermitidis, Nocardia asteroides,
Actinomyces fumigates*

Toxin-mediated CNS disease - --
Clostridium tetani (tetanus) H3
Clostridium botulinum

Otitis externa H4
– *S. epidermidis*
– *S. aureus*
– *P. aureuginosa*

– *Candida albicans*

Otitis media
– See 'common cold'
causes

– **S. pneumoniae**
– **H. influenzae**
– *S. pyogenes*
– *S. aureus* H5

Parotitis H6
– Mumps

Encephalitis H2
NB: mostly unknown cause
– **HSV (most common)**
– CMV
– Rabies & lyssavirus
– Arboviruses (insect-borne)
– HIV
– West Nile virus

– Creutzfeldt–Jakob disease

– *Toxoplasma gondii*
– *Trypanosma* spp.

– *Cryptococcus neoformans*

– *Treponema pallidum*
– *Mycoplasma pneumoniae*
– *Borrelia burgdorferi* (Lyme)

NB: MMR & polio – less common
due to vaccination

Conjunctivitis/eye infection
– Adenovirus   – Cocksackie A24
– VSV   – HSV
– Enterovirus 70   – *N. gonorrhoeae*
                    – *C. trachomatis*
Outer eye
– *S. aureus*
– *S. pneumoniae* H7

Endocarditis
– *Streptococcus* spp.
– *S. aureus*
– *S. epidermidis*
– *Enterococcus* spp.

– *Candida* H8
– Other rarer causes

FIGURE III.6 Head and neck infections (+ endocarditis) (coordinates H1–H8).

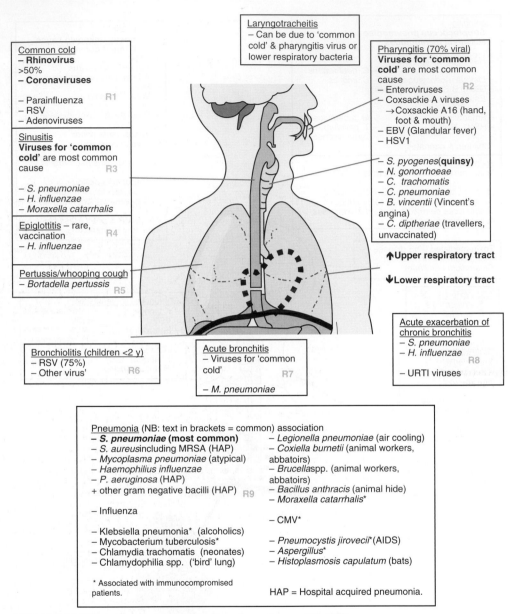

Laryngotracheitis
– Can be due to 'common cold' & pharyngitis virus or lower respiratory bacteria

Common cold
– Rhinovirus
>50%
– Coronaviruses

– Parainfluenza   R1
– RSV
– Adenoviruses

Pharyngitis (70% viral)
Viruses for 'common cold' are most common cause
– Enteroviruses   R2
– Coxsackie A viruses
→Coxsackie A16 (hand, foot & mouth)
– EBV (Glandular fever)
– HSV1

– *S. pyogenes*(**quinsy**)
– *N. gonorrhoeae*
– *C. trachomatis*
– *C. pneumoniae*
– *B. vincentii* (Vincent's angina)
– *C. diptheriae* (travellers, unvaccinated)

Sinusitis
Viruses for 'common cold' are most common cause   R3

– *S. pneumoniae*
– *H. influenzae*
– *Moraxella catarrhalis*

Epiglottitis – rare, vaccination   R4
– *H. influenzae*

↑Upper respiratory tract

↓Lower respiratory tract

Pertussis/whooping cough
– *Bortadella pertussis*   R5

Acute exacerbation of chronic bronchitis
– *S. pneumoniae*
– *H. influenzae*   R8
– URTI viruses

Bronchiolitis (children <2 y)
– RSV (75%)
– Other virus'   R6

Acute bronchitis
– Viruses for 'common cold'   R7
– *M. pneumoniae*

Pneumonia (NB: text in brackets = common) association
– S. pneumoniae (most common)
– *S. aureus*including MRSA (HAP)
– *Mycoplasma pneumoniae* (atypical)
– *Haemophilius influenzae*
– *P. aeruginosa* (HAP)
+ other gram negative bacilli (HAP)   R9

– Influenza

– Klebsiella pneumonia* (alcoholics)
– Mycobacterium tuberculosis*
– Chlamydia trachomatis (neonates)
– Chlamydophilia spp. ('bird' lung)

* Associated with immunocompromised patients.

– *Legionella pneumoniae* (air cooling)
– *Coxiella burnetii* (animal workers, abbatoirs)
– *Brucella*spp. (animal workers, abbatoirs)
– *Bacillus anthracis* (animal hide)
– *Moraxella catarrhalis**

– CMV*

– *Pneumocystis jirovecii**(AIDS)
– *Aspergillus**
– *Histoplasmosis capulatum* (bats)

HAP = Hospital acquired pneumonia.

FIGURE III.7 Respiratory tract infections (coordinates R1–R9).

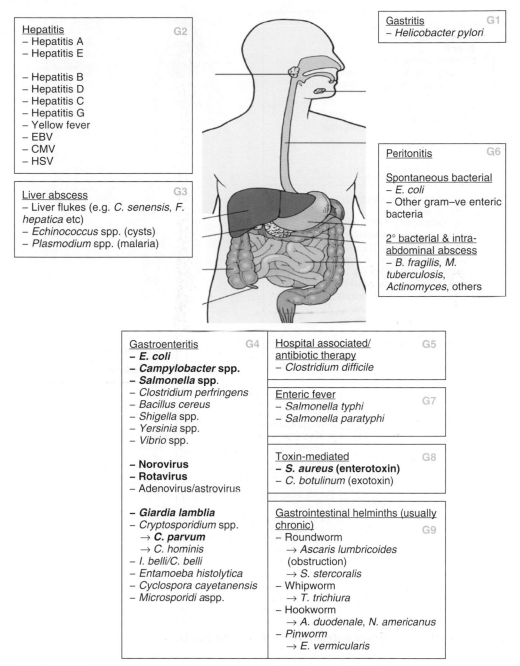

Hepatitis   G2
– Hepatitis A
– Hepatitis E

– Hepatitis B
– Hepatitis D
– Hepatitis C
– Hepatitis G
– Yellow fever
– EBV
– CMV
– HSV

Liver abscess   G3
– Liver flukes (e.g. *C. senensis, F. hepatica* etc)
– *Echinococcus* spp. (cysts)
– *Plasmodium* spp. (malaria)

Gastritis   G1
– *Helicobacter pylori*

Peritonitis   G6

Spontaneous bacterial
– *E. coli*
– Other gram–ve enteric bacteria

2° bacterial & intra-abdominal abscess
– *B. fragilis, M. tuberculosis, Actinomyces*, others

Gastroenteritis   G4
– **E. coli**
– **Campylobacter spp.**
– **Salmonella spp.**
– *Clostridium perfringens*
– *Bacillus cereus*
– *Shigella* spp.
– *Yersinia* spp.
– *Vibrio* spp.

– **Norovirus**
– **Rotavirus**
– Adenovirus/astrovirus

– **Giardia lamblia**
– *Cryptosporidium* spp.
   → **C. parvum**
   → *C. hominis*
– *I. belli/C. belli*
– *Entamoeba histolytica*
– *Cyclospora cayetanensis*
– *Microsporidi* aspp.

Hospital associated/ antibiotic therapy   G5
– *Clostridium difficile*

Enteric fever   G7
– *Salmonella typhi*
– *Salmonella paratyphi*

Toxin-mediated   G8
– **S. aureus (enterotoxin)**
– *C. botulinum* (exotoxin)

Gastrointestinal helminths (usually chronic) G9
– Roundworm
   → *Ascaris lumbricoides* (obstruction)
   → *S. stercoralis*
– Whipworm
   → *T. trichiura*
– Hookworm
   → *A. duodenale, N. americanus*
– Pinworm
   → *E. vermicularis*

FIGURE III.8 Gastrointestinal system infections (coordinates G1–G9).

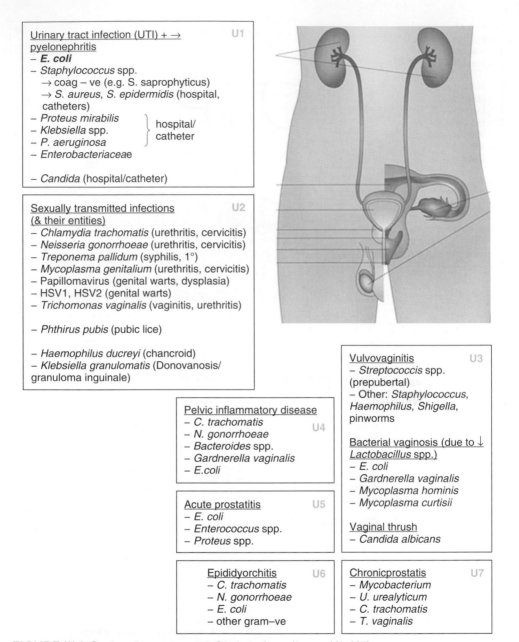

Urinary tract infection (UTI) + →   U1
pyelonephritis
- ***E. coli***
- *Staphylococcus* spp.
 → coag − ve (e.g. S. saprophyticus)
 → *S. aureus*, *S. epidermidis* (hospital,
 catheters)
- *Proteus mirabilis* ⎫ hospital/
- *Klebsiella* spp.   ⎬ catheter
- *P. aeruginosa*   ⎭
- *Enterobacteriacea*e

- *Candida* (hospital/catheter)

Sexually transmitted infections   U2
(& their entities)
- *Chlamydia trachomatis* (urethritis, cervicitis)
- *Neisseria gonorrhoeae* (urethritis, cervicitis)
- *Treponema pallidum* (syphilis, 1°)
- *Mycoplasma genitalium* (urethritis, cervicitis)
- Papillomavirus (genital warts, dysplasia)
- HSV1, HSV2 (genital warts)
- *Trichomonas vaginalis* (vaginitis, urethritis)

- *Phthirus pubis* (pubic lice)

- *Haemophilus ducreyi* (chancroid)
- *Klebsiella granulomatis* (Donovanosis/
granuloma inguinale)

Vulvovaginitis   U3
- *Streptococcis* spp.
(prepubertal)
- Other: *Staphylococcus,
Haemophilus, Shigella,*
pinworms

**Bacterial vaginosis (due to ↓
Lactobacillus spp.)**
- *E. coli*
- *Gardnerella vaginalis*
- *Mycoplasma hominis*
- *Mycoplasma curtisii*

Vaginal thrush
- *Candida albicans*

Pelvic inflammatory disease
- *C. trachomatis*
- *N. gonorrhoeae*   U4
- *Bacteroides* spp.
- *Gardnerella vaginalis*
- *E.coli*

Acute prostatitis   U5
- *E. coli*
- *Enterococcus* spp.
- *Proteus* spp.

Epididyorchitis   U6
- *C. trachomatis*
- *N. gonorrhoeae*
- *E. coli*
- other gram−ve

Chronicprostatis   U7
- *Mycobacterium*
- *U. urealyticum*
- *C. trachomatis*
- *T. vaginalis*

FIGURE III.9 Genitourinary system infections (coordinates U1–U7).

Common/important bacterial skin infections
Cellulitis
– *S. aureus*   S1
– *Streptococcus pyogenes*
– Other: oral flora (bites), faecal flora

Impetigo/school sores
– *S. pyogenes*
– *S. aureus*

Necrositing fasciitis & synergistic bacterial gangrene
– *S.aureus* & *S. pyogenes* + many other mixed bacteria (e.g. *Proteus*, *Enterobacter*, *Pseudomonas*, *Clostridium*)

Other infections caused by *S. aureus* & *S. pyogenes*
– Wound infections
– Erysipelas
– Scalded skin syndrome (*S. aureus* toxin)
– Folliculitis, boils, carbuncles

Acne   S2
– *Propionibacterium acnes*

Other bacterial skin infections   S3
Mycobacterium
– *M. leprae* (leprosy)
– *M. mannum* (water)
– *M. ulcerans* (chronic, painless skin ulcers)
– *M. tuberculosis* (cutaneous TB)

Viral skin infections   S4
– Papillomavirus
– Molluscum contagiosum
Systemic virus w/skin involvement
– HSV
– VSV
– Dengue
– Coxsackie virus
– Parvovirus
– Measles, rubella (rare now)

Parasites (often cause skin infection by   S5
burrowing action)
– *Leishmania* spp.
– Schistosoma (swimmers itch)

– Hookworms
– *Onchocerca volvulus* (river blindness)

Other
– *Sarcoptes scaibiei* (scabies)
– Larvae of ticks, lice, mites etc

Fungal skin infections   S6
– Pityriasis versicolour
– White piedra
– Black piedra
– Tinea nigra

Tinea: T. capitis, barbae, corporis, cruris, pedia, unguium, onychomycosis
– Multiple species can cause these fungal infections

Candida
Sporothrix schenckii

FIGURE III.10 Skin infections (coordinates S1–S6).

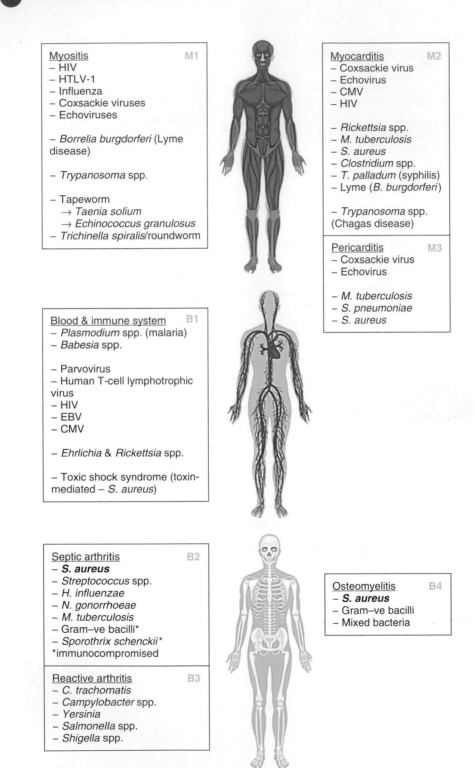

Myositis   M1
– HIV
– HTLV-1
– Influenza
– Coxsackie viruses
– Echoviruses

– *Borrelia burgdorferi* (Lyme disease)

– *Trypanosoma* spp.

– Tapeworm
  → *Taenia solium*
  → *Echinococcus granulosus*
– *Trichinella spiralis*/roundworm

Myocarditis   M2
– Coxsackie virus
– Echovirus
– CMV
– HIV

– *Rickettsia* spp.
– *M. tuberculosis*
– *S. aureus*
– *Clostridium* spp.
– *T. palladum* (syphilis)
– Lyme (*B. burgdorferi*)

– *Trypanosoma* spp. (Chagas disease)

Pericarditis   M3
– Coxsackie virus
– Echovirus

– *M. tuberculosis*
– *S. pneumoniae*
– *S. aureus*

Blood & immune system   B1
– *Plasmodium* spp. (malaria)
– *Babesia* spp.

– Parvovirus
– Human T-cell lymphotrophic virus
– HIV
– EBV
– CMV

– *Ehrlichia* & *Rickettsia* spp.

– Toxic shock syndrome (toxin-mediated – *S. aureus*)

Septic arthritis   B2
– **S. aureus**
– *Streptococcus* spp.
– *H. influenzae*
– *N. gonorrhoeae*
– *M. tuberculosis*
– Gram–ve bacilli*
– *Sporothrix schenckii**
*immunocompromised

Osteomyelitis   B4
– **S. aureus**
– Gram–ve bacilli
– Mixed bacteria

Reactive arthritis   B3
– *C. trachomatis*
– *Campylobacter* spp.
– *Yersinia*
– *Salmonella* spp.
– *Shigella* spp.

FIGURE III.11 Muscle, joint/bone, blood and immune system infections (coordinates M1–M3, B1–B4).

APPENDIX IV

ANTIBIOTICS

Paul Watson and Joseph M O'Brien

TABLE IV.1 Aminoglycosides

MEDICATION	INDICATIONS	DOSE	RENAL ADJUSTED DOSE?	RESTRIC-TIONS	BRAND NAMES
Gentamicin	• Surgical prophylaxis • UTI • Endocarditis • Empirical treatment for severe Gram negative infection • *P. aeruginosa* infection	See Chapter 23	Yes	Yes, ID approval	N/A
Tobramycin	• *P. aeruginosa* infection • Serious infections resistant to other antibacterials • Severe Gram negative infections	IM/IV – dependent on CrCl >60 mL: 5–7 mg/kg D 30–60 mL: 4–5 mg/kg D <30 mL seek specialist advice	Yes, see left	Yes, ID approval	Tobra-Day

TABLE IV.2 Carbapenems

MEDICATION	INDICATIONS	DOSE	RENAL ADJUSTED DOSE?	RESTRICTIONS	BRAND NAMES
Meropenem	• Multi-resistant Gram negative infections • Febrile neutropenia • Meningitis • LRTIs in cystic fibrosis	Febrile neutropenia/ cystic fibrosis: 1–2 g IV TDS Meningitis: 2 g IV TDS	Yes, reduce dose if CrCl <50	Yes, ID approval	Merrem

TABLE IV.3 Cephalosporins

MEDICATION	INDICATIONS	DOSE	RENAL ADJUSTED DOSE?	RESTRICTIONS	BRAND NAMES
Cefaclor	• Otitis media (mainly paediatric) • LRTI from *H. influenzae* • Bacterial sinusitis	PO 250–500 mg PO TDS	Yes	No	Keflor
Cefepime	• *P. aeruginosa* infections • Febrile neutropenia	IM/IV 1–2 g BD	Yes	Yes, ID approval	N/A
Ceftazidime	• *P. aeruginosa* infections	1–2 g IV TDS	Yes	Yes, ID approval	Fortum
Ceftriaxone	• Empirical treatment of: severe CAP and HAP, orbital cellulitis and bacterial meningitis • Intrabdominal sepsis and prophylaxis where penicillin/gentamicin not indicated • Prevention of meningococcal disease • Septicaemia	1 g IV daily	No	Yes, ID approval	Rocephin
Cefuroxime	As for Cefaclor + gonococcal infection	PO 250–500 mg BD Gonococcal infection: 1 g once only	If severe renal impairment, yes	No	Zinnat
Cephalexin	• Staphylococcal + streptococcal infections • UTI • Epididymo-orchitis	250–500 mg PO QID	If severe renal impairment, yes	No	Keflex Ibilex Cilex Ialex
Cephazolin	• As for cephalexin + surgical prophylaxis	1–2 g IV every 6–8/24	Yes	No	Cefazolin

TABLE IV.4 Glycopeptides

MEDICATION	INDICATIONS	DOSE	RENAL ADJUSTED DOSE?	RESTRICTIONS	BRAND NAMES
Teicoplanin	• MRSA + MRSE infections • Recurrent *C. difficile* not responding to metronidazole • Surgical prophylaxis for patients having prosthetic inserted with previous MRSE/MRSA • Persistent VRE infection	<u>Severe septicaemia:</u> 6–12 mg/kg every 12/24 for 3 doses, then 6 mg/kg Daily <u>Septic arthritis:</u> 12 mg/kg every 12/24 for 3 doses then 12 mg/kg D	CrCl: 40–60 mL/min: usual doses for the first 3/7, then usual dose every 2 days (or ½ dose D) <40 mL/min: usual doses for the first 3/7, then usual dose every 3/7	Yes, ID approval required	N/A
Vancomycin	• MRSA infections • *C. difficile* resistant to metronidazole • Surgical prophylaxis in patients having implantation of prosthesis with previous MRSE/MRSA	See Chapter 23	Yes	Yes, ID approval required	Vancocin

TABLE IV.5 Lincosamides

MEDICATION	INDICATIONS	DOSE	RENAL ADJUSTED DOSE?	RESTRICTIONS	BRAND NAMES
Clindamycin	• Toxoplasmosis • Bacterial vaginosis • Anaerobic infections • Alternative in patients with allergy to penicillins and cephalosporins	150–450 mg PO TDS every 6–8/24	No	Yes, ID approval required	Cleocin Dalacin

TABLE IV.6 Macrolides

MEDICATION	INDICATIONS	DOSE	RENAL ADJUSTED DOSE?	RESTRICTIONS	BRAND NAMES
Azithromycin	• Chlamydial • Streptococcal URTI • CAP • Pertussis	Chlamydial infection: PO 1 g single dose CAP: 500 mg IV D, then convert to oral as soon as possible 500 mg initial dose then 500 mg D for 2/7, then 250 mg for 4/7	No	No	Zithromax Zedd
Clarithromycin	• H. Pylori eradication therapy • LRTI • Pertussis	PO 250–500 mg BD H. pylori eradication: 500 mg PO BD for 7/7	If CrCl <30 then ½ dose	No	Clarac Clarithro Klacid
Erythromycin	• LRTI • Legionnaires' disease • Campylobacter enteritis • Chlamydia	PO 250–500 mg 6–8/24 Severe pneumonia: IV 0.5–1 g every 6/24	If severe renal impairment, yes	No	E-mycin
Roxithromycin	• URTI + LRTI • Skin infections	PO 150 mg BD or 300 mg D Severe hepatic impairment: 150 mg D	No	No	Rulide Roxar Biaxsig

TABLE IV.7 Nitroimidazoles

MEDICATION	INDICATIONS	DOSE	RENAL ADJUSTED DOSE?	RESTRICTIONS	BRAND NAMES
Metronidazole	• C. difficile • Intra-abdominal infections • Lung abscess • Surgical prophylaxis • H. pylori eradication • Anaerobic infections • Giardiasis	Surgical prophylaxis: 500 mg IV prior to skin incision or 400 mg PO 1–2/24 prior C. difficile: PO 400 mg TDS for 10/7 Severe infections: 500 mg IV 8/24	No For hepatic impairment reduce dose to ½ or ⅓	No	Flagyl Metrogyl Metronide

TABLE IV.8 Penicillins

MEDICATION	INDICATIONS	DOSE	RENAL ADJUSTED DOSE?	RESTRICTIONS	BRAND NAMES
Amoxicillin	• Bronchitis • CAP • Bacterial otitis media • Gonococcal infection • Epididymo-orchitis, UTI • Non-surgical prophylaxis of endocarditis • H. pylori eradication	PO 250–500 mg TDS or PO 1 g BD H. pylori eradication: PO 1 g BD Severe infection: IV 1 g 6/24 (as alt. to ampicillin)	No	No	Maxamox Alphamox Amoxil Cilamox Yomax
Amoxicillin with clavulanic acid	• HAP • Epididymo-orchitis • UTI • Bites • Acute sinusitis • Acute cholecystitis (after IV Rx)	Dosage made on amoxicillin dose PO 500–875 mg BD for 5–10/7	No Contraindicated in patients with jaundice	No	Augmentin DF
Ampicillin	• Exacerbation chronic bronchitis • Gonococcal infection, UTI • Non-surgical prophylaxis endocarditis • Intra-abdominal sepsis and prophylaxis	IV/IM 500 mg–1 g every 4/24	CrCl <10 IV/IM 1–2 g BD or D	No	Ampicyn Austrapen Ibimicyn

Benzylpenicillin	• Bacterial endocarditis • Meningitis • Aspiration and CAP • Syphilis	IV 0.6–1.2g every 4–6/24	If severe renal impairment, yes	No	BenPen
Flucloxacillin	• Staphylococcal skin infections • Osteomyelitis • Septicaemia • Surgical prophylaxis	1–2 g IV QID (acute) 500 mg–1 g PO QID (step-down, or less severe infections)	If severe renal impairment, yes	No	Flupen Staphylex Flucil
Piperacillin + Tazobactam	• Mixed aerobic + anaerobic infection • Febrile neutropenia	Based on piperacillin dose: 2–4 g every 6–8/24 Typical dose: 4.5 g IV TDS	Yes, reduce frequency	Yes, ID approval	Tazocin
Ticarcillin + clavulanic acid	Same as Tazocin	Based on ticarcillin dose: 3 g every 4–6/24 Typical dose: 3.1 g IV TDS	CrCl and dose: 30–60: 2 g 4/24 10–30: 2 g 8/24 <10: 2–3 g 12/24	Yes, ID approval	Timentin

TABLE IV.9 Quinolones

MEDICATION	INDICATIONS	DOSE	RENAL ADJUSTED DOSE?	RESTRICTIONS	BRAND NAMES
Ciprofloxacin	• Shigellosis • Complicated UTIs • Bone or joint infections • Epididymo-orchitis • P. aeruginosa infection • Prevention of meningococcal disease • Typhoid • Prostatitis • Febrile neutropenia	PO 250–500 mg BD IV 200–300 mg 8–12/24 <u>Bone and joint infections:</u> PO 750 mg BD <u>Prevention of meningococcal disease:</u> PO 500 mg as single dose	CrCl <30 ½ dose	Yes, ID approval	Ciprol Cifran Ciproxin C-flox
Moxifloxacin	• CAP • Bacterial sinusitis resistant to other agents • Acute exacerbations of chronic bronchitis • Severe complicated skin infections • Multi-resistance TB	PO/IV 400 mg D	No	Yes, ID approval	Avelox
Norfloxacin	• Resistant uncomplicated UTIs • Shigellosis • Campylobacter • Prostatitis • Prophylaxis in cirrhotic patients with GI haemorrhage	<u>Resistant UTI:</u> Uncomplicated 400 mg 12/24 3/7 Relapsing 400 mg 12/24 10–14/7 <u>Campylobacter:</u> 400 mg 12/24 for 5/7 <u>Prostatitis:</u> 400 mg BD for 28/7 <u>Prophylaxis in cirrhosis with GI haemorrhage:</u> 400 mg BD for 7/7	CrCl <30: reduce to 400 mg D	Yes, ID approval	Roxin Nufloxib

TABLE IV.10 Tetracyclines

MEDICATION	INDICATIONS	DOSE	RENAL ADJUSTED DOSE?	RESTRICTIONS	BRAND NAMES
Doxycycline	• CAP • Exacerbation of chronic bronchitis • Acute bacterial sinusitis • Chlamydial PID • Chronic prostatitis	100 mg PO BD (treatment dose) 50 mg PO daily (prophylactic dose) 100 mg PO D (malaria prophylaxis)	Not recommended in severe renal impairment	No	Doxy Doxylin

TABLE IV.11 Other antibiotics

MEDICATION	INDICATIONS	DOSE	RENAL ADJUSTED DOSE?	RESTRICTIONS	BRAND NAMES
Trimethoprim	• Empirical treatment for uncomplicated UTIs • Epididymo-orchitis • Prostatitis	300 mg PO D Women: 3/7 course Men: 14/7 course	CrCl 15–30: 3/7 days, then halve dose 10–15: halve dose	No	Alprim Triprim
Trimethoprim + sulfamethoxazole	• Treatment and prevention of PCP • Atypical pneumonia • Shigellosis • Prevention and treatment of pertussis	800/160 mg PO daily (prophylaxis) 1.6 g/320 mg PO BD (treatment dose) <u>Severe infection:</u> 800/160 mg PO BD twice weekly (respiratory prophylaxis)	Not recommended in severe renal impairment	No	Resprim Forte, Bactrim DS

INDEX

Page numbers followed by "*f*" indicate figures, "*t*" indicate tables, and "*b*" indicate boxes.

E

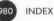